The Bacteriology of Tuberculosis

The Bacteriology of TUBERCULOSIS

Egons Darzins, M.D.
RESEARCH SCIENTIST, ANOKA STATE HOSPITAL

UNIVERSITY OF MINNESOTA PRESS
Minneapolis

Printed in the United States of America
at the North Central Publishing Company, St. Paul

Library of Congress Catalog Card Number: 57-8918

PUBLISHED IN GREAT BRITAIN, INDIA, AND PAKISTAN BY
THE OXFORD UNIVERSITY PRESS, LONDON, BOMBAY, AND KARACHI

TO MY TEACHERS AND FRIENDS AT THE

University of Latvia (1919–1944)

Rockefeller Foundation, New York

Pasteur Institute, Paris

Robert Koch Institute, Berlin

University of Marburg am Lahn

State Seruminstitute, Copenhagen

Brazilian Institute for Tuberculosis Research, Bahia

University of Minnesota, Minneapolis

Anoka State Hospital, Anoka

Preface

IN SPITE of great advances in the treatment and cure of tuberculosis, there are still millions of tuberculous people spread over the surface of the earth. Chemotherapy, the use of antibiotics, and surgery still leave resistant cases in which the disease continues to progress steadily. And while some problems in the bacteriology of tuberculosis have been solved, others – some previously unknown – have arisen. The survival of tubercle bacilli in organisms treated with antibiotics and chemotherapeutics, the relation of the cord factor to pathogenicity, the role of chromogenic bacilli in the pathogenesis of tuberculosis, the cultivation of tubercle bacilli from paucibacillary material – these are some of the new problems.

In the course of the past twenty years many works in the field of the bacteriology of tuberculosis have been published, dispersed in both well-known and less familiar periodicals all over the world. Before further advance in tuberculosis research can be made, it is necessary to summarize the results already achieved; this is one of the aims of this book. Another of my objectives is to point out unsolved problems in the bacteriology of tuberculosis and to indicate recently developed experimental methods for the study of tubercle bacilli.

Their limited knowledge of foreign languages and the pressure of time often make it difficult for the younger generation of scientists to trace the development of problems. Yet we really know a problem only when we are acquainted with its history. When scientists lack such historical background, apparently new contributions often turn out to be a repetition of work done previously. The avalanche of such repetitive work is rolling on and increasing in size. If it were possible to direct all this wasted energy upon previously untrod paths, the achievements would increase in value and the flood of publications would diminish. These considerations led me to present the material of this book in historical sequence, although through such an approach some well-known names will lose their priority as propounders of certain discoveries.

Preface

In my attempt to follow work in the bacteriology of tuberculosis up to this very day, I was forced to consider yet unfinished work. In such cases, as Claude Bernard has pointed out, it is only possible to gather the raw facts. These data will often be contradictory, but they may serve as centers for the generation of new ideas and work.

The number of persons, institutions, and editors who have in various ways been helpful to me in preparing this manuscript has, over the years, grown so great that it is impossible to mention all of them here; but I am deeply grateful for their friendly aid. The reader will find some of their names in the text itself. I would, however, like to express my particular gratitude to the personnel of the University of Minnesota Library for tireless assistance in collecting material for the manuscript and to the personnel of the University of Minnesota Press.

E. Darzins

Anoka, Minnesota
October 1957

Contents

Part Three. The Isolation and Identification of the Tubercle Bacillus

Part Four. The Types and Pathogenicity of the Tubercle Bacillus

Part Five. Experimenting with the Tubercle Bacillus

PART ONE

Morphology and Cytology of the Tubercle Bacillus

I

Tubercle Bacillus as a Unicellular Organism

ROBERT KOCH (1882), in his paper on the discovery of the cause of tuberculosis, described the tubercle bacillus, stained with methylene blue and counterstained with vesuvin, in the following terms (p. 222): "The bacteria made visible through this procedure are somewhat peculiar in aspect. They have the shape of a rod and, because of this form, belong to the group of bacilli. They are very thin and one-fourth to one-half as long as the diameter of a red blood cell; sometimes they reach a greater length and are as long as the whole diameter of a red cell. Under certain conditions, the bacilli produce spores already in animal organism; some bacilli contain several spores, in most cases there are two to four of them; oval in form, they are distributed, in uniform intervals, along the axis of the bacilli."

The picture of the tubercle bacillus given by Koch was confirmed by the later and more efficient staining methods of Ehrlich and Ziehl-Neelsen. The tubercle bacillus belongs to the genus *Mycobacterium.* Three variants, *Mycobacterium tuberculosis* var. *hominis, bovis,* and *avium,* cause tuberculosis in mammals.

Early Upholders of the Unity of the Cellular World

Early investigators regarded the bacterial cell as a living unit endowed with the same constituents as the cells of higher plants and animals. These early upholders of the unity of the cellular world reached their conclusions by means of the incomplete data they got from the observation of living cells. Schottelius, as early as 1888, used reagents to determine the differences in chemical composition of the bacterial cell structures. He observed in the cells of *Bacillus anthracis* a dark central body in the transparent protoplasm which he called a "nucleus" to designate its central position. He affirmed that the cell division of these bacilli is preceded by the division of the central body, and expressed the hope that further investigations

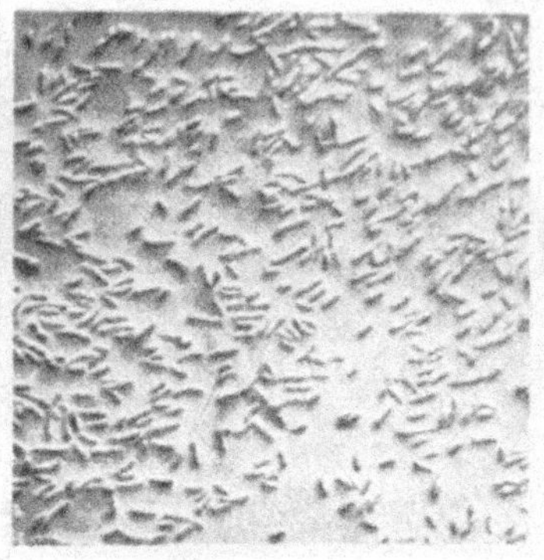

Figure 1. Unstained tubercle bacilli; oblique illumination; × 1,000 (Lembke and H. Ruska, 1940).

would furnish additional information about the nature of the central body.

Two works, by Ernst (1889) and Babes (1889), advanced the knowledge of the internal structure of the bacterial cell to the point that there was practically no progress in later works till new tools of investigation were created. The significance of the work of Ernst and Babes in bacterial cytology has been overlooked by the latest reviewers of this field.

Ernst demonstrated, by means of simple procedures, the nuclear nature of granules of the bacterial cell. He showed that these granules are not vacuoles, nor are they of fatty nature because they are not dissolved by fat solvents. The cell granules, like any other nuclear substance, were stained in deep violet by hematoxylin. By treating these cell granules with pepsin and hydrochloric acid, Ernst showed that the granules are less resistant to enzyme digestion than are bacterial spores. He observed that the granules take part in the formation of spores and that the division of the granules takes place prior to cell division. The sum of these observations enabled Ernst to conclude that the granules in the bacterial cells are of nuclear nature.

Besides nuclear bodies, fat and glycogen granules were discovered in the bacterial cell. Grimme (1902) found that a large number of the granules of bacterial cells were dissolved in hot water or by diluted acids and that they disappeared under unfavorable conditions of nutrition and reappeared when the conditions improved. Grimme named such granules "volutin" and regarded them as the stored food of the cell. This view was accepted by Fisher in 1903 and by Guilliermond (1910).

The clear concept of the first unitarians, Ernst and Babes, who regarded the bacterial cell, like the cells of higher living forms, as endowed with the nuclear substance but living independently, was obscured by the mosaic of observations that followed.

The works and discussions of later investigators mostly took the form of a controversy about the presence of volutin in bacterial cells and especially in tubercle bacilli. The presence of volutin in tubercle bacilli was affirmed by Babes (1910), Guilliermond (1910), and Hollande and Crémieux (1928), but denied by Kirchensteins (1922), Lewis (1941), and others.

Some investigators described the nucleus of the bacterial cell as a separate body which can be differentiated from the cytoplasm, fat, and volutin (A. Meyer, 1912). For others, the nucleus in the bacterial cell was made up of chromidial granules dispersed in the cytoplasm (Guilliermond, 1933), or the bacterial cell was devoid of any structures at all. According to this last view, the morphologic elements seen in the cells were created by the action of external agents upon the colloids of the cytoplasm (Wámoscher, 1930).

Opponents of the Theory of the Unity of the Cellular World

The hypothesis that the cell of the tubercle bacillus is composed of living units endowed with properties different from those of the whole bacillus emerged from the discussions of the nature of the formations seen in the tubercle bacillus by Koch. He identified these as spores, although it was early recognized that these bodies are not comparable to the spores of ordinary bacilli. The sensitivity to heat of the tubercle bacillus was alone sufficient to refute such an assumption. For some authors, the bodies were simple granules (Metschnikoff, 1888); others identified them as fat droplets (Grimme, 1902), volutin (A. Meyer, 1912), or as nuclear substances (Feinberg, 1900; Guilliermond, 1908; Eisenberg, 1909; Kirchensteins, 1921, 1922).

Spengler (1905a) approached the problem of the role of the bodies in the tubercle bacilli from a new angle. According to him, the tubercle bacillus is composed of living units, the *Splitter*. Their size is in the limits of microscope resolution, and they are acid-resistant but cannot be stained by the Ziehl-Neelsen technique. These *Splitter* are capable of reproducing new bacilli and may cause tuberculosis.

Much (1907 a, b), by applying to the tubercle bacilli Gram staining with successive iodine treatment and decolorization of the preparation with an alcohol-acetone mixture, was able to reproduce granules in the inside of the bacilli as well as scattered around them. These granules, according to Much, cannot be stained by the Ziehl-Neelsen technique but may generate new tubercle bacilli.

The work of the Brazilian investigator Fontes stimulated new interest in the cell structure of tubercle bacilli. In his first publication (1909), Fontes related how he had applied double staining to the bacilli, namely Ziehl-Neelsen's carbolfuchsin staining and the Gram treatment. In this way he tried to differentiate the pathogenic tubercle bacilli, containing Much granules, from the apathogenic ones without these granules. In his second paper (1910a), Fontes described the multiplication through division of these granules in the inside of a cell and on its outside and applied the term "virus" to these formations. In another paper (1910b), Fontes described the application to the tubercle bacillus of the well-known method of separating the virus from the substrate by filtering the material through a bacterial filter. He inoculated a guinea pig with the filtered caseous material and transplanted the organs of this animal into a fresh one. When after five months of observation the animal was killed, the autopsy revealed the infiltration of round cells, granules, and occasional acid-fast bacilli in the lymph nodes and the lungs.

After years of oblivion, the early works of Fontes were rediscovered by Vaudremer (1923). He repeated Fontes' filtration experiments and confirmed the development of acid-fast bacilli on media and in animals inoculated with these filtrates. Vaudremer's article provoked a great quantity of research. The filtrability of the tubercle bacillus or the tuberculous virus (the *ultravirus tuberculeux* of the French authors) and the new disease produced by it were described.

An attempt to deprive the tubercle bacillus of its position as a member of the well-separated group of mycobacteria and to connect it with non-acid-fast saprophytic microorganisms was made by Ferrán (1905). He described non-acid-fast members in the chain of evolution of acid-fast bacilli. These findings have been upheld by Kahn (1929), among others.

Gardner (1929), Oerskov (1932), Brieger and Fell (1946), and Roth (1949) reinvestigated these assertions but could not confirm them. The classical acid-fast form of the tubercle bacillus was not lost and non-acid-fast forms were not generated in the development process of tubercle bacilli. Wyckoff (1934) used micro-motion photography to study the reproduction of tubercle bacilli and found that the bacilli multiply by transverse division. This division continues for a long time after the growth in length of the bacilli has stopped. Because of this, old cultures contain an abundance of short rods. In the tubercle bacilli he found no evidence of any cyclic life phenomena.

After thirty years of strenuous efforts to disintegrate the cell of the tubercle bacillus into invisible fragments and to attribute to these parts the characteristics of a "tuberculosis virus" – characteristics not revealed by the whole bacillus – no tangible results have been achieved. The great amount of work dedicated to the problem of the filtrability of the tubercle bacillus has yielded very few scientific facts. The critically controlled experiments have not revealed any form of tuberculosis in which the disease was provoked by a virus or by non-acid-fast bacilli or in which the bacillus of Koch was not at work.*

* A complete account of the filtrability of tubercle bacilli and of the virus problem was given by L. Nègre in A. Calmette, *L'infection bacillaire et la tuberculose chez l'homme et chez les animaux* (Masson, Paris, 1936), pp. 93–122.

Tubercle Bacillus as a Unicellular Organism

The works of Spengler, Much, Fontes, and many others who regarded the tubercle bacillus as composed of living units, created great expectations and promised great contributions to the understanding and prevention of tuberculosis. As with time these expectations faded, the *Splitter* and granules became the object of purely academic interest.

A new era dawned when the exact methods of physics and chemistry were applied to research on the cell. The investigation of bacterial cells in ultraviolet light, with an electron microscope, and by means of the histochemical and enzyme methods produced a considerable advance in the knowledge of the cytology of bacterial cells and particularly of the cytology of the tubercle bacillus. This type of investigation showed that the bodies in the bacterial cell are of nuclear nature and are connected with the assimilation, growth, and inheritance of the cell.

II

Physical Methods for Identifying Cell Structures

Ultraviolet Light Microscopy

THE resolving power of a microscope is inversely related to the wave length of the illuminant used; that is, the resolving power increases with decreasing wave length. For this reason, short-wave microscopy could be a considerable advance over earlier methods of penetrating into fine structures of the cellular world. But the practical realization of short-wave microscopy presented difficulties with respect to the source of the short-wave light and the material to be used for the lenses of the microscope and the slides. Light with a wave length of less than 300 mμ is ultraviolet, and ultraviolet light cannot penetrate glass. Köhler (1904) overcame these difficulties by using a homogenic linear light source of 275 mμ wave length which produced blue and violet monochromatic light from cadmium electrodes and by using a quartz objective and slides of mountain crystal. Finally, he attached a photographic device to this ultraviolet light microscope.

The investigation of the structure of the cell – particularly the bacterial cell – was the branch of biology that profited most from ultraviolet microscopy. Köhler himself took the first step in this direction. Living objects in particular attracted his attention. From photographs of the dust cells of the wings of a butterfly and the cells of a triton he concluded that the absorption phenomena of ultraviolet light in the structures of organic tissue are of special importance. (*"Ein hervorragendes Interesse bieten die Absorptionserscheinungen, die die organischen Gewebe diesem Licht gegenüber zeigen."*) The absorption of ultraviolet light was considerably greater in the nuclei than in the cytoplasm of the cells studied. Chromatin, the component of the nucleus, which in an ordinary light microscope is less transparent and which eagerly takes up the basic dyes, was also less transparent to ultraviolet light.

After the work of Köhler, important contributions in the field of the physical analysis of cell structures by means of ultraviolet light were made by Caspersson (1936, 1939, 1940, 1950) and his co-workers. The absorption of ultraviolet light by organic and inorganic compounds had been studied before Caspersson by Dhéré (1906). Dhéré's experiments showed that the radiations of wave lengths 274.8 mμ and 239.4 mμ are absorbed by a 1:10,000 solution of nucleic acid. It was known that the hydrolysis of nucleic acid produces phosphoric acid, carbohydrate, purine, and pyrimidine bases. Phosphoric acid and carbohydrate in the experiments of Dhéré did not absorb ultraviolet light, the absorption of ultraviolet light by nucleic acid being caused by its content of purine and pyrimidine bases. These investigations had shown the specific absorption maximum of nucleic acid to be in the region of 260 mμ wave length.

Caspersson developed the method of microscopic photometry, which permits the measurement, under a microscope, by means of a photoelectric cell, of the amount of different wave lengths transmitted by different parts of a cell. Two groups of substances in the cell showed strong absorption of ultraviolet light. The proteins, especially those containing cyclic amino acids, such as tryptophan and tyrosine, had this property, although the absorption of another group of substances, nucleic acids, dominated the phenomenon (see Fig. 2). The absorption of nucleic acids in the region of 260 mμ wave length was so high, and the absorption of other substances in comparison with it so low, that the absorption of these other substances can be disregarded. The conjugated double bonds in pyrimidine of desoxyribonucleic acid of the nuclei, caused this high absorption of ultraviolet

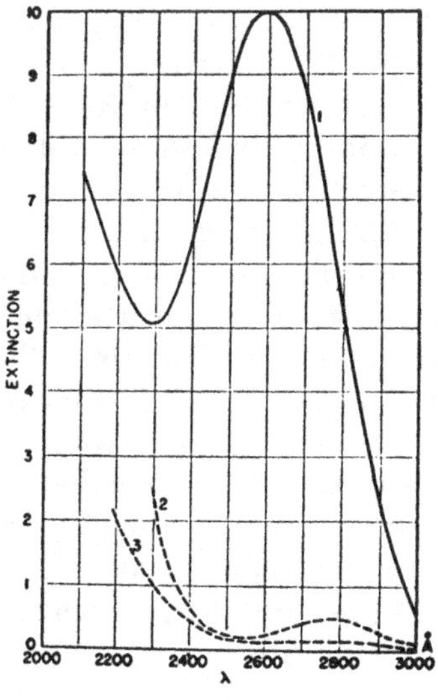

Figure 2. Comparison of absorption of ultraviolet light by nucleic acid and protein. 1. Thymonucleic acid, 0.5 per cent concentration. 2. Serum albumin, 0.5 per cent concentration. 3. Protamine sulfate, 5 per mill concentration. (Caspersson, 1950.)

light. Even a very high protein concentration cannot produce, at 260 mμ wave length, an absorption comparable to 5 per cent nucleic acid solution.

The shape of the absorption curve is often typical of a determined substance, so that the qualitative differentiation of substances was possible.

Monosaccharides and polysaccharides gave no signs of absorbing ultraviolet light. The absorption of lipids and fatty substances was low; even the drops of fat of more than 10 mμ in diameter were completely transparent to ultraviolet light. Some of the complex salts of inorganic compounds showed selective absorption of ultraviolet light, but Caspersson attributed the whole absorption of ultraviolet light in cells to the nucleoproteins. (Complete information about the ultraviolet absorption spectra of proteins and amino acids was given by Beaven and Holiday, 1952.)

The concentration of nucleic acids in the cytoplasm of cells during their growth is subject to considerable change. Caspersson and Schultz (1939) compared ultraviolet light absorption in the cytoplasm of rapidly growing cells with that of resting cells. They found that growing cells absorbed highly ultraviolet light. The resting cells had low absorption – and it was not of the nucleic acid type but of the protein type – with the maximum toward the 300 mμ wave length.

The cells engaged in intense growth produce large quantities of nucleic acids. The liver cells of a chick embryo, during rapid growth of the organism, contain a high concentration of ribonucleic acid in their cytoplasm. At this period the cytoplasm is intensively stained with basic dyes. The same phenomenon is observed in rapidly growing parts of plants. When the growth has ceased, the nucleic acid concentration in the cell is low and the cell is only slightly stained by the basic dyes (Caspersson, 1950). It must be assumed that the high concentration of nucleic acids in the cell is correlated with the growth of the cell and not merely with some other metabolic activity. This conclusion is supported by the observation of similar activities in yeast cells.

In the cytoplasm of resting yeast cells only ultraviolet light–absorbing grains of volutin can be seen. Caspersson and Brandt (1941) and Brandt (1942) observed that these volutin grains composed of ribonucleic acid disappear when the growth of the cell starts. At the same time the basophilic staining properties and the ultraviolet light absorption of the cytoplasm increase. Volutin of the cytoplasm is used up to synthesize the ribonucleotides, which in turn participate in the synthesis of the proteins.

The connection between genes and nucleic acids was revealed by the investigations of Hollaender and Emmons (1946). The fungus *Trichophyton mentagrophytes,* when irradiated with ultraviolet light, produced mutants. The maximum mutation of the fungus was obtained with a radiation of 265 mμ wave length, which coincides with the maximum absorption of nucleic acids.

Progressing tuberculosis in guinea pigs brings about a decline in the amount of ribonucleic acid in the epithelial cells of the bronchi and in the cells of the kidney and spleen. Treatment of the animals with streptomycin or isoniazid restores the normal distribution of ribonucleic acid in the cells. Particularly rich in ribonucleic acid are the fibroblasts, macrophages, and rapidly growing cells in tuberculous lesions that are healing (Averbakh, 1956).

Bacteria in ultraviolet light. Köhler (1904) observed ultraviolet light–absorbing substances in the cells of bacteria and yeast.

Ultraviolet light microscopy was used by Barnard (1925, 1930) to investigate virus particles invisible through the ordinary light microscope. The ultraviolet light photographs of the cell content of large bacilli (*Megatherium*) in the living state convinced Barnard that bacteria possess nuclei which undergo mitotic division.

Gates (1930) studied the action of monochromatic light on bacteria (*Staphylococcus, Escherichia coli*) and found that the maximum of destructiveness was confined to the radiations between 260 and 270 mμ. He concluded that the radiations of this region must be absorbed by some essential substances of the cell (see p. 67).

Wyckoff and Ter Louw (1931) investigated, in ultraviolet light, five-hour-old living cells of *Bacillus subtilis.* Young, rapidly growing cells did not contain structures that could be detected by ultraviolet light microscopy. The older cells became granulated and the amount of granulation increased with the increase of the age of the cells. No indications of formed nuclei in the cells were found.

Piekarski (1939) found that the cells of the spore-forming *Bacillus subtilis* contain bodies which have the same ultraviolet light absorption maximum as thymonucleic acid. These bodies were 0.15 μ–0.2 μ in diameter, as compared to the 1 μ–1.2 μ diameter of the spores, and underwent division, but no chromosome formation was seen in them.

Prudhomme, Rouyer, and Staub (1946) found that the absorption maximum of *Escherichia coli* and paradysentery bacteria was at 260 mμ, and the minimum at 245 mμ. The absorption spectra of all microorganisms studied were identical; they were the same even in dead bacteria.

Considerable work on ultraviolet light–absorbing structures of microorganisms was done by Malmgren and Hedén (1947). By means of the method devised by Caspersson, these authors investigated in both Gram-positive and Gram-negative bacteria (*Escherichia coli, Bacillus cereus, Corynebacterium diphtheriae,* etc.) the quantitative distribution of nucleic acids during their growth cycle. In all organisms investigated the highest content of cell nucleic acids was reached at the end of the lag phase or at the beginning of the growth phase. The bacteria contained two types of nucleic acid, one of the ribose, the other of the desoxyribose type. The ribose nucleic acid was present in cells in the form of ultraviolet light-absorbing cytoplasmic granules. The desoxyribose nucleic acid granules of the nuclei underwent fission, and were identified as the functional counterpart of the chromatin of the metazoan cell. Ultraviolet light absorption, enzyme digestion, and Feulgen reaction of bacterial cells indicated that the nucleic acid systems are connected with bacterial growth, with protein synthesis, and with gene production and that they form one functional cell unit. These findings were in agreement with the findings on metazoan cells (Caspersson, 1948; Abolins, 1948).

Fluorescence Microscopy

Fluorescence is the property that some substances have of emitting light under the influence of excitants. Well known are the cases of emission of light by substances irradiated with a visible light (photoluminescence), under the action of Röntgen rays, and the cases of luminescence which accompany chemical reactions (phosphorescence). The fluorescent light emitted by a substance is largely independent of the nature of the excitant. The fluorescence spectra of platinum salts are identical, whether provoked by Röntgen rays or by ultraviolet light (H. Lehmann, 1913). The emission of light takes place when the energy applied to a substance is absorbed and transformed into radiation. The light of short waves, such as ultraviolet of 300 mμ or less, or blue light of wave lengths between 300 mμ and 450 mμ, can provoke fluorescence. The emitted fluorescent light is always of longer wave length than the excitant light. When ultraviolet light is the excitant, the fluorescent light will be blue; when blue light is the excitant, the fluorescent light may be green, yellow, or red. Long light waves do not cause fluorescence. The intensity of fluorescence is proportional to the intensity of the excitant. Only a fraction of the excitant energy absorbed in a substance is emitted as fluorescent light. Because of this, the excitant light used in fluorescence microscopy must be rich in short light waves.

A particle in a light microscope is recognized on the basis of its color or because of the refraction of light coming from an outside source. In a fluorescence microscope the fluorescent particle itself emits light, which is provoked in it by an outside excitant. Köhler (1904), working with the ultraviolet microscope, observed the fluorescence of biological objects. This fluorescence of objects was one of the major obstacles in the application of ultraviolet light microscopy to research in biology, although Köhler early recognized that the fluorescence of objects might be utilized in research (Ellinger, 1940). The work of H. Lehmann (1913) created the necessary basis for fluorescence microscopy. He said: "In order to observe the traces of fluorescence it is necessary to have an appliance permitting the irradiation of objects with very strong and pure ultraviolet light. This could be achieved by the use of appropriate ray filters." He proposed the use of a solution of copper sulfate to filter off the visible light. This solution is sufficiently penetrable for short light waves from 300 mμ to 450 mμ. As a source of ultraviolet light, Lehmann used the light of an electric arc. To eliminate the disturbing action of ultraviolet light, which, penetrating into the microscope and into the eye of the observer, makes the lens of the eye intensely fluorescent, he introduced a second filter in the form of a coverslip made of glass impenetrable to ultraviolet light but permitting the passage of the green and red light emitted by the fluorescent object. Under these conditions, the pure fluorescent light of the object was seen on the dark background of the microscope and Lehmann even obtained color photographs on Lumière color plates.

Most fluorescent biologic objects emit only a pale blue light; only a few of them (chlorophyll, porphyrins) produce bright green, yellow, or red fluorescence. von Prowazek (1914) had the idea of endowing non-fluorescents with fluorescence by impregnating them with fluorescent chemicals. Further work in this direction was done by Haitinger and Hamperl (1933). In systematic studies, they discovered the important fluorescent compounds or "fluorochromes," in their terminology, such as auramine, berberine sulfate, acridine compounds, and natural plant extracts (*chelidonium*).

A dye rapidly loses its hue when diluted with an inert substance (water, tissues, etc.), but a fluorescent substance conserves its fluorescence at high dilutions: only the tint of fluorescence changes. Fluorescent substances often emit enough light of a specific color to be recognized even when highly diluted. Because of this property, the fluorescence procedure is an analytical method of high sensitivity for the optical identification of self-fluorescent substances or bodies impregnated with fluorochromes.

The fluorescence microscope. The field in the fluorescence microscope appears dark to the human eye, unless it contains fluorescent objects. In the presence of such objects, luminous particles can be seen in the dark field.

In most medical examinations, green, yellow, or red fluorescence is useful. Such fluorescence may be provoked by blue light of short wave length. An excitant of this kind is far less destructive to the living objects than is ultraviolet light, and the ordinary glass lenses of the microscope may be used with such light. When the blue fluorescence of an object is desired, the ultraviolet light source and quartz equipment must be used.

Daylight and the light of an incandescent bulb are unsatisfactory as light sources in fluorescence microscopy. In blue light fluorescence microscopy, high amperage, low voltage filament lamps may be used. In ultraviolet light fluorescence microscopy, light rich in ultraviolet radiation, such as the light emitted by carbon or mercury arc lamps, is employed.

Recently these lamps, which are not easy to manipulate, have been successfully replaced by tungsten filament bulbs.

To recognize fluorescent particles in a dark field, lenses of relatively low power may be used. This is one of the advantages of the fluorescence microscope over the light microscope. A binocular microscope cannot be used in fluorescence microscopy because the presently known light sources are insufficient for this purpose. Fluorite lenses are fluorescent; so is cedar oil. Pure paraffin oil or synthetic immersion oil may be used instead.

Filters. The light emitted by a fluorescent lamp does not consist of pure blue and violet radiations, but also contains heat rays of the red spectrum. To eliminate these undesirable radiations, the light is filtered through a blue filter.

Blue or ultraviolet light, after having stimulated the object to fluorescence, and having passed through the object, is filtered off by means of a yellow filter. Lehmann used a yellow cover-glass to filter off this undesirable light; at present yellow eyepiece filters are used instead. Glass manufacturers produce filters that transmit fluorescent light of approximately 520 mμ wave length.

Fluorochromes. The impregnation of nonfluorescent objects with fluorochromes is in principle equivalent to the staining of an object, although the fluorochromes may be colorless and the treated object may not change its tint. The accumulation of fluorochrome in an object leads to the appearance of a kind of fluorescence that, in contrast to the natural fluorescence of objects, is called secondary or induced fluorescence.

Most fluorochromes are organic compounds and, according to their chemical nature, are called cathodic, anodic, or neutral. In cathodic fluorochromes the cations are responsible for the fluorescence, in anodic fluorochromes the anions. The dissociation of cathodic fluorochromes takes place in the acid region; in the neutral region the dissociation decreases, and in the alkaline region the cathodic fluorochromes are not dissociated. Contrary to this, the anodic fluorochromes are dissociated in the alkaline region. With the change of dissociation in different regions, the fluorochromes change the hue of their fluorescence.

Haitinger and Hamperl (1933) observed the particularly strong fluorescence of tissue nuclei treated with berberine sulfate. Fluorescence microscopy was vigorously revived when Hagemann (1937, 1938) introduced the diphenylmethane dye auramine as a fluorochrome for impregnating acid-fast bacilli.

The fluorescence of auramine can be provoked not only by ultraviolet light but also by blue and violet light with a wave length 334 mμ to 480 mμ (Keller, 1938). The first absorption maximum of auramine is at 360 mμ; the second at 450 mμ (Levaditi *et al.*, 1948). Experiments with a mercury lamp showed that the visible line at 435.8 mμ is the most effective excitant of auramine fluorescence.

The wave length of light emitted by auramine in gelatin was found to be from 540 mμ to 650 mμ. This spectral region includes the yellow-green band of wave length 560 mμ, where retinal sensitivity is the greatest (Graham, 1943).

The fluorescent efficiency of auramine – the ratio between the amount of light absorbed and the amount of light emitted – was determined to be approximately 0.02 per cent. There is hope that a dye with higher fluorescent efficiency will be discovered and thus the efficiency of fluorescence microscopy will be increased (Graham, 1943).

Absorption of fluorochromes in the cells. In order to acquire secondary fluorescence, a cell must absorb a fluorochrome, the uptake of which depends on the isoelectric point of the proteins in the cell cytoplasm. In most cases this point is between *p*H 2 and *p*H 5. The cathodic fluorochromes are highly dissociated between *p*H 2 and *p*H 5; their absorption by cytoplasm is highest in this *p*H range. Of practical importance are the cathodic fluorochromes which are dissociated when dissolved in distilled water.

Fluorescence microscopy in biology. In medicine, fluorescence microscopy is frequently associated with the search for tubercle bacilli, although this method has developed into an effective tool of research in many branches of biology.

The intravital fluorochroming of cells and tissue found application in botany, zoology, and bacteriology. Fluorescence microscopy was successfully used in the histology of nerve connections by Hirt in 1939, for the fluorochroming of whole animals, such as frogs and mice by Asher in 1947, to study various problems of pathology, such as the formation of amyloid (Chiari in 1947), or cancerogene substances (Cowdry in 1943); in biochemistry it was applied to the identification of vitamins (Popper, 1940), porphyrins, sex hormones (Burkl, 1954), and in the study of many other problems. Accounts of the application of fluorescence microscopy in various fields of biology were given by Ellinger (1940), by the Russian scientist Petrovskaia (1948), and others.

Fluorescence microscopy of tubercle bacilli. Fluorescence microscopy was first applied to the bacteriology of tuberculosis by Kaiserling (1917). Working with the luminescence microscope of Lehmann, Kaiserling tried to differentiate strains of tubercle bacilli according to their fluorescence.

Hoffmann (1921) used the dark-ground illumination technique to observe the yellow-green fluorescence of tubercle bacilli stained with carbolfuchsin according to the Ziehl-Neelsen method. He recommended this procedure for recognizing tubercle bacilli in sputum. This good head start made by fluorescence microscopy, however, was undermined by observations about related phenomena. The play of light seen in objects irradiated with ultraviolet light and observed through the screen of Wood attracted a great deal of attention on the part of investigators.

Hagemann (1937) observed preparations treated with auramine through the low-power objective of a fluorescence microscope of total magnification 180 diameters. Under these conditions the tubercle bacilli were seen as brilliant red spots in a dark field.

Auramine is endowed with high fluorescent capacities, and easily impregnates acid-fast bacilli so strongly that decolorizing with acid and alcohol does not remove the fluorochrome from them.

Lembke and H. Ruska (1940) investigated with a fluorescence microscope the avian type of tubercle bacilli treated with berberine sulfate. The cytoplasm in some of the cells contained a considerable quantity of granules. These granules showed particularly strong fluorescence, comparable to that of the nuclei of the cells of higher forms of life.

Kölbel (1952, 1953) carried on a comparative study of the morphology of the internal structure of tubercle bacilli impregnated with auramine, and of bacilli stained by the Ziehl-Neelsen method. The observation of the same objects, successively treated according to the first and the second technique, confirmed that both procedures reveal identical structures, although the Ziehl-Neelsen staining procedure deformed the objects more than the fluorochroming method. Fluorescence microscopy revealed in the colonies of avian tubercle bacilli cells of different intensity of fluorescence (Figs. 3 and 4). The strongly acid-fast cells, when impregnated with auramine, showed bodies of bright fluorescence, whereas the fluorescence of

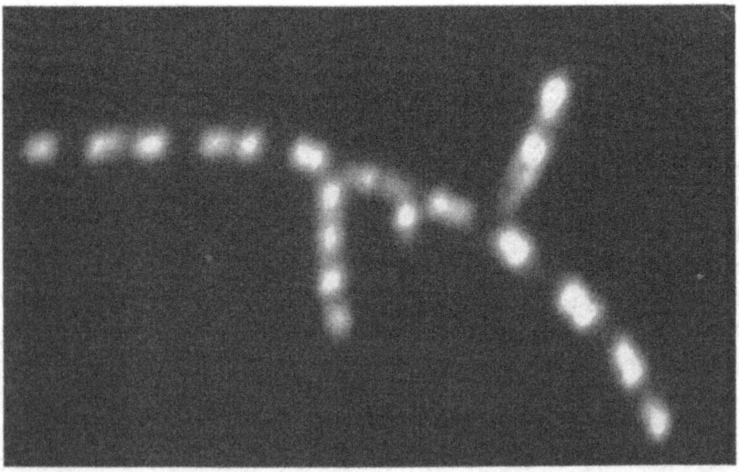

Figure 3. Mycobacterium tuberculosis, avian type, branching form and granules; fluorescence microscopy; stained with auramine; × 8,000 (Kölbel, 1952).

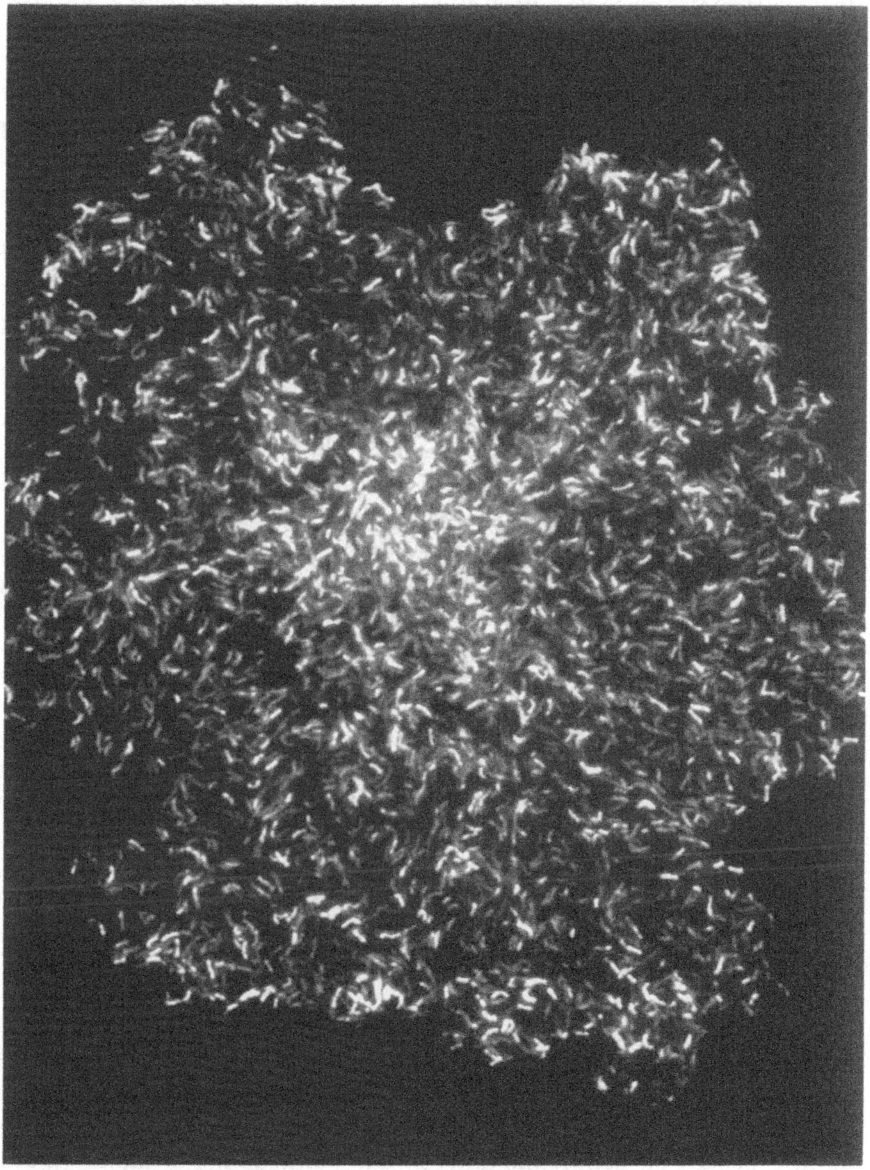

Figure 4. Colony of *Mycobacterium tuberculosis*, avian type; fluorescence microscopy; stained with auramine; tubercle bacilli of different intensity of fluorescence; × 1,200 (Kölbel, 1952).

the feebly acid-fast cells was scarcely perceptible. Branching cells were seen.

The investigations of Krieg (1954a) showed that when corynebacteria are fluorochromed with acridine orange (1:5,000), polar metachromatic granules of metaphosphate, which have red fluorescence, and intermediate nuclear bodies of green fluorescence, are clearly visible. In the cells of tubercle bacilli and in the cells of *Mycobacterium phlei* the relations were not so simple. The young cells of these acid-fast bacilli, after fluorochroming with acridine orange, were found to contain a nuclear substance in the shape of a spiral, which later, by means of fragmentation, produced nuclear bodies. These bodies had green fluorescence and became visible after the cells had been treated with hydrochloric acid or enzyme. They were not identical with the metaphosphate bodies revealed by the electron microscope, but it is possible that the metaphosphate bodies originate from the nuclear bodies after the latter have absorbed metaphosphate.

Fluorescence and the reducing power of living and dead cells. Plating and colony counts are the ordinary procedures for establishing the proportion of living cells in a bacterial population.

An early attempt to observe the structure and the function of a living cell was made by the intravital staining of cells. Pfeffer was the initiator of these works in 1886. The problem has not yet been completely solved. The investigations of Strugger (1940, 1949) revealed one important cause for the death of intravitally stained cells.

When a cell is intravitally stained with an ordinary stain to a degree where the results can be seen in an ordinary microscope, the concentration of the stain in the cell reaches such a high level that the noxious effect of the stain on living cytoplasm is inevitable. Some fluorochromes, detectable by the fluorescence microscope at high dilutions, do not show any noxious influence on the living cytoplasm. In this regard the fluorochrome acridine orange has attracted special attention on the part of investigators such as Bukatsch and Haitinger (1940), Strugger (1940), and Krieg (1954a).

Acridine orange has a particularly strong affinity with protoplasm. This fluorochrome showed important accumulation differences in living and dead cells (Strugger, 1940). Because of these differences, the living protoplasm has green, the dead one copper-red fluorescence. The differences in fluorescence are caused by the difference in permeability of the ectoplasm of cells. Below the isoelectric point of the cytoplasm the cells accumulate small quantities of acridine orange and their fluorescence is green, whereas above the isoelectric point the selective permeability of the cell wall is destroyed and the cytoplasm accumulates considerable amounts of acridine orange, producing red fluorescence. In an experiment by Kölbel (1947) a 0.2 per cent suspension of living yeast cells took up 1.5 per cent of

Figure 5. The accumulation of acridine orange in living and dead yeast cells. I. Living cells. II. Dead cells. Abscissa: time of action of acridine orange. Ordinate: accumulated acridine orange expressed as percentage of weight of treated yeast cells. (Kölbel, 1947.)

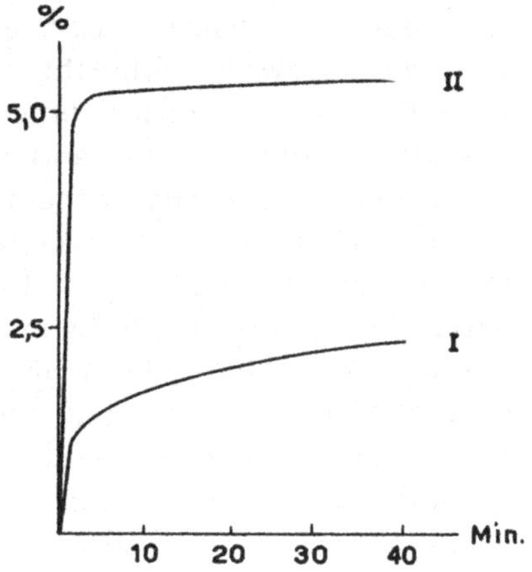

the dye from an 0.5×10^3 M/liter acridine orange solution; the same suspension of dead yeast cells absorbed 5.1 per cent acridine orange from this solution (Fig. 5).

Gärtner (1943) applied the acridine orange fluorochroming method to the study of the action of sulfonamides on *Escherichia coli* and on the typhoid group of microorganisms. The killed bacteria showed red, the living ones green fluorescence.

Strugger (1949) studied the intravital fluorochroming of tubercle bacilli with acridine orange. The human type of bacilli were treated for five minutes with a 1:1,000 solution of acridine orange. The fluorescence of living bacilli was green, that of heat-killed bacilli red. The viability of tubercle bacilli was unaffected by the acridine orange.

The investigations of C. H. Schneider (1944) revealed that the results of the fluorochroming of tubercle bacilli cannot be interpreted as simply as those yielded by fluorochroming Gram-negative bacteria. Living tubercle bacilli (avian type), when treated for one hour with alcohol, retained their green fluorescence. These bacilli, planted on Petragnani's medium, did not grow and, injected into guinea pigs, did not produce infection. The death of alcohol-killed bacilli was not revealed by a change in their fluorescence. According to Bertalanffy, Masin, and Masin (1956), the cells of malignant tumors, unlike normal cells, show intense orange-red fluorescence in the cytoplasm and yellow in the nuclei when stained with acridine orange.

Kölbel (1951) reported that differentiation between dead and living tubercle bacilli was not always possible by means of acridine orange and he affirmed that this was due to the difference in the concentration of lipids in the cells which accumulated different concentrations of fluorochrome.

According to Krieg (1954b), the cells that show red fluorescence are dead, but not all cells that have green fluorescence are living; after careful fixation in corrosive sublimate, many cells are dead but nonetheless have green fluorescence when fluorochromed with acridine orange.

MacVandiviere, Gentry, and Willis (1952) investigated the possibility of utilizing the capacity of the living cells to reduce colorless tetrazolium salt to red formazan, discovered by Kuhn and Jerchel (1941), in order to determine the viability of tubercle bacilli. The quantity of reduced tetrazolium is supposed to be in direct relation to the viability of the cells.

Two strains of tubercle bacilli (BCG and R_1Rv) were used in the experiment of MacVandiviere *et al.* Several tubes of Dubos' Tween 80–albumin medium were inoculated with decreasing quantities of bacilli. A colony count on the Löwenstein-Jensen medium was made on each tube. To the bacilli one ml. of the 0.25 per cent solution of 2,3,5-triphenyltetrazolium chloride solution was added. After the incubation of the mixture for two hours at 37°C., acetone was added to the suspension and the extracted color was read on a colorimeter with a 550 mμ color filter.

The tubes containing living bacilli assumed a deep red tint, whereas the tubes with killed bacilli remained colorless. The readings, plotted on semilogarithmic paper, gave a straight line and indicated that the degree of reduction of tetrazolium salt was the function of amount of living cells in the medium.

Neotetrazolium (from 0.01 to 0.25 per cent) added to the solid medium produced dark blue or purple colonies of tubercle bacilli. The addition of streptomycin to tubercle bacilli sensitive to the drug inhibited the reduction of tetrazolium salt.

Kopper (1952) studied the reducing power of *Escherichia coli* on 2,3,5-triphenyltetrazolium chloride and found that a linear relation exists between the number of live bacteria in the suspension and the amount of tetrazolium reduced. The optimum reduction was at *p*H 7.5 for young cells. In the absence of sodium chloride, tetrazolium was not reduced, but a concentration of sodium chloride over 1 per cent inhibited the reduction. The incubation for twenty minutes of resting cells of *Escherichia coli* with various substances, such as glucose, peptone, and broth, increased the reducing power of *Escherichia coli.* This effect was most pronounced with glucose. (Glycerol was not tested.) Compounds that did not increase the reducing power of bacteria were unable to support their growth.

The use of fluorescence microscopy in the detection of mycobacteria will be discussed later (see p. 191).

Phase Contrast Microscopy

After the optical work of Ernst Abbe, research on the improvement of the microscope was concentrated on the resolving power of the objective.

The optical conditions of the transparent object itself, which could contribute to an increase in the resolving power of the microscope, however, were largely neglected.

The human eye, when focusing on an object, recognizes differences in dimension, shape, brightness, and color. A transparent and unstained object is recognized when its light refraction or absorption is different from that of the surrounding medium. The difficulty of observing unstained bacteria under a microscope is due chiefly to the transparency of these organisms, which is usually equal to that of the liquid in which they exist.

A new approach to the problem was indicated by Zernike (1934), who described the phase contrast microscope and its theory.* Phase contrast microscopy is based on two properties of the light wave, its phase and its amplitude. When a light wave passes through a transparent object, it is slowed down and is out of phase in contrast to the surrounding light which did not pass the object. Under these conditions two light waves enter the microscope, one retarded by the object, the other unaffected in its passage through the surrounding medium. As they continue their journey, these waves combine and form the image in the microscope. The human eye and the photographic plate are sensitive to differences in the amplitude of the light waves (distance from crest to depression of the wave) but not to differences in their phases. When the amplitude of the light waves passing through the object and of those passing through the surrounding medium are equal, there is no contrast between the image of the object and its background; i.e., the object in the microscope is invisible. The phase contrast microscope changes the phase differences of the light waves into amplitude differences.

Köhler and Loos (1941) indicated that the chief field where phase contrast microscopy could find useful application was the study of unstained transparent biological objects. The photographs of unstained kidney and epithelial cells taken by these scientists through a phase contrast microscope can hardly be distinguished from pictures of carefully stained preparations. The cell wall, the nuclei, and the protoplasmatic inclusions were clearly reproduced in the phase contrast photographs, whereas pictures of identical preparations taken by means of an ordinary microscope showed only vague outlines of cells – without showing any internal structures. The same differences in contrast were shown by Michel (1941) in unstained pictures of chromosomes.

Knöll (1944) recognized that phase contrast microscopy, which transforms small differences in the refraction of unstained objects into strong

* For general discussions of phase contrast microscopy, see A. H. Bennett, H. Osterberg, H. Jupnik, and O. W. Richards, *Phase microscopy. Principles and applications* (Wiley, New York, 1951); and A. G. Hansen, A. Römiger, and K. Michel, *Das Phasenkontrastverfahren in der Medizin* (Vandehöck and Ruprecht, Göttingen, 1952).

light contrasts, would be particularly helpful to the study of fine structures and the reproduction of unstained, living cells. His observations on three-month-old cells of *Escherichia coli, Proteus vulgaris,* and other bacteria revealed that in old cultures only a few rods showed uniformly high cytoplasm density and were living, and that all other cells were gray and dead. During growth and reproduction the cell structure was subject to considerable changes. The cell interior consisted of dark and bright zones, and the number of bright zones was as high as 32 in the cells. The nuclear bodies were localized in the bright zones, the dark zones were occupied by cell cytoplasm. (See also the findings of Stempen (1950), Knöll and Zapf (1951), and others.) The division of nuclear bodies occurred without being immediately followed by the division of the cytoplasm, producing polynucleoid cells.

Richards (1948), in his survey of the application of phase contrast microscopy to bacteriology, indicated that under a phase contrast microscope the living bacteria show sharp edges and thin cell walls. The bacilli studied *(Bacillus cereus)* had paired bodies in the nonsporulating cells, similar to those observed by Robinow (1942, 1949) in stained bacilli.

Tulasne (1949) using a phase contrast microscope, attempted to answer the question whether nuclear bodies, seen in the bacterial cells after their fixation, acid or enzymatic digestion, and staining, are not artifacts created as a result of the treatment. *Proteus vulgaris* and *Escherichia coli* were grown on a thin layer of agar between the slide and the cover-glass and examined by a phase contrast microscope. The unstained and living cells showed sharp edges and one or more bodies in the form of rods were seen in their interior. The division of these bodies was later followed by the division of the cells.

Stempen (1950) indicated that earlier methods of cytology had involved the study of dead cells, and that the fate of their nuclear bodies had been to a great extent reconstructed by logic. But with the phase contrast microscope, it was possible to demonstrate and to follow up the fate of the nuclear bodies in young, living cells of *Escherichia coli* and *Proteus vulgaris* and to compare the obtained results with those yielded by the study of fixed and stained cells. One-hour-old cells were fixed in vapors of osmium tetroxide, hydrolized in hydrochloric acid, and stained with basic fuchsin. The images obtained in the light microscope were compared with those revealed in the living cells of the same culture by the phase contrast microscope. The dark-phase contrast microscope showed light and dark areas in the living cells. Compared with the hydrolized and the stained cells, the light areas in the living cells occupied the positions of the dark bodies in the hydrolized cells, and the dark areas of the living cells were identical with the light cytoplasmic areas of the stained cells. Therefore it must be concluded that in living cells the light areas represent the location of the nuclear bodies and the dark areas that of the cytoplasm. (Under a light–phase contrast microscope the picture is reversed.)

The nuclear bodies in the living cells of *Escherichia coli* never have the appearance of dumbbells, as was stated by Robinow (1942). Probably in Robinow's experiments the hydrolysis of the cells had removed some portions of the nuclear bodies, which caused them to look like dumbbells.

Eisenstark, McMahon, and Eisenstark (1950) from their investigations with the electron microscope, the phase contrast microscope, and by nuclear staining of the cells of *Azotobacter*, reached the conclusion that the bodies in the bacterial cells revealed by the different methods of investigation have the same location, and probably are of nuclear nature.

Knöll and Zapf (1951) studied the structural changes in the nuclear apparatus of multiplying and resting cells of *Escherichia coli, Proteus vulgaris*, and other Gram-negative bacteria. Untreated living cells grown on agar were investigated with a dark-phase contrast microscope, and the cells, after staining according to the Piekarski-Robinow and Romanowsky procedures, were observed in a light microscope. Feulgen reaction tests were also performed on them. In the early stages of development the rods of *Escherichia coli* showed cellular homogeneity and appeared gray in the phase contrast microscope. The differentiation of the cell protoplast started after the cultures had been incubated at 37°C. for one to two hours: two dark polar bodies, separated by a light intermediary zone, appeared in the cells; in the light zone a dark streak, starting out at the periphery of the zone, progressed toward the center of the cell. This dark streak progressively increased in width, so that at last the cells had two bright zones and three dark ones: two dark zones at the poles, one in the middle of the cell, with the bright zones lying between. As the growth process continued at 37°C., the central dark zone increased in width, and, in 30 to 60 minutes, an indentation appeared in the cell wall; the indentation progressed inward so that in 90 to 120 minutes after the indentation had appeared, two new cells were formed (see Fig. 6).

In the logarithmic phase the majority of the cells have two light and three dark zones and this structure must be regarded as the normal appearance of the bacterial cell; the cells with four light zones are the mature, dividing cells, and the cells with one light zone and two dark polar bodies are the resting cells.

The Feulgen reaction and the treatment of cells according to the Piekarski-Robinow method showed that the light areas of the cells as seen in the phase contrast microscope are the areas where the nuclear bodies are located, the dark zones being the areas of the cytoplasm.

The nuclear phenomena described were seen in all bacteria studied and were taken to represent the general course of the bacterial life cycle, which starts with the growth of the resting cell and ends with the division of the

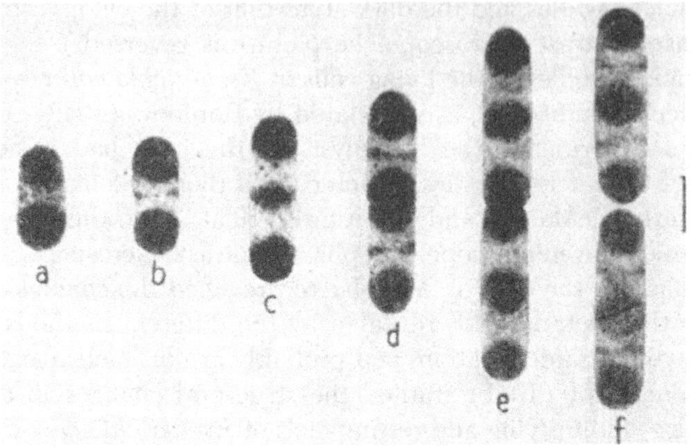

Figure 6. Scheme of division of *Escherichia coli*; phase contrast microscopy. a. Resting cell. b, c. Logarithmic phase. Light areas: nuclear bodies. Dark areas: cytoplasm. Vertical line at right = 1μ. (Knöll and Zapf, 1951.)

cell; as in the higher cells, the division of the nuclear bodies located in the light areas precedes the division of the cell protoplast proper.

Phase contrast microscopy of mycobacteria. Phase contrast microscopy was also applied to the study of the cytology and the development of mycobacteria.*

Richards and Wade (1948) studied the morphology of *Mycobacterium leprae.* Bacilli from human lesions appeared in the form of rods. Many among them contained polar and occasionally central nuclear bodies. Free-lying granules were also seen.

Bassermann (1952) indicated that the Feulgen-positive granules in tubercle bacilli are easier to observe by means of the phase contrast microscope than with the ordinary microscope. Brieger and Glauert (1952) investigated an avian strain of tubercle bacilli. The bacilli were observed in living state in cover-glass cultures grown in chick embryo extract. The phase contrast microscope revealed cell details not seen with the ordinary microscope. The bacilli produced two forms of growth, the rod form and the mycelial form. The media, inoculated with short rod-shaped bacilli up to 1μ in length, developed, in five to seven days of incubation, filaments from 8 to 10μ in length. In five days the mycelial branches became dense and gave rise to a formation of cords (see p. 295). In twenty days the filaments broke up into rods. The density of bacillary cells varied. The bacilli showed polar densities. The structure of the bacilli revealed great similarity to the pictures obtained by the Piekarski-Robinow staining method. Krieg (1954a) found alternate dark and bright bodies in the cells

* For a further discussion of phase contrast microscopy as applied to the detection of mycobacteria, see p. 191.

of mycobacteria and corynebacteria. The dark bodies were metaphosphate granules, the light ones nuclear bodies. In the case of the absence of metaphosphate granules, the cell structure of these bacilli was identical to that of *Escherichia coli,* consisting of light nuclear and dark cytoplasmic areas.

In his latest survey, Richards (1954) collected 205 papers published during 1950–1954 on the application of phase contrast microscopy in the studies of microorganisms, cells, and tissues.

Electron Microscopy

The electron microscope was developed by E. Ruska, Knoll, and von Borries (1932) in the laboratories of the Technische Hochschule in Berlin. At the same time work was being done in this field in Berlin at the Allgemeine Elektrische Gesellschaft laboratories (Brüche, 1932), in Belgium by Marton, and in England by Martin *et al.* In this country the electron microscope was developed in the laboratories of the Radio Corporation of America.*

Electrons are particles emitted by the cathode and carrying negative charges. Their mass is approximately 1/1,840 that of the hydrogen nucleus. In the straight path from their source, the electrons are easily scattered or stopped by solid or gaseous obstacles, such as glass or air. All work with electrons must therefore be carried out in a vacuum. Busch came to the conclusion in 1926 that the magnetic or electric field acts on the electrons as a glass lens acts on a light beam. The electrons can be deflected from their trajectory and focused. The laws of optics may be applied to explain the behavior of electrons in magnetic or electric fields.

The principal parts of the light microscope are present in the electron microscope, which operates in the same manner as the light microscope. The position of the source of light in the electron microscope is the reverse of that of a light microscope. The electron beam, produced in cathode from tungsten filament is directed downwards. The beam of electrons passing through the magnetic or electric field of the condenser is focused on the object. Entering the field of the objective, the image of the object is formed in the same manner as in the light microscope. The image is magnified once more by the projection coil and thrown onto the fluorescent

* For a more extensive study of the historical background and the question of the priority of the invention of the electron microscope, see von Borries and E. Ruska (1938, 1948).

For general information on electron microscopy, see M. von Ardenne, *Elektronen-Übermikroskopie* (Springer, Berlin, 1940); C. Grégoire, *Microscope électronique et recherche biologique* (Masson, Paris, 1950); C. E. Hall, *Introduction to electron microscopy* (McGraw, New York, 1953); B. Jirgensons and M. E. Straumanis, *A short textbook of colloid chemistry* (Wiley, New York, 1954); L. Marton, *The electron microscope in biology* (37), 1943, 12, 587; A. B. Novikoff, *Electron microscopy: cytology of cell fractions* (212), 1956, 124, 969; and R. W. Wyckoff, *Electron microscopy, technique and applications* (Interscience, New York, 1949).

screen. On this screen the image may be observed or photographed, the photographic plate being sensitive to electrons.

According to de Broglie in 1924, although the nature of the electron is corpuscular and different from that of light, the high speed electrons have a wave motion similar to that of light. The velocity of electrons increases with the increase of the voltage applied, but their wave length shortens with the increasing velocity. The wave length of electrons is inversely proportional to the square root of the voltage applied and can be calculated by the formula of de Broglie:

$$\lambda = \sqrt{\frac{150}{V}} \times 10^{-8} \text{ cm.}$$

where *V* is the voltage used.

At high voltage the velocity of electrons may reach ⅔ that of light. When electron velocities of 60 or more kilovolts are used in an electron microscope, the electron wave length will be 1/100,000 that of light. According to Abbe a powerful light microscope will reveal particles 1/5,000 mm. in diameter; when rapid electrons instead of light are used in a microscope, particles smaller than 1/1,000,000 mm. in diameter will be reproduced. The electron microscope permits the linear magnification by 100,000 diameters or more of a suitable object.

In an electron microscope, the object, depending upon the thickness and density of its parts, either scatters or absorbs the electrons. These properties of the object determine the electron image of the object. The image in an electron microscope consists of the general pattern of the dark and light parts of the object without any specific structural details. The contrast of the image is increased by using a small aperture in the objective. The decrease in the aperture diminishes the resolving power of the microscope. Because of this, the resolving power of the electron microscope is smaller than one would expect from the wave length of the electrons used in the microscope. In compensation, the small aperture increases the depth of focus so that the object in an electron microscope can be clearly seen even if it is considerably displaced in the direction of the axis of the electron beam. (See Table 1 and Fig. 7.)

Preparation of objects for investigation. As electrons are of corpuscular nature, they have no significant penetrating power and are absorbed by objects of 0.1 μ thickness. The slides for the electron microscope cannot be of glass. Supporting membranes penetrable by electrons must be used instead of glass slides.

The first successful solution to this problem was found by H. Ruska (1939). A drop of collodion dissolved in amyl acetate was deposited on a large water surface and, spreading across it, produced a 10 mμ-thick

Table 1. Comparable Parts and Properties of the Light and Electron Microscopes

Light Microscope	Electron Microscope
Parts	
Light source	Electron source
Condenser lens	Magnetic condenser
Objective lens	Magnetic objective
Eyepiece	Image projector
Observation screen	Second-stage magnified image
Photographic plate	Photographic plate
Properties	
Wave length: 800 mμ–200 mμ	Wave length: about 0.5 mμ
Penetrating power: great	Penetrating power: small
Contrast formed by refraction and absorption of light	Contrast formed by electron scattering and absorption
Contrast enhanced by staining, dark-field illumination	Contrast enhanced by impregnation with J, W, Os, and by shadowing
Focal depth: small	Focal depth: great
Resolving power: 200 mμ	Resolving power: 2 mμ

Figure 7. Image formation in light microscope and in electron microscope.

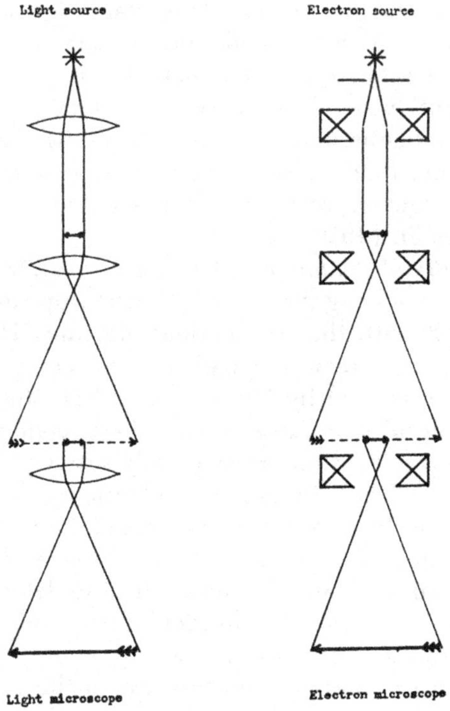

film quite invisible on the water's surface. Such a film of cellulose is sufficiently resistant to support the objects and also sufficiently transparent for the electrons to penetrate. Hillier, Knaysi, and Baker (1948) introduced the technique of growing microorganisms directly on the cellulose film itself. By their method, the film of collodion is spread over the surface of the water covering an agar medium. When the water is removed the film settles on the agar surface and may be inoculated with a diluted suspension of microorganisms. At a convenient stage of growth the desired areas of film are cut out and investigated with an electron microscope. There are reports that this cultivation procedure produces famine conditions for streptococci and distorts their cellular structure (Hennessen, Grün, and Lindner, 1950). Collodion film may also be used for the cultivation of bacteria on liquid media. In our experiments, the cultivation of tubercle bacilli on collodion film floating on the surface of the liquid medium was easily realizable. After one week of incubation, the young colonies of tubercle bacilli could be seen with the naked eye.

Klieneberger-Nobel's (1950) method of cultivating microorganisms one cell layer deep under a glass or film cover may be of use in electron microscopy.

Objects suitable for investigation with an electron microscope can be obtained from tissue sections a fraction of a micron thick, as shown by von Ardenne in 1939. The rotary high-speed microtome was invented for such sections (Claude and Fullam, 1946); even the conventional microtome was adjusted for such use (Pease and Baker, 1948), and new instruments were devised (Watson, 1953). Ultrasonic waves were applied to disintegrate the tissue into fine fibrils penetrable by electrons (Wuhrmann *et al.*, 1946). The method of growing thin tissue cultures suitable for investigation with an electron microscope was described by Martin and Tomlin (1950).

Metal shadowing. Any particle can be seen when its dimensions exceed the resolving power of the microscope and when it produces enough contrast with the surrounding medium. The contrast of a particle may be increased by impregnating it with compounds of heavy metals. This method was used by Husemann and H. Ruska (1940) with glycogen, whose molecules, because of their loose connections, scatter few electrons, and their images are consequently scarcely visible through an electron microscope. These investigators obtained contrast-rich pictures of the molecules when they transformed glycogen into a para-iodobenzoyl compound containing 40.6 per cent iodine. This "staining" of the preparations with a stainless chemical allowed them to determine the dimensions of the glycogen molecules. The fixation of preparations with phosphotungstic or osmic acid also increases the contrast.

An important step forward in the electron microscopy of transparent objects was made when the method of metal shadowing was introduced – a method well known in the mirror industry (see Fig. 8). H. O. Müller (1942) applied this procedure to measure in an electron microscope the dimensions of the shell structures of the *Pleurosigma angulatum.* A filament of a heavy metal, when vaporized in a vacuum, scatters particles which in most cases settle down on the side of the object which has been turned toward the source of the metal. Behind the object is a zone without a metal layer, which in a microscope appears as the shadow of the object. When the length of the shadow and the angle of the metal deposit are known, the height of the object may be calculated ($h = s \tan \alpha$).

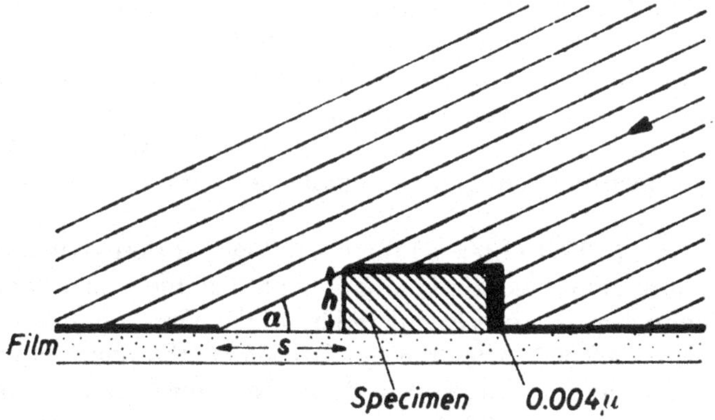

Figure 8. Metal shadowing. s. Length of shadow. h. Height of specimen. a. shadowing angle. $h = s \tan \alpha$.

This method of depositing metals on the surface of an object greatly increased the value of the electron microscope in biology when Williams and Wyckoff (1945, 1946) introduced this procedure to produce contrast-rich images and indicated suitable metals for shadowing. The deposited metal mirror must not have a structure of its own, must not alter the surface of the object, and must scatter the electrons strongly enough to produce a contrast-rich image. Tungsten, palladium, chromium, gold, and other metals are used for shadowing.

When the deposit of a metal on an object is made at a suitable angle, the metal layer is of different thickness and produces varying shades of opacity which greatly increases the contrast of the object and gives the impression of a three-dimensional image.

Sources of error in the interpretation of images. Electrons carry a great amount of energy. When absorbed by the object, the liberated energy rapidly raises the temperature of the object. To prevent this, the object must be thin and highly transparent. In a high vacuum the drying of the object proceeds rapidly and under the impact of electrons the organic substance is destroyed. These obstacles greatly restrict the use of the electron microscope in biology. The shading of the object from electrons partially eliminates these difficulties, so that von Ardenne (1941) was able to follow for many hours the germination of bacterial spores under an electron microscope.

Changes in the object under the impact of the energy of electrons may cause errors in the interpretation of the pictures obtained. The formation of pseudostructures in preparations for the electron microscope was called to the attention of investigators. The bombardment of tubercle bacilli with rapid electrons for 30 seconds produced vacuoles in the nuclear bodies of the bacilli. Prolonged bombardment caused shrinkage of the cells, the disappearance of the granules, and the evaporation of the background material. Bessis, in 1948, observed filaments in electron microscopic pictures of thrombocytes, which he recognized as artifacts. Angulo, Watson, and Olarte (1950) indicated that some particles which, when viewed through an electron microscope, resemble elementary bodies, are in reality crystals.

C. L. Smith (1953) observed the breakdown of desoxyribonucleic acid under deuteron and electron bombardment. The molecular weight of dry desoxyribonucleic acid was calculated by Fluke, Drew, and Pollard (1952) to be about 6,000,000. After the bombardment, the units into which the desoxyribonucleic acid was broken down were much smaller, their molecular weight being about 2,100.

The exposure of cells to the beam of electrons changes their physical and chemical properties. After such exposure they became resistant to hydrolysis by hydrochloric acid and to cytolysis by distilled water. The collodion film and embedding media, after they had been treated with electrons, were insoluble in the usual solvents and resistant to high temperature. In such cases the fixation of the objects by electrons is obviously due to deep changes in their molecular structure (Hillier, Mudd, Smith, and Beutner, 1950).

The electron microscope in biology. The electron microscope revealed the structure of the microcosm far beyond the resolving power of the light microscope. In microbiology the electron microscope found a wide application in virology and in the study of cell morphology and structure.

The first micrographs of electron microscopic images of the colon-typhoid bacteria, the smallpox virus (Paschen's corpuscles), and the virus of ectromelia of the mouse and of myxoma of the rabbit were obtained by von Borries, E. Ruska, and H. Ruska (1938). The dimensions of these structures were about 10 $m\mu$, only twice as large as an egg albumin molecule. Kausche, Pfankuch and H. Ruska (1939) produced electron micrographs of the tobacco mosaic virus and of the potato-X virus. These were rodlike structures, 150 mμ–300 mμ long, and 15 mμ in cross section. The micrography of molecules of hemocyanin, the protein of snail blood, was obtained. Their size was 2.10^{-5} mμ, in accord with the earlier determination of their size by physical methods (von Ardenne, 1940). Stanley and Anderson (1942) examined five different proteins by an electron microscope. The molecules of the bushy stunt virus and of *Limulus polyphemus* hemocyanin appeared to be spherical in shape and approximately 20 mμ–26 mμ in diameter. The shadowing of purified hemocyanin, prepared by the ultracentrifugation of the blood of *Limulus*, showed spherical molecules (Williams and Wyckoff, 1945). An account of the results obtained with the electron microscope in the study of macromolecules was given by Wyckoff (1951).

The first investigation of bacterial cells with an electron microscope was made by Piekarski and H. Ruska (1939). Cultures of cocci, sarcina, and bacilli, four to twenty-four hours old, appeared very poor in internal structure, often homogeneous and dark in appearance. The non-spore-forming bacterial cells were richer in structural elements. The young cells showed polar thickening; the old ones had thick central formations. The dividing cells revealed four cytoplasmatic bodies. Not all cell formations that were seen in the electron microscope could be identified on the basis of light microscope examinations of stained preparations.

Mudd and Lackman (1941) and Mudd, Polevitzky, Anderson, and Chambers (1941) studied some details of bacterial cells with the electron microscope. *Streptococcus*, *Bacillus subtilis* and *Bacillus anthracis* were chosen as test objects. All cells showed a rigid outer membrane or a cell wall. The cytoplasm retracted from the cell wall or escaped after the injury of the cell, leaving the empty cells in the form of "ghost cells." The supposed presence of a nucleus similar to those found in higher forms was questioned by these investigators. The bacterial cell wall which covers the cell from the outside was observed by Knaysi (1929) under a light microscope and seen in section experiments of isolated cells by Wámoscher (1930).

Johnson (1944) investigated with an electron microscope the process of division of the young cells of *Bacillus cereus* grown on agar. The several stages of cell division were apparent. A slight notch in the protoplast in the cell wall end indicated that the process was in an early phase. In the later stages the cell wall and the cytoplasm were drawn out between the two dividing cells. These dividing cells remained for some time connected with the cytoplasmic bridge (plasmodesmid). (See Fig. 9.)

Khodukin (1948) gave a general account of the application of the electron microscope to microbiology.

Chapman and Hillier (1953) made thin (less than 0.1 μ) cuts through seven-hour-old cultures of *Bacillus cereus* and investigated these preparations with an electron microscope. The cells were found to be covered

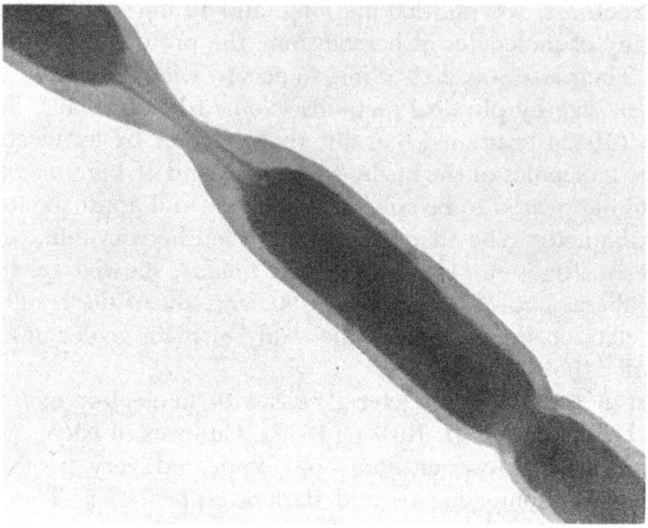

Figure 9. Electron micrograph of *Bacillus cereus*; several stages in cell division are shown in the central and adjacent cells; the sharply defined bridge (plasmodesmid) is enclosed by the drawn-out cell walls (Johnson, 1944).

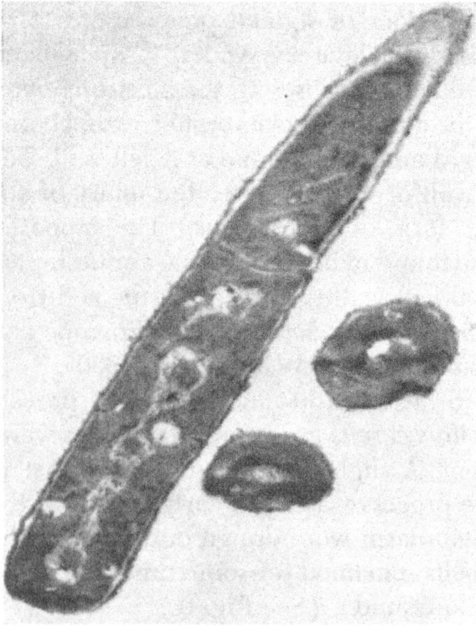

Figure 10. Electron micrograph of an ultrathin section of *Bacillus cereus*, × 59,500. The cells are covered with the cell wall, which contains dark granules. The formation of the transverse septum can be seen in the lower cells. The nuclear material in the cytoplasm has the form of a light knotty cord, suggesting different stages of division. Vacuoles can be seen in the form of light round bodies. (Chapman and Hillier, 1953.)

with a cell wall that was approximately 20 mμ thick and contained vacuoles that were 0.2 mμ in diameter. As Figure 10 shows, the configuration of the nuclear material suggested that it was dividing, but there were no indications of chromosomes or structures identical to mitotic figures. The distribution of nuclear material was not axial and no organelles identical to mitochondria were seen.

Electron microscopy of the tubercle bacillus. Among the obstacles encountered in the investigation of tubercle bacilli with an electron microscope was the difficulty of preparing a uniform, single-cell suspension of tubercle bacilli. As is well known, it is particularly difficult to break down the human type of tubercle bacilli to a single-cell suspension. The grinding of a culture particle in a mortar followed by the filtration or centrifuging of the suspension was of some help. The cultivation of tubercle bacilli in liquid media containing dispersing agent Tween 80 was not helpful. As Knaysi, Hillier, and Fabricant (1950) discovered, under these cultivation conditions tubercle bacilli produce large quantities of a mucoid substance. This substance is very slightly transparent to the beam of electrons, and particles of this substance, which cover the surface of tubercle bacilli, can produce images of cellular structure.

The first electron microscope images of tubercle bacilli were obtained in 1939 in the laboratories of the Technische Hochschule, Berlin (von Borries, 1952).

von Borries and E. Ruska (1939) published electron micrographs of the avian strain of tubercle bacilli magnified 26,000 times. The cytoplasm of these bacilli contained dark bodies of different sizes.

The first thorough investigation of tubercle bacilli with an electron microscope was made by Lembke and H. Ruska (1940), who studied the avian type of bacilli grown on Petragnani medium. The culture consisted of rods containing up to eight large bodies in their cytoplasm. The size of the bodies was 300 mμ–350 mμ; they were dark in appearance under the electron beam. Besides these large bodies, there were much smaller, more transparent ones of 20 mμ–50 mμ in diameter. No division of these bodies was observed. There was a third type of bodies, transparent inclusions, well separated from the cytoplasm wall, which were identified as vacuoles. The cell wall (membrane) was seen, but the *Hülle,* which earlier workers presumed to exist around the cell, was not detected (see p. 185).

Mudd and Lackman (1941) and Mudd, Polevitzky, Anderson, and Chambers (1942) observed, in the opaque cytoplasm of tubercle bacilli, dense granules from 70 mμ–230 mμ in diameter. The cells were covered with a thin cell wall. Rosenblatt, Fullam, and Gessler (1942) in their studies of tubercle bacilli in the electron microscope (see Fig. 11), confirmed many earlier observations and added some new data, particularly concerning the internal structure of bacilli. The bacilli varied in size. The size of the strain H37 subcultured at Columbia University varied from 4.3 μ x 0.4 μ to 1.0 μ x 0.2 μ; the same strain obtained at the American Trudeau Society laboratory contained bacilli varying in size from 1.8 μ x 0.6 μ to 1.0 μ x 0.3 μ. The bacilli were predominantly rod-shaped; curved rods or

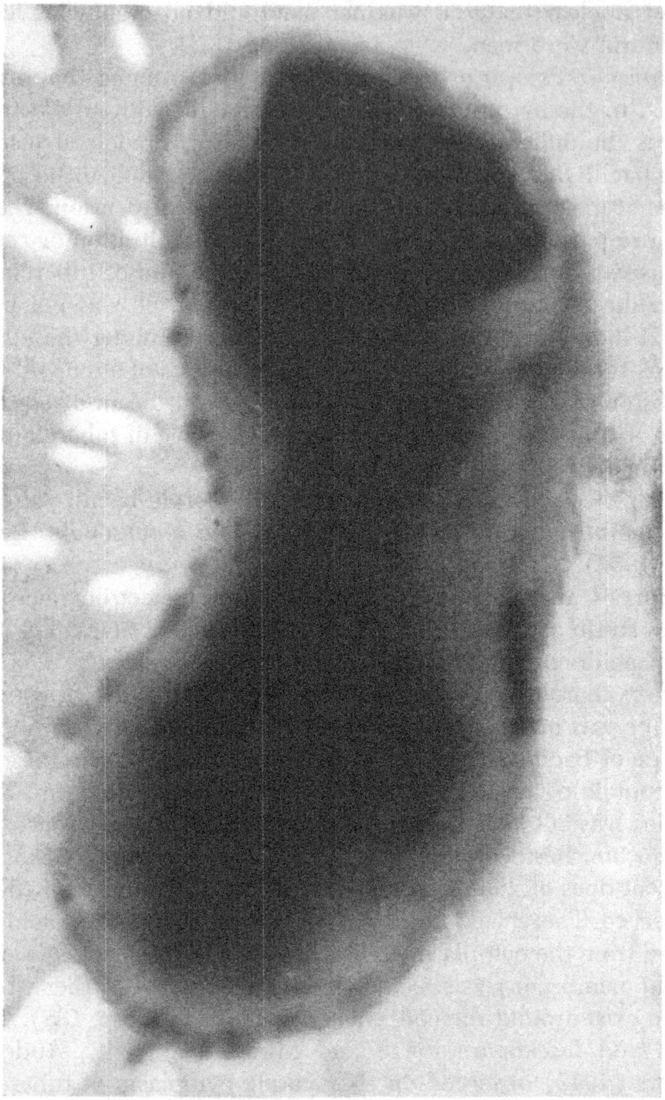

Figure 11. Electron micrograph of *Mycobacterium tuberculosis,* human strain (Trudeau), × 105,000. The bacilli are straight, curved, or bean-shaped rods with rounded ends; they measure 1.5 μ × 0.6 μ. Relatively thick (0.03 μ) cell wall (membrane) is uniformly present; it contains granules. Internal structure of the bacilli consists of granular cytoplasm which contains one or more dense nuclear bodies. The light spaces between the nuclear bodies give the bacilli a beaded appearance. Large and small vacuoles can be seen.
(Rosenblatt, Fullam, and Gessler, 1942.)

branching bacilli were not seen. The cell wall (membrane or capsule in the terminology of these authors) was always present; sometimes it was as thick as 0.03 μ and contained granules. The internal structure showed dense nuclear masses within the granular cytoplasm. These bodies varied in size; most of them were located at the end of the bacillus. When there were many of these bodies in the cell, they were distributed along the axis of the bacillus. The density of the cytoplasm varied; it contained many granules and vacuoles of different sizes. The bacilli of the bovine type investigated were shorter than the human strains, their average size being 1.0 μ in length, and 0.5 μ in width. Electron microscopy did not reveal any significant structural differences between saprophytic and pathogenic acid-fast bacilli.

Wessel (1942) investigated the cells of the human type of tubercle bacilli and observed the presence of a cell membrane. The cytoplasm of the bacilli contained vacuoles and two types of granules. One type of granule was resistant to electron radiation, the other disappeared under its impact. According to Lembke (1947), in old cultures of tubercle bacilli the granular structure of the bacilli increases and a mass of free granules besides the intact bacilli can be seen on their outside. These granules showed a light absorption maximum between 253.7 and 275 mμ, identical to that of the bacilli.

More facts about the morphologic structure of tubercle bacilli were revealed by the recent investigations of Knaysi, Hillier, and Fabricant (1950). Because of its unusual transparence to the electron beam, a strain of avian tubercle bacilli was used (Fig. 12). The cells were cultivated on collodion film deposited on the surface of an agar medium. The growth of tubercle bacilli on the film proceeded in the first days in one cell layer, and it was possible to investigate this layer in the electron microscope or, after the bacilli had been stained, in a light microscope. These cultures can also be investigated with a phase contrast microscope.

These investigations confirmed earlier findings in regard to the assumption that the cytoplasm of young cells is dense, that the basic dyes stain it deeply and uniformly, and that it contains vacuoles and hyperchromic bodies. The cell protoplast was seen surrounded by a 0.023 μ thick and ductile cell wall. The cytoplasm itself was covered with a thin cytoplasmic membrane which closely adhered to the cell wall. Both the cytoplasm and the cytoplasmic membrane were transparent to electrons and contained a great number of rodlike granulations or micelles 0.005 to 0.03 μ in size, like those observed in other bacteria. The rodlike granulations were also seen scattered in the cytoplasm and exhibited high surface activity, accumulating on the internal surfaces of the cell and probably forming the membranes around the vacuoles. The cytoplasmic membrane was clearly revealed in tubercle bacilli when they were subjected to disintegration un-

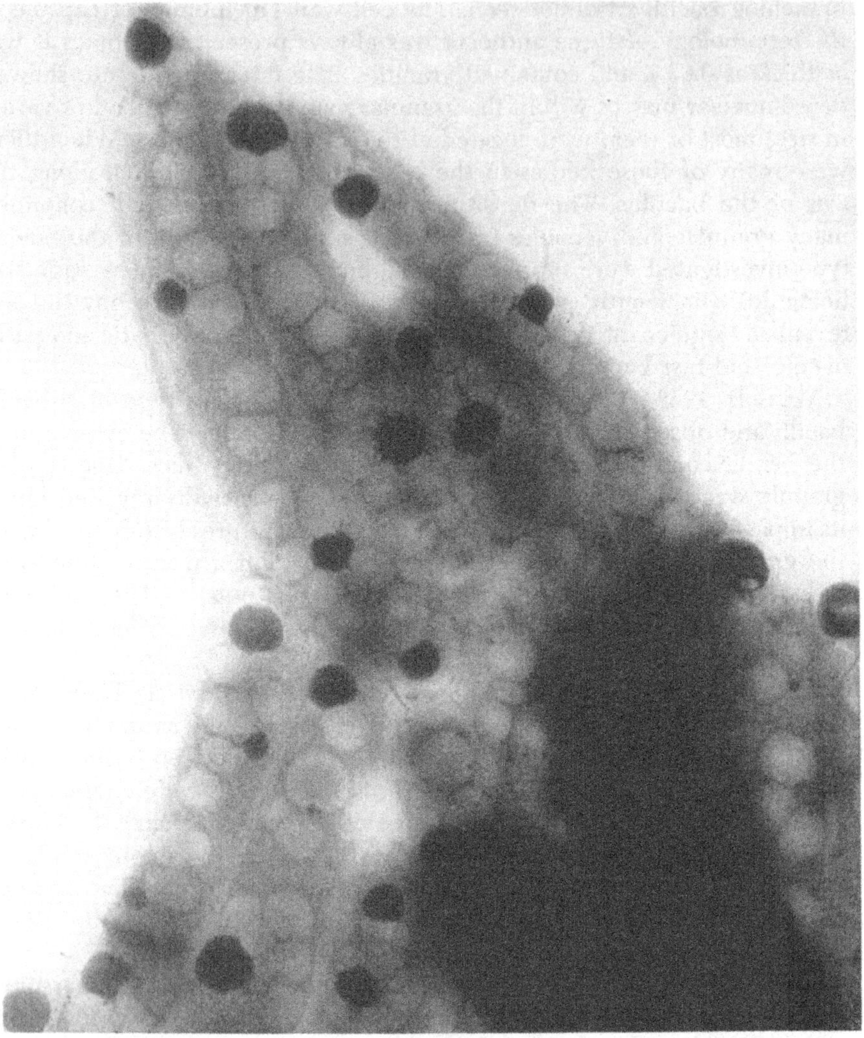

Figure 12. Electron micrograph of tubercle bacilli, avian strain, 21 × 5 hours at 37°C., × 42,500. Cytoplasm, nuclear (phosphate) bodies, vacuoles, cytoplasmic membrane, and cell wall are seen. Some cells and nuclear bodies are in various stages of division. In the cytoplasm the rod-like micelles (mitochondria?) can be seen. Many vacuoles contain amorphous material. Some vacuoles are deformed because of turgor pressure. (Knaysi, Hillier, and Fabricant, 1950.)

der a strong electron bombardment. The cytoplasm disintegrated first under such treatment, the membrane resisted longer.

In the cytoplasm of the bacilli, bodies of two different types were located. The first ones were spheroids of high density to the electron beam.

Their number in the cell varied from one to five; their dimensions in young cells were from 0.3 to 0.4 μ. In the old cultures most of the cells had central bodies of 0.8 to 1.0 μ diameter. Similar to the phenomena observed in the cells of *Escherichia coli* and other microorganisms, these large bodies of old cells originated from the smaller ones and, as they grew up, they reached larger dimensions and came to occupy a great part of the cellular space. These large bodies of old cells consisted of cortex and stroma. The cortex was stained in violet, the stroma in red by Romanowsky strain. In young cells some of the small bodies showed elongation and appeared paired. This may indicate that they were dividing.

The other type of bodies located in the cytoplasm of tubercle bacilli were the sap vacuoles. It was difficult to observe them in the light microscope, but they were promptly revealed by the electron microscope. Vacuoles did not stain with basic dyes and were highly transparent to the electron beam. They were separated from the cytoplasm by a wall and their transparent content could become opaque to the electron beam.

The division of the cells of tubercle bacilli was seen in these young cultures. In the equatorial zone of the cell, on the inner side of the cell wall, a double cell plate was formed. The growth of this plate proceeded till the mother cell was divided into two daughter cells. The separation of newly formed cells occurred between these plates, which then covered the poles of the right and the left cells. Before the cytoplasm divided, the division of cellular bodies was observed.

The electron microscope did not reveal any principal differences between the structures of pathogenic and saprophytic mycobacteria. Saprophytic *M. phlei* and *M. smegmatis* were rod-shaped, round-ended cells, their dimensions being 1.5 μ x 0.5 μ. The big round cellular bodies were located in the poles of the cells, the smaller ones being distributed in their cytoplasm.

In an electron microscope it was not possible to observe any differences between the surface of virulent and avirulent bacilli. No kind of layer around the cells of pathogenic bacilli was observed, and no indications of "life-cycle" or "filtrable forms" of mycobacteria were found (Werner, 1951).

The work of H. Ruska, Bringmann, Neckel, and Schuster (1952) added further knowledge to the field of the cytology and cytochemistry of tubercle bacilli. These authors pointed out that a relation exists between the structure of the cell and the age of the cell. The first structural differentiation in the cell of *M. avium* Chester grown at 37°C. appeared in 140-hour-old cultures. Subpolar in the short cells were seen two dark bodies without any structure, varying from 30 to 200 mμ in diameter. As the cell increased in length, the number of cytoplasmic bodies also increased. This increase in the number of bodies was particularly great between the twenty-fourth and the twenty-eighth day of growth, so that finally cells containing 12 to 15 bodies were not rare. The largest bodies, which measured 350 mμ x 700 mμ, lost their round form and stretched out along the axis of the cell. In three-month-old cells the substance of the dark bodies had disappeared and the empty cells were left.

In an early stage of development, the cell cytoplasm showed bright spots. In fifteen to twenty-five days these spots developed into round or oval vacuoles. Between the vacuoles in the cytoplasm dark micrograules were scattered. (See Figs. 13 and 14.)

In old or extracted cells a very fine cell wall was observed. There was

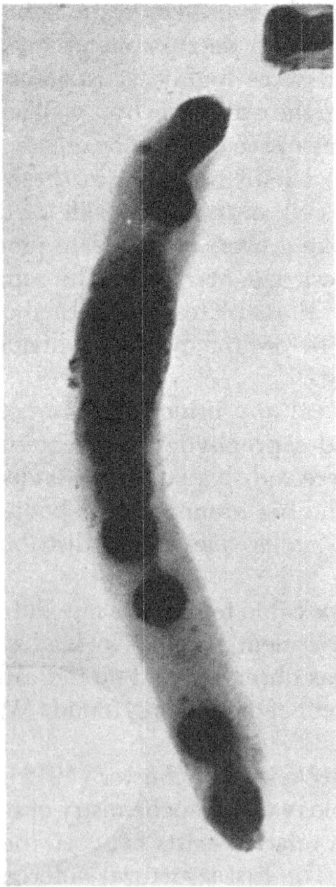

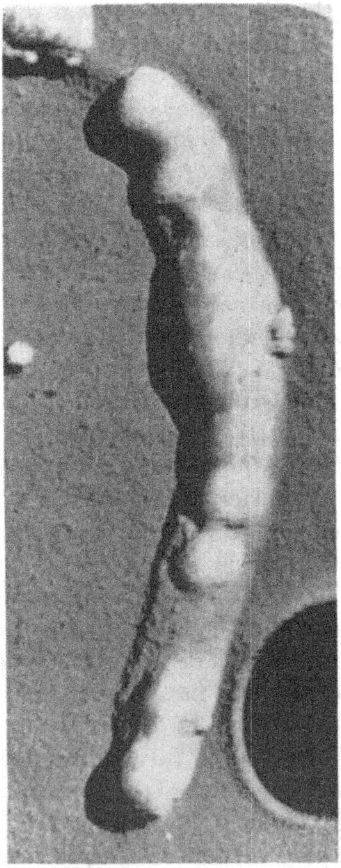

Figure 13. Electron micrograph of *M. avium* Chester; culture 23 days old, $\times$ 20,000, before shadowing. The dark phosphate granules and opaque lipid vacuoles are revealed. (H. Ruska, Bringmann, Neckel, and Schuster, 1952.)

Figure 14. The same bacillus after shadowing with tungsten; the granules are revealed as exceeding the surface of the cell.

no probability that the large amounts of lipids of the bacilli could be localized in this thin membrane and that it might play the role of *Hülle* as had been suggested by earlier authors.

The investigations of H. Ruska *et al.* (1952) demonstrated that after the extraction of tubercle bacilli by means of Carnoy's solution, the vacuoles were lost; the fixation of cells with vapors of formaldehyde and following extraction of cells with alcohol-chloroform or petrol ether brought about the disappearance of vacuoles, while the nuclear bodies remained unaffected. The authors concluded that the vacuoles are the reservoirs of cell lipids. Through the separation from the cytoplasm, these substances accumulate in the vacuoles.

The morphology of Bacille Calmette-Guérin (BCG) and the influence of freezing and drying on BCG were studied by means of an electron microscope by C. I. Reed, Rosenthal, and Reed (1948). The bacilli were grown on bile potato, the presence of bile permitting easy dispersion of the bacilli in liquid. Chromium shadowing was applied to the bacilli. The predominant form of the bacilli was that of a slightly curved rod with rounded poles. Only in two bacilli of the several thousand studied were ramifications seen. The average dimensions of the bacilli were from 2.5 to 3.5 μ in length and 0.6 μ in width. The internal structure of BCG in isotonic salt solution consisted of pale cytoplasm with spherical masses in the extremities of the bacilli. These masses were also irregularly distributed in the cytoplasm. Free granules were seen outside the bacilli.

Bishop, Suhrland, and Carpenter (1948) investigated, with an electron microscope, the structure of *Mycobacterium leprae murium* and of human *M. leprae*. Material from the leproma was minced, ground, and centrifuged. After fixation with osmium tetroxide, dark cellular bodies were seen located at the poles of the bacilli. They occupied 30 to 50 per cent of the cell volume. Nuclear material was more widely distributed throughout these cells than in the other species of mycobacteria. The cell wall was visible. Boiling the material in a 0.05 *N* sodium hydroxide solution for fifteen minutes partially destroyed the cell bodies and revealed small dense polar bodies in the transparent cytoplasm.

X-Ray Microscopy

The use of X-rays in microscopy would considerably clarify those obscure problems of research to which light and electron microscopes are of no avail. If it were possible to build an X-ray microscope, one would have an instrument that would be handicapped neither by the limited resolving power characteristic of the light microscope nor by the lack of penetration power of the electron microscope. The impossibility of focusing X-rays, however, is an obstacle which has so far made the construction of such an instrument practically impossible. The works of Kirkpatrick (1950), at Stanford University, on X-ray focusing and image formation by means of X-ray deflection in mirrors coated with metal, are encouraging.

X-ray structure of tubercle bacilli protein. The X-ray structure of bacterial protein is not influenced by the composition and the *p*H of the media, or by the temperature of cultivation. However, the intensity of X-ray diffraction depends on the concentration of proteins in the sample investigated. Bacilli grown on media rich in protein or polypeptides will produce accentuated X-ray reflexes, although the size of polypeptide chains and their arrangement in the molecule will not be altered. Any change in the polypeptide chains of a molecule would indicate the formation of a new protein.

Table 2. The Size of Polypeptide Chains of Tubercle Bacilli, Yeast, and Egg Albumin, Calculated with Bragg's Law from Their X-ray Images

Object	Lateral Distance	Depth Distance
Mycobacterium tuberculosis....	1.05 mμ	0.422 mμ
Saccharomyces cerevisiae......	1.10	0.455
Egg albumin.................	1.10	0.467

Source: Lembke and Lück (1950–1951).

Bacterial protein revealed a diverse arrangement of polypeptide chains in the molecule. The molecules with a linear arrangement of chains and of fibrous structure, and those with an irregular chain arrangement, produce characteristic pictures of X-ray diffraction. In the case of unarranged protein chains, the X-ray pattern has the shape of circles or rings. In the image of a bacterial protein there may be two or three such rings.

A study of tubercle bacilli by means of X-ray diffraction was performed by Fournier (1949). His diagrams were constructed according to the method of Debye and Scherrer. Humid bacilli were spread on collodion film and covered with another collodion membrane. The images formed by human strains consisted of two rings with the interreticular distance of 0.4 and 0.5 mμ and another weak ring at 1 mμ distance. In the BCG strain one ring of 0.4 mμ was seen. Saprophytic bacilli produced a very vague ring. Paraf, Desbordes, and Fournier (1950) found that the ring of 0.4 mμ was always present in all mycobacteria, unlike the ring of 0.5 mμ, which was well developed in pathogenic strains but not found in saprophytic strains.

According to Lembke and Lück (1950–1951), most bacteria have two X-ray diffraction rings, one of them 0.45 mμ in diameter, indicating the depth distance, another 1.0 mμ, showing the lateral distance from one polypeptide chain to another (see Table 2).

In tubercle bacilli the distance between the chains of their polypeptides is the smallest, the greatest distance being between the chains of yeast polypeptides. The significance of this peculiarity in the structure of protein molecules of tubercle bacilli is not known.

The X-ray pictures of tubercle bacilli protein show few specific details.

III

Biological Methods for Identifying Cell Structures

Differential Staining: Romanowsky Method

THE young bacterial cell, when treated with a basic dye, is uniformly and deeply stained. The stain prevents the observer from looking into the interior of the cell. On the other hand, a stain with a specific affinity to chromatin, which would stain cytoplasm in a color different from that of the nucleus, would be capable of indicating the presence or absence of a nuclear substance in the cell.

Romanowsky (1891) started his study of malaria with the intention of finding a combination of dyes that would stain the nuclei and the cytoplasm in different colors. A mixture of basic methylene blue and acid eosin showed promise of producing a neutral stain with the desired properties. This mixture stained the red blood cells a deep red, the nuclei of white blood cells and of all other cells a deep red-violet, and their cytoplasms a light blue. Some parts of the malaria parasite in red blood cells became red-violet, and Romanowsky concluded that these formations of the parasite cell must be of nuclear or chromatinic nature. The thirty-five colored drawings of the malaria parasite that accompanied the work of Romanowsky showed, for the first time, the now well-known polychromic picture of the malaria parasite in red blood cells.

Ziemann (1898), in a systematic study, indicated the causes for the occasional failure of the Romanowsky procedure, and made the procedure independent of chance. After testing the method in higher cells of plants and animals, Ziemann applied it to the investigation of the nucleus in yeast, mold, and bacterial cells. In the cells of *Saccharomyces cerevisiae, Torula, Oidium, Aspergillus, Spirillum,* and in water bacilli, Ziemann observed the same stained formations as in the higher cells: blue protoplasm and red-violet grains. Ziemann called these red-violet formations of the bacterial cell the "chromatin granules." He was not able to see these formations in the cells of the typhoid, coli, subtilis, and tubercle bacilli. Zettnow (1899) confirmed the findings of Ziemann and was of the opinion that the internal part of the body of the bacterial cell is mostly made up of nuclear substance. He coined the word "ectoplasm" to designate the outer layers around the central nuclear substance of the cell.

A further step ahead in the study of the internal structure of bacterial cells by means of the Romanowsky staining method was taken by Feinberg (1900). By a simple procedure he showed that the Romanowsky stain, in a concentrated solution, made alkaline and applied hot (80°C.) for 3–4 hours, reveals, in all bacterial cells investigated (*Escherichia coli*, corynebacteria, tubercle bacilli, etc.), red or red-brown granules.

The analogy between the staining results of the bacterial cells and the results obtained from the higher cells permitted Feinberg to conclude that the bacterial cells, like the higher cells, are made up of cytoplasm and nuclear formations (*Kerngebilde*).

Dobell (1908) investigated the structure of the *Bacillus flexilis, Treponema*, and other bacilli from the intestines of a frog. A large number of red-stained granules was seen inside the organisms.

The investigations of Michaelis (1901) clarified the origin of the specific staining properties of the Romanowsky staining mixture. He found that methylene blue easily produces decomposition derivatives. One of the oxidation products of methylene blue is methylene azure. The methylene azure molecule is characterized by the sulfo group (SO_2) in the place where the methylene blue molecule has the S-atom. The solution of methylene blue is blue; the solution of methylene azure is red. Methylene azure has specific affinities with chromatinic bodies and causes their red hue. Methylene azure is present in old alkaline solutions of methylene blue and is responsible for the metachromatic staining properties of these solutions.

Michaelis' later investigation (1947) disclosed further factors involved in the metachromatic staining properties of the basic dyestuffs, such as methylene blue. The basic dyes produce polymers in solutions. In higher concentrations high polymers, with the absorption band displaced toward shorter wave length (γ-band), are formed, shifting the blue color toward purple or even pink.

Giemsa (1902) found that methylene azure alone does not lead to the red staining of chromatinic bodies, and that the presence of eosin in the solution is necessary. He observed that dried azure and eosin, when redissolved in alcohol, do not lose their original staining properties. This discovery greatly facilitated the use of the azure-eosin stain in the investigations of infections caused by Protozoa in tropical countries. In his publications, Giemsa correctly used the term "Romanowsky staining" to designate the specific staining of nuclear structures with azure-eosin. But as the azure-eosin became commercialized, the name of Romanowsky was largely replaced by that of Giemsa.

The investigations of Brachet (1940) revealed that the selective staining of a tissue with the methyl green and pyronin mixture of Unna-Pappenheim is caused by the nucleic acid content of the cell. The nucleic acids in a cell, because of their acidic character, readily combine with basic dyes. When the cells are stained with a mixture of methyl green and pyronin, the nuclear bodies are stained green, and the basophilic elements of cytoplasm eagerly take up the pyronin and acquire a red hue. When the ribonucleic acid in the cytoplasm is dissolved by means of acid or enzyme (see p. 45), the staining properties of the cytoplasm are lost, but the nuclei retain their green color. It must be concluded that methyl green in the Unna-Pappenheim mixture is capable of staining the polymerized desoxyribonucleic acid of the nuclei but fails to stain the ribonucleic acid in the cytoplasm, which is stained red by pyronin. Jeener and Brachet (1943) observed that toluidin blue has specific polychromatic affinities with ribonucleic acid.

Bertalanffy and Bickis (1956) applied fluorescence technique and acridine orange staining to differentiate ribonucleic acid from desoxyribonucleic acid. They found that the ribonucleic acid in the cytoplasm gives a bright red fluorescence, and the desoxyribonucleic acid of the chromatin fluoresces green.

Acid Hydrolysis

A further advancement in the use of staining methods for studying the structure of bacterial cells occurred when Piekarski (1937) applied Feulgen's acid hydrolysis procedure to demonstrate the presence of nuclear formations in the cytoplasm of the cells.

The cytoplasm of young cells has a strong affinity with basic dyes. The deep stain of the cytoplasm makes the observation of the internal cell structure impossible. Before staining, Piekarski treated the cells for five to ten minutes with *N* hydrochloric acid at 60°C. The ribonucleic acid of the cell cytoplasm was hydrolyzed and dissolved, but the desoxyribonucleic acid of the nuclear bodies resisted and remained unchanged by this treatment. When the cells treated with hydrochloric acid were stained with methylene blue or Romanowsky stain, well limited and deeply stained bodies were revealed in the faintly tinged cytoplasm.

Piekarski observed that after the division of the cells of Gram-negative bacteria, there remained only one central body in each cell, while there had been two bodies before the division. The positive Feulgen reaction of these bodies, and their division, which occurs before the division of the cells, seemed to indicate that the properties of these bodies were the same as the properties of the nuclei of higher cells. However, there is actually no proof that these bodies of bacterial cells are similar in structure and function to the nuclei of the metazoan cell. To distinguish these bacterial bodies from nuclei, Piekarski named them "nucleoids."

Neumann (1941) confirmed the presence of Feulgen-positive bodies in bacterial cells.

The technique of Piekarski as refined by Robinow (1942, 1949) yielded irrefutable proofs of the presence of nuclear structures in the bacterial cells. In the young cells, volutin granules and droplets of fat are mostly absent and do not prevent the observation of the internal structure of the cell. After the fixation of the cells with osmium tetroxide and after hydrolysis, the nucleoids (or nuclear bodies, in the terminology of Robinow) were well colored and exposed in a colorless cytoplasm, with the aid of Romanowsky stain. The nuclear bodies had the shape of dumbbells; they divided and gave rise to two or more bodies in the multiplying bacilli. The transverse septa separating the cells were generated from the inner surface of the cell wall, and by growing inward, separated the cells.

Peshkov (1945) after carrying out acid hydrolysis and staining the cells of colon-typhoid bacteria with Romanowsky stain, obtained good pictures of nucleoids. After their fixation in Carnoy's liquid and a double staining with Romanowsky stain and light green stain, red-violet nuclear bodies were seen in the green cytoplasm. The results obtained by Piekarski, Robinow, and Peshkov were confirmed by Tulasne (1947) and others.

The Piekarski-Robinow method was used by Klieneberger-Nobel (1947) to investigate the "chromosomes" in alternating filaments and short forms of *Proteus vulgaris*, and by Bisset (1948) to study the nuclear bodies in myxobacteria and *Azotobacter*.

Mudd and Smith (1950) showed that electron microscopy is most rewarding when used simultaneously with other methods of investigation.

The density and the thickness of an object determine the differences in electron scattering and produce contrast in the electron microscope. Microcolonies of *Escherichia coli* and of *Salmonella typhosa*, grown for 2½ hours on collodion films overlying nutrient agar and fixed in osmium tetroxide vapors, showed, in an electron microscope, uniformly dark cells with lighter intermediate regions. The additional treatment of these cells with *N* hydrochloric acid and staining completely reversed the picture (see Figs. 15 and 16). After the treatment the highly electron-scattering cytoplasm had lost its density and had become transparent, but the light vesicular bodies, seen in the untreated cells, had retained their density and position in the cells and acquired the appearance of dark bodies in light cytoplasm. These were the nuclear bodies of desoxyribonuclein, which is not attacked by hydrochloric acid. The ribonuclein of the cytoplasm was dissolved as a consequence of treatment with the acid. Other microcolonies of *Escherichia coli* grown on collodion film were prepared for investigation

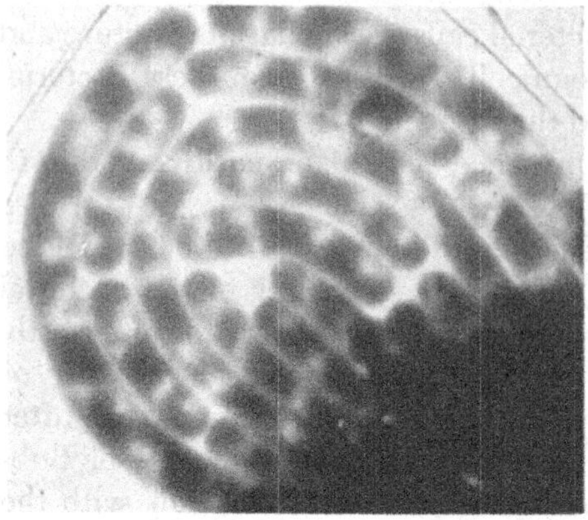

Figure 15. Electron micrograph of microcolony of *Escherichia coli* grown on collodion film for 2½ hours; fixed in osmium tetroxide vapors; × 11,000 approximately (Mudd and Smith, 1950).

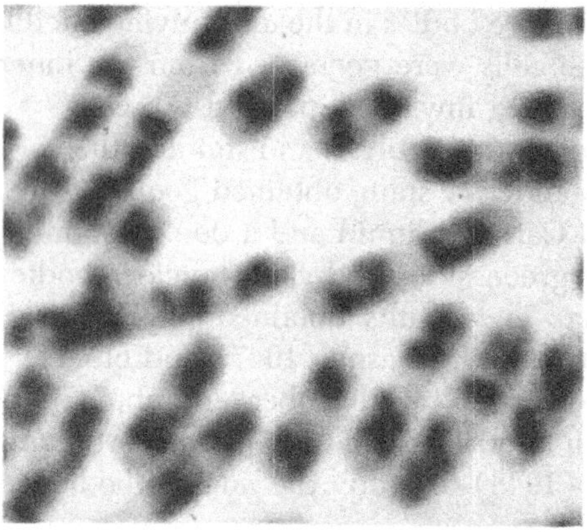

Figure 16. Microphotograph of *Escherichia coli* cells grown for 1¼ hours, fixed in osmium tetroxide vapors, treated with *N* hydrochloric acid and formaldehyde, stained with 0.3 per cent basic fuchsin for 3 minutes; light microscope, × 6,000 approximately (Mudd and Smith, 1950).

with a light microscope. The bacteria were fixed in osmium tetroxide vapors, treated with hydrochloric acid and formaldehyde, and then stained with basic fuchsin. The cells showed dark, stained bodies in their light cytoplasm. The comparison between electron pictures of cells of *Escherichia coli* fixed with osmium tetroxide with pictures of cells treated additionally with hydrochloric acid and with other cells treated with hydrochloric acid, mordanted with formaldehyde (A. G. Smith, 1950), stained with basic fuchsin, and observed in a light microscope, revealed striking similarities in internal structure and an identical location of nuclear bodies.

Electron micrographs of identical sites of *Escherichia coli*, grown on collodion film, taken before fixation in osmium tetroxide and after the fixation and shadowing with chromium, were presented by Mudd, Smith, Hillier, and Beutner (1950). Clear images of nuclear bodies, which had the form of irregularly shaped vesicular areas, were seen in the young cells. In fixed and metal-shadowed cells the nuclear sites were visible through the chromium coating and appeared as dark areas in light cytoplasm. (In positive prints, the nuclear bodies are seen as light spots in dark cytoplasm; in negative prints the picture is reversed, the nuclear sites appearing as dark bodies in light cytoplasm.)

The position of the nuclear bodies in electron micrographs of unfixed and fixed cells corresponds to the position and image of these bodies seen in living cells by the means of a phase contrast microscope (Tulasne, 1949; Stempen, 1950).

A. G. Smith (1950) investigated the structure of *Escherichia coli* by means of a modified Piekarski-Robinow technique. The cells revealed fine rodlike or round nuclear bodies. Distinct doubling of nuclear bodies before cell division was observed, and cells containing 2, 4, 8, or 16 nuclear bodies were not rare. In the cells of *Bacillus megatherium* the nuclear bodies presented a complicated picture, because chromatin had not been distributed regularly as in the cells of *Escherichia coli,* but rather in the form of irregular masses. Vacuoles could be seen in nearly every cell.

Bringmann (1954) presented some objections to the generalizations of the preceding interpretations of the electron micrographs of bacterial cells. If the light areas seen in bacterial cells by means of an electron microscope and revealed, after acid treatment and staining, as dark bodies, are the nuclear substance, Bringmann said, then desoxyribonuclein would have to fill up most of the cell space. According to Bringmann, the nuclear bodies of mycobacteria are not vesicular but solid in structure.

Enzyme Methods

Nucleases. Nucleases are enzymes which depolymerize nucleic acids and form mononucleotides. Ribonuclease depolymerizes ribonucleic acid and converts it into soluble and diffusible products. Desoxyribonuclease depolymerizes and makes soluble desoxyribonucleic acid. The temperature optimum for the action of these enzymes is about 60°C. and the *p*H optimum is about 7.5. These enzymes occur in animal and plant tissues.

The specific action of enzymes constitutes an important analytical tool. An unknown enzyme can be identified when its specific action on a known structure of substrate is established and, vice versa, an unknown structure of the substrate can be identified when the enzyme of a known and specific action reacts to it.

Enzyme digestion methods for the study of tissue structures were early used in cytology. Ernst (1889) used them to investigate the nature of the bodies in the bacterial cells. He observed that these bodies are less resistant to the action of pepsin and hydrochloric acid than are the bacterial spores (see p. 4). Unfortunately pepsin and trypsin have no specific action on the nuclear structures; nuclear bodies are digested like other proteins, although Miescher claimed that the pepsin digestion of nucleoproteins is only partial.

Sachs (1905) precipitated the enzyme nuclease from the juice of the pancreas by means of ammonium sulfate and showed that this enzyme is not identical with trypsin.

Enzyme analysis of cell compounds was considerably advanced by Oes (1908) who observed that the rapidly growing young cells of root endings and sprouts of seeds contain an enzyme which, at temperatures of 32°–40°C., dissolves the chromatin of nuclei. The alkaline reaction of the medium was favorable, the acidic one unsuitable for the nucleic acid–splitting action of this enzyme. This enzyme, the nuclease, also dissolved the chromatin of cells fixed in alcohol, but the cell membrane and the nucleolus were not attacked.

van Herwerden (1913, 1914–1915, 1918) produced evidence that the basophilic staining properties of the cells depend on their nucleic acid content. She obtained purified nuclease by precipitating the spleen juice with acetic acid. The cells digested with the nuclease had lost their basophilic properties. The specific action of this enzyme on structures rich in nucleic acids, such as frog sperm and the nuclei of blood cells, was observed. van Herwerden's attempts to digest, by means of this enzyme, the volutin granules of yeast cells were unsuccessful.

Dubos and MacLeod (1938) discovered an enzyme in animal tissue which was active on yeast nucleic acid. The pneumococci treated with this extract lost their affinity to the basic dyes and became Gram-negative. The enzyme ribonuclease attacked ribonucleic acid between *p*H 5.5 and *p*H 9.5 and rendered this substance soluble in mineral acid. Ribonuclease did not decompose the desoxyribonucleic acid (Dubos and Thompson, 1938). The ribonuclease and desoxyribonuclease were crystallized by Kunitz (1940, 1948).

Brachet (1940) and Jeener and Brachet (1943) reported that the basophilic properties of yeast cells are caused by the compounds of phosphoric acid, i.e., by their nucleic acid content. This view was supported by the observation that, after the treatment of animal or yeast cells with ribonuclease, the basophilic properties of the cytoplasm were lost but the staining properties and the Feulgen reaction of nuclei, caused by the desoxyribonucleic acid, remained unaffected.

A considerable amount of research on cell structures was carried out by means of chemical and enzyme methods, by a group of French investigators headed by Boivin. The French authors use the term *noyau,* that is "nucleus," to designate the nuclear formations of the bacterial cell.

Boivin and Vendrely (1943) showed that microorganisms are even richer in nucleic acids that the thymus or the sperm of the fish. The nucleic acids are localized in the small nuclear bodies, in the form of desoxyribonucleic acid and in the cell cytoplasm mainly as ribonucleic acid. The bacteria (dry weight) contain 50 to 70 per cent protein and 10 per cent nucleic acids. Further quantitative studies of ribonucleic and desoxyribonucleic acids in the bacterial cell were made by Vendrely and Lehoult (1946). The acids were extracted from the cells with a cold solution of 5 per cent trichloracetic acid, followed by a hot trichloracetic acid extraction at 90°C. These consecutive treatments made it possible to extract the total content of both acids. In the extract obtained, a separated dosage of ribonucleic and desoxyribonucleic acid was made.

As Table 3 shows, approximately 10 per cent of the dry weight of microorganisms consists of ribonucleic acid and 3 to 4 per cent is made up of desoxyribonucleic acid.

Table 3. Ribonucleic and Desoxyribonucleic Acid Contents in 100 Parts of Dry Bacteria

Micro-organism	Total Nitrogen	Total Protein	Nucleic Acid	Desoxy-ribonucleic Acid	Ribo-nucleic Acid	Desoxyribonucleic Acid ÷ Nucleic Acid
Staphyloccus (strain 72)......	13.95	75.50	11.57	2.82	8.75	0.24
Salmonella typhosa (strain D_1)	14.61	78.50	12.84	3.72	9.12	0.29
Escherichia coli (strain C_1)	14.40	76.80	13.12	4.40	8.72	0.34

Source: Vendrely and Lehoult (1946).

The extraction of bacterial cells (staphylococci, coli) with *N* hydrochloric acid at 60°C., according to the procedure of Piekarski, released only 7.5 per cent of the total content of desoxyribonucleic acid; the remainder could only be extracted with trichloracetic acid at 90°C. Contrary to this, with hydrochloric acid at 60°C., it was possible to extract the total quantity of ribonucleic acid from the cells. The differences in the solubility of these two nucleic acids in hydrochloric acid explain the success of Piekarski and Robinow in demonstrating the presence of the nuclear bodies in a cell. The ribonucleic acid that impregnates the cytoplasm and strongly binds the basic dyes is soluble in hydrochloric acid; when it has been dissolved, the cells become transparent and the nuclear bodies, containing insoluble desoxyribonucleic acid in hydrochloric acid, become visible when stained (Vendrely and Lipardy, 1946).

Tulasne and Vendrely (1947) treated fixed bacteria successively with a purified preparation of ribonuclease and desoxyribonuclease. After the treatment of bacteria with ribonuclease, the affinity of cytoplasm with the basic dyes was lost, but the chromophilic nuclear bodies were left untouched in the cells. When, after the treatment with ribonuclease, the cells were subjected to the action of desoxyribonuclease, the nuclear bodies were also lost; only the protein skeleton of the cells of poor colorability remained.

Vendrely-Randavel (1949) found that the action of ribonuclease and desoxyribonuclease on the cells of the liver, the pancreas, and the kidney of a mouse was equal to its action on the cells of microorganisms. Welsch and Nihoul (1948) indicated that in order to reveal the nuclear bodies in a cell, the ribonucleic acid of a cytoplasm can be extracted not only by means of acids, but also by the action of alkalies (*N* sodium hydroxide). (A general account of the works of the French investigators was given by Boivin, 1948.)

P. Boquet and Lehoult (1948) found that the venom of some snakes, chiefly *Vipera ruselli*, hydrolyzes nucleic acids. After the action of this venom the cytoplasm of *Escherichia coli* had lost its basophilic properties, but the nuclear bodies remained fully visible. The heated venom had no action on the bacterial cytoplasm.

In the electron microscope the definite structure of desoxyribonucleic acid can be seen. The spherical units are organized in a network of fibrils (Liquier-Milward, 1953). As a result of the action of crystalline ribonuclease on yeast and on pig liver cells, 60 to 70 per cent of the nucleotides present in the substrate were liberated as low molecular, rapidly dialyzable compounds. All preparations contained nondialyzable residue which resisted enzymatic digestion. A weak alkali produced complete hydrolysis of mononucleotides (Magasanik and Chargaff, 1951). The hydrolysis of ribonucleic acid, by means of ribonuclease or by alkali, produces cyclic nucleotides (Markham and Smith, 1952). Part of the polynucleotides of high molecular weight remains unattacked by ribonuclease. This enzyme liberates only the pyrimidine bases from nucleic acid (Vignais, 1953). Hoffman (1951) indicated that it is impossible to completely remove ribonucleic acid from the bacterial cells by the conventional technique. Ribonucleic acid is present in the cortex of the intracellular bodies of *Lactobacillus.* Although the significance of intracellular bodies in bacteria still remains obscure, the presence in these bodies of ribonucleic acid does not rule out their nuclear nature.

It was observed by Levene in 1909 that nucleic acids contain pentose sugar ribose. Chargaff and Moore (1944) and Chargaff and Saidel (1949) showed that the extraction of tubercle bacilli with alkalies yields glycogen and nucleic acids. Vischer, Zamenhof, and Chargaff (1949) recognized that the sugar obtained from the nucleic acids of tubercle bacilli and yeast is identical with 2-desoxyribose of thymus nucleic acid. The research done by these authors also revealed the presence of the pyrimidines cytosine (6.8 per cent) and thymine (32 per cent) in the desoxyribonucleic acid of tubercle bacilli. The purines adenine and guanine contained in this acid of tubercle bacilli were determined as being 3.9 and 10.1 per cent respectively. These works definitely established that some important cell constituents of tubercle bacilli are identical with those of cells of higher plants and animals.

Desoxyribonucleic acid is in its composition characteristic of the species from which it is derived. There are no differences among the desoxyribonucleic acids obtained from different tissues of the same species. The macromolecules of desoxyribonucleic acid probably differ in no more than the sequence of a few of their component nucleotides (Chargaff, 1951).

In the higher forms of life the nuclei of cells contain unchanging amounts of desoxyribonucleic acid (Boivin, Vendrely, and others). As was shown by Caldwell and Hinshelwood (1950) the desoxyribonucleic acid content of the cells of *Bacterium lactis aerogenes* is nearly constant despite variations in cell size. This may indicate that there is a connection between cell division and the desoxyribonucleic acid contained in the cells.

Nucleic Acids in Some Other Cell Functions

There must be chemical or physical differences in the cell structure which account for the different behavior of bacteria when submitted to Gram staining. The conversion of Gram-positive organisms to the Gram-negative state was realized by treating them with acids or alkalies, or by the action of their autolytic enzymes. Churchman (1927) observed that when a small amount of aqueous solution of gentian violet was added to a thick suspension of a young culture of *Bacillus anthracis,* a large number of the cells changed their staining property from Gram-positive to Gram-negative.

Henry and Stacey (1943) rendered Gram-positive bacilli Gram-negative by extracting them at 60°C. with a 2 per cent aqueous solution of bile salts. Both the treated cells and the material in the extract were Gram-negative. This material was precipitated by alcohol and consisted essentially of magnesium ribonucleate. The extracted substance, when added to the treated bacilli, rendered the organisms Gram-positive. The union of both parts was possible under reduced conditions carried out with 1 per cent formalin solution. The treated bacilli, if exposed to air, became irreversibly oxidized and the recombination of both parts did not occur. It was not possible to restore the Gram-positive properties of extracted cells by means of desoxyribonucleate or to transform naturally Gram-negative organisms into Gram-positive ones by treating them with magnesium ribonucleate. The magnesium ribonucleate extracted from the cells was not endowed with the specificity of any type. Extracts of one species of

Gram-positive bacilli restored Gram-positive properties in extracted cells of other species.

Bartholomew and Umbreit (1944) used crystalline ribonuclease, prepared according to Kunitz to remove the Gram-positive properties of *Saccharomyces, Bacillus subtilis, Bacillus cereus,* and other organisms. After 15 to 60 minutes of action by the enzyme, the cells were Gram-negative. The Gram-positive properties of the cells reside in the outer layer or ectoplasm of the cell. The combination of ribonucleic acid with proteins and carbohydrates of the cells involves basic groups of arginine and the groups of sulfhydryl, which are autoxidizable in air and also combine with iodine. These groups, when oxidized, prevent the recombination of magnesium ribonucleate with the cell. The magnesium ribonucleate, in combination with the protein of the outer layer of the cell, reacts chemically with gentian violet and iodine and was recognized as being responsible for the Gram-positive staining properties of the cell.

For their optimal growth, Gram-positive bacilli need about ten times more magnesium than Gram-negative bacteria. Gram-positive bacilli fail to grow when the concentration of magnesium is as low as 0.6 part per million, whereas this concentration of magnesium can maintain the maximal growth of Gram-negative bacteria.

In the absence of ionic magnesium in the medium, Gram-positive bacilli grow in the form of long filaments (M. Webb, 1949, 1953). These filaments revert to their normal form when cultured in a medium containing magnesium. The growth of bacilli is not affected, but the cell division is impeded. The oxygen consumption of filamentous cells of *Bacillus cereus* was only one third that of normal cells (Nickerson and Sherman, 1952).

The essential steps in the Gram procedure are the staining of bacilli with a stain of the pararosaniline class (methyl, crystal, gentian violet), "mordanting" the stained bacilli with iodine, and decolorizing the preparation with alcohol. When Gram staining is applied to acid-fast bacilli, the iodine treatment is not necessary; the stain is retained without iodine treatment. In such cases all other Gram-positive bacilli will lose the stain when decolorized. This basic difference between the staining properties of mycobacteria and Gram-positive bacilli led some authors (Kretschmer, 1934) to the conclusion that acid-fast bacilli do not possess genuine Gram-positive properties.

The role of nucleic acids in the transformation of bacterial types was discovered by F. Griffith (1928). Mice succumbed when inoculated with the living avirulent R strain of pneumococci type II, together with heat-killed pneumococci type III (S). Cultures of heart blood revealed the presence of pneumococci type III. The transformation of types of pneumococci, which never occurs spontaneously, was then performed *in vitro* (Dawson and Sia, 1931). Avery, MacLeod, and McCarty (1944) isolated from the pneumococci the transformation-inducing agent, which they identified as desoxyribonucleic acid.

Katunuma and Nakasato (1954) extracted desoxyribonucleic acid from streptomycin-resistant avian tubercle bacilli and added this extract to Sauton's medium. A sensitive strain cultured on this medium became streptomycin-resistant.

Fraenkel-Conrat and Williams (1955) announced that they had succeeded in splitting the infectious tobacco mosaic virus into two noninfectious parts of protein and ribonucleic acid. The union of both parts reconstituted an infectious virus. If the results of Fraenkel-Conrat's and Williams' experiments are confirmed, their significance for the understanding of life phenomena will have to be determined.

IV

Chemical Methods for Identifying Cell Structures

Feulgen Reaction

THE high affinity of chromatin to basic dyes was attributed to the acid compounds of chromatin, and chiefly to its large nucleic acid content. The staining process of the nucleus itself was regarded as a process of salt formation between the acid and the base. If this were the case, the staining properties of the nucleus would not necessarily point out chromatin. Indeed, the cartilage and the mucus are equal to chromatin in their Romanowsky staining properties. The notion of chromatin was morphologic rather than chemical. The discovery of a reaction which would specifically point out chromatin would be of great value in identifying the cell structures equivalent to those of the nuclei of higher plants and animals.

The nucleic acids are complex constituents of the cell but do not have any specific properties which might be used for their histochemical identification. Among the decomposition products of nucleic acid are some which give specific color reaction and will indicate the presence of nucleic acid.

Feulgen and Rossenbeck (1924) discovered that the nucleic acid of the type of desoxyribonucleic acid, when subjected to mild hydrolysis with *N* hydrochloric acid, and then treated with fuchsin decolorized by sulfurous acid (Schiff's reagent) produces a red-violet color. Schiff's test is used in chemistry to detect aldehydes. In the presence of aldehydes the color of the fuchsin in Schiff's reagent is restored. It must be assumed that by hydrolysis the nucleic acid is split and the aldehyde groups are set free. The reacting groups may be those of desoxyribose, the carbohydrate of desoxyribonucleic acid. Because of the aldehyde nature of the reaction, Feulgen and Rossenbeck called it "nucleal reaction." It is also known as the Feulgen reaction. The nucleal reaction is not equivalent to the staining of the nucleus, for the reagents employed in the process are colorless;

this microchemical color reaction is more like a spot test of the chemist done inside the cell (Mirsky, 1943). The basophilic staining properties of the chromatin of the nucleus and the nucleal reaction are both due to the same component of the nucleus as nucleic acid.

The isolation of desoxyribonucleic acid from rye germs was performed by Feulgen, Behrens, and Mahdihassan (1937), and its location exclusively in the nuclei of the cells recognized.

Although ribonucleic acid was discovered by Hammarsten as early as 1894, the isolation of ribonucleic acid from rye germs and the determination of its location in the cytoplasm of the cells was performed in Feulgen's laboratory by Behrens only in 1938. The Feulgen reaction is positive with the nuclei but negative with the cytoplasm of the cells. This is the most important specific property of the Feulgen reaction, one that is instrumental in revealing the presence of desoxyribonucleic acid in the chromatin of nuclei, whereas it remains itself negative in a cytoplasm containing ribonucleic acid but devoid of desoxyribonucleic acid.

In their first report, Feulgen and Rossenbeck stated that they were not able to obtain the nucleal reaction with yeast cells and bacteria. They believed that the nucleic acids of the plant nucleus are different from those of the animal cells. A further investigation of this problem by Voit (1925, 1927), in Feulgen's laboratory at Giessen, revealed that the investigated bacteria – *Bacillus subtilis, Escherichia coli, Pseudomonas aeruginosa*, and others – showed positive Feulgen reaction when treated in thick layers. Tubercle bacilli of the bovine type grown on egg media also produced a positive nucleal reaction. These microorganisms, when grown on synthetic media in the absence of desoxyribonucleic acid, showed positive nucleal reaction; their cells were able to synthesize the desoxyribonucleic acid from other ingredients of the medium.

The Brazilian investigators da Cunha and Muniz (1929) observed Feulgen stained formations in *Treponema duttoni* and in young cultures of *Bacillus anthracis* after their fixation with osmium tetroxide. These authors used the term "nuclear" instead of "nucleal reaction" (*réaction nucléaire*) to designate the Feulgen reaction. This orthographic change had far-reaching consequences. "Nucleal reaction" indicates the aldehyde nature of one compound of the nucleus, the nucleic acid; "nuclear reaction" on the other hand, designates the presence of the morphologic element of the higher cells, the nucleus.

The findings of Voit were confirmed by Neumann (1930). Imšenecki (1936) investigated the Feulgen reaction of some bacteria (micrococci, *Proteus, Bacillus mycoides*, and others). The sediment of these microorganisms after hydrolysis and treatment with Schiff's reagent showed intensive nucleal reaction, but the bacterial cells themselves remained unstained and no Feulgen-positive structures were discovered in them.

Stille (1937) was able to obtain positive Feulgen reaction in Gram-positive bacterial cells (*Bacillus subtilis, Bacillus mesentericus,* yeast cells, and others). The cells were either uniformly stained or the stain was localized in determined spots in the cells. In the latter case, the cytoplasm of the bacilli remained unstained. Stille found that the substratum used to cultivate the bacilli has no influence on the Feulgen reaction but that the duration and the temperature at which the hydrolysis of the cells was performed influences the result considerably. The desoxyribonucleic acid could be so profoundly split that the resulting fractions became water-soluble, penetrated from the nuclear bodies into the cytoplasm of the cells, and produced diffused staining.

Guilliermond (1933) observed that the Feulgen reaction was uniformly positive in the nuclear bodies and cytoplasm of the *Bacillus subtilis* and *Bacillus megatherium.* He regarded this observation as a confirmation of his view of the dispersed state of bacterial nuclei.

The bacilli investigated by Stille had in their cells at least two Feulgen-positive bodies of 0.3 μ–0.4 μ diameter. At the beginning of the division of the cell, four bodies shaped like dumbbells were formed in each cell. The division of the cytoplasm re-established the original number of two bodies in each daughter cell. In spore-forming bacilli the Feulgen-positive body entered into the spore. Piekarski (1937, 1940) found in the cells of Gram-negative bacteria *(Escherichia coli, Salmonella paratyphi)* Feulgen-positive bodies separated from the cytoplasm.

The mentioned investigations demonstrated the uniform presence of Feulgen-positive bodies in Gram-positive and Gram-negative bacteria.

The Feulgen reaction has been used for the quantitative determination of desoxyribonucleic acid in the cells. Ris and Mirsky (1950) used the microscope and the photoelectric tube to measure the intensity of Feulgen reaction in the cells.

Feulgen Reaction and Romanowsky Staining of Tubercle Bacilli

After Ernst (1889) had indicated the presence of a nuclear substance in microorganisms (see p. 4), the tubercle bacillus was subjected to study by means of the Romanowsky staining method and the Feulgen reaction.

The first attempts to stain tubercle bacilli with a Romanowsky stain were made by Ziemann (1898) and Zettnow (1899). Both were unsuccessful. Feinberg (1900) found that the Romanowsky stain reveals the presence of red or red-brown granules in the cytoplasm of tubercle bacilli. In tubercle bacilli, these nuclear formations made up only a small fraction of the cell body, but resisted the decolorizing action of alcohol. The work of Feinberg was accompanied by good drawings of stained tubercle bacilli.

A rude attack on Feinberg's work by Zettnow (1900) on the grounds of an unjustified feeling that his priority had been ignored, has caused the work of Feinberg to fall into disregard.

The Brazilian scientist Fontes (1933) observed that the Feulgen-positive substance in the cells of tubercle bacilli was in the form of fine dust, scattered throughout the cyanophile cell substance.

The Russian investigators Epstein, Ravitsch-Birger, and Svinkina (1935) found that a great many tubercle bacilli, when treated by the Romanowsky method, remained unstained. In an attempt to stain all of them, the authors applied to the bacilli, for one hour, a fixation of Carnoy's liquid (a mixture of chloroform, alcohol, and acetic acid), and afterwards treated them with carbon disulfide (CS_2). After this treatment, the tubercle bacilli, when stained according to the Romanowsky method or with toluidin blue lithium, showed cellular inclusion bodies. The Romanowsky solution stained these bodies in red-violet color, and their Feulgen reaction was positive.

Brieger and Robinow (1947) studied both bacillary and mycelial strains of avian tubercle bacilli to investigate whether the nuclear structures present in ordinary bacteria could be detected in tubercle bacilli. In tubercle bacilli, as in ordinary bacteria, there was close parallelism between the Feulgen reaction results and those obtained with acid hydrolysis and by means of Romanowsky staining. Feulgen reaction was positive to the bodies revealed by Romanowsky staining, indicating that these bodies are of nuclear nature.

Malek and Sterzl (1948) used the statistical method to study comparatively the cellular structure of tubercle bacilli as revealed by different staining procedures. The slides, prepared from the same cultures, were stained according to the Ziehl-Neelsen, Much, and Piekarski-Robinow methods respectively and Feulgen reaction was performed on them. The number and location of granules counted in bacilli stained by different procedures were nearly the same in all preparations. The different staining procedures revealed the same structures.

Epstein *et al.* called Feinberg's drawings, which revealed for the first time the structure of tubercle bacilli stained according to Romanowsky, "naive." When one compares Feinberg's drawings, made in 1900, with those of Kirchensteins, made 22 years later, or with those of Fontes, made 34 years after Feinberg's, no improvement in structural details or in execution can be seen in the works of the later authors.

The Romanowsky stain has become part of the ordinary outfit of the tubercle bacilli cytologists. The absence of progress in the investigation of cell structures by means of the Romanowsky staining method was due to the limitations of the Romanowsky or other staining methods in this field. The Romanowsky stain reveals the chromatin substance in the cells, and the Feulgen reaction confirms the nuclear nature of this substance, but these methods are not specific enough to determine whether the bodies in the bacterial cells are similar to the nuclei of higher cells. Neither the Romanowsky stain nor the Feulgen reaction reveals, in nuclear bodies, morphologic structures, physiologic or genetic transformations comparable to those of the nuclei of higher cells.

Metaphosphoric Acid and Nuclear Bodies

The presence of metaphosphoric acid in yeast cells was discovered by Liebermann (1890). During the chemical separation from the cells he obtained it as a barium salt, $Ba(PO_3)_2$, and believed that it was a constituent of the yeast nucleic acid. The presence of metaphosphoric acid in yeast cells was confirmed by Kossel (1893), but he rejected Liebermann's conclusion that metaphosphoric acid of yeast cells has its origin in the nucleic acid of these cells. Kossel showed that the properties of the phosphoric acid in the nucleic acid of the yeast cells are different from those of the metaphosphoric acid. Thus the presence of metaphosphoric acid in yeast cells was confirmed, but its origin and its significance for the cells remained unknown.

von Prowazek (1908) indicated that some substances ("lecithin") of the cell are, like nuclear bodies, stained by nuclear stains (hematoxylin, azure-eosin), and contain phosphoric acid in the form of metaphosphoric acid. Because of this, concluded von Prowazek, not all substances in the cell stained by nuclear stains must necessarily be chromatin. Reichenow (1909–1910) found in the cells of *Haematococcus pluvialis* granules which he identified as volutin. When this coccus was cultivated in media not containing phosphoric acid, the volutin granules gradually disappeared and, with the progressive loss of phosphorus content, the cells' property of retaining nuclear stains (methylene blue, hematoxylin) was also gradually lost. Reichenow concluded that the staining properties of these bodies must be attributed to their phosphorus compounds. van Herwerden (1918) cultivated cells of *Ustilagineae* and *Torulaceae* on a medium containing glycine and asparagine and did not observe in these cells any grains of volutin. When she transplanted these cells on a medium containing phosphate, volutin grains appeared. By that time there was no doubt that volutin is a phosphorus-containing compound, probably a nucleic acid. The basophilic properties of the yeast cells decreased when the cells were grown in the absence of the compound of phosphoric acid. The addition of phosphates led to the reappearance of the basophilic properties of the cytoplasm.

Brachet (1940, 1953) confirmed these observations. The addition of phosphate to the yeast cells grown in the absence of this substance produced a strong increase in the ribonucleic acid content of the cells. Schmidt, Hecht, and Thannhauser (1946) found that the amount of non-lipid phosphorus in 100 g. of moist weight of phosphorus-starved baker's yeast was 160 mg.; but, after two hours of incubation in *M*/10 sodium phosphate solution, the phosphorus content reached 1,250 mg. per 100 g. After the yeast cells were treated with alcohol, the phosphate formed in the cells could be extracted with cold water. The extracted phosphoric compound was determined to be metaphosphate.

The investigations of König and Winkler (1948) revealed that dark bodies, observed with an electron microscope in the cells of diphtheria, tubercle, and other bacilli, when heated for several hours in a vacuum furnace at 350°C., did not show any changes in appearance. These bodies did not even change after a strong bombardment with electrons or after they had been extracted with ether and acetone. From these results König and Winkler concluded that the dark bodies in the cells of diphtheria and tubercle bacilli are of inorganic nature. These bodies dissolved after five minutes of treatment with 2 per cent of lactic or acetic acid. The cellular bodies of the human and the avian types of tubercle bacilli were soluble in diluted acids after they had been treated with ether. A chemical analysis of the dissolved bodies of diphtheria and coli bacilli revealed the presence of calcium and phosphate ions. The addition of calcium phosphate to the diphtheria media produced bacilli far richer in cellular bodies than the bacilli grown on cultures without phosphate. Inorganic calcium phosphate is not stained by methylene blue; presumably the calcium and phosphate in the cellular bodies are bound with some organic substance and thus can only be stained electively.

Ebel (1949), by means of differential hydrolysis, determined the amount of metaphosphoric acid in microorganisms. *Escherichia coli* and staphylococci do not contain metachromatic granules and did not produce any significant amount of metaphosphoric acid after hydrolysis. The yeast cells cultivated on malt agar contained 20 to 25 per cent of this acid. The pathogenic strains of *Corynebacterium diphtheriae* with abundant metachromatic granules in their cells, when treated with hydrochloric acid at 60°C., lost their granules and also their metaphosphoric acid content. When cultivated on ordinary agar, the metachromatic granules and the metaphosphoric acid of *Corynebacterium diphtheriae* disappeared.

Tubercle bacilli, too, when grown in a liquid medium rich in phosphates, contain a considerably greater amount of intracellular granules than the bacilli grown in a medium of low phosphate content. It must be concluded that metaphosphoric acid is the constituent of volutin of yeast cells and of the metachromatic granules of *Corynebacterium diphtheriae.* Minck and Minck (1949) indicated that the localization of metachromatic granules, their form, and their staining properties, have nothing in common with the nuclear bodies of microorganisms. (These investigators, like most French authors, use the term "nucleus" to designate the nuclear bodies.)

The metachromatic granules, unlike the nuclear bodies, do not resist the action of ribonuclease. Minck and Minck indicated that the metachromatic granules may be the condensation products of ribonucleic acid impregnated with metaphosphoric acid.

Wiame (1949) reported that two types of metaphosphates are found in yeast cells. One is soluble in cold, the other in hot trichloracetic acid. The solutions of these phosphates give a metachromatic reaction with toluidin blue. Metaphosphate precipitates the protein; the yeast cells rapidly and reversibly transform the metaphosphate into orthophosphate. The change in color of toluidin blue from blue to purple indicates the presence of metaphosphate. In the case of Wiame the toluidin reaction was positive at a $10^{-4}M$ concentration of metaphosphate.

The investigations of H. Ruska, Bringmann, Neckel, and Schuster (1952) revealed that the impregnation of nuclear bodies of tubercle bacilli with phosphates starts during the early stages of the development of the cell. The Feulgen reaction of desoxyribonucleic acid in the nuclear bodies was independent of the presence or absence of phosphates. The treatment of bacilli with an acid mixture of alcohol and chloroform (Carnoy's solution) dissolved the phosphate of nuclear bodies and the bodies were no longer detectable by an electron microscope. The obtained extract was investigated for the presence of phosphates. The Ba^{++}, Pb^{++}, and silver nitrate produced precipitate in the extract. These reactions indicated the presence of metaphosphate and pyrophosphate in the solution. Ruska *et al.* tried to estimate the quantity of metaphosphate in the nuclear bodies of tubercle bacilli by preparing solutions of metaphosphoric acid which, when mixed with silver nitrate, would produce a precipitate of the same intensity as that obtained in the extract of tubercle bacilli. These estimations showed that 1 g. dry weight of tubercle bacilli contained 11 mg. of $(PO_3^-)n$, which means that about 36 per cent of the total phosphate content of the nuclear bodies of tubercle bacilli was in the form of metaphosphate.

It is a well-known fact that the large nuclear bodies in the cells of tubercle bacilli can be destroyed by a strong beam of electrons. The drops, 0.05 μ–1 μ in diameter, prepared from protein, starch, and ribonucleate, showed no change under the most intense action of electrons, but the solutions of orthophosphate or metaphosphate disintegrated under these conditions. Nucleic acid was not destroyed under the action of electrons, but when mixed with metaphosphate (80 per cent ribonucleate and 20 per cent sodium metaphosphate), the mixture decomposed just like nuclear bodies charged with metaphosphate.

The investigations of Meissner and Kropp (1953) revealed that the total phosphorus content of tubercle bacilli, dried at 60°C., was 0.9 to 1.9 per cent, and that one half of this quantity was in the form of an organic compound and the other half of inorganic phosphate. The uptake of isotopes P^{31} and P^{32} by tubercle bacilli showed that the rate of uptake of P^{32} was up to twenty times higher than that of P^{31}. This difference in the speed of uptake was lost when the isotopes were transformed into compounds of orthophosphoric acid by boiling with mineral acid. These authors found that isotope P^{32} was the mixture of orthophosphates and metaphosphates and, because the metaphosphate was selectively and more rapidly taken up by tubercle bacilli than the compound of orthophosphoric acid, the rate of disappearance of P^{32} was higher than that of P^{31}. In a further work, Meissner and Diller (1953) indicated that the impregnation of nuclear bodies with metaphosphates is not a property of tubercle bacilli alone, but of other microorganisms (corynebacteria, *Actinomyces*) as well. According to these authors, microorganisms accumulate metaphosphate by transforming orthophosphate, or acquire it directly from the medium. According to Schmidt *et al.* (1946), the transformation of orthophosphate into a meta-compound is an enzymatic process, and this transformation takes place not in the nuclear bodies themselves, but in the cytoplasm of bacilli, the nuclear bodies being the places where metaphosphate accumulates. The increase of metaphosphate coincides with the appearance of nuclear bodies in the bacilli. This selective accumulation of phosphates is an active process, and the metaphosphate represents the source of energy of the tubercle bacilli (see p. 86).

Mitochondria of Tubercle Bacilli

Mudd, Winterscheid, DeLamater, and Henderson (1951) interpreted the granules in the cytoplasm of mycobacteria as mitochondria identical to those encountered in the cells of higher organisms.

The cytoplasmic granules or mitochondria were isolated from mammalian tissues by differential centrifugation in a relatively pure state. A study made of the mitochondria of animal cells by means of an electron microscope revealed that the largest of them are 2.0 μ x 0.48 μ in size; the other fraction consisted of smaller particles, from 60 μ to 200 mμ (Claude, 1941, 1944; Claude and Fullam, 1945). Both fractions contained nucleoprotein. Mitochondria derived from water homogenates of rat liver, separated as "large granule" fractions, consisted of spherical bodies ranging from 0.5 μ to 0.2 μ in diameter (Hogeboom, Schneider, and Pallade, 1947).

It was shown that the enzymatic activities of the cell, such as succinic dehydrogenase, histohematin (cytochrome) oxidase, adenosine triphosphatase, and the enzymes of Krebs' cycle were connected with the fraction of "large granule" (Schneider, 1946; Hogeboom, Schneider, and Pallade, 1947; Kennedy and Lehninger, 1948).

Georgi, Militzer, Burns, and Heotis (1951) obtained cell-free lysate from thermophile bacilli after treating them with lysozyme. Most enzymes of these bacilli were encountered in an insoluble cell fraction, separated from the lysate by centrifugation. This fraction consisted of spherical bodies which were not the spores of the bacilli. These granules, like the mitochondria, were the site of the bacilli's enzymatic activities. Malic dehydrogenase, histohematin oxidase, histohematin 3 (cytochrome c), and other enzymes were found concentrated in these granules.

Some biological stains are known to reveal the enzyme activities of the mitochondria. Michaelis (1900) showed that Janus green B initially stains the mitochondria blue-green, but that later, as the cell activity progresses, the hue of the stain changes to red. In another test, it was found that mitochondria reduce tetrazolium to red formazan.

Mudd, Winterscheid, DeLamater, and Henderson (1951) studied, with an electron microscope, the enzymatic properties of the cell granules of *Mycobacterium thamnopheos,* H37Rv, and other strains of acid-fast bacilli grown on collodion film. Mudd *et al.* observed in the granules, located in the poles and along the cell axis, the reduction of Janus green B and the progression of green color to red and colorless. These granules were stained when treated with acid hematin and Harman's stain, which are regarded as specific for mitochondria. Other tests (Nadi reaction) were also performed, and these granules gave positive tests. In the first publication, Mudd *et al.* (1951) say that mitochondria have smooth spheroidal to ellipsoidal contours and that, when the granules have been volatilized by intense electronic bombardment, definite limiting surface membranes are left over. This description and the electron micrographs included in the paper unmistakably indicate that the authors had identified the nuclear bodies as the mitochondria of acid-fast bacilli.

In their further work, Mudd, Brodie, Winterscheid, Hartman, Beutner, and McLean (1951) examined other organisms in the light of the same criteria as applied to the investigation of mycobacteria. The granules of *Escherichia coli, Bacillus megatherium,* and other organisms were found to have the various characteristics of the mitochondria of mycobacteria. These granules were localized in electron-scattering places of bacterial cells but differed from the nuclear bodies in that their Feulgen reaction was negative and that their presence was not revealed by the nuclear staining methods.

Winterscheid and Mudd (1952) reported their views on the nature of mitochondria and the nuclei of mycobacteria at a meeting of the Histochemical Society. In communicating the data known from the abovementioned publications, these investigators affirmed that there are enough data to differentiate two types of granules in mycobacteria, and labeled these two types as mitochondria and nuclei. According to Winterscheid, the difference between these cell granules resides in the positive Janus green reaction and negative Feulgen reaction in the mitochondria and in the positive Feulgen reaction and negative Janus green stain in the nuclei. According to Mudd, the evidence for the presence of a nucleus in a bacterial cell rests on a stronger basis than some cytochemical or staining evidences. The observations of DeLamater (1951) about the presence of chromosomes and the occurrence of mitosis and nuclear fusion in the bacterial cells were regarded as further proof of the presence of a nucleus in the bacterial cell.

In their later publications, Mudd (1953a, b) and Winterscheid and Mudd (1953) emphasized the differences between the mitochondria and the nuclei (nuclear bodies) of the bacterial cells. According to these investigators, the mitochondria can be differentiated from the nuclear bodies, not only by means of the above-mentioned staining and cytochemical reactions, but also by staining the cells with a diluted old solution of Löffler's methylene blue or carbolfuchsin. In preparations stained with methylene blue, the cytoplasm appeared light blue, the nuclear bodies were dense blue, and mitochondria were red-violet. The nuclear bodies were usually proximal in position to the mitochondria. In these publications of Mudd *et al.*, as in their earlier works, the nuclear bodies are called nuclei.

Hollande and Crémieux (1928) did not detect any mitochondria in the cells of tubercle bacilli; Mudd *et al.*, called these observations faulty. H. Ruska (1954) also questioned the existence of mitochondria in tubercle bacilli.

The reducing potential of triphenyltetrazolium is —80 mV., that of flavine enzymes —60 mV. The flavine enzymes are able to reduce triphenyltetrazolium. It must be concluded that triphenyltetrazolium indicates the presence of reducing flavine enzymes. Probably because of this no correlation was found between the reducing centers and the location of nuclear bodies in bacteria (Hahn, 1952).

The Action of Physical, Chemical, and Biological Agents on the Bacterial Cells as Observed with the Electron Microscope

The action of heat on the bacterial cells was investigated by means of an electron microscope by H. Ruska (1942). Streptococci, after they had been boiled for a short time, gave signs of a considerable shrinkage of cytoplasm and the separation of cytoplasm from the cell wall. Salton and Horne (1951) heated a suspension of *Escherichia coli* from 55° to 100°C. and observed the changes in the cells with an electron microscope. Considerable granulation and shrinkage of cytoplasm occurred when the temperature was below 70°C.; between 70° and 100°C. the rupture of the cell wall took place.

Mudd (1943) investigated the action of germicidal and antibacterial substances on the *Salmonella typhosa*. The bacilli, exposed to the salts of silver, lead, mercury, and nickel, showed that the cytoplasm but not the cell wall had been selectively darkened as a result of its shrinkage and coagulation. The same organism, exposed to homologous rabbit antiserum, showed as a result of antigen-antibody action the formation of films on the surface of the flagella and on the cell walls of bacteria.

The largest and most important group of these investigations deals with the action of antibiotic and antituberculous substances on the bacterial cells.

Gärtner (1943) investigated the action of sulfonamides on the *Salmonella typhosa* and *Escherichia coli*. Observations with an electron microscope revealed direct damage to the bacterial cells. In extreme cases of cell damage the outflow of cytoplasm from the cell and the destruction of the cytoplasm was observed. Kellenberger and Werner (1948) investigated the action of streptomycin on *Bacillus subtilis*. Extreme shrinkage of cytoplasm and succeeding extrusion of it from the cell were seen.

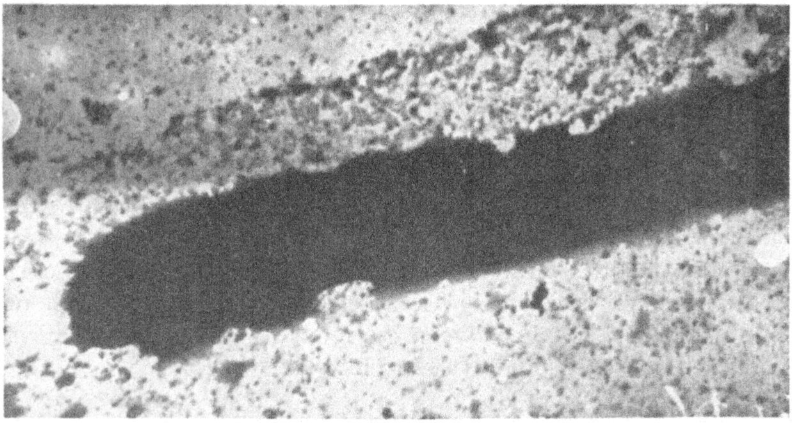

Figure 17. Bacillus cereus incubated for 10 hours at 37°C. on the surface of agar containing 0.07 μg. tyrothricin per ml.; shows action on the cell wall, disintegration of the cell; × 6,000 (Johnson, 1944).

Johnson (1944) investigated the action of tyrothricin on the *Bacillus cereus*. The corrosion of the outer cell portions and the disintegration of the cell took place.

Tubercle bacilli. Ruziczka and Orth (1950) investigated the action of thiosemicarbasones Tb I and Tb VI on the H37Rv strain of tubercle bacilli grown on Hohn's medium. One fourth of a 25 mg. tablet of compound was deposited on the inoculated medium. After seven days of incubation the drug was surrounded by large clear zones without growth. The bacilli of these zones were small and fine, their cell content being not homogeneous but granular; in some cases the cytoplasm had retracted from the cell wall. The same authors (1952) studied the action of streptomycin, neomycin, and *para*-aminosalycilate (FR7) on tubercle bacilli, using the previously described method. After eight days of action by these drugs, the bacilli appeared as they would be in a six-month-old culture. The bacilli seemed little influenced by the presence of 1 μg. per ml. of streptomycin; 5 μg. produced granular development, 10 μg. dissolved the cell wall and cytoplasm of the bacilli.

Bringmann (1953) reported that the avian strain of tubercle bacilli, under the action of thiosemicarbasones, streptomycin, and PAS, showed undisturbed growth but that the division of the cells was stopped.

The Russian investigators Tschertkova and Buinov (1953) studied the action of streptomycin, PAS, and Tb I on the morphologic changes of different strains of tubercle bacilli. Bacilli were cultivated on Sauton's liquid medium; the tested substance was added to the medium. After six days of action by three units of streptomycin, the bacilli were swollen; the cytoplasmic bodies had been transformed into a formless mass. After nine days of contact with streptomycin, only loose fibers and granules were left over: 0.1 mg. of PAS in 100 ml. of the medium produced lysis of the bacilli. The combined action of streptomycin and PAS was stronger than the action of either compound alone.

Brieger, Cosslett, and Glauert (1953) studied the action of 10 and 100 μg. per ml. of streptomycin and of isoniazid on avian tubercle bacilli, grown on collodion film on Dubos' medium. The cultures containing streptomycin grew slowly; 100 μg. of streptomycin per ml. arrested the growth of bacilli in the mycelian stage. The action of isoniazid on bacilli was different. The concentration of 10 μg. per ml. of this drug had hardly any visible effect on the bacilli; the doses of 20 μg. and more per ml. arrested the elongation of the bacilli; the bacilli lost their transparency and appeared as dense, oval bodies.

Braunsteiner, Mlczoch, and Zischka (1953) investigated the action of isonicotinic acid hydrazide (Rimifon) on tubercle bacilli cultivated in Dubos' medium containing Tween 80 and 10 μg. of the drug per ml. The cultures were investigated after six, twelve, and twenty-four hours of action of the drug. The greatest effect of the drug on the bacilli was observed after twelve hours of action and consisted in increased transparency of the cells, retraction of cytoplasm from the cell walls, plasmolysis, and the formation of empty "ghost" cells. After twenty-four hours of action the bacilli could no longer be cultivated.

V

The Bacterial Cell and the Metazoan Cell

Summary

THE nucleus is an isolated body in the cytoplasm of a cell. The presence of an organized nucleus composed of nucleolus, chromosomes, and genes will indicate the appurtenance of a cell to a higher form of life. Although the notion of nucleus is more morphologic than chemical, some general criteria of distinction between the organized nucleus, nuclear bodies, and other cell organelles should be indicated.

The nucleus of higher forms of life is present in the cytoplasm at all conditions of nutrition, at any age, and at any stage of cell development. The disappearance of the nucleus means the death of the cell. The nucleus divides before the cell divides, acquires a specific tint when stained according to Romanowsky, and produces positive Feulgen reaction; it is further characterized by high ultraviolet light absorption at 260 $m\mu$ wave length and by its high desoxyribonucleo-protein content.

As the many works mentioned have shown, when these criteria are applied to the bodies found within a bacterial cell, one must recognize that a great many of these bodies, as well as the bodies found in tubercle bacilli, satisfy most, if not all, of the criteria for nuclear structures.

Knaysi (1929, 1938), Piekarski (1939), H. Ruska (1941), Robinow (1945), Mudd (1949, 1950), Stempen (1950), and other investigators compared the cell structures of *Escherichia coli* and other bacteria as they appeared when stained conventionally, when hydrolyzed and then stained according to Romanowsky, and when either investigated after their death with conventional, ultraviolet, and electron microscopes or in their living state with a phase contrast microscope. These studies showed that every bacterial cell has one or more bodies which are stained like chromatin with the Romanowsky stain, produce positive Feulgen reaction, and have the maximum ultraviolet light absorption at 260 $m\mu$. These bodies are revealed in an electron microscope and they divide, as seen in the phase contrast microscope, prior to the division of the cell body. Malek and Sterzl

(1948) compared the results of different methods of discovering nuclear bodies in tubercle bacilli. The Ziehl-Neelsen, Much, and Piekarski-Robinow staining methods and the Feulgen reactions were tried out on specimens taken from the same material. The different procedures revealed bodies localized in the same parts of the bacterial cells.

Table 4 summarizes what is actually known about the cytology of the tubercle bacillus. The investigations of tubercle bacilli in their stained or unstained state, by means of a light microscope and according to conventional methods, revealed in them all the essential cytologic elements of the higher cells, such as the cell wall, the cytoplasm, the nuclear bodies, the granules, and the vacuoles. The Romanowsky staining procedure, when applied to bacilli hydrolyzed with acids or specific enzyme, exposed bodies hidden by the intensively stained ribonucleic acid of cytoplasm. These bodies, which contain the desoxyribonucleic acid and are capable of producing positive Feulgen reaction, are of nuclear nature. Through the application of ultraviolet and electron microscopy to the study of the cell structures of tubercle bacilli, additional information on the size and shape of bacilli, their cell wall, cytoplasmic membrane, nuclear bodies, and the granules and vacuoles of the cytoplasm were obtained. The observation of bacilli through a phase contrast microscope confirmed the presence of these cytologic elements in the living cells of tubercle bacilli and refuted the objections that these formations may be artifacts formed within the cell through the intervention of chemical or physical agents during the preparation or investigation of the specimens. The greatest significance of these observations resides in the fact that they confirm the invariable presence of a nuclear substance in the bacterial cells and also in tubercle bacilli.

The work done by Caspersson and co-workers, by Malmgren and Hedén (1947), and by others contributed considerably to the understanding of the role of ribonucleoproteins and desoxyribonucleoproteins in the cells of higher forms, as well as in the yeast and bacterial cells. These investigations indicated the possible connection between bacterial nucleoprotein and the synthesis of proteins, the cell growth, and heredity as this is known in the higher cells.

These findings confirmed the observations and opinions of the early cytologists – whose tools were imperfect microscopes and a few stains – namely, that the nuclear substance is universally present in the cells and is the symbol of the unity of the cellular world.

Refined and powerful tools of investigation are at the disposal of modern cytologists, whose aspirations are not confined to the confirmation of the identity of the building scheme of the cellular world. Rather, they collect data to prove the exact identity in structure, multiplication, and heredity

Table 4. Morphology and Cytology of the Tubercle Bacillus

Cytologic Elements	Light Microscopy, Unstained or Conventionally Stained Specimens	Ultraviolet Light Microscopy	Fluorescence Microscopy	Phase Contrast Microscopy	Electron Microscopy
Shape and size	Rod shaped; ¼–½ diameter of the red blood cell	Granular rods	Yellow-red rods, granular	Rods of sharp edges, granular	Granular rods of 4.3 x 0.4–1.0 x 0.2μ or 1.8 x 0.6–1.0 x 0.3μ
Cell wall	Thin, elastic membrane with thickened areas; stains metachromatically. Black when silver impregnated				Thin, 0.023–0.03μ, ductile, contains rodlike granulations of 0.005–0.03μ
Hülle	Presumed. Not demonstrated				Absent
Cytoplasmic membrane	Very thin, surrounding cytoplasm. Sudan, protein, lipoid, positive				Clearly seen, especially in disintegrated cells
Cytoplasm	Very dense, uniformly dark when stained with basic dyes. Contains bodies, granules, vacuoles	Absorption weak or absent	Granular	Variable density	Granular, variable density
Nuclear bodies	Two or more hyperchromic bodies, polar or along the cell axis. Not of fatty or waxy nature. Not spores. Division observed. Nucleoids, nuclei	Strong absorption at 260 mμ wave length	Bodies of red and green fluorescence	Nuclear bodies located in the same regions as seen in the stained specimens. Light nuclear and dark cytoplasmic areas	Initially transparent then dark (phosphate) 1–15 in number, subpolar or along the cell axis. In young cells 30–350 mμ; in old 800 mμ in diameter. In young cells paired. Divide before division of cytoplasm
Granules	Spores, *Splitter*, granules, virus				Cytoplasmic granules. Mitochondria. Microgranules
Vacuoles	In cytoplasm; do not stain with basic dyes			Highly transparent; the content may be opaque. Chief deposit of fatty substances	
Cell division	Notch in the cell wall, retraction of cytoplasm. Membrane between the daughter cells			Division of nuclear bodies, then notch in the cell wall. Formation of double cell plate between daughter cells	

as Revealed by Different Methods of Investigation

Acid Hydrolysis, Romanowsky Staining	Enzyme Hydrolysis, Romanowsky Staining	Feulgen Reaction	Authors
			Koch (1882); Hagemann (1937); Richards and Wade (1948); Brieger and Glauert (1952); von Borries and E. Ruska (1939); Lembke and H. Ruska (1940)
			Knaysi *et al.* (1929, 1950); Mudd *et al.* (1942); Rosenblatt *et al.* (1942); Darzins (1926)
			Ehrlich (1882); Bienstock (1886); H. Ruska *et al.* (1952)
		Positive	Knaysi *et al.* (1929, 1950)
Staining properties lost	Staining properties lost	Negative	Knaysi *et al.* (1929, 1950); Piekarski (1937); van Herwerden (1913); Fuelgen (1924); Brachet (1940); Mudd *et al.* (1942); Wessel (1942); Knaysi *et al.* (1950)
Red-violet bodies along the cell axis or subpolar	Red-violet bodies along the cell axis or subpolar	Red-violet bodies or dust along the cell axis or subpolar	Feinberg (1900); Voit (1925, 1927); Knaysi *et al.* (1929, 1950); Fontes (1933); Epstein *et al.* (1935); Piekarski (1939); Lembke and H. Ruska (1940); Mudd *et al.* (1942, 1950); Brieger and Robinow (1947); Brieger and Glauert (1952); H. Ruska *et al.* (1952); Kölbel (1952); Krieg (1954)
			Koch (1882); Spengler (1902, 1905); Much (1907, 1908); Fontes (1909, 1910); Vaudremer (1923); Lembke (1947); Reed *et al.* (1948); Mudd *et al.* (1951); H. Ruska *et al.* (1952)
			Knaysi *et al.* (1929); Rosenblatt *et al.* (1942); Mudd *et al.* (1942); Knaysi *et al.* (1950); H. Ruska *et al.* (1952)
			Knaysi *et al.* (1929, 1950)

of the bacterial cell with the metazoan cell. Some of these scientists attempt to bridge the gap in knowledge which at the present time separates the bacterial cell from the metazoan cell by using similar designations for the structures and phenomena only apparently alike in both cells. To Piekarski, the bodies seen in a bacterial cell were nucleoids; to Feulgen, the color reaction of desoxyribonucleic acid and Schiff's reagent was a nucleal reaction. Now the nucleoids are called nuclei or chromosomes, and the nucleal reaction is nuclear reaction (Barnard, Boivin, Klieneberger, Bisset, DeLamater, and others).

The Sexuality of Bacterial Cells

The sexuality of higher cells is one of the differences between these cells and bacterial cells.

Bisset (1949) described in *Escherichia coli* a life cycle resembling that of myxobacteria. The vesicular nucleus was located in a microcyst, which was formed by a process suggesting sexual conjugation of the cells. Lembke (1950–1951) observed with an electron microscope images in *Escherichia coli* resembling chromosomes, and a mitotic process similar to that of higher cells. The diameters of these formations, which were located in the extremities of the cells, were approximately 0.02 μ. DeLamater (1951) observed that methylene blue and thionine, when treated with sulfurous acid, are capable of staining the nuclei intensively. By dehydrating the object in deeply cooled (−20°C.) alcohol and acetone, DeLamater obtained preparations in which the structures of the bacterial cell interior were not distorted by treatment. DeLamater described the nuclear cycle of *Bacillus megatherium* as subject to the typical mitotic process. The metaphase spindle with haploid chromosomes was seen, and also the other phases of the process. Later, DeLamater and Mudd (1951) were more reserved in interpreting the nuclear phenomena of *Bacillus megatherium.* These authors indicate that a photograph of a cell records only one optical section of the cell, whereas the cell is three-dimensional. It becomes apparent that the axis of the nuclear bodies occurs at random in relation to the axis of the cell. The authors recognized that the "divisional stages can be confusing because of the variation of their axis," and that "the hazards of misinterpretation are large."

Knöll and Zapf (1951) attempted to investigate, with the phase contrast microscope, the influence of penicillin and colchicin on the growth and multiplication of Gram-negative bacteria. The addition of 15 units of penicillin per ml. to the medium produced giant cells in which rapid division of the nuclear zones and retarded division of cytoplasm occurred but mitotic cell division was not seen. The addition to the medium of sublethal doses of colchicin (diluted 1:1,000), which is a spindle poison capable of arresting the mitotic cell division in metaphase, had no effect on the division of the bacterial cells. Knöll and Zapf concluded that phase contrast microscopy did not reveal any indications of the existence of mitosis in bacterial cells.

Chapman and Hillier (1953) investigated with an electron microscope ultrathin sections from the dividing cells of *Bacillus cereus*. Structures that could be identified as chromosomes, mitotic figures, or mitochondria were not found (see p. 32). All attempts to prove the existence in bacterial cells of sexual process or mitosis comparable to that of higher cells, by means of the electron microscope or the phase contrast microscope, or by the use of physiologic and cytologic methods of revealing cell structure, must at present be recognized as unsuccessful. From the phylogenetic point of view, it is perhaps too hopeful to expect the presence of mitosis in bacterial cells, since the existence of mitosis has not yet been demonstrated even in cells of a higher organization, such as the yeast cells.

According to Dienes (1946), the multiplication of bacteria by binary fission does not provide the possibility of new combinations and rearrangements of heritable characteristics. Dienes accepts the fact that the discovery of L forms in the cultures of *Streptobacillus moniliformis* by Klieneberger (1955) opened a new way to the understanding of bacterial sexuality. Klieneberger regarded these tiny living organisms as symbionts of *Streptobacillus*. Dienes observed in *Proteus* the formation of large bodies in the zone of contact between two cells. This phenomenon suggested the sexuality of the process, a sexuality comparable to that of the conjugation and production of sexual cells in the fungi.

The Spanish investigator Xalabarder (1953) centered his attention mainly on the problems of the reproduction and pathogenicity of mycobacteria. According to him, the reproduction of mycobacteria is a cyclic process, producing L forms. Large bodies in the form of cysts were formed, containing filtrable elements of mycobacteria. The conjugation of the nuclear bodies occurs as an element of the cycle.

In spite of the analogy existing between bacterial nuclear protein formations and the nuclei of higher cells, a great cleft separates these formations. The inferiority in organization and function of the bacterial cell compared with the organization and function of metazoan cell is sensed by many investigators. "The micrographs show the presence of bodies which reasonably correspond to our conception of a bacterial nucleus; one should still always realize that all proof that one is dealing with structures worthy of the name of nucleus, is completely lacking" (Iterson, 1947).

Piekarski (1950) has summarized our actual knowledge of the bacterial nucleoids and the properties separating them from the nuclei of higher forms of life. The nucleus has the following properties: (1) it always arises from the nucleus and never from the cytoplasm (*omnis nucleus ex nucleo*); (2) it divides by the karyokinetic process, forming chromosomes and the spindle; (3) it contains desoxyribonucleic acid, which is localized chiefly in the chromosomes; (4) it contains a Feulgen-positive substance which forms the genes; (5) the nuclei are dominant in the sexual process, in the course of which they fuse and form the generation nucleus of a new individual.

Recently various Russian investigators headed by Lepeshinskaia (1952) attempted to demonstrate the acellular origin of cells. The Akademia Nauk (Academy of Sciences, U.S.S.R.) in 1952 officially approved this hypothesis. Later, in 1953, the same Academy recognized that "there was not a sufficiently critical examination of the obtained data but too enthusiastic a devotion to theoretical schemes."

In bacteria the nuclear bodies are constantly present, and they (1) arise by dividing and never from the cytoplasm; (2) contain desoxyribonucleic acid; (3) are Feulgen-positive. The nuclear bodies of bacterial cells differ from the nuclei of higher cells in morphology. The nuclear bodies have neither a nucleolus nor a nuclear membrane; the bacterial nucleoids do not divide by the karyokinetic process, they do not form chromosomes, and the nucleoids do not fuse in sexual process to produce a generation nucleus. (Piekarski admits the possible existence of some kind of sexuality in bacteria.)

Piekarski and Pontieri (1956) examined ultrathin sections of the cells of *Bacillus subtilis* and *Escherichia coli* in the electron microscope and concluded that the division of nuclear substance in these cells is not identical with the mitosis of higher cells.

It is no longer possible to separate bacteria from the cells of higher forms of life on the ground that they are organisms without nuclei, but this does not imply that the morphologic, physiologic, and genetic properties of bacterial nuclei are identical with those of the nuclei of metazoan organisms. To indicate these differences, one is justified in giving to the bacterial nuclei names that differentiate them from the nuclei of higher cells.

The absence in the bacterial cell of a nucleus comparable to that of higher cells does not imply the absence of sexuality in the bacterial cell. The recent unitarians tried to find in bacteria a nucleus and sexual cycle comparable to that of the higher cells. The geneticists have approached the problem from a different angle. They have abandoned the search in the bacterial cell for formations identical to the chromosomes or figures of mitotic division that are characteristic of the higher cell. In bacteria, the genes must not necessarily be organized in chromosomes. The genes are the material carriers of the inheritable properties, and the essence of the sexual process is the exchange of genes and the creation of a new individual different in many respects from the parents.

The induction in cells of new properties different from those of the parent cells was performed in *Neurospora* by means of irradiation (X-rays, atomic radiation). By the action of drugs on the tubercle bacilli and other bacteria, streptomycin- and isoniazid-resistant strains were created, and by means of desoxyribonucleic acid the transformation of the types of pneumococci was achieved. The formation of such cells with heritably transmissible new properties is in essence equal to the formation of cells with new properties in the sexual process.

By means of X-ray irradiation, heritably stable mutants of *Escherichia coli* K-12 requiring for their growth biotin (B—) but not requiring threonine (T+) were obtained (Tatum and Lederberg, 1947). When these cells were grown together with the mutants not requiring biotin (B+) but requiring threonine (T—), new cells not requiring biotin or threonine (B+, T+) were obtained. To explain the formation of these cells with new properties, the crossing over (transduction) of genetic material from one cell into another must be postulated (Lederberg and Tatum, 1951; Lederberg, 1955, Hotchkiss, 1955).

According to Lederberg and Tatum, mating in the form of rapid conjugation and separation of the parent cells is the most probable form of sexual process in these cells. No sexual cells or gametes, but the genes or soluble substances of desoxyribonucleic acid character participate in the process. Lederberg and Tatum admit that the morphologic basis of the bacterial sexual process is still obscure.

Wollman and Jacob (1955) studied the kinetics of recombination in bacteria. These authors found that the period of contact necessary to produce the recombination was slow enough to afford the possibility of disrupting the mating process by the mechanical separation of the pair of cells. The cells separated by means of agitation before ten minutes' contact were prevented from forming new recombinants. After ten minutes' contact the number of recombinants increased rapidly, reaching its maximum after fifty minutes of contact.

Descending the organizational ladder of the living world and leaving the highly organized animal, plant, and bacterial cells behind us, we enter the world of living macromolecules, where the cellular organization of the nuclear substance may be absent. Crystalline plant viruses of ribonucleoprotein are known, as well as the viruses of desoxyribonucleoprotein (vaccinia).

The gene is a macromolecule of desoxyribonucleoprotein. In what way the desoxyribonucleic acid controls the properties of the living organism and how desoxyribonucleoprotein, penetrating into other living cells, can induce their mutation or produce new hereditable properties, are questions that are yet to be answered.

For additional information on structure of bacterial cell see the sixth symposium of the Society for General Microbiology, *Bacterial anatomy* (Cambridge University Press, Cambridge, England, 1956), and K. A. Bisset, *The Cytology and Life-History of Bacteria* (Williams & Wilkins, Baltimore, 1955).

PART TWO

Sources of Energy and Growth of the Tubercle Bacillus

VI

Oxidation, Fermentation, and Growth of the Tubercle Bacillus

TO LIVE means to consume energy. The living organism does not create energy but uses the energy of the sun (as found in green plants) or gets it by transforming the chemically bound energy of foodstuffs. The tubercle bacillus, like all other living cells devoid of chlorophyll, is unable to utilize the radiant energy of the sun. The process of breaking down complex compounds into simple ones permits the organism to use the energy thus liberated. The breakdown of foodstuffs is performed by means of oxidation or fermentation. As Lavoisier recognized in 1770, respiration, like combustion, is a process of oxidation, and the external similarity between respiration and combustion is clearly brought out in the facts that both processes involve the exchange of gases, the uptake of oxygen, and the elimination of carbon dioxide. These energy-yielding transformations, according to the second law of thermodynamics, are irreversible. By lowering through stepwise reactions the energy level of the system, free energy is gained, and the entropy increased.

The anaerobic breakdown of foodstuffs (fermentation) is a poor source of energy in comparison to the aerobic oxidation of foodstuffs. Tubercle bacilli by means of aerobic oxidation break down glucose to water and carbon dioxide, and the energy stored in glucose is rendered available to bacilli. The oxidation of glucose yields

$$C_6H_{12}O_6 + 6\ O_2 \rightarrow 6\ CO_2 + 6\ H_2O - 673 \text{ kg.-cal}/M$$

The fermentation of glucose to lactic acid produces

$$C_6H_{12}O_6 \rightarrow 2\ C_3H_6O_3 - 54 \text{ kg.-cal}/M \text{ (approx.)}$$

The rest of the energy stored in glucose remains in the waste products of fermentation (alcohols, aldehydes, etc.). In order to obtain sufficient energy by means of such a poor procedure as fermentation, the cell must transform great quantities of substance and utilize a considerable amount of the gained energy to accomplish this work. In its work the anaerobic cell has one advantage over the aerobic organism: it is independent of any external supply of oxygen.

According to Warburg (1956), in cancer cells, unlike normal cells, metabolism is characterized by the prevalence of glycolysis over respiration.

Green plants synthesize organic matter from inorganic substances and lead a life that is independent (autotrophic) of the organic world; the chemo-autotrophs, although devoid of chlorophyll, can utilize the energy gained through simple chemical transformations (Winogradsky, 1887). All other forms of life without chlorophyll live on the energy stored in organic compounds (heterotrophs).

There are two ways by which chemically bound energy can be utilized: (1) by being transformed into heat and the heat into work (steam engine), or (2) by the direct transformation of the energy into work. Live organisms utilize energy in the second way. Only a fraction of available energy is converted into work; the bulk of it is lost in engine and living organism alike. The transformation of energy into work is understandable if the process is examined from the point of view of Nernst's theorem of heat (Báron and Pólányi, 1913).

Linhart (1920) calculated the energy transformations in the process of nitrogen fixation by *Azotobacter* from the thermodynamic equation:

$$\triangle F = \triangle H - T\triangle S$$

where $\triangle F$ stands for the free energy gained, $\triangle H$ for the amount of energy available in the process, T for the absolute temperature, and S for the entropy – the energy lost in the process.

$\triangle F$, the energy freed in the process, indicates whether the process may take place spontaneously. In the case of negative $\triangle F$, the process is exergonic; the energy is liberated and made available to the organism. If $\triangle F$ is positive, the process is endergonic; it is tied up with the increase of energy in the system and may be performed only if the energy is supplied by an outside source. In the case of photosynthesis the sun is such a source. Meyerhof (1916), in his study of the oxidation of nitrite by Winogradsky's nitrifying bacteria, found that the process goes on according to the equation

$$NaNO_2 + O = NaNO_3$$

and that 5 per cent of the liberated energy is utilized by the nitrifying organism. Ruhland demonstrated in 1924 that bacteria under optimal conditions utilize 26.4 per cent of the energy liberated in the oxidation of hydrogen. In the oxidation process of sulfur by *Beggiatoa* this amount is 8.3 per cent. (See the reviews by Baas-Becking and Parks, 1927, and J. Hirsch, 1931.)

Oxidation, Fermentation, and Growth

The synthetic processes of heterotrophs are far less than their energy-producing processes. As shown by Hirsch (1926) in his study of the metabolism of *Vibrio comma*, the relation

$$\frac{\text{assimilation}}{\text{dissimilation}}$$

is always less than one. The cell needs considerably less energy in the absence of cell divisions than in the case of rapid cell divisions. Obviously a dividing cell consumes a considerable amount of energy (Nickerson and Sherman, 1952).

Respiratory System of Mycobacteria

The bulk of the energy consumed by an aerobic cell is obtained by the oxidation of metabolites. The oxidizing enzymes, i.e., the oxidases, were taken to be the catalysts of intracellular or protoplasmatic oxidation reactions, occurring without any rise in the temperature of the environment. The power to transform inert molecular oxygen into an active state of peroxide, so that it will react with the inert substrate, was attributed by Bach to these oxidases. It was difficult to make this oxidase theory conform with the known facts. For one thing, there are many substances, such as formaldehyde and oxalic acid, which are easily oxidized *in vitro*, but resist oxidation in a living body; on the other hand, some compounds which are resistant *in vitro*, such as acetic and higher fatty acids, are promptly oxidized in the organism.

A different concept of biological oxidations was suggested by Wieland (1912, 1922). According to him, the hydrogen atoms of the substrate or of the donor are activated or made mobile by the enzyme dehydrogenase. When there are acceptors of hydrogen, the transfer of the atoms takes place. The process is simultaneously one of oxidation and of reduction. In the case of aerobic respiration, oxygen is the acceptor of hydrogen. In the absence of oxygen, when respiration is of the anaerobic type, other substances are capable of acting as hydrogen acceptors. In the presence of palladium black which activates hydrogen, and of methylene blue which acts as a hydrogen acceptor, alcohol is oxidized to acetaldehyde and to acetic acid, even though the absence of oxygen is complete. For every Mol of acetic acid produced, two Mols of methylene blue are decolorized, or hydrogenated. This combustion without oxygen (*sauerstofflose Verbrennung*, Wieland) is not oxidation in the strict chemical sense, but the dehydrogenation of the substrate:

$$\underset{\text{ETHYL ALCOHOL}}{CH_3CH_2OH} + \underset{\text{METHYLENE BLUE}}{M} \rightarrow \underset{\text{ACETALDEHYDE}}{CH_3COH} + \underset{\text{LEUCOMETHYLENE BLUE}}{MH_2}$$

Sources of Energy, Growth of Bacillus

The two seemingly distinct catabolic processes, aerobic respiration and anaerobic fermentation, are, in essence, alike. The definition of Pasteur, "*La fermentation est la vie sans air,*" remains unchanged in the light of these discoveries.

Respiration and fermentation are processes of catalytic oxido-reduction. After oxidation or fermentation a substrate has lost all or part of its stored energy. In 1931, Braun demonstrated that the respiration or fermentation processes will take place in the living organisms when (1) the hydrogen of the donor is activated by catalysts (dehydrogenases) and transferred to the acceptor, so that oxidation and reduction can occur simultaneously; (2) the process liberates the amount of energy necessary for the growth of a cell; (3) the transformations create a compound which may be used to build up the cell.

Thunberg (1917), from the standpoint of the oxidation theory of Wieland, investigated the biologic processes and demonstrated, by means of methylene blue reduction reaction, the presence of dehydrogenases in animal tissue, higher plants, and microorganisms.

Another theory of oxidation or respiration was advanced by Warburg in 1924 which in some points resembles that of Bach. According to Warburg, the uptake of molecular oxygen by a living substance is the function of iron catalysis, and molecular oxygen never combines directly with the combustible material of the cell but is transferred to it by the intermediary action of the organic iron compound. Molecular oxygen oxidizes the ferrous iron of the cell compound to ferric iron, which is reduced by the cell substrate to the original ferrous form, the cycle proceeding without interruption. Through the change of valence of iron the oxygen is made available to the respiring cell.

MacMunn (1886), examining with a spectroscope the cell content of very different species of the animal kingdom (Mollusca, Arthropoda, Reptiles, Birds, Mammals), discovered in their cells a pigment with identical absorption bands in its spectrum. This pigment he called "histohematin." He observed reduced and oxidized forms of it and expressed the opinion that it has a respiratory function, which consists in taking up the oxygen of blood hemoglobin and transferring it to the tissues. MacMunn states that the pigments "combine with the oxygen conveyed to them in the blood, and hold it for the purposes of metabolism." The oxidation of metabolites does not take place in the blood but in the interior of the cells. He indicated the way in which the oxygen of blood hemoglobin is transferred to the protoplasm of the cells. The name histohematin indicates its structural and functional relation to the hematin of blood. MacMunn recognized that the union of histohematin with oxygen is much more stable than that of hemoglobin with oxygen. Histohematin can be reduced by ammonium sulfide but cannot be reoxidized by a current of air or a stream of oxygen.

Fischer and Hilger (1924) discovered hematin in yeast cells. Keilin (1925) confirmed the findings of MacMunn and demonstrated the universal presence of histohematin in the cells of animals and plants. Unfortunately, he changed the name of histohematin to "cytochrome." As was pointed out by Warburg (1948), Keilin replaced a name that indicates the chemical constitution and relationship of the pigment with an unspecific term which does not distinguish "cytochrome" from the other pigments of the cell Palladin and his co-workers investigated, in a series of works, the respiratory system of plant cells and showed that some pigments of the cells act as acceptors of hydrogen and have a respiratory function (Palladin and Lowtschinowskaia, 1914).

Histohematin is characterized by four absorption bands in its spectrum. MacMunn designated the absorption bands of histohematin by 1, 2, 3, 4; Keilin changed their designation to a, b, c, d. The precision of MacMunn's work may be illustrated by a comparison of his values for the wave length of absorption bands of histohematin with those of Keilin's cytochrome (see Table 5).

Table 5. Wave Lengths of the Absorption Bands of Histohematin and Cytochrome (in mμ)

Histohematin (MacMunn, 1886)		Cytochrome (Keilin, 1925)	
Absorption Band	Wave Length	Absorption Band	Wave Length
1	613–591 (or 593)	a	614–593
2	569–560	b	567–561
3	556–548.5	c	554–546
4	536–516 (approx.)	d	531–513

The absorption spectrum of histohematin disappears in an aerated suspension of yeast cells; after the cessation of aeration, it reappears within a few instants. The spectrum is visible in the cells of a working insect muscle; it disappears in a resting one. It is evident that the spectrum belongs to the reduced pigment; it disappears in the oxidized one. The histohematin is reduced in yeast cells at 18° to 20°C. in 6–8 seconds; at 0° to 2°C., the reduction is delayed till 70 seconds. The function of histohematin is inhibited by potassium cyanide, narcotics, and alcohol.

Histohematin is present in aerobic microorganisms and mostly absent from anaerobic ones. The top yeast used in bakeries contains histohematin in abundance, it is scarce in the bottom yeast of beer; the first type of yeast consumes ten times more oxygen than the second (Meyerhof, 1925).

Histohematin, like hemoglobin, is a porphyrin pigment; it is formed by the combination of porphyrin with the nitrogenous base. Histohematin, as a derivative of porphyrin, contains iron in the molecule and gives a positive peroxidase (benzidine) reaction. The histohematin 3, in a water extract of yeast cells, was purified by Theorell (1938). It is a heat-stable hematin and protein compound of molecular weight 13,000, containing 0.43 per cent iron.

Ferric iron of oxidized histohematin can be reduced by chemicals to ferrous iron. The reduced ferrous histohematin is not reoxidized by molecular oxygen outside the cell, but the oxidation occurs easily in a living cell. Histohematin itself does not react with cyanide, although its oxidation in cells is blocked by cyanide. These observations suggest that the oxidation of reduced histohematin is catalyzed by some cyanide-sensitive enzyme. Keilin and Hartree (1939) recognized the hematin nature of this enzyme, which he named cytochrome oxidase. The right name for this enzyme would be histohematin oxidase. This enzyme is thermolabile, it is a compound auto-oxidizable by molecular oxygen, and it unites with HCN, H_2S, and CO. These gases unite with the iron of the enzyme and block the transfer of oxygen to histohematin. In this respect, cyanide is a most powerful agent; at a $M/10{,}000$ concentration it can inhibit respiration.

In the aerobic acetic acid *Bacterium pasteurianum* it is possible to observe with a spectroscope in the yellow region of 592 mμ wave length, the absorption bands of histohematin oxidase. The absorption bands of proper histohematin of this bacterium are localized in the green region at 550 mμ–560 mμ. The bulk of histohematin oxidase of a rat liver is localized in the large granules (mitochondria, from 0.5 μ to 0.2 μ in diameter) of the cell cytoplasm (W. C. Schneider, 1946; Kennedy and Lehninger, 1948). (See p. 61.)

In a living cell histohematin undergoes reversible reduction and oxidation and, by means of histohematin oxidase, the molecular oxygen participates in respiration.

The respiratory system of the aerobic cell is made up of histohematin dehydrogenases, histohematin oxidases, catalases, nucleotides. The cyclic process by which histohematin is reduced and then oxidized provides the mechanism of aerobic respiration. The respiration of the anaerobic microorganisms rests on dehydrogenation (Frei, 1935).

Warburg's theory of respiration was seemingly in contradiction with that of Wieland-Thunberg. The battle about the mechanism of activation of molecular oxygen in respiration which raged for two decades between Wieland, Willstätter, Euler, and Keilin on one side, and Warburg and his pupils on the other, was waged with the finest tools that science could provide, and its final result was a considerable enlargement of our knowledge of this obscure but fascinating problem of biology.

Keilin and Hartree (1939) summarized the situation on the battlefield in the following terms: Wieland-Thunberg's system of dehydrogenases and

Warburg's system of oxidase and histohematin are both essential to respiration.

Histohematin of Mycobacteria

Yaoi and Tamiya (1928) described the histohematin in tubercle bacilli grown on glycerol agar and on a broth medium. All four absorption bands of histohematin were seen; most distinct among them was band 2. These investigators observed the absorption band at 630 mμ, and concluded that it was caused by the presence of methemoglobin in the bacilli. Warburg and Negelein (1933) showed that this band is that of auto-oxidizable histohematin oxidase, which reacts with cyanide and carbon monoxide.

Table 6. The Respiratory System of Tubercle Bacilli *

M. tuberculosis or Its Products	Media of Cultivation	Absorption Bands of Histohematin (mμ)				Histohematin Oxidase	Peroxidase	Catalase	Hematin	Coproporphyrin
		1	2	3	4					
H37Rv	Egg, glycerol agar, synthetic media	590 600	565	550	529.6	+	+++		+	
Bovine, BCG, avian strains	Glycerol broth, synthetic media	590 600	555		526.0	–	+	+	++	
Human strain 14 days old and younger	Glycerol broth					–	–	+	–	
Alcoholic extract of tubercle bacilli										+

Source: Yaoi and Tamiya (1928); Frei, Riedmüller, and Almasy (1934); Grove and Walker (1951); Andrejew and Rosenberg (1952).

* Minus sign indicates absence of the substance. Plus signs indicate presence, in varying degrees.

Frei, Riedmüller, and Almasy (1934) investigated the respiratory systems of a considerable number of pathogenic microorganisms, including tubercle bacilli of human, bovine, and avian types. They did not find histohematin 3 in the bovine and avian bacilli.

As Table 6 shows, all the elements of the aerobic respiratory system – histohematin, histohematin oxidase, peroxidase, catalase, and coproporphyrin – were found in tubercle bacilli. The differences in their amount are great. The origin of these variations and their significance for the cell of the tubercle bacilli, however, have not yet been understood. (For the role of catalase see p. 293.)

Fujita and Kodama (1934) found that the absorption bands of the histohematin of bacterial cells have a location in the spectrum that is different from the location of the same bands in the muscle cells of an insect. The bacterial absorption bands were particularly strong between 460 and 490 mμ.

Todd (1949) described the histohematin of different saprophytic mycobacteria (*M. phlei, M. smegmatis*). Andrejew and Rosenberg (1952), contrary to the observations of Frei *et al.*, found that human, BCG, and avian strains of mycobacteria have three absorption bands of histohematin. When air was passed through a dense suspension of mycobacteria for five hours, the absorption bands disappeared. These bands reappeared ten to twenty minutes after the air current was stopped. The absorption bands reappeared earlier and were brighter when glycerol, lactate, glucose, and succinate were present in the medium. The absorption spectrum of tubercle bacilli and *M. phlei* was similar to that of the yeast cells.

In some saprophytic mycobacteria (*M. smegmatis, M. stercoris*), coproporphyrin was discovered. This compound was detected in tubercle bacilli by Dhéré, Glücksmann, and Rapetti (1933). Porphyrins are present in hemoglobin and chlorophyll. Uroporphyrin was found in urine, coproporphyrin in the feces. Grove and Walker (1951) isolated coproporphyrin from the alcoholic extract of tubercle bacilli. The function of these pigments in tubercle bacilli is unknown.

E. G. Ball (1934) studied the influence of phthiocol, the pigment isolated from tubercle bacilli by Anderson, on the respiration of tubercle bacilli. Phthiocol's prismatic crystals are water soluble; their melting point is at 173°–174°C. Phthiocol is yellow in acid solution and reddish in alkaline. The part this substance plays in the respiration of tubercle bacilli is not known. Odier (1949) investigated the role of phthiocol (methyl-2-naphthoquinone) in different mycobacteria (*M. tuberculosis, M. phlei*) and recognized it as the growth factor of mycobacteria. Natural pigments may have some significance in the metabolic processes of mycobacteria. Carotenoids slow down the growth of *M. phlei* (Darzins, 1939). Turian (1950) identified, among pigments of *M. phlei* grown on a glycerol medium, a carotenoid which had the properties of a weak acid, chemically related to astacin. In the heavy tuberculosis of the Brazilian frog, the *gia*, the peritoneal nodules are of brown-yellow color (Darzins, 1952).

Goth (1945) showed that aspergillic acid inhibits the growth of the H37Rv strain of tubercle bacilli at a dilution of 1:80,000 when grown in the absence of iron. When grown on Long's synthetic medium containing 5 mg. ferric ammonium citrate per 100 ml., aspergillic acid formed an insoluble red complex with iron. In this case no inhibition was observed, not even at a dilution of 1:20,000 of aspergillic acid. It was assumed that the inhibiting action of aspergillic acid on the tubercle bacilli was due to the interference of aspergillic acid with the functioning of the iron-containing enzyme system of mycobacteria.

Some auxiliary respiratory pigments of microorganisms are known. One of them, pyocyanine, the blue pigment of *Pseudomonas pyocyanea*, was synthesized by Wrede (1930). Bacteria are capable of reducing it to colorless leucobase, which is reoxidized to the blue form by the oxygen in the air. Friedheim (1931), using the Barcroft-Warburg manometric technique, showed that pyocyanine itself does not consume oxygen but added in a *M*/5,000 concentration to the suspension of *P. pyocyanea*, increases the oxygen consumption of these bacteria up to 440 per cent. In anaerobic bacilli, pyocyanine does not have this effect.

Other Sources of Energy

Mycobacteria also dispose of energy gained in other transformations. Through the elimination of one molecule of water from each molecule of phosphoric acid, the polymerization products of phosphoric acid, the polyphosphates, are formed. Thilo and Rätz (1949) attributed the ring structure to trimetaphosphate. As was shown by H. Ruska and others (see p. 60), tubercle bacilli start to take up phosphate early, transforming it into metaphosphate and accumulating it in the nuclear bodies.

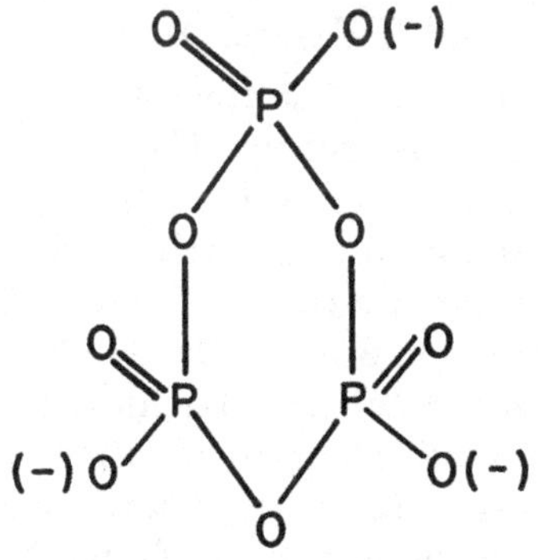

TRIMETAPHOSPHATE

The metaphosphate metabolism in mycobacteria was investigated by Winder and Denneny (1954, 1956). According to these authors, the phosphorus-containing compounds vary in different strains of mycobacteria and are influenced by the cultivation conditions. Inorganic polyphosphate was the chief phosphorus compound found in mycobacteria. Metaphosphate was found to be the reservoir of phosphate. It was partly used up during the growth of bacilli or in the course of phosphorus starvation. The heat of formation of gram-formula weight of orthophosphoric acid (H_3PO_4) is 303.13 kg.cal.; for metaphosphoric acid (HPO_3), it is 224.90 kg.-cal. Both acids are built up of the same elements, but metaphosphoric acid is richer in energy, because only part of the energy is eliminated during the formation of the compound. The difference (303.13 — 224.90) is 78.23 kg.-cal., which represents the energy stored in the cells in the form of metaphosphate. The difference between the amounts of energy stored in these two compounds is also expressed by their heat of solution. The gram-formula weight of orthophosphoric acid dissolved in water evolves 2,700 kg.-cal. of heat, that of metaphosphoric acid, 9,749 kg.-cal. The living cell can transform metaphosphate into orthophosphate and use the energy liberated in the process. In 1928 Kitasato investigated the hydrolysis of metaphosphates. The hydrolysis of polyphosphates of yeast was studied by Mattenheimer (1951). The enzymes active in these processes were obtained from yeast cells and animal organs. These enzymes are active at *p*H 7 to *p*H 9 and only in the presence of magnesium ions.

Meyerhof, Shatas, and Kaplan (1953) prepared an enzyme extract of yeast which hydrolyzed trimetaphosphate to orthophosphate. The hydrolysis caused a decrease in free energy in the compound at more than 21,000 cal/*M*. Thus the authors have demonstrated the high energy content of the P—O—P bond of trimetaphosphate.

Influence of Oxygen Tension on the Respiration and Growth of Tubercle Bacilli

Respiration, the external manifestation of cellular metabolism, was first studied in higher animals and plants. The early bacteriologic technique permitted only a rough estimation of the gas exchange of microorganisms. The investigation of respiration was much facilitated by the development of the manometric technique by Haldane, Barcroft, and Warburg (see reviews by Umbreit, Burris, and Stauffer, 1951; Dixon, 1951).

The exchange of gases in tubercle bacilli does not differ qualitatively from the gas exchange in other microorganisms, but the rate of exchange in tubercle bacilli is low. The first analytic study of gas exchange in tubercle bacilli was made, at the suggestion of Koch, by Hesse (1893). Hesse used Hempel's burette to analyze the gases and observed that the oxygen content in the cultures of tubercle bacilli grown on glycerol agar diminished, and that the concentration of carbon dioxide increased. During the growth period of bacilli considerably less carbon dioxide was formed than the oxygen uptake would permit. Part of the oxygen was incorporated in the substance of the bacilli, concluded Hesse.

The investigation of gas exchanges in tubercle bacilli grown on glycerol agar made by Moore and Williams (1909) corroborated the findings of

Hesse. Carbon dioxide accumulated and oxygen diminished in the cultures of these workers. The atmosphere in the airtight tubes of tubercle bacilli cultures contained 18.7 per cent carbon dioxide and no oxygen. According to Moore and Williams (1909, 1911) the tubercle bacillus grows only when a certain amount of oxygen is contained in the atmosphere. The tubercle bacillus does not grow in the complete absence of oxygen or under the partial pressure of oxygen amounting to 80 per cent of the atmosphere.

The studies of the respiration of tubercle bacilli by Novy and Soule (1925) showed that the tubercle bacillus can develop under different oxygen tensions. In hermetically sealed tubes the bacilli die rapidly. In the experiments of Novy and Soule, tubes with 10 ml. of glycerol agar were inoculated with tubercle bacilli and then sealed with a blast-lamp. The volume of air in the three sets of tubes was approximately 40, 90, and 140 ml. After 37 days of incubation at 37°C., the tubes containing 40 ml. of air gave no evidence of growth, the tubes with 90 ml. of air showed slight but distinct growth, while the tubes with 140 ml. of air exhibited a fair growth. The growth was proportional to the air supply. The tubes inoculated and closed with sealing wax or paraffin showed no growth, although growth began when minute openings in the sealing wax appeared and the leakage of air started. A dry rubber stopper does not hold a vacuum, but stoppers boiled in glycerol sealed the tubes airtight and did not permit the growth of bacilli.

A study of the influence of decreased oxygen tension on tubercle bacilli cannot be made in vessels of insufficient volume. In small jars, oxygen will be consumed during the growth of bacilli and the concentration of oxygen will fall below the level necessary for growth. In the experiments of Novy and Soule, the influence of 6, 3, 1, and 0.5 per cent (volume) oxygen concentrations on the growth of tubercle bacilli was investigated. To furnish the 100 ml. of diluted oxygen necessary for growth, a 2 liter container was used to study the influence of a 6 per cent oxygen concentration. In the experiments with 0.5 per cent oxygen concentration a jar with a capacity of 20 liters was employed. Under these conditions it was found that the growth of tubercle bacilli in atmosphere containing 6 per cent oxygen was as good as in ordinary air, but a further decrease in oxygen concentration resulted in decreased speed of growth. The thin oxygen atmosphere diminished considerably the respiration rate and the growth intensity of the bacilli. The cultures growing in 5.31 per cent oxygen needed 5 weeks, the cultures growing in 0.5 per cent oxygen 7 weeks, to reduce the oxygen concentration to zero. These differences were due to the mass action of oxygen. The tubercle bacillus cannot grow in the total absence of oxygen; it can, however, grow slowly under an oxygen tension as low as 3.5 mm., which is sufficient to bring about the growth of some anaerobic microorganisms.

The absolute amount of oxygen consumed by tubercle bacilli growing in the presence of different oxygen tensions, contrary to differences in their respiration rate and growth speed, was practically the same, that is, about 100 ml. per culture. This indicates that the respiratory quotient,

$$\frac{CO_2 \text{ eliminated}}{O_2 \text{ consumed}},$$

is constant under different oxygen tensions. In the presence of a small quantity of oxygen, tubercle bacilli use only a small part of their respiratory system, but the mechanism of oxygen fixation and carbon dioxide production remains the same as in the presence of a large amount of oxygen, when the full respiratory system is at work. The cell of the tubercle bacillus is an efficient factory; under a heavy crisis of raw material supply it closes most of its sections, and those remaining turn out a small quantity of the product, which is of the old high standard.

Loebel, Shorr, and Richardson (1933a) showed that, in a virulent human H37Rv strain deprived of oxygen for two days on Long's synthetic medium, the respiration decreased by two thirds. In the following three or four days of anaerobiosis the bacilli died. The saprophytic *Mycobacterium phlei* survived the anaerobic exposure at least up to the thirty-fifth day. After 20 days on Long's medium, in containers closed with rubber hoods, 97.5 per cent of the acid-fast saprophytic bacilli were dead, but aerated cultures in the same time contained only 60 per cent dead bacilli (Andrejew, 1946a).

Kempner (1939) studied the respiration of the H37Rv strain of tubercle bacilli under different oxygen tensions. The Barcroft-Warburg technique was used, and bacilli, grown on a solid medium, were suspended in a phosphate buffer of *p*H 7.4. The suspension contained from 7 to 15 mg. dry weight of bacilli per ml. During the experiment the tubercle bacilli gave no signs of growth. The increase in oxygen concentration from 20 to 100 per cent produced only about a 6 per cent increase in respiration. When the concentration of oxygen was diminished, the organisms manifested a reduction in respiration. Kempner's study of the effect of a reduced oxygen tension on the respiration of tubercle bacilli (compared with the rate of respiration in air) is shown in the accompanying tabulation.

Amount of Oxygen	*Reduction in Respiration*
5.0%	20.4%
2.0	58.0
1.1	70.0

The data of Kempner confirmed the findings of Novy and Soule (1925) and showed that the respiration rate of tubercle bacilli changes under increased or decreased oxygen tension, but the respiratory quotient of bacilli remained 0.75 under varying oxygen tensions. The affirmation of Kempner that, according to Warburg, the respiration rate of cells remains unchanged under different oxygen tensions (the law of "all or nothing") is based on an erroneous interpretation of Warburg's German text. To Warburg, respiration always means the uptake of oxygen and the elimination of carbon dioxide (*Gaswechsel*), although sometimes he speaks of oxygen consumption only. Warburg indicated as early as 1914 that, as Henze had concluded before him from experiments on the respiration of sea urchin eggs, "there is no alteration in the exchange of gases (*Gaswechsel*) connected with changes in the concentration of oxygen" (Warburg, 1914a). Warburg is the discoverer of the constancy of the respiratory quotient of cells.

The recent measurement of the respiratory quotient of tubercle bacilli made by Heplar (1953) indicates that some change in this quotient may take place at low oxygen tensions. Ten strains of mycobacteria cultivated in a Tween-albumin liquid medium produced, under 1 per cent oxygen tension, a slight increase in the respiratory quotient compared with that in air. The cause of this increase remains unknown; it may be due to some glycolytic process of the bacilli.

When small plantings of tubercle bacilli initiate growth, their need for oxygen is very slight. Cohn (1944) before and after the inspissation of an egg medium, placed it for four hours in vacuum, planted on it 0.00001 mg. of tubercle bacilli, and filled the vessels with an inert gas, nitrogen. A slight growth still occurred. When nitrogen had been passed over a glowing copper gauze and through a sodium pyrogallate solution in order to remove the last traces of oxygen, no growth occurred.

The merit of Buc (1924) is that he clarified the conditions necessary for the growth of tubercle bacilli in a liquid medium. He showed that in the soft Veillon's agar, thoroughly inoculated with tubercle bacilli, the colonies do not appear on the surface of the medium, but in the "first centimeters below the surface." This observation was later corroborated by B. Lange (1932), Häflinger (1939), and Second and Chatelain (1951). The growth rate of the tubercle bacilli reaches its maximum when the oxygen concentration is between 12 and 14 per cent by volume of the atmosphere, which corresponds to partial oxygen pressures of 91 and 106 mm. Hg. This oxygen concentration is in the range of partial oxygen pressure in alveolar air of the lungs at sea level (97.1 mm. Hg, Camroe and Dripps, 1944). In an infected human or animal body the pulmonary tissue is often the localization of the tubercle bacilli. In an infected body anaerobic conditions exist only rarely although the diffusion of oxygen may be very restricted in the centers of caseous necrosis or in calcified tuberculous lesions.

Rich and Follis (1942) attempted to determine the influence of continuous low oxygen tension of three or four weeks' duration on the development of tuberculosis in 106 animals (rabbits and guinea pigs). In the animals exposed to an atmosphere with an oxygen content not higher than

9 to 10 per cent, the development of infection was markedly inhibited in comparison to the control animals kept in the same room at a normal oxygen level.

Olson, Scott, Hanlon, and Mattern (1952) produced alterations of the pulmonary arterial circulation in 31 monkeys and then infected the animals with pathogenic tubercle bacilli. The tuberculous process was more severe on the side of the systemic-pulmonary anastomosis. Unfortunately these experiments are not conclusive because of unknown distribution of tubercle bacilli in the altered circulatory system of the animals.

In the tuberculous cavities of the lungs, which communicate, by means of the draining bronchi, with the outside, the atmosphere of the cavity is suitable to the growth of tubercle bacilli. It contains 16 to 19 per cent oxygen and 1 per cent carbon dioxide (Coryllos and Birnbaum, 1930). The fibrous capsule of the cavity and the outside air pressure which governs the cavity prevent it from collapsing. The internal necrotic layer of the cavity, which is rich in nutritive substances, is the breeding place of tubercle bacilli (Canetti, 1946, 1955). As these cavities may remain open during the whole life of a person, they produce and eliminate enormous quantities of tubercle bacilli along with their necrotic material. (They are also the chief place of production of streptomycin-resistant bacilli.) When the cavity is not connected with the outside, its internal conditions are different; the percentage of carbon dioxide in its atmosphere increases to 5 per cent, but the oxygen content may go down to 1 per cent or disappear completely (Coryllos and Birnbaum). These semianaerobic conditions in a cavity saturated with water have some resemblance to the conditions existing in the closed vessel of tubercle bacilli cultures, where the tubercle bacilli are dying rapidly. Adams and Vorwald (1934) saw tuberculous cavities, produced experimentally in the lung of a dog, disappear when, after a silver nitrate cauterization, a total occlusion of the corresponding bronchi developed.

The respiration of tubercle bacilli deprived of foodstuffs and put on a starvation regime in a physiological salt solution, decreases progressively, and is very low after a few days of starvation. The addition of foodstuffs restores the respiration. The full restoration of oxygen consumption was possible after 15 days of starvation but the restoration was incomplete after 34 days of starvation (Loebel, Shorr, and Richardson, 1933b). This ability of the tubercle bacilli to cut down a considerable part of their respiration and to burn up slowly the food reserves of the cell under unfavorable external conditions is one of the most important factors in their survival. Such severe food restrictions as in the experiments of Loebel *et al.*, where only sodium chloride and water were available to the bacilli, occur rarely in natural conditions, and the survival time of tubercle bacilli would be considerably longer if some food were available to them. In the experiments of Mannsfeld (1937), carried out in my laboratory in Riga, human tubercle bacilli in water from the city canal remained alive for three months when exposed to light and air at room temperature, and for three and a half months in the darkness of a cellar.

Contrary to the observations showing the fragility of tubercle bacilli under anaerobic conditions are the findings of T. S. Potter (1935) revealing that human and avian types of tubercle bacilli, when subjected to the high vacuum of 10^{-6} mm. Hg and completely dried, conserved their viability for two years, as was proved by inoculation into guinea pigs. The tubercle bacilli showed an extraordinary resistance when deprived of oxygen and humidity. The vital staining of tubercle bacilli with acridine orange also demonstrated their exceptional resistance to drying: fixed on a slide, they remained alive for many hours (Strugger, 1949).

These contradictions are only apparent. Tubercle bacilli die rapidly in cultures under anaerobic conditions in the presence of humidity. Tubercle bacilli can live for months or even years, if dried and kept in the absence of humidity. In the absence of oxygen but in the presence of water some anaerobic cellular processes destroy the viability of the bacilli. Completely dried and kept under these conditions, the bacilli reach a state of anabiosis in which the external functions of life are apparently lost but the viability is conserved.

Novy and Soule also determined the influence of increased oxygen tension on the growth of tubercle bacilli. Tubercle bacilli probably do not encounter any increased oxygen concentrations in nature so that the results of the studies of their behavior under *decreased* oxygen tension are of much greater importance. Tubes of glycerol agar, inoculated with tubercle bacilli (strain H37Rv), were filled with 30, 40, 60, and 100 per cent oxygen (by volume). All the cultures consumed oxygen, and growth resulted in all tubes. The speed of the oxygen consumption and the intensity of growth under *increased* oxygen concentration depends on the oxygen concentration in the tubes. Growth in tubes containing 40 to 50 per cent oxygen was more rapid and abundant than in tubes containing ordinary air. In cultures where the oxygen concentration was above 50 per cent, growth was greatly impeded, but even in the presence of 100 per cent oxygen some growth occurred. In a jar with 40 per cent oxygen the cultures consumed, in 55 days, 239 ml. of oxygen and produced 203 ml. of carbon dioxide, as compared to the 182 ml. of oxygen consumed and the 151 ml. of carbon dioxide produced in ordinary air (20.93 per cent oxygen). According to Bance (1942), every liter of Sauton's medium produced in 63 days 10.966 g. dry mass of tubercle bacilli per liter. To form this quantity of bacilli, 33.18 g. of oxygen was used, and from this quantity of oxygen 18.38 g. were utilized to form 25.272 g. of carbon dioxide, the remaining amount of 14.80 g. was fixed by the culture.

The Influence of the Bacterial Strain, Its Age, and the Composition of the Medium on the Respiration of Tubercle Bacilli

The respiration rate of tubercle bacilli under constant oxygen pressure and temperature varies with the strain, its age, and with the composition of the medium. Loebel *et al.* found that the respiration rate of an H37 strain of bacilli on Long's medium was highest on the eighth day and that it began to decrease rapidly after the fifteenth day. In general, however, the respiration of tubercle bacilli is at a low level, namely only from 1/20 to 1/50, that of pneumococci.

Table 7. The Respiration Rate of Different Strains of Tubercle Bacilli of Different Ages at 38°C.

Strains of Tubercle Bacilli	Oxygen Consumed: 15-Day-Old Cultures	Oxygen Consumed: 45-Day-Old Cultures
239 H	5.0 cmm/hr	2.5cmm/hr
R1	7.8	0.3
L2	4.0	1.0

Source: Andrejew (1947).

Table 8. Gas Exchange of Tubercle Bacilli, Strain H37, at 37°C. and 760 mm. Hg

Medium	Age of Culture in Days	CO_2 Produced	O_2 Consumed	Respiratory Quotient
Glycerol agar	27	124 ml.	149 ml.	0.83
Glucose agar	26	26 ml.	25 ml.	1.0

Source: Novy and Soule (1925).

Zetterberg (1949) also stated that the oxygen consumption of tubercle bacilli diminishes as their age increases.

The chief reason for the decrease in the respiration rate of bacilli is their increased death rate in the cultures. Initially the incubation temperature of 38°C. favors the growth and respiration of bacilli, afterwards it is the cause of their accelerated death. The oxygen uptake of tubercle bacilli also largely depends on the foodstuffs at their disposal. The oxygen uptake of tubercle bacilli growing on Long's synthetic medium is two or three times that of bacilli growing in the liquid egg yolk medium of Besredka. The conversion of firm ingredients of Long's medium to bacillary substance requires more energy than the conversion of organic, energy-rich substances of egg yolk.

In 27 days a culture on glycerol agar consumes six times more oxygen and produces approximately five times more carbon dioxide than a culture on glucose agar in 26 days. The respiratory quotient of tubercle bacilli grown on glycerol agar approximates the theoretical value of 0.85; on glucose agar the value was 1.0.

Uga (1935), by means of the Haldane manometric technique, investigated the oxygen uptake of 11 pathogenic human strains of tubercle bacilli and did not find any difference between their respiratory quotient and that of tubercle bacilli of bovine and avian types (respiratory quotient 0.8281 to 0.8325). He did not find any quantitative differences in the oxygen consumed by pathogenic and apathogenic strains of mycobacteria under 5 to 40 per cent oxygen tension.

Rate of Growth and Generation Time of Tubercle Bacilli

As early as 1887, Buchner, Longard, and Riedlin pointed out that a bacterial culture containing *c* multiplying cells can produce, after the first cell division *c*.2 cells, after the second, *c*.2.2 cells, and after *n* generations, $c.2^n$ cells. If the final number of cells is *d*, then:

$$c.2^n = d$$

$$2^n = \frac{d}{c}$$

$$n = \frac{\log d - \log c}{\log 2}$$

where *n* is the number of generations produced in the unit of time, or the growth rate of bacilli. The time needed to produce one generation is called the generation time (*G*) of an organism:

$$G = \frac{T}{n}$$

where *T* is the time and *n* the number of generations produced in this time.

A mathematical formulation of the rate of growth and generation time can be regarded as correct only under the presumption that every cell in the culture will divide. If, for instance, only 80 per cent of the cells divide, the formula would be

$$n = \frac{\log d - \log c}{\log 1.6}.$$

The generation time cannot be calculated with accuracy unless the total count and the count of viable organisms is known (Wilson, 1922).

When the medium is suitable for growth, the rate of growth will be constant, and the number of organisms at *T* time after the inoculation of *c* organisms into the medium will be:

$$\log d = \log c + KT$$

where *K* is the velocity constant of the rate of growth (Kohn and Harris, 1941). From the above formula *K* was derived:

$$K = \frac{\log d - \log c}{T}$$

The last formula may be used to calculate the rate of growth or the rate of death of the bacterial culture when processes follow a uniform and consistent course (Migaki and McCulloch, 1949).

An outline for a relatively simple method of determining the rate of growth of bacteria was given by Ingraham (1933). From her studies of the bacteriostatic action of gentian violet she concluded that the earlier methods of estimating the dye sensitivity of an organism, which consisted in finding the lowest possible concentration of dye that would inhibit growth, were unsatisfactory because they were not quantitative. The rate of growth, the number of generations of organisms produced in a given unit of time, could not be established by the earlier methods.

The time necessary for the bacteria to produce turbidity or apparent growth in a constant quantity of liquid medium depends on the size of the inoculum. When the time necessary to produce turbidity is plotted against the logarithm of the number of cells inoculated, an ascending line will be obtained and the change in the rate of growth, due to the influence of dye or other factors in the medium, will change only the slope of the line.

Youmans and Youmans (1949, 1951) applied these findings to devise a method for quantitative estimation of the growth rate of small tubercle bacilli inocula. The practice of earlier workers, which consisted in inoculating the media with graded suspensions of bacilli varying from 10^{-2} to 10^{-10} mg. and determining the smallest inoculum capable of producing a culture regardless of the time factor, did not provide quantitative data on the speed of multiplication of bacilli. The lack of such data accounts for the lack of information about the suitability of media for the initiation of the growth of a small number of tubercle bacilli.

Information about the rate of growth can be obtained on the grounds that different quantities of the same bacilli inoculated in an equal amount of a medium of the same composition and cultured under equal conditions would have the same rate of growth. The time of visible appearance of growth will depend on the amount of bacilli inoculated. A linear relationship will be obtained when the time of the first appearance of growth of each inoculum is plotted against the number or the logarithm of the number of bacilli inoculated. The slope of the ascending straight line obtained will indicate the rate of growth of the bacilli. The presence of growth-impeding or growth-favoring factors in the medium will be reflected in the size of the inoculum formed at the same time. In cases of rapid growth the visible size of the inoculum will be formed earlier than when growth is delayed. The slope of the ascending line will be steep in the first case, whereas in the second case it will be slanting. According to Youmans, the generation time is equal to

$$G = \frac{\log 2}{K}$$

where K equals the reciprocal of the slope of lines.

Hershey demonstrated, in 1941, that in growing cultures increase in cell mass must be distinguished from increase in the number of cells. The estimation of growth rate according to the Ingraham-Youmans method is based chiefly on the increase in bacillary mass during the growth period.

Youmans and Youmans inoculated suspensions containing from 10^{-1} to 10^{-8} mg. tubercle bacilli (wet weight) into tubes of modified Proskauer and Beck's synthetic medium. The growth of bacilli in basal medium with 0.2 per cent of bovine albumin (Fraction V) and in basal medium containing 10 per cent bovine serum was studied comparatively. The tubes were examined daily for the appearance of granular growth on the bottom of the liquid. The detection of bacterial mass formed on the bottom of the containers inoculated with different quantities of bacilli will signify that the growth of the inoculum has produced an approximately equal mass of tubercle bacilli, i.e., the smallest possible amount of bacilli that can be seen with the naked eye. Youmans and Youmans (1949) estimated this amount to be approximately 0.5 mg. in five ml. of medium. The generation time of tubercle bacilli H37Rv in basal medium was found to be 19.9 hours, in albumin Fraction V medium 17.3 hours, and in a medium containing bovine serum 14.4 hours (Fig. 18). On the solid egg media the generation

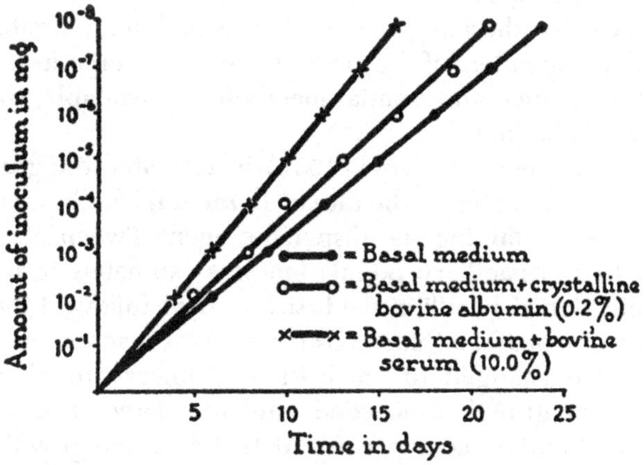

Figure 18. The rate of growth of tubercle bacilli, H37Rv, in three different media (Youmans and Youmans, 1949).

time of the tubercle bacilli was calculated to be approximately 24 hours. The generation time of the H37Rv strain of tubercle bacilli on Löwenstein-Jensen medium was found to be 18 hours, on Petragnani's medium, 24 hours (Gutiérrez-Vázquez, 1956). Only two or three inocula (10^{-2}, 10^{-4}, 10^{-6} mg.) in the liquid medium were necessary in order to establish the slope of the line and to calculate the rate of growth.

The method of Ingraham-Youmans was successfully used by Scholer (1951, 1952) to determine the role of the different components of Dubos' medium in the growth of tubercle bacilli (see p. 245), by Youmans and Youmans (1951) to calculate the generation time of tubercle bacilli in infected mice (see p. 353), and by Abramson (1952) to investigate the influence of chick embryo extract on the growth on tubercle bacilli (see p. 378).

Linear Growth of Tubercle Bacilli

Plating the cells and counting the colonies reveals that bacterial multiplication goes on with different speed in different phases of growth. It starts with the lag phase which is followed by the logarithmic or exponential phase when the cell number increases rapidly. The logarithmic phase terminates in the standstill of multiplication and the decline of the number of living cells in the culture (the stationary phase and the phase of decline). Thus, under ordinary conditions of cultivation, the growth curve would assume the form of a distorted bell, with a steep left side of increase and a slanted right side of decrease.

Monod (1949) described another type of growth curve for which he coined the name "linear growth." The curve of increase of the number of bacteria in these cases appears as a straight line function of time. As Monod indicated, growth will stop when an essential nutrient, which the organism is not capable of synthesizing, present in the medium in limited quantities, is exhausted, independent of the amount of other metabolites. If a constant, limited supply of such an essential metabolite is available, the increase in cell number will be linear.

Fisher, Kirchheimer, and Hess (1951) investigated the growth curve of tubercle bacilli inoculated at the rate of 10 million bacilli per ml. in Dubos' liquid medium, containing the dispersing agent Tween. The increase in the density of the bacillary population was estimated turbidimetrically. The multiplication of bacilli in the first four days followed the logarithmic rate until the rate of 100 million cells per ml. was reached. At that time the logarithmic rate changed to an arithmetic linear growth pattern. The arithmetic linear growth proceeded until the sixteenth day, when there were about 850 million cells per ml. At that time the growth entered the stationary phase.

In their further work, Fisher, Kirchheimer, and Hess (1952) studied

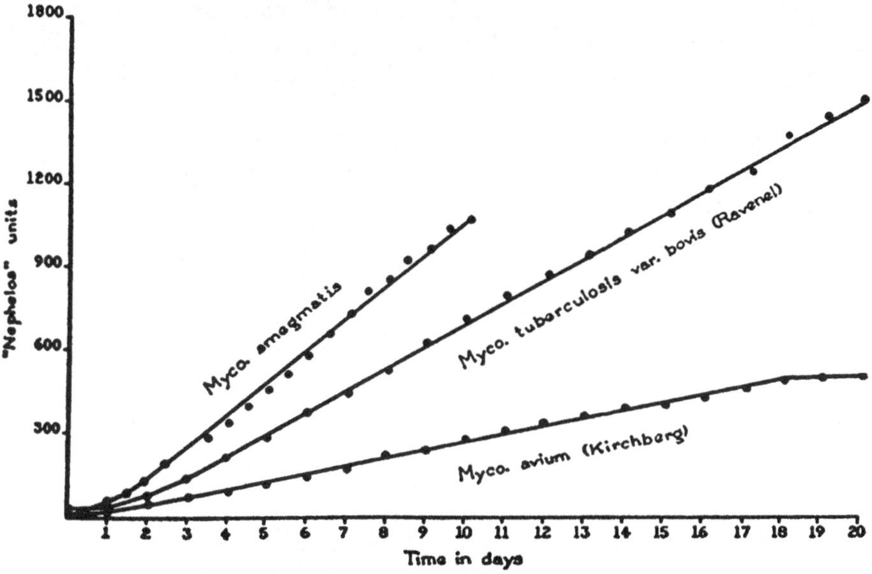

Figure 19. The linear growth of mycobacteria (Fisher, Kirchheimer, and Hess, 1952).

the growth pattern of fifteen different strains of pathogenic and apathogenic mycobacteria in liquid media. All of them exhibited growth of the linear type.

The linear type of growth is observed in heavily inoculated cultures and is probably absent in cases where small inocula are used. According to Fisher *et al.*, the linear growth occurs not only in the cultures of tubercle bacilli grown in liquid media containing dispersing agent Tween, but also in the liquid media without Tween.

The cause for the transformation of the speedy logarithmic growth rate into the pattern of slow arithmetic linear rate of growth was seen in the inhibiting conditions originating in the cultures, such as the depletion of oxygen or nutrients (Monod, 1949; Fisher *et al.*, 1952).

Volk and Myrvik (1953) presented data which may be interpreted as being in support of the view that the cause of the linear growth of microorganisms in liquid media is the depletion of oxygen supply. Cultures of pathogenic *M. tuberculosis*, saprophytic *M. phlei* and *M. smegmatis*, *Micrococcus lysodeikticus*, and *Sarcina lutea* were grown in a modified Dubos medium containing 0.04 per cent Tween. One part of the cultures was incubated under stationary conditions, another part of them was incubated and aerated constantly by shaking in a rotary shaker. The increase in the density of the bacterial population was determined turbidimetrically. The shaken cultures of mycobacteria, like the cultures of micrococci and sarcina, showed logarithmic growth; linear growth was obtained only in the cultures that had not been shaken. The depletion of oxygen in the liquid medium caused the growth pattern to change from the logarithmic to the linear type.

The growth of tubercle bacilli that had been placed on a shaker was faster than the growth of bacilli that had not been subjected to shaking (Miller and Roessler, 1956).

VII

The Action of Fatty Acids, Salicylates, and Benzoates on Tubercle Bacilli

Fatty Acids

RESPIRATION, growth, and reproduction are different phases of cellular life and are of different significance to it. Respiration may go down to a very low level, as occurs in the bacterial spores, but its total cessation would mean death to the cell. These findings led to the erroneous conception that the contrary is also true, that is, that any increase in respiration signifies increased growth or reproduction of the cell. There is no growth and reproduction without respiration, but increased respiration of the cell does not necessarily entail better growth and greater reproduction. The reproduction of a cell, which follows its growth, depends on undisturbed, normal respiration. It is easier to disturb the growth and reproduction than the respiration of the cell. Growth and reproduction cease long before respiration is abolished. Under the influence of bacteriostatic substances the cell continues to respire when growth and reproduction stand still. Growth and reproduction take place when the cell is young, when food is abundant and adequate, and cease in old, starving, or poisoned organisms.

The influence of different substances on the respiration of pathogenic human tubercle bacilli, strain H37, grown on Long's synthetic medium, was studied by Loebel, Shorr, and Richardson (1933b). These authors used the Barcroft-Warburg manometric technique and for several days "starved" bacilli, kept suspended in saline and sodium phosphate buffer at *p*H 7.4, to avoid the interference of foodstuffs with the respiration and also to prevent the multiplication of the bacilli. Glycerol, introduced into the medium in the amount of 0.005 per cent of the medium, increased the respiration of the bacilli. To raise the rate of respiration to the glycerol level 0.1 per cent of glucose had to be added to the medium. Glycerol was the most important source of energy for the tubercle bacilli. The stimulation of the respiration of tubercle bacilli by sodium lactate was rather unique. For a short period it increased the respiration even more than did glycerol. Fatty acids, soaps of higher fatty acids, blood serum, total milk fat, and caseous material stimulated the respiration, but oleate reduced it by 30 per cent. Levulose and other carbohydrates, and salts of iron and magnesium had no influence on the respiration of tubercle bacilli. These authors took for granted the fact that the increased respiration of the bacilli is due to the assimilation of the added substances.

Nakamura (1938) investigated the influence of different compounds on the respiration of two human, BCG, the bovine, and the avian strains of mycobacteria. The bacilli were grown on Lockemann's synthetic medium and the Barcroft-Warburg technique was used to estimate their respiration. Changes in the *p*H of the medium did not have any significant effect on the respiration. The respiration was not influenced by the addition of carbohydrates (glucose) and amino acids to the medium, with the exception of glycine, alanine, and glutamic acid, which led to a slight increase in respiration. Among alcohols only glycerol caused a considerable increase in respiration. The sodium salts of organic acids (citric, formic, tartaric, malic, succinic), in a 1 per cent solution, did not have any influence on the respiration.

Bernheim (1941), using tubercle bacilli of the bovine type suspended in phosphate buffer at *p*H 6.7, confirmed the findings of Loebel *et al.* (1933a) in regard to the stimulation of the respiration of tubercle bacilli by sodium salts of higher fatty acids. This stimulation of the oxygen uptake was small in comparison with the effect of the sodium salts of lower fatty acids (acetic, propionic, butyric, valeric) on the oxygen consumption of tubercle bacilli. The increase in oxygen uptake was proportional to the concentration of these substances in the medium. Like Nakamura (1938), Bernheim did not observe an increase in the oxygen uptake of tubercle bacilli after carbohydrates and amino acids had been added to the medium. In his experiments glycerol did not increase the respiration. According to Bloch (1944), because of incomplete homogenization and insufficient washing, the tubercle bacilli in the experiment of Bernheim were not completely liberated from their nutrients. They continued to respire at a high level and no increase in respiration due to the addition of glycerol could be observed.

The discovery of the action of oleic acid on the growth and respiration of microorganisms has a fascinating history. In his study of acne, Fleming (1909) observed that fatty secretions of the sebaceous glands stimulate the growth of the acne bacillus (*Corynebacterium*) isolated by him from skin lesions. Oleic acid, added in the amount of 0.1 per cent to glycerol agar, had the same favorable action on the growth of the acne bacillus.

The role of oleic acid as a growth factor of microorganisms was greatly clarified by Mueller and his co-workers. In his first report in 1939, Mueller expressed the belief that the growth-stimulating factor of diphtheria bacilli in blood serum is of vitamin nature. His further work (Cohen, Snyder, and Mueller, 1941) showed that the growth factor is present not only in blood but also in milk and casein. This factor was extracted from casein with acetone, ether, and alcohol, and identified as oleic acid. The growth factor occurs in casein because of the presence of small amounts of butterfat in commercial casein. Casein hydrolyzate, added to the basal medium, also favored the growth of *Clostridium tetani* (Feeney, Mueller, and Miller, 1943).

Schrell, Thomas and Peterson (1949) observed that oleic, linoleic, and ricinoleic acids (as oleates) are able to take the place of biotin in promoting the growth of *Clostridium sporogenes* in the basal medium. Pollock, Howard, and Boughton (1949) found that a satisfactory growth of *Corynebacterium* did not occur in the basal medium but was promoted by the addition of hydrolyzate of casein, oleic acid, or linoleic acid (in reality their sodium soaps). All saturated fatty acids tested (palmitic, staric, lauric) had no effect on the growth of *Corynebacterium*, which, however, was promoted by purified Tween 80. From this observation the authors conclude that *Corynebacterium* can utilize the oleate in the esterified form of Tween 80. (Dubos and co-workers indicate that Tween 80, even when purified, liberates oleic acid in the medium.) Boughton and Pollock (1952) report that the "tail" of oleic acid can be shortened by at least two C-atoms without influencing its growth-stimulating effect on *Corynebacterium*; the addition of two C-atoms to the oleic acid annihilates this property. The double bond in the molecule of oleic acid can be moved from the 9 – 10 position to 11 – 12 and 6 – 7, but not so far away as 4 – 5, without reducing the activity of the acid.

In their study of the influence of fatty acids on the respiration of mycobacteria, Franke and Schillinger (1944) expressed their results by the quotient of oxygen uptake:

$$Q_{O_2} = \frac{\text{cmm. } O_2}{\text{mg. bacilli} \times \text{hours}}$$

The effect of $M/50$ solutions of fatty acids on the quotient of oxygen uptake of *Mycobacterium lacticola* is shown in the accompanying tabulation.

Without added acids	19	α, β oleic acid added	47
Stearic acid added	44	Oleic acid added	3
Oxystearic acid added	33	Chaulmoogric acid added	8

Oleic and chaulmoogric acids brought about a strong inhibition of respiration. The unsaturated fatty acids – oleic, linoleic, and linolenic – stopped the oxygen consumption of tubercle bacilli respiring in glycerol broth in the following dilutions: oleic acid, 1:10,000; linoleic acid, 1:15,000; linolenic acid, 1:30,000.

Franke, Lee, and Kibat (1949) reinvestigated the action of sodium salts of unsaturated fatty acids on the respiration of *Mycobacterium phlei* and *M. rubrum*, using the Barcroft-Warburg manometric technique. The action of unsaturated acids was compared with the oxygen uptake of auto-respiring mycobacteria and with the action of saturated acids on these organisms.

The oxygen uptake of *M. phlei* under the action of unsaturated oleic and chaulmoogric acids was strongly reduced, when compared with the action of saturated stearic acid or even with the auto-respiration of the bacilli. The *cis* forms of the acids were less active in reducing the respiration of the bacilli than the *trans* forms. With the increase in the number of the double bonds in the molecule the inhibiting action of the compound was increased. The double bond – not the ring – in cyclic chaulmoogric acid inhibits the respiration (Franke, Lee, and Kibat, 1949).

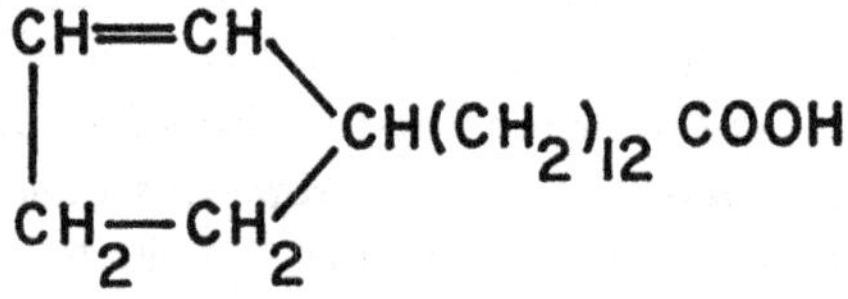

CHAULMOOGRIC ACID

Weitzel (1952) did not attribute the action of chaulmoogric acid on the growth of tubercle bacilli to the double bond in the molecule of the acid but to its ring structure. Franke and Schillinger (1944) regard the inhibitory action on the respiration of unsaturated fatty acids and of the saturated acids of chain lengths between C_{10} and C_{14} as a characteristic feature of acid-fast bacilli. The inhibition of respiration of tubercle bacilli is proportional to the concentration of the acid in the medium. According to C. T. Gray (1949), 500 μg/ml. of oleate produce complete inhibition of respiration, 250 μg. partially inhibit the respiration, but 75 μg. stimulate the respiration of mycobacteria. Oginsky, Smith, and Solotorovsky (1950) investigated the influence of saturated fatty acids on the respiration and on the metabolism of tubercle bacilli (Kirchberg strain) grown in Dubos' Tween-albumin medium. Under the action of 2 micrograms per ml. of lauric, palmitic, and stearic acids, added to the suspension of bacilli, the respiration of the bacilli increased for a few hours, then ceased altogether. The same concentration of myristic acid (C_{14}), when added to the bacilli, inhibited the respiration.

The action of fatty acids on the respiration of mycobacteria follows some general rules. The lower fatty acids, down to C_6, strongly enhance respiration. The higher saturated acids have some enhancing influence on the respiration. The saturated acids from C_{10} to C_{14}, in some concentrations, inhibit the respiration as strongly as the unsaturated acids. According to the rule of Traube, fatty acids, if dissolved in water, lower the surface tension in proportion to the length of their carbon chains.

Oginsky *et al.* were unable to verify the presence in the medium of respiring tubercle bacilli of acetoacetate, citrate, *cis*aconitic or *trans*aconitic acids as intermediates of the oxidation of fatty acids. The attempts to increase the stearic acid oxidation by tubercle bacilli through the addition of oxalacetate, aspartic acid, or asparagine also ended in failure. All endeavors to demonstrate that fatty acids are the metabolites of tubercle bacilli were unsuccessful. In their work on fatty acids as metabolites of tubercle bacilli, Youmans and Youmans (1954a) inoculated tubercle bacilli (strain H37Rv) into a modified Proskauer-Beck's medium in which fatty acids in doses of 1.0 to 0.000004 per cent replaced glycerol as a source of carbon. The rate of growth was established by the small inocula technique (see p. 94). Of the fatty acids tested, only the caprylic and capric acids permitted growth at a rate comparable to that of glycerol. Acetic, propionic, butyric, and caproic acids were also utilized as carbon sources, but the growth of bacilli was not so rapid as with caprylic and capric acids. It was found that there was for each fatty acid a narrow range of concentration where the growth of small inocula occurred. Fatty acids of low molecular weight stimulated the growth of tubercle bacilli more than those of high molecular weight. The action of oleic acid on the growth of tubercle bacilli could not be established with certainty because of irregular results obtained.

McJunkin (1923–1924) discovered that living tubercle bacilli, incubated for seven days at 37°C. in oleic acid, were rendered non-acid-fast. Injected into guinea pigs, they did not produce infection. This observation was corroborated by Boissevain (1926), who showed that saturated acids (stearic) do not have any action on tubercle bacilli, but that the action of unsaturated acids increases in the following order: oleic, linoleic, linolenic. All these acids have the intact $-COOH$ group; oleic has one, linoleic two, and linolenic three double bonds in their molecules. The ability of these acids to deprive tubercle bacilli of their acid-fastness depends on (a) the long carbon chain, (b) the $-COOH$ group, (c) the double bond, and (d) the solubility in water of the acids. The water solubility of unsaturated fatty acids increases with the number of double bonds in the acids. The sodium salts of these acids did not, in the experiments of Boissevain, destroy the acid-fastness of tubercle bacilli, nor did they, after 24 hours of action, eliminate the pathogenicity of the bacilli.

The destruction of acid properties ($-COOH$ group) and the saturation of double bonds in the acid through heating lead to the disappearance of the bactericidal properties of the acid (Hettche and Weber, 1940). The ability of acids to dissolve bacilli increases with the augmentation of their iodine number (tested on staphylococci by A. Hirsch, 1947). Living tubercle bacilli are dissolved by oleic acid, but not so the bacilli killed by formaldehyde (Solomidès, 1946).

The bactericidal action of fatty acids upon mycobacteria was observed by Stanley, Coleman, Greer, Sacks, and Adams (1932). These investigators found that the bactericidal action of fatty acids has a relation to their molecular weight, reaching its maximum in acids of 15 and 18 carbon atoms. The inhibition of respiration runs parallel to the bactericidal activity of the acids (Bergström, Theorell, and Davide, 1946). A concentration of oleic acid in the synthetic medium, when as low as $1:10^{-7}$, causes the inhibition of the growth of small inocula of human tubercle bacilli (Dubos, 1946). These findings were corroborated by Malek and Malkova (1948).

Unsaturated fatty acids are absorbed by tubercle bacilli, and the bactericidal activity of the unsaturated fatty acid solution is considerably decreased after the removal of the added suspension of tubercle bacilli from the solution (Bergström, Theorell, and Davide, 1946). The better growth of large inocula as compared to small inocula was attributed to the removal from the medium of fatty acids by the large inocula of tubercle bacilli (Davis, 1948).

The action of sodium ricinoleate on the growth of an avian strain of tubercle bacilli in Sauton's medium was studied by Luzzati (1952). After the addition of 20×10^{-6} ml. of this soap to a suspension of bacilli, the partial lysis of the bacilli occurred and their reproduction ceased. This phenomenon was chosen as a means of determining the action of different fatty acids on the growth of bacilli. The concentration of acid needed to produce lysis and to stop the reproduction of bacilli decreased with the increase of the length of the carbon chain of the acid added and had to be highest in sodium myristate (C_{14}). The adsorbability of fatty acids by wax extracted from tubercle bacilli reaches the maximum in the fatty acids of 14 carbon atoms, which also have the greatest growth inhibiting effect. The total inhibition of the growth of tubercle bacilli was obtained when 6×10^{-6} g. of sodium oleate per ml. were added to the medium containing 10^8 bacilli per ml. The growth ceased when each bacillus had absorbed 2.5×10^{-13} g. of sodium oleate. No considerable differences were found between the uptake of sodium oleate by living and dead bacilli (Luzzati, 1954).

Weitzel (1952) investigated the influence of natural fats, the double bond, and the position and number of double bonds in the molecule of fatty acids on the growth of H37Rv and other strains of tubercle bacilli cultivated on Hohn's egg medium and on the synthetic liquid medium containing 2 and 5 per cent serum.

The triglycerides *in vitro* have a restricted growth-inhibiting action on tubercle bacilli. In Hohn's egg medium the bacteriostatic action of the natural fats (butter, coconut fat, olive oil) on the H37Rv strain of bacilli was not higher than in the dilution 1:1,000. Only chaulmoogric oil, linseed oil, and dog fat had a higher but irregular bacteriostatic action. There does not seem to be any relation between the iodine number of natural fats and their bacteriostatic action on mycobacteria. The growth-inhibiting action of C_{18} – acids was uniformly feeble; the increase in the number of double bonds in the molecule is accompanied by an increase in the growth-inhibiting action, but no difference in action between the linoleic acid with two unsaturated bonds and linolenic acid with three unsaturated bonds in the molecule was observed.

Salicylates and Benzoates

Bernheim (1940, 1941) observed that the addition of one mg. per ml. of sodium salicylate (ortho-hydrobenzoate) to a strain of tubercle bacilli of the avian type suspended in a buffer solution of *p*H 6.7 more than doubled the oxygen consumption of the bacilli. Benzoate also increased the oxygen uptake but para- and meta-hydrobenzoates and methylsalicylate were without effect. (See Fig. 20.) Acetylsalicylate was active after the acetyl group had been hydrolyzed. *Para*-aminobenzoate had no action on respiration. In the range of 0.1 to 0.2 mg. per ml. the increase of oxygen uptake was proportional to the concentration of salicylate and benzoate in the medium.

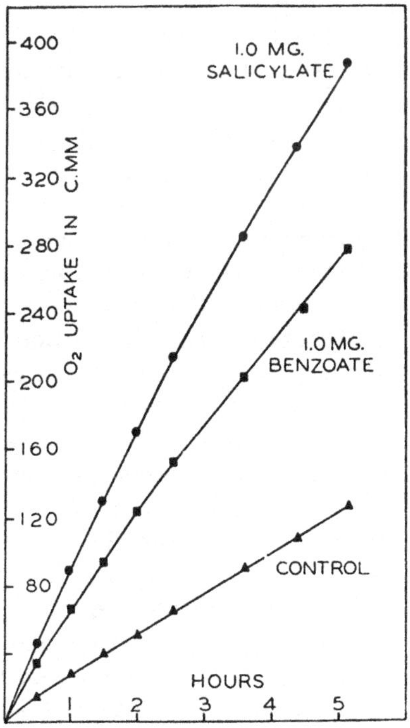

Figure 20. The effect of sodium salicylate and benzoate on the oxygen consumption of tubercle bacilli (Bernheim, 1940).

The addition of 0.05 *M* potassium cyanide inhibited the increase of oxygen uptake by salicylate or benzoate, the removal of KCN restored it. Citral, heptaldehyde, isovaleraldehyde, anisaldehyde, benzaldehyde, and furfural also increased the respiration rate of tubercle bacilli. The last two compounds were most active. Ethyl alcohol had no effect on the respiration, but the higher alcohols (propyl, butyl, amyl, and *iso* forms) increased the oxygen consumption. The respiration of non-acid-fast microorganisms was not influenced by salicylates and benzoates.

The work of Loebel, Shorr, and Richardson (1933b) (see p. 99) revealed the increase of oxygen uptake in tubercle bacilli under the action of fatty acids, soaps, and caseous material. According to the views of these authors, the increased respiration indicates the assimilation of the added substance. These views were shared by Bernheim and his co-workers. Fitzgerald, Bernheim, and Fitzgerald (1948) announced that even the pathogenic strain H37Rv is capable of developing adaptive enzymes and utilizing benzoic acid as the source of carbon instead of asparagine. Roulet and Zeller (1948) considered the increase in the oxygen uptake of mycobacteria in the presence of peptides (glycyl-L-leucine, glycyl-L-tyrosine, etc.) in the medium as a proof of the presence in mycobacteria of enzymes decomposing these substances. According to J. Lehmann (1946a), the oxygen uptake of pathogenic mycobacteria only can be increased by salicylate and benzoate. This observation was to some extent corroborated by Fitzgerald and Bernheim (1947). An increase in the oxygen uptake of pathogenic strains of tubercle bacilli under salicylate was also observed by Desbordes and Fournier (1950).

The study of Andrejew (1951) confirmed the effect of salicylate and benzoate on the respiration of tubercle bacilli and showed that this stimulation of respiration is produced in young, rapidly growing bacilli suspended in phosphate buffer and is without any influence on twenty-day-old bacilli, or bacilli suspended in a liquid nutritive medium. According to Andrejew a nine-day-old BCG strain under benzoate and salicylate acted exactly like a pathogenic strain. The same results were obtained with the nonlethal human strain H37Ra. Pope (1952) confirmed the findings of Andrejew. (The strain BCG is not apathogenic. See p. 303.)

Stanier *et al.* (1950) investigated the oxidation of simple aromatic compounds by *Pseudomonas fluorescens*. The manometric technique was used to estimate the oxygen uptake. Pyrocatechol was found to be an intermediate product of the metabolism of these compounds by *Pseudomonas*. Wagner (1951) using the manometric technique and following Loebel's and Bernheim's conception of the metabolism of benzoate by mycobacteria, studied the metabolism of twenty aromatic compounds in *M. smegmatis*. In conformity with the findings of Bernheim, Wagner observed the development of adaptive enzymes as early as 20 minutes after the bacilli had been in contact with the solution of benzoic acid. Only three (benzoic acid and its derivatives) of the twenty compounds studied produced a slight increase in the oxygen uptake of *M. smegmatis.* This increase in oxygen consumption was taken to be an indication of the utilization of the compound in bacilli. Since pyrocatechol showed a similar slight increase in oxygen uptake, it was accepted as the intermediate substance in the metabolism of benzoic acid in mycobacteria. The quantitative estimation of benzoic acid revealed that the decrease or disappearance of this substance took place only when large amounts (10–20 g.) of young cells of mycobacteria were added to the solution of benzoic acid.

The purpose of the work of Gale (1952) was identical with that of Wagner, namely to determine the intermediate substances of metabolism of benzoic acid in mycobacteria. Gale found that the BCG strain formed adaptive enzymes for the oxidation of benzoic acid. The cells of *M. butyricum* adapted to benzoate had a reduced lag period when catechol was added and formed ketone bodies from benzoate (Rothera test was transiently positive). No direct identification of the intermediates was made. Bernheim (1953), in conformity with these observations, suggested that the oxidation of benzoic acid proceeds, in mycobacteria and *Pseudomonas* alike, through catechol and pyrocatechol.

The search for substances that would inhibit the extra oxygen uptake of tubercle bacilli under the action of salicylate or benzoate was started by Saz and Bernheim (1941). The Woods-Fildes theory (1940, 1941) of competitive enzyme inhibition was assumed as the guiding hypothesis. According to Woods and Fildes, the sulfonamides, because of their structural analogy with *para*-aminobenzoic acid, which is the growth factor of microorganisms, are capable of replacing it and inhibiting the growth. (See review of R. J. Henry, 1947.) It was expected that substance that inhibits the extra oxygen uptake of mycobacteria under the influence of salicylate or benzoate might be of value as a chemotherapeutic agent in the treatment of tuberculosis. Saz and Bernheim discovered that 2,3,5-triiodobenzoate caused a marked inhibition of the extra oxygen uptake of tubercle bacilli under the influence of salicylate. The problem was further studied by J. Lehmann (1946a, b). Investigating more than fifty derivatives of salicylic and benzoic acid as to their inhibiting effect on the growth of tubercle bacilli, he found *para*-aminosalicylic acid (PAS) to be the most effective growth inhibitor of the BCG bacilli. *Para*-aminosalicylic acid, added in a concentration of 10^{-5}M (1 in 650,000 or 0.15 mg. per 100 ml.) to the medium, brought about a 50 to 75 per cent growth inhibition of the culture. These findings were confirmed by Youmans (1946b); according to his experiments, PAS from 0.019 and up to 0.156 mg. per cent inhibited the growth of twelve strains of tubercle bacilli, including strains resistant to streptomycin. Vennesland, Ebert, and Bloch (1948) found that 1.2 micrograms per ml. of PAS in Dubos' medium inhibit the growth of the H37Rv strain (Fig. 21).

Para-aminosalicylic acid, streptomycin, and sulfonamides have little effect on the respiration of tubercle bacilli (J. Lehmann, 1946a; Zetterberg, 1949; Andrejew, 1951; Bernheim, DeTurk, and Pope, 1953). Streptomycin has a strong bacteriostatic effect on pathogenic tubercle bacilli. According to Youmans and Feldman (1946), less than one microgram of streptomycin inhibits the growth of tubercle bacilli. Moderate concentrations of strepto-

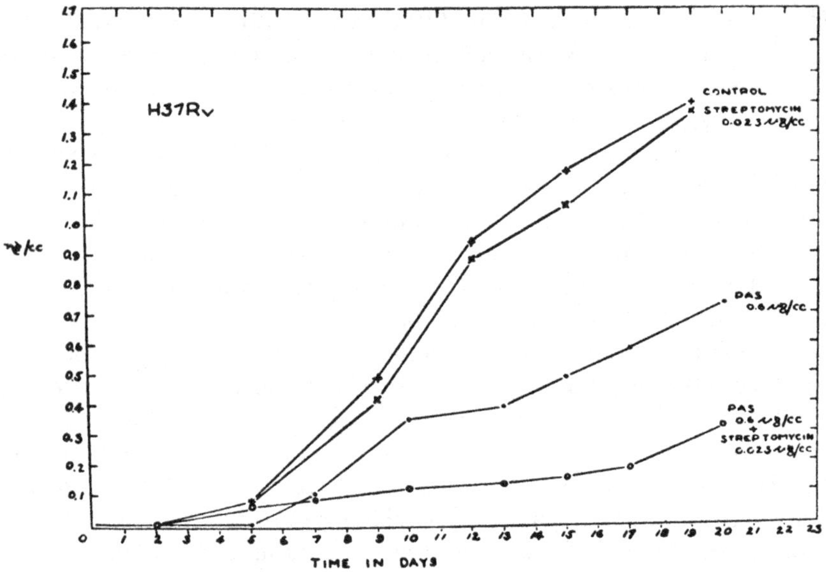

Figure 21. The effect of various concentrations of streptomycin, PAS, and streptomycin and PAS combined on the growth of tubercle bacilli, H37Rv (Vennesland, Ebert, and Bloch, 1948).

mycin inhibited the growth of tubercle bacilli in the presence of a noninhibiting concentration of PAS, and the action of PAS was enhanced by the addition of noninhibiting concentrations of streptomycin to the medium. The bacteriostatic effect of *para*-aminosalicylic acid was nullified when the amino group was moved into the *ortho* or the *meta* position or when the place of NH_2 in the compound was taken by NO_2. Substitutions in the amino group by CH_3 or stearic acid reduced only slightly the bacteriostatic effect of PAS. When the hydroxy group in the *ortho* position was replaced by CH_3, the activity was retained, but not when it was replaced by NH_2 or Cl. *Para*-aminosalicylic acid was nontoxic to rats when given along with food during one to two months in a concentration of 5 per cent.

Table 9. The Influence of Sodium Salts of Fatty Acids on the Growth of Tubercle Bacilli *

Variations of Sauton's Medium	Growth
Complete (control)	xxx
Without glycerol	0
With ¼ glycerol of control	x
With ¹⁄₁₀ glycerol of control	x
Complete, with palmitate	xxx
Complete, with oleate	0
Without glycerol, with palmitate	0
Without glycerol, with oleate	0
With ¼ glycerol of control, with palmitate	0
With ¼ glycerol of control, with oleate	0

Source: Cutinelli (1941).
* 0 = no growth; x = meager growth; xxx = vigorous growth.

Enhanced Respiration of Tubercle Bacilli as Related to Growth

The contradictory nature of fatty acids, salicylate, benzoate, and other substances which stimulate the oxygen uptake of mycobacteria but inhibit their growth, encouraged investigators to study these substances. Cutinelli (1941), H. Bloch (1944), Oginsky *et al.* (1950), Luzzati (1952), and Bernheim *et al.* (1953) looked for an answer to the basic problem of how the increase or inhibition of the respiration of tubercle bacilli influences their growth. J. Lehmann (1946a) observed that if Bernheim's interpretation of the "benzoic and salicylic" effect is true, the benzene ring of these compounds must be split by the bacilli. Compounds with the ring structure, such as phenylalanine, tryptophan, imidazole are not metabolized by tubercle bacilli (Long, 1921–1922).

The manometric studies of Cutinelli (1941) showed that, in Sauton's medium, capric acid increases the respiration of tubercle bacilli by 250, stearic by 185, and palmitic by 120 per cent, and that, as far as respiration is concerned, the fatty acids can even take the place of glycerol in the composition of the medium. In the further experiments of Cutinelli, glycerol in Sauton's medium was replaced by equimolar quantities of fatty acids so as to test whether these acids, instead of glycerol, could be used by tubercle bacilli as growth and building material. These experiments showed that fatty acids, which may increase the respiration of tubercle bacilli, are not utilized by the bacilli as building material and do not support the growth of the bacilli. Palmitic and oleic acids cannot even partially replace glycerol in Sauton's medium (see Table 9).

The work of Bloch further clarified the problem. Bernheim (1940, 1941) showed that benzaldehyde, furfural, and sodium salicylate increase the respiration of tubercle bacilli. The investigations of Bloch revealed that none of these substances was capable of replacing glycerol in the medium or promoting the growth of tubercle bacilli. Bloch recognized that the increase in the respiration of tubercle bacilli under the influence of these substances takes place only within narrow concentration limits. In a slightly increased concentration the substance that formerly promoted respiration inhibits respiration. These observations by Bloch (1944), on aldehydes and sodium salicylate, are in agreement with those of Franke and Schillinger (1944), who found that only within certain limits of concentration do fatty acids promote the respiration of tubercle bacilli.

Substances of opposite action – which would inhibit the respiration but promote growth – are not known. All respiration-inhibiting substances also inhibit growth (Bloch, 1944; Zetterberg, 1949).

Bloch divided substances into three categories according to their influence on the respiration and growth of tubercle bacilli: (a) substances that increase respiration and are capable of replacing glycerol in the medium (glucose);* (b) substances that increase respiration but are not capable of replacing the glycerol in media (stearic acid, Cutinelli, 1941); (c) substances that increase the respiration, inhibit growth, and are not capable of replacing glycerol in media (sodium salicylate, benzoate, aldehydes, etc.) – which also, in higher concentrations, inhibit respiration.

In our studies, the synthetic medium prepared according to Bernheim, containing 10 mg. per 100 ml. of sodium salicylate instead of asparagine, did not permit the growth of tubercle bacilli (strain H37Rv).

A number of Erlenmeyer flasks containing 12 ml. of our synthetic medium with added salicylate were inoculated with equal fragments of pellicle of *Mycobacterium phlei.* After seven days of growth at 37°C. the bacilli were collected, washed three times with distilled water, dried in an oven at 80°C. and over phosphorus pentoxide in vacuum, and weighed. The results are shown in the accompanying tabulation, which shows that sodi-

Amount of Salicylate Added to the Medium (mg. per 100 ml.)	*Dry Weight in Grams of the Bacilli Collected from 12 ml. of the Medium (Average from 3 Experiments) Cultures of 168 Hours at 37°C.*
5	0.0220
10	0.0217
20	0.0052
0	0.0363

um salicylate considerably undermines the growth of saprophytic *M. phlei* and, in a concentration of 20 mg. per 100 ml., can inhibit it altogether. The oxidation of glucose by *M. phlei* in the presence of salicylate is stopped

* At present there are no known substances that can fully replace glycerol in media for tubercle bacilli. Glucose is the second best after glycerol.

(see p. 112). Salicylate and the related compounds inhibit the oxidative enzymes of Krebs cycle in kidney and liver homogenates; α-ketoglutaric dehydrogenase and succinic dehydrogenase are inhibited to the greatest extent (Kaplan, Kennedy, and Davis, 1954).

The growth of a cell is not possible without an increased uptake of nitrogen. Only a few (proteins and glycerol) of the presently known substances simultaneously increase the respiration and the nitrogen intake of tubercle bacilli. Bernheim, DeTurk, and Pope (1953) studied the nitrogen assimilation of tubercle bacilli in connection with their increased oxygen uptake under the action of different substances. The resting cells of five strains of BCG were suspended in a buffer solution of *p*H 6.7 and their respiration estimated by the Barcroft-Warburg technique. The nitrogen was determined as ammonia. The addition of $(NH_4)_2SO_4$ to the suspension of bacilli did not affect the auto-respiration of the bacilli. No assimilation of nitrogen occurred without the addition of glycerol to the medium. The assimilation of nitrogen was roughly parallel to the amount of glycerol added.

As Table 10 shows, there are many substances (glycerol, succinic acid, sodium acetate, dinitrophenol) which are capable of increasing the oxygen uptake of BCG, but only a few of them can increase at the same time the assimilation of nitrogen. The substances that increase the nitrogen assimilation are succinic acid, sodium pyruvate, and sodium acetate, with malonate immediately following glycerol. In regard to the increase of oxygen

Table 10. The Effect of Various Substances on Oxygen Uptake and Ammonia Assimilation by Resting BCG Bacilli, Strain 8420, in the Presence of 1 mg. $(NH_4)_2SO_4$ Containing 214 Micrograms N, in 210 Minutes, at *p*H 6.0 and 37°C.

Substance	Amount Added (mg./ml.)	Extra O_2 Uptake (cmm.)	Nitrogen Assimilated from NH_3 (micrograms)
Due to autorespiration			126–159
Glycerol	1	569	166
Succinic acid	1	793	182
Sodium pyruvate	1	321	177
Malonic acid	1	193	153
Oxalic acid	1	0	126
Sodium acetate, anhydrous	1	372	189
Propionic acid	1	367	132
Caprylic acid	1	475	74
Oleic acid	1	137	117
PAS	0.5	478	95
Aureomycin	0.05	284	91
Streptomycin	0.05	420	125
2,4-dinitrophenol	0.05	841	66
Sodium fluoride	0.5	711	7

Source: Bernheim, DeTurk, and Pope (1953).

uptake and the simultaneous increase of NH_3-assimilation, only succinic acid surpasses glycerol. Some of these data contradict the observations of earlier authors: Long (1921–1922), Kondo (1924, 1925), Braun (1942), and Schaefer *et al.* (1949) did not observe any growth stimulation of tubercle bacilli by succinate and pyruvate; Nakamura (1938) did not obtain stimulation of respiration by succinate. Acetate was known to stimulate growth and respiration (Braun *et al.*, 1924; Kondo, 1924, 1925; Bernheim, 1941; Schaefer, 1948). *Para*-aminosalicylic acid, streptomycin, and fatty acids (especially caprylic and oleic) reduce the nitrogen uptake of tubercle bacilli.

Conclusions

As the foregoing shows, some substances metabolized by mycobacteria, such as glycerol, increase their oxygen uptake. These observations led to the inference that substances that increase the oxygen uptake of mycobacteria are metabolized by mycobacteria (Loebel, Shorr, and Richardson, 1933a; Nakamura, 1938; Bernheim, 1940).

This conjecture caused considerable controversy, because facts accumulated indicating that the increase in oxygen uptake in mycobacteria in the presence of some poisonous substances cannot be attributed to the assimilation of these substances by mycobacteria (Warburg, 1914a; Cutinelli, 1941; Lehmann, 1946a; Bernheim, DeTurk, and Pope, 1953).

The procedure generally used to determine the changes in oxygen uptake of mycobacteria under the action of an added substance is the manometric method. This method, however, does not indicate the changes in the amount of metabolized substance. A substance capable of increasing the oxygen uptake may be metabolized or this very substance may increase the uptake of some other compound present in the growth substrate of bacilli; in these cases the decrease in the amount of the substances metabolized must be demonstrated by quantitative analysis. This was our leading thought when investigating these problems.

Agitated *M. phlei* rapidly oxidize glucose. This observation led us to apply the shaking technique, which we had introduced for the purification of tuberculous material, to the study of the action of sodium salicylate and oleate on glucose oxidation in *M. phlei*.

The laboratory strain of *M. phlei* was adapted to grow on our liquid medium (see Table 32) with glucose as chief source of carbon. Pellicles of *M. phlei* collected after 72 hours of growth at 37°C. were washed and dispensed at the rate of 150 mg. (wet weight) into sterile bottles of 500 ml. capacity containing 200 glass beads and 5 ml. of 100 mg. per 100 ml. glucose solution with or without sodium salicylate. The bottles were shaken in a Kahn shaker at 275 strokes per minute. After 1, 2, and 3 hours of shaking the amount of glucose remaining in the bottles was estimated by

Nelson's micromethod. Readings were made in an Evelyn photoelectrometer with a filter transmitting light of 660 mμ wave length. We had previously established that glucose in a water solution remains unchanged when shaken in air or in the atmosphere of carbon dioxide or nitrogen. The oxidation of glucose takes place when it is shaken in air in the presence of living *M. phlei*. The kinetic energy of shaking increases the catalytic burning of glucose on the surface of living mycobacteria.

The amount of glucose oxidized by 1 mg. of *M. phlei* in 1 ml. of 100 mg. per 100 ml. glucose solution during one hour of shaking was accepted as the quotient expressing the oxidative power of mycobacteria in the given moment of shaking:

$$Q_{gluc} = \frac{\text{mg. per 100 ml. glucose oxidized}}{\text{mg. mycobacteria} \times \text{hours of shaking} \times \text{ml. 100 mg. per 100 ml. glucose solution}}$$

The course of glucose oxidation in shaking experiments in the presence and in the absence of sodium salicylate is shown in Table 11. The glucose

Table 11. Course of Glucose Oxidation in *Mycobacterium phlei* Shaken in 100 mg. per 100 ml. Glucose Solution with and without Sodium Salicylate for 1, 2, and 3 Hours

	Without Salicylate			With 1 mg./ml. Salicylate		
Hours of Shaking	Average from 5 Experiments	Standard Deviation	Q_{gluc}	Average from 3 Experiments	Standard Deviation	Q_{gluc}
One	44.6	±5.40	0.059	23	±2.95	0.030
Two	17.0	±7.07	0.011	20	±7.57	0.013
Three	8.0	±1.79	0.004	16	±2.83	0.007

oxidation quotient of *M. phlei* shaken without salicylate drops from 0.059 to 0.004 from the first to the third hour of shaking. In the presence of salicylate the rate of glucose oxidation after one hour of shaking is only half as high as without salicylate (quotient 0.030), and, as the shaking continues, the rate of glucose oxidation drops less than when glucose is shaken without salicylate. In the third hour of shaking, due to the narcotic action of salicylate, the rate of glucose oxidation in the presence of salicylate is not increased and remains approximately twice as high as in the exhausted cells shaken without salicylate (quotients 0.007 and 0.004 respectively). This leaves the impression that glucose oxidation in *M. phlei* increases under the action of salicylate. The rate of glucose oxidation in bacilli in the presence of salicylate does not reach the oxidation level of fresh bacilli. Salicylate not only reduces the oxidative power but also diminishes the harvest of cultures of *M. phlei* (see p. 110).

Sodium oleate, when present in a glucose solution, strongly reduces the oxidative power of *M. phlei*. The addition of blood serum (5 per cent) to a glucose solution containing oleate restores the oxidative power of *M. phlei* to the level of controls shaken without oleate.

Long hours of work during several weeks are needed to follow up the amounts of glucose utilized in *M. phlei* in cultivation experiments. The same goal can be reached in a few hours by means of the shaking technique.

VIII

Sources of Carbon

Glycerol

NOCARD and Roux (1887) discovered that the addition of glycerol to the agar medium stimulates the growth of tubercle bacilli highly. Th. Smith (1904–1905) observed that there exists some difference between the ways the human and bovine types of tubercle bacilli react to glycerol. Both types consume glycerol, but most human strains, after several weeks of incubation, acidify the glycerol broth, whereas most bovine bacilli alkalize it. If bacilli are grown on broth without glycerol, these differences are not revealed; the reaction is alkaline in both cases.

Siebert (1909), like Th. Smith, attributed the acidification of glycerol broth under the influence of growing tubercle bacilli to the production and release into the media of some acids; and he found that neutralizing these acids by adding sodium hydroxide or marble stimulated the growth of bacilli.

There exists a very pronounced difference between mycobacteria and non-acid-fast bacteria with respect to their glycerol and carbohydrate metabolism. Mycobacteria completely oxidize glycerol and glucose to water and carbon dioxide, and there is no accumulation in the medium of partly oxidized acidic or alkaline cleavage products which would account for the changes in the *p*H of the medium. The accumulation of these products (alcohols, acids) in media brings the growth of other microorganisms to an early standstill, while the growth of mycobacteria goes on for weeks (Dingle and Weinzirl, 1932). The acidification of glycerol media may be the result of the withdrawal of some alkaline constituents from the medium by growing tubercle bacilli (Wedum, 1936). Friedemann and Seibert (1939) investigated the acidification of media containing glycerol, and like Merrill (1930) did not discover any lactic acid formation in media where tubercle bacilli had grown. The cause of this acidification phenomenon is still unknown.

The problem of the optimal concentration of glycerol in the media, its influence on the production of the bacillary mass, and other aspects of glycerol metabolism, were studied by many authors. Siebert (1909) found that tubercle bacilli utilize relatively large quantities of glycerol. One strain of tubercle bacilli, in 75 days of growth, reduced the concentration of glycerol in broth from 3.7 per cent to 1.12 per cent, another strain to 1.53 per cent. The complementary addition of glycerol and the neutralization of the medium increased the yield of bacilli by about 2.8 times. The highest harvest of bacilli was from 16-day-old cultures, after that time the weight of bacilli in the culture diminished, and after 119 days was 33 per cent smaller than after 16 days of growth. Tiffeneau and Marie (1912) observed that a culture of tubercle bacilli consumed, in ten months of growth, 15 grams of glycerol. Frouin and Guillaumie (1924a) studied the utilization of glycerol by tubercle bacilli in a synthetic medium in which asparagine was the sole source of nitrogen. In an acidic medium of *p*H 6.0–6.5 the increase in weight of bacilli collected after 20 days of incubation was parallel to the increase in the glycerol concentration in the medium, but glycerol, in a concentration of 2 to 4 per cent, produced approximately the same amount of bacilli, by weight. Similar results were obtained by Long and Finner (1927), who reported that 100 ml. of a synthetic medium, containing 0.5 per cent glycerol, produced, in four weeks, 0.13 g. bacilli (dry weight); when the glycerol content of the medium was raised to 5 per cent, the weight of the bacilli went up to 0.95 g., and at 6 per cent, it reached 1.44 g. No increase in the harvest was obtained by a further increase of the glycerol concentration in the medium. These observations were corroborated by Goyal (1936). The weight of bacilli collected from the medium was augmented when the glycerol concentration was increased from 1 to 6 per cent, but diminished when the concentration was above 6 per cent. A quantitative estimation of the glycerol consumption and the increase of weight of tubercle bacilli obtained in Long's synthetic medium was made by Friedemann and Seibert (1939). The glycerol consumption and the dry weight of bacilli harvested increased rapidly and reached the maximum in 3.5 weeks of cultivation. Thereafter the weight of collected bacilli diminished but considerable amounts of tuberculin appeared in the medium.

It was supposed that the fatty substances of the tubercle bacillus are derived from proteins of the medium. As E. R. Long and Finner (1927) showed, the concentration of glycerol in the medium and the lipid content of tubercle bacilli are in some relation. Tubercle bacilli produced 10.4 per cent chloroform-soluble lipids when grown on Long's synthetic medium containing 0.5 per cent glycerol, but 27.6 per cent when the glycerol concentration of the medium was 12.5 per cent. Long and Campbell (1922–1923) produced data showing that the glycerol in the medium must be the progenitor of the acid-fast properties of tubercle bacilli.

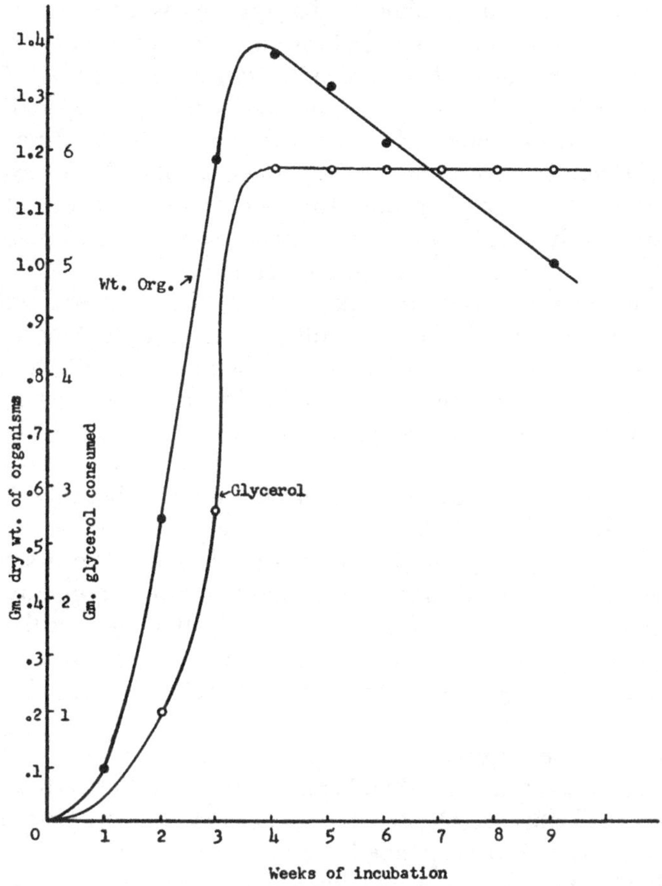

Figure 22. Glycerol consumption and increase in dry weight of harvested tubercle bacilli (Friedemann and Seibert, 1939).

Isotopic carbon in the studies of Long, Anderson, Rittenberg, Karnovsky, and Henderson (1955) revealed important facts about the pathway of assimilation of carbon in tubercle bacilli. Three carbon sources of tubercle bacilli were studied: glycerol, acetic acid, and carbon dioxide. Compounds containing labeled carbon in different positions were prepared and incorporated in Long's synthetic medium. Tubercle bacilli were inoculated on the surface of the medium and after six weeks of growth the cultures were collected and analyzed.

Glycerol was labeled with C^{14} in the alpha position

$$C^{14}H_2OH \cdot CHOH \cdot CH_2OH$$

and in the beta position

$$CH_2OH \cdot C^{14}HOH \cdot CH_2OH$$

The cultivation experiments showed that glycerol is a source of energy as well as a source of building material for all major constituents of tubercle bacilli. Labeled carbon of both positions was utilized by bacilli. Fifteen per cent of labeled glycerol carbon appeared as carbon dioxide, 15 per cent was incorporated in lipids and in the body of the bacilli, 2 per cent was found in proteins of tuberculin, and 4 per cent in soluble polysaccharides. The rest of the labeled carbon, approximately 50 per cent, was found to be incorporated in the metabolic compounds of low molecular weight such as sugars and amino acids of the culture medium.

The radioactive isotopes, principally those of phosphorus and carbon, are important tools in experimental tuberculosis. The problems of growth of mycobacteria *in vitro*, the behavior and the fate of bacilli in an infected body, and the mode of action of chemotherapeutics are some of the fields of research where the isotopes have been used successfully. For further information and bibliography see the review of Lebeurre (1956).

The coefficient of glycerol utilization (the relation between the weight of carbon fixed by bacilli and the carbon of glycerol consumed) is about 0.47. About half of the glycerol utilized is used to build bodies of tubercle bacilli, the other half is oxidized and converted into carbon dioxide.

The protein utilization and ammonia production by mycobacteria decreases when glycerol or glucose is present in the medium. (On this protein-sparing role of glycerol and carbohydrates, see Kendall, Day, and Walker, 1914).

Glycerol has the effect of an antiseptic substance on mycobacteria. In a 6 per cent glycerol solution tubercle bacilli died within two to four weeks. The presence or absence of oxygen did not influence this phenomenon. In the absence of glycerol, suspended bacilli survived for many weeks (Boissevain, 1943). This action of glycerol on mycobacteria is masked by egg media and by an abundant inoculum of fresh bacilli. On nutrient agar, inoculated sparsely with six-week-old *M. butyricum* and incubated at 37°C., growth starts in 24 hours; on agar containing 3 per cent glycerol, growth appears in 72 hours; on agar with 6 per cent glycerol, in 120 hours (Darzins, 1948).

Although ethylene glycol and glycerol have many common properties, ethylene glycol is not utilized by tubercle bacilli (E. R. Long, 1921–1922), and does not enhance their respiration (Nakamura, 1938). In a concentration of 5 to 7 per cent, propylene glycol inhibits the growth of tubercle bacilli (Bazzicalupo, Portella, and Contieri, 1951).

Glycerol injected subcutaneously into animals is partly oxidized, partly eliminated through the kidneys. Like ethylene glycol, it produces hemorrhagic nephritis. Minra found, in 1911, that propylene glycol in an animal organism is detoxified and eliminated in combination with glucuronic acid.

Sources of Carbon

Glucose

Nocard and Roux (1887) stated that glucose enhances the growth of tubercle bacilli but cannot replace glycerol; Kühne (1894), and Proskauer and Beck (1894) also observed that glucose cannot substitute for glycerol in a medium. In the two human, two bovine, and one avian strains of mycobacteria studied, no differences in the utilization of glucose were found (Gamble and Herrick, 1922).

In neutral or alkaline media the utilization of glucose increases at high concentrations (Frouin and Guillaumie, 1923b). The increase of glucose in a medium augments the speed of growth of tubercle bacilli. In four weeks of growth in a synthetic medium containing glucose, 1.4 g. of bacilli were obtained; the same medium without glucose produced the same quantity of bacilli in eight weeks. The production of bacilli is mainly influenced by the glucose in the first four weeks of growth.

Tubercle bacilli (human, bovine, and avian types), growing on media containing glucose instead of glycerol, turn the medium alkaline (Kendall, Day, and Walker, 1914; Gamble and Herrick, 1922; Frouin and Guillaumie, 1923b; Novy and Soule, 1925; Weinzirl and Knapton, 1927).

The influence of glucose concentrations on the growth and weight of the cultures of tubercle bacilli in a synthetic medium with 0.5 per cent asparagine as the source of nitrogen was investigated by Frouin and Guillaumie (1923b). The weight of harvested bacilli increases with the increase of the glucose concentration in the medium: 0.478 g. of glucose in 100 ml. of the medium produced 0.194 g. of dry bacilli; 4.032 g. of glucose in the same medium produced 0.452 g. of bacilli. The increase in the bacillary harvest does not keep pace with the increase in glucose concentration: a tenfold increase of sugar (from 0.478 to 4.032) produces only two to three times more bacilli. To produce 1 g. of bacilli in a medium containing 0.478 g. per cent glucose, 2.37 g. of glucose were utilized; in the same medium containing 4.032 per cent glucose, 5.84 g. of this substance were necessary to produce 1 g. of bacilli. When increased over the optimal concentration level of 1 or 2 per cent, glucose is burned up by bacilli without being used in the synthesis of their bodies. These findings of Frouin and Guillaumie were later corroborated by many authors (Loebel, Shorr, and Richardson, 1933a; Schaefer, Marshak, and Burkhart, 1949).

There are great differences between the lipid content of tubercle bacilli grown on glycerol or on glucose broth. From bacilli grown for nine weeks on glycerol broth, 25.20 per cent lipids could be extracted by chloroform; from those grown on glucose, 7.5 per cent (Vaillant, 1906). These findings were confirmed by Allilaire and Fernbach (1920), who found 60 to 80 per cent less fatty substance in bacilli grown on a glucose medium than in bacilli grown on a glycerol medium. The addition of glucose to a medium containing glycerol did not increase the level of the alcohol-soluble fats of bacilli (Frouin, 1921). Glycerol is used up by tubercle bacilli at the same rate when glucose is present in the medium as when glucose is absent (Henley, 1929).

According to Stephenson and Whetham (1922, 1924), one gram of glucose in *Mycobacterium phlei*, grown on a synthetic medium, leads to the formation of 0.0189 g. protein nitrogen and 0.028 g. of lipid material. It was possible to account for all carbon of glucose utilized by *M. phlei* during a 21-day growth period to within the limits of 0.5 to 1.0 per cent.

Carbon respired as carbon dioxide	67.66%
Carbon found in organisms	25.84
Carbon remaining in media	7.09

Table 12 summarizes the differences in growth and metabolism of tubercle bacilli on glycerol and glucose media.

Other Alcohols, Carbohydrates, and Amino Acids

Besides glycerol and glucose many other alcohols and carbohydrates have been investigated as possible sources of carbon for tubercle bacilli. Proskauer and Beck (1894) observed that the monosaccharides mannose

Table 12. Glycerol and Glucose in the Media for Tubercle Bacilli

	Glycerol	Glucose	Author
Utilized	By all strains	Not by all strains	Merrill (1931); Loebel *et al.* (1933a); Model (1933); Fitzgerald and Bernheim (1947)
Optimum concentration	No optimum, not above 6%	1%	Nocard and Roux (1887); Proskauer and Beck (1894); E. R. Long *et al.* (1927); Schaefer *et al.* (1948, 1949)
*p*H optimum	6.5–7.5	Acidic range	E. R. Long (1919); Frouin and Guillaumie (1928)
Final *p*H of the medium	Acidic	Alkaline	Th. Smith (1905, 1910); Gamble and Herrick (1922); Weinzirl and Knapton (1927)
Amount activating respiration	0.005%	0.1% No activation	Loebel *et al.* (1933a) Cutinelli (1940); Edson and Hunter (1943)
Oxygen uptake per tube when grown for 26 days at 37°C., 750 mm. barometric pressure	153 ml.	31 ml.	Novy and Soule (1925)

Table 12—*continued*

	Glycerol	Glucose	Author
CO_2 production per tube, when grown for 26 days at 37°C., 750 mm. pressure	127 ml.	52 ml.	Novy and Soule (1925)
CO_2 production from synthetic medium in 23 days	164 ml.	293 ml.	Merrill (1930)
Ml. of CO_2 dissolved in 10 ml. of medium after 26 days of growth of tubercle bacilli	0.38	3.27	Novy and Soule (1925)
Consumption of CO_2 when fermented by propionic acid bacteria	Considerable	Slight	Wood and Werkman (1940)
Respiration quotient	0.836	0.992	Novy and Soule (1925)
Heat of combustion kg.-cal. per gram molecule	397	673	
Influence on some apathogenic mycobacteria			
Increase of growth	Meager	Good	Pinner (1932)
Increase of respiration	Small	Three to four times	Edson and Hunter (1943)
Microliter of oxygen consumed per mg. dry weight of *M. phlei*/hour in Warburg technique, Substance 0.02 *M.*	8.2	25.3	Edson and Hunter (1947)
Growth promotion	Glycerol better than glucose		Nocard and Roux (1887); Kühne (1894); Proskauer and Beck (1894); Bloch (1947); Youmans *et al.* (1953)
	Glycerol and glucose equal		A. S. Griffith (1907); Massol and Breton (1911)
		Glucose better than glycerol	Vaillant (1906); Merrill (1930); Dubos (1947)
Dry weight of bacilli from 100 ml. of broth (grams)			
Washed	0.463	0.243	Calmette, Massol, and Breton (1909)
	0.95	0.22	E. R. Long and Finner (1927)
	1.149	0.555	Frouin and Guillaumie (1928)
	1.350	0.250	Model (1929)
Not washed	0.859–2.178	1.307–2.347	Vaillant (1906)
When autoclaved at 120°C.	Not altered	Noxious caramelization products	Proskauer and Beck (1894); Dubos (1946)

Table 12—*continued*

	Glycerol	Glucose	Author
When mineral salts in medium increased	Considerable increase of harvest	Slight increase of harvest	Frouin and Guillaumie (1928)
Favorable influence of iron on growth	In acidic and neutral media	In acidic media	Frouin and Guillaumie (1928)
Wetting of tubercle bacilli	Wetting	No wetting	Darzins (1953)
Production by tubercle bacilli of yellow pigment from *p*-aminosalicylic acid	Abundant	Inhibited	Mayer and Crane (1950)
Amount of carotenoid pigment produced by *M. phlei* from 100 ml. of medium	550 gamma units/g.	100 gamma units/g.	Ingraham and Steenbock (1935)
Final dissimilation products	H_2O and CO_2	H_2O and CO_2	
Intermediate dissimilation product	Pyruvic acid (?)	Pyruvic acid(?)	

and fructose, the disaccharides lactose and maltose, and the trisaccharide raffinose, in a 1 per cent solution in a synthetic medium, did not support the growth of tubercle bacilli. When these carbohydrates were introduced into the medium together with 1.5 per cent glycerol, they were utilized by the tubercle bacilli.

The same has been said about dulcitol, *iso*-dulcitol, and mannitol. The statement of Proskauer and Beck that "the above mentioned disaccharides and raffinose must be regarded as good growth material for tubercle bacilli and this must be especially said of cane sugar," created a confusion which has persisted to our day.

Frouin and Guillaumie (1923a) reported that human, bovine, and avian strains in a synthetic medium containing 0.5 per cent glycerol utilized in one month of growth lactose, maltose, saccharose, and trechalose. According to Kondo (1925), methyl, ethyl, and amyl alcohols, mannitol, and carbohydrates (with the exception of glucose) were not utilized by tubercle bacilli. Tubercle bacilli of cold-blooded animals (fish, frog), as well as saprophytic smegma and timothy bacilli, utilized ethyl alcohol as a source of carbon when nitrogen was available in the medium (E. R. Long, 1921–1922).

Weinzirl and Knapton (1927) stated that the human, bovine, avian, fish strains, and saprophytic *M. phlei*, *M. smegmatis*, and *M. butyricum* produced progressive alkalinity when grown on media containing dextrose, mannitol, and lactose. Apparently the strains are unable to utilize these substances. All strains produced acidity in media containing glycerol. Merrill (1930, 1931) found that the *p*H curves of media are of little value in determining whether carbohydrates are utilized. The direct quantitative determination of carbohydrate could be of value. All fourteen strains of mycobacteria studied utilized glycerol; ten of them utilized glucose; in the case of H37 the utilization of glucose was doubtful. Fructose, galactose, arabinose, maltose, lactose, sucrose, raffinose, inulin, mannitol, ethyl alcohol, salicin, sodium lactate, and sodium citrate were not metabolized. One strain used sodium acetate.

Model (1933) found that the tubercle bacillus utilizes levulose when grown on a medium containing glycerol. Without glycerol, levulose was not metabolized. Similar results were obtained by Wedum (1936). He found that human, bovine, and BCG strains in Long's synthetic medium, in the presence of glycerol, metabolized glucose, mannose, fructose, galactose, arabinose, xylose, and maltose, but not lactose. In the experiments of Loebel *et al.* (1933a) and Nakamura (1938), of all carbohydrates and alcohols tested, only glycerol produced a significant increase in the growth and the respiration of tubercle bacilli.

From these observations some conclusions can be drawn: for one, glycerol is metabolized by all strains of mycobacteria; furthermore, glucose is the carbohydrate metabolized by most mycobacteria, but not by all. No other carbohydrates are metabolized by human and bovine strains of mycobacteria. The situation is different when carbohydrate and glycerol are simultaneously present in the media. Under these conditions many carbohydrates are metabolized by mammalian strains of mycobacteria. The reasons for this peculiar course of carbohydrate metabolism of mycobacteria have not yet been discovered (see acetate, p. 131).

Recently an account of the carbohydrates and the polyhydric alcohols utilized by human strain H37Rv was given by Youmans and Youmans (1953). They studied the utilization of 24 compounds in a synthetic medium with concentrations ranging from 0.016 to 4.0 per cent. Only three of the compounds studied, glycerol, glucose, and maltose, permitted the growth of *M. tuberculosis* var. *hominis*, strain H37Rv, regardless of the size of the inoculum (see Table 13). These findings are in concordance wtih the data of Proskauer and Beck, Kondo, and Merrill. The observations of Nocard and Roux, Kühne, Proskauer and Beck, to the effect that glucose, contrary to the opinion of Merrill (1930) and Dubos (1947) is inferior to glycerol in growth promotion, were confirmed by Youmans and Youmans. These authors expressed the suspicion that the apparent growth promotion by maltose could in reality have been brought about by the glucose present in that substance as impurity.

We still do not know a substance which can replace glycerol in media for tubercle bacilli; even human and horse sera are not capable of success-

Table 13. Assimilation by *Mycobacterium tuberculosis* (H37Rv) of Carbohydrates and Polyhydric Alcohols (Concentrations from 0.016 to 4.0%)

Compound	Metabolized	Not Metabolized
Monosaccharides		
Pentoses		
D(−) arabinose		x
L(+) arabinose		x
D(+) xylose		x
D-ribose		x
D(−) lyxose		x
L(+) rhamnose		x
Hexoses		
D(−) glucose	x	
D(+) mannose		x
D(−) galactose		x
Fructose		x
Disaccharides		
D(+) maltose (?)	x	
Lactose		x
Sucrose		x
Trisaccharides		
D(+) raffinose		x
Polysaccharides		
Inulin		x
Polyhydric alcohols		
Glycerol	x	
Trimethylene glycol		x
Propylene glycol		x
Triethylene glycol		x
L-arabitol		x
Sorbitol		x
Mannitol		x
Dulcitol		x

Source: Youmans and Youmans (1953).

fully carrying out the functions of glycerol (Bloch, Matter, and Suter, 1947).

In Dubos' liquid medium containing Tween 80, citrate, and albumin, a turbidimetric estimation revealed levulose, galactose, and arabinose as being superior to glucose in promoting the growth of *M. avium* (Ackart and Murray, 1951).

The growth of human (H37), bovine, and avian strains of tubercle bacilli is not possible in media containing amino acids DL-alanine, histidine, tryptophan, tyrosine, but no glycerol. These amino acids neither served the tubercle bacilli as sources of carbon nor of nitrogen.

Intermediate Pathway of Glycerol and Glucose Metabolism in Mycobacteria

The source of energy of the tubercle bacillus outside the living organism is glycerol or glucose. The utilization of glucose by living cells is a more completely understood process than the utilization of glycerol. The breakdown of glucose in the cells takes place with the intermediation of anaerobic glycolysis. The first step in this direction is the phosphorylation of glucose. The enzyme hexokinase in the presence of coenzyme adenosine triphosphate catalyzes this process. The ester linkage between phosphoric acid and the hydroxyl group of glucose is established through the elimination of water. The energy bound in adenosine triphosphate is the main immediate source of energy at the disposal of the cell in its synthetic work. The breakdown of glucose through phosphorylation leads to the formation of a highly reactive keto acid, pyruvic acid, which is the chief intermediate compound in further transformations. In the process of the breakdown of glucose one molecule of glucose produces two molecules of pyruvic acid and consequently results in the over-all gain of two energy-rich phosphate bonds. Each of them yields 12 kg.-cal. per gram molecule, if hydrolyzed. The formation of energy-rich phosphate is possible only when phosphoric acid is available to the cell. Warburg and Christian, Bücher, Kunitz, and others isolated and purified the enzymes involved in these reactions.

Apparently different in their essence, the processes of fermentation and respiration have common initial steps. Both of them start as phosphorylation reactions which lead, in both cases, although in different ways, to pyruvic acid.

Most of the intimate processes of the aerobic breakdown of glycerol and glucose by mycobacteria and the enzymes catalyzing these processes are only partially known and therefore it is at present impossible to give a coherent picture of the glycerol and glucose intermediate pathway in mycobacteria. The assimilation of nutrients by mycobacteria is performed with such a high efficiency that partially oxidized metabolites do not accumulate in the medium.

The tubercle bacillus cannot grow in the absence of oxygen but, notwithstanding this fact, anaerobic metabolic processes are not excluded from the intermediate metabolism of the tubercle bacillus. The search for an anaerobic phase among the metabolic processes of tubercle bacilli was the objective of many investigations. The anaerobic breakdown of glucose by human bacilli was investigated by Loebel, Shorr and Richardson (1933a). These authors followed the hypothesis that the final breakdown products of glucose by mycobacteria will be lactic acid:

$$C_6H_{12}O_6 = 2C_3H_6O_3$$

Two methods were used to determine the quantity of the expected lactic acid. The quantity of carbon dioxide produced as a consequence of the neutralization of the resulting lactic acid by sodium bicarbonate was determined by means of the Barcroft-Warburg manometric technique; and in addition, the attempt was made to perform direct chemical identification of lactic acid. Both methods yielded very low values of lactic acid production of tubercle bacilli from anaerobic glycolysis. Compared with the anaerobic glycolysis of Type 1 pneumococci, the values produced by tubercle bacilli were only six hundredths of the values obtained in pneumococci. The yield of lactic acid was not increased when glycerol, arabinose, inositol, levulose, glycerophosphate, and caseous material were added to the culture of tubercle bacilli. The energy derived by tubercle bacilli through anaerobic glycolysis was less than 0.5 per cent of that gained by them through aerobic respiration in Long's synthetic medium. Ebina and Nakamura (1937) confirmed the data of Loebel *et al.* and found that the anaerobic breakdown of glucose by mammalian and avian variants of tubercle bacilli and by saprophytic *M. phlei* and *M. smegmatis* was extremely low.

The investigations on the aerobiosis of tubercle bacilli were carried on with living, multiplying bacilli (Buc; Novy; Soule); not multiplying, washed suspensions of bacilli (Warburg); and starved suspensions of bacilli (Loebel *et al.*). The starvation of mycobacteria on a sodium chloride–phosphate solution reduces the auto-respiration of the bacilli and permits one to see the influence of an added substance on the respiration. The auto-respiration diminishes in two to six hours, although the viability of bacilli is retained up to 55 days. In all these investigations the action of integral bacterial cells on glycerol or glucose was studied. It can be expected that new light will be cast on the intermediate metabolism processes of tubercle bacilli by the study of the action of the juice of disintegrated bacilli or of the cell-free enzyme extracts of these bacilli. These methods were successfully applied to the study of the life processes of the cells of higher plants and animals. By crushing the cells with glass or sand or freezing them in liquid air and afterwards letting them thaw, attempts were made to extract the enzymes from mycobacteria. (Franke and Schillinger, 1944). In 1951, Geronimus, Faine, Whiteside and Edson found that the cell-free extracts of *M. smegmatis* and *M. phlei* take up, *in vacuo*, oxygen in the presence of hexosediphosphate and methylene blue. The oxygen consumption in the presence of methylene blue as hydrogen acceptor was probably caused by the oxidation of the phosphate. These observations revealed the possible presence, in mycobacteria, of the chief enzymes aldolase, triosephosphatase, dehydrogenase, enolase of anaerobic breakdown of carbohydrates, and suggested the possibility that in mycobacteria the assimilation of glucose and glycerol can be carried out not only by the aerobic, histohematin-governed system, but also by the Embden-Meyerhof anaerobic fermentation pathway.

Glycerol dehydrogenase was obtained from *Escherichia coli* in the active state by Asnis and Brodie (1953). The cell-free extract of *Escherichia coli* was heated to destroy any other oxidative enzymes present in the solution. The heat-stable dehydrogenase was purified by precipitation with ammonium sulfate. Oxidation of glycerol was specifically DPN-linked, and resulted in the production of dihydroxyacetone in 1:1 M ratio with the DPN^+ reduced.

It is not necessary to assume that the anaerobic breakdown of glycerol has a different pathway than the fermentation of glucose. The fermentation of glucose as well as of glycerol can yield energy-rich phosphate bonds:

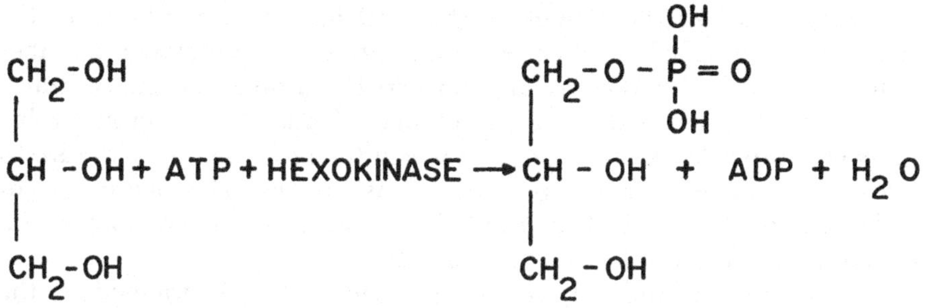

GLYCEROL ADENOSINE TRIPHOSPHATE α-GLYCEROPHOSPHATE ADENOSINE DIPHOSPHATE

The formed glycerophosphate liberates three kg.-cal. per gram molecule of energy, if hydrolyzed. In principle, there probably are no differences in the first steps of the breakdown of glucose and glycerol in mycobacteria. The differences between the assimilation of glucose and glycerol by tubercle bacilli seem to be quantitative rather than qualitative in nature. The surface of tubercle bacilli is water-repellent and the uptake of glucose solutions by tubercle bacilli largely depends on the concentration of this substance or on the osmotic pressure in the medium (Loebel *et al.*, Schaefer). Glycerol is capable of wetting the surface of tubercle bacilli and of penetrating into the fatty surface of mycobacteria.

A direct proof that glycerol is phosphorylated by mycobacteria is lacking, but the presence of enzymes of Embden-Meyerhof scheme (aldolase, enolase, dehydrogenase) in acid-fast bacilli indicates this possibility. An attempt was made to capture the quickly vanishing glucose and glycerol intermediate metabolism members of mycobacteria with the aid of poisons inhibiting the activities of intervening enzymes. The respiration of mycobacteria is cyanide-sensitive; addition of 0.001 *M* of cyanide to the bacilli abolishes their respiration; arsenite added to mycobacteria abolishes the oxidation of ketonic bodies (pyruvate, oxalacetate) and that of fatty acids; iodacetate inhibits the oxidation of fatty acids, glucose, and glycerol. The cell suspension of *M. phlei* and *M. smegmatis* vigorously oxidizes the added pyruvic acid and acetate. The addition of arsenite to the suspension of mycobacteria abolishes the oxidation of pyruvic acid and only slightly depresses the respiration of the bacilli. This leads to the accumulation of pyruvic acid in the medium (Edson and Hunter, 1943; Lindsay, O'Donnell, and Edson, 1950). The acetone-treated *M. phlei*, in the presence of lactate, vigorously consumes oxygen, but does not oxidize pyruvate to acetate. Under anaerobic conditions and with methylene blue as hydrogen acceptor the acetone powder of *M. phlei* catalyzes the dehydrogenation of lactate to pyruvate, indicating that pyruvate is an intermediate product in the anaerobic assimilation of lactate (Edson, 1947).

Pyruvic acid, $CH_3COCOOH$, is the most important substance of the intermediate metabolism of carbohydrates, fats, and proteins. Like other ketoacids, it is highly reactive and participates in diverse chemical transformations. Pyruvic acid is the end product of a long chain of anaerobic glycolytic processes and the point at which the processes enter the Krebs cycle of aerobic or oxidative pathway of assimilation. This phase of alcoholic fermentation is well understood, a great many of the enzymes involved having been isolated. (See Stotz, 1945.)

The fate of anaerobically formed pyruvic acid is determined by the existing circumstances. Under aerobic conditions pyruvate is easily oxidized to acetic acid:

$$\underset{\text{PYRUVIC ACID}}{CH_3COCOOH} + \tfrac{1}{2}O_2 = \underset{\text{ACETIC ACID}}{CH_3COOH} + CO_2$$

The acetone powder of *M. phlei* contains an enzyme which catalyzed the reaction (Edson and Hunter, 1947):

$$\underset{\text{LACTIC ACID}}{CH_3CH(OH)COOH} + O_2 = \underset{\text{ACETIC ACID}}{CH_3COOH} + CO_2 + H_2O$$

The fate of the acetate formed in an organism was investigated by Wieland and Rosenthal in 1943. They demonstrated that the aerobic formation of citric acid takes place with the intermediation of the condensation of oxalacetate and acetate in kidney tissue. These observations were confirmed by Stern and Ochoa (1949) on the basis of their experiments with the cell-free filtrates of the tissue. The formed acetate is oxidized in the reactions of the Krebs cycle. The existence of some similar steps of pyruvic acid metabolism in mycobacteria was revealed by the investigations of Lindsay, O'Donnell, and Edson (1950). Under undisturbed conditions pyruvate is oxidized to acetate by *M. ranae*. The breakdown of the formed acetate is stopped if iodacetate is added to the suspension of mycobacteria, and the trapped acetate accumulates in the medium.

Some enzymes of the Krebs cycle were discovered in mycobacteria which, in stepwise reactions, lead to the formation of α-ketoglutarate: aconitase, isocitric dehydrogenase, oxalsuccinic carboxylate, α-ketoglutaric dehydrogenase, malic dehydrogenase, fumarase, and succinic dehydrogenase. These enzymes are not purified. (See Edson, 1951.)

The phosphorylation reactions of glucose, fructose, and glycerol, as well as some other enzyme reactions, take place in the presence of magnesium ions. In the absence of magnesium the oxidative phosphorylation in mammal and insect mitochondria was reduced, although respiration was not influenced (Sacktor, 1954).

Besides phosphorylation, another way of carbohydrate assimilation is at work in mycobacteria. Glucose disappears from the solution when shaken in a Kahn shaker (275 strokes per minute) in the presence of air or oxygen and living mycobacteria. Glucose solution containing 1 mg. of glucose per ml. loses approximately half of its glucose content when shaken for 3 hours with 30 mg. *M. phlei* (wet weight). This is the result of the oxidation of glucose on the surface of mycobacteria, which acts as a living catalyst. This reaction occurs in the absence of inorganic phosphorus and it does not produce fructose compounds, indicating the absence of phosphorylation (our unpublished data).

Organic Acids

The possibility that organic acids may be growth stimulants and sources of carbon to tubercle bacilli has been investigated many times. Only in a few instances is there full agreement about the role of these acids in the growth of tubercle bacilli. Proskauer and Beck (1894) stated that magnesium citrate considerably stimulates the growth of tubercle bacilli. This observation was supported by many later investigators and it is easy to verify its correctness.

Tubercle bacilli of cold blooded animals (fish, frog) as well as saprophytic smegma and timothy bacilli utilized propionate and pyruvate as sources of carbon when nitrogen was available in the medium (E. R. Long, 1921–1922). Kondo (1925) found that four human and two bovine strains, in two months of growth, did not utilize the salts of formic, propionic, butyric, lactic, succinic, malic, tartaric, and citric acids, added to a synthetic medium in a 0.5 per cent concentration.

Bance (1942) reported that tubercle bacilli grown on Sauton's medium containing 2 g. of citric acid per liter did not use more than 1 g. of the acid. Although the amount of citric acid consumed was small, the presence of the acid in the medium was indispensable to the growth of bacilli. The flasks of Sauton's medium without citric acid, inoculated with BCG strain of tubercle bacilli, did not produce a pellicle, whereas the medium containing citric acid produced it regularly. Edson and Hunter (1943) indicated that citric acid effectively reduces the lag phase and promotes the growth of small inocula of *M. phlei.* Citric acid is not oxidized by *M. phlei* but is utilized during the growth by tubercle bacilli, and finally disappears from the medium (Friedemann and Seibert, 1939).

Since the publication of the study of Proskauer and Beck (1894), citrates have become an inseparable part of synthetic media (Sauton, 1912; Long and Seibert, 1926; Kirchner, 1932; and others). Confusion arose when some investigators started to regard citrates not as a growth-stimulating agent of mycobacteria, but as a source of carbon. This conception of the role of citrates in synthetic media was criticized by many investigators (Finlayson, 1946; Schaefer, 1948). Model (1929) advanced a different explanation of the role of citrates in the media. According to him, the salts of magnesium, added to a broth containing ammonia and phosphates, produce an ammonium-phosphate-magnesium compound insoluble in water, which precipitates out of the solution. The added citrate dissolves the salts of magnesium and calcium, and leaves the magnesium phosphate in the solution where it is available to mycobacteria.

The identification of citric acid as a member of the Krebs cycle, however, threw different light on the role of citric acid as a metabolite of mycobacteria. The breakdown of fatty acids in an animal organism starts with the oxidation of β-carbon (called β-oxidation by Knoop in 1904) and the formation of C_2-acetic acid units ("active acetate"). In the continuation of the process the acetic acid reacts with oxalacetic acid to form citric acid. (See reviews by Breusch, 1948; Green, 1949). With the increase in length of the carbon chain of fatty acids their tendency to form acetoacetate in a homogenate of rat liver diminishes. Saturated fatty acids from C_{14} to C_{17} and unsaturated oleic, línoleic, and linolenic acids are oxidized to CO_2 (Kennedy and Lehninger, 1949).

Gözsy and Szent-Györgyi (1934) pointed out that the respiration of ground pigeon breast muscle tissue is highly stimulated if succinate or formate is added to it. The action of these substances must be catalytic, as they are not utilized in the reaction. The investigations of Szent-Györgyi and co-workers in 1937 showed that the chief intermediary agents of pigeon breast muscle tissue respiration are the dicarboxylic (succinic, fumaric, oxalacetic, malic) acids. Between these acids oxidation-reduction reactions take place. These reactions are thermodynamically possible.

Krebs and Johnson (1937) discovered that the respiration of ground pigeon breast muscle begins to fall off after 20 to 40 minutes of high activity. If citrate is added to the mash, the falling off is prevented or delayed. The extra oxygen uptake of ground tissue is far greater than can be accounted for by the oxidation of citrate. The stimulation of respiration by citrate is higher if carbohydrates, glycogen, hexosediphosphate, and α-glycerophosphate are added. This suggests that the citrates catalyze the oxidation of carbohydrates. Citric acid is metabolized in the organism (Östling, 1931), and the breakdown of it has anaerobic and oxidative pathways. Under aerobic conditions citric acid was a poor substitute for carbon dioxide, but in the absence of oxygen it was a good substitute in the culture of *Aerobacter aerogenes.* (Ajl and Werkman, 1949). Citric acid in an animal organism is completely consumed and metabolized as a simple sugar (Thunberg, 1953). The physiologic breakdown of citric acid and the connection between its dissimilation and the course of oxidation of carbohydrates was indicated by Martius and Knoop (1937). Citric acid, regarded as a substituted malic acid, through aconitic and isocitric acids, leads to α-ketoglutaric acid. The latter is metabolized to pyruvic acid through the intermediation of succinic and oxalacetic acids. Thus citric acid enters the pathway of carbohydrate metabolism.

Sources of Carbon

Acetic acid is not metabolized by tubercle bacilli when supplied as the sole source of carbon (Long, 1921–1922) but it is utilized when other sources of carbon are present in the medium. According to Kondo (1925), tubercle bacilli do not metabolize any salts of organic acids except for acetates. Although sodium lactate (Loebel *et al.*, 1933a) and acetate (Bernheim, 1941) stimulate for a short period the respiration of tubercle bacilli even more than glycerol, their inadequacy to support the growth of tubercle bacilli was established by Long (1921–1922) and Kondo (1925). The strain of tubercle bacilli studied by Bloch, Matter, and Suter (1947) did not grow on acetate, although this substance highly stimulated the respiration of bacilli.

Similar to the above observation of Long are those of Schaefer (1948). In a Dubos' medium containing Tween 80 and albumin Fraction V the pathogenic human tubercle bacilli developed well when sodium lactate and sodium acetate in a 0.1 per cent concentration were the source of carbon. These compounds were not utilized as sources of carbon in media without Tween 80 and albumin. Sodium acetate containing isotopic carbon in the methyl group ($C^{13}H_3COONa$) and in the carboxyl ($CH_3C^{13}OONa$) were prepared by Long, Anderson, Rittenberg, Karnovsky, and Henderson (1955) and incorporated into Long's synthetic medium. During the growth of the cultures carbon dioxide was produced from both labeled radicals, more from $-C^{13}OONa$ than from $C^{13}H_3-$. C^{13} was found in the bodies and lipids of the tubercle bacilli, in the soluble proteins of tuberculin and in polysaccharides. The experiments confirmed the earlier findings that acetic acid in the presence of another source of carbon can serve as a building material for the fats, proteins, and carbohydrates of tubercle bacilli.

Dubos (1950b) presented data indicating that some organic acids in a relatively low concentration *in vitro* may exert a bacteriostatic and even a bactericidal action on tubercle bacilli and suggested that diminished oxygen tension favorably influences this action by acids. Dubos found that particularly active in this respect is lactic acid, for in a 0.01 *M* concentration it destroyed tubercle bacilli within two days. Other aliphatic acids—acetic, propionic, and butyric—had a similar but weaker action. The hypothesis was advanced that conditions equivalent to the above (low concentration of organic acids and diminished oxygen tension) may be at work in the infected body and may play some role in tuberculous infection and resistance to tuberculosis. The views of Dubos were shared by J. Hirsch (1952) who indicated that caseous areas become acidic in relation to the surrounding tissue. The retention of carbon dioxide and the accumulation of organic acids in the infected areas favor the destruction of tubercle bacilli. These acids are mostly unsaturated (Čmelik, 1952).

The influence of acids, alcohols, aldehydes, chemotherapeutics, antibiotics, and stimulants on the growth and respiration of *M. tuberculosis* or other mycobacteria (when stated), according to the findings of different authors, is shown in Table 14.

Hydrocarbons and Related Substances

The work of Söhngen (1913) is generally accepted as a decisive proof of the utilization of hydrocarbons of the general formula C_nH_{2n+2} (gasoline, kerosene, paraffin oil, hard paraffin) as a source of carbon by microorganisms. As the medium for the cultivation of these microorganisms, Söhngen used a solution of mineral substances. To this liquid about 1 per cent of hydrocarbons was added. Hard paraffin was melted and added in the form of drops. The flasks were inoculated with soil particles from a garden and incubated at 20, 28, and 37°C. To separate the microorganisms growing in the liquid, the cultivation was carried out on a solid agar medium in Petri dishes. As a source of carbon, kerosene was added in a small dish, on filter paper, or on the lid of the Petri dish. This procedure allowed the separation, in a pure culture, the saprophytic mycobacteria utilizing hydrocarbons as a source of carbon (*M. phlei, M. mölleri, M. album, M. hyalinum*, and others) from the other microorganisms.

The work of Söhngen was verified by Büttner (1926), who studied especially the utilization of hydrocarbons by *M. phlei, M. lacticola, M. friburgense*, and others, when pure paraffin was the source of carbon. After 5 days of incubation at 37°C., growth started.

Haag (1926) indicated that the utilization of hydrocarbons by mycobacteria depends on the double bonds in the compounds. The double bonds are indicated by the iodine number. The higher the number, the more rapid the growth of mycobacteria. In hydrocarbons with high melting point the iodine number is low, the growth of mycobacteria is slow.

Zobell (1946), in a review of this problem, indicated that about a hundred different species of microorganisms, and about ten species of mycobacteria among them, are capable of decomposing hydrocarbons. These species are widely distributed in the soil, particularly in such as has been soaked with oil, in marine sediments, and on plants. The criteria for the estimation of the utilization of hydrocarbons by microorganisms are (a) the disappearance of hydrocarbon from the medium, (b) the production of carbon dioxide, (c) the formation of acid, (d) the multiplication of microorganisms, and (e) the consumption of oxygen. The presence of oxygen is necessary to these microorganisms. Carbon dioxide, organic acids, and unsaturated compounds are products of the decomposition of hydrocarbons by microorganisms.

The possible utilization of hydrocarbons as a source of carbon by pathogenic mycobacteria was investigated by Morellini and by Saz. Morellini (1937) affirmed that the growth of a human variant of tubercle bacilli is

Table 14. Influence of Organic Acids, Alcohols, Aldehydes, Chemotherapeutics, Antibiotics, and Stimulants on the Growth and Respiration of *Mycobacterium tuberculosis* and Other Mycobacteria

Compound	Growth	Respiration	Author
	Organic Acids (Sodium Salts)		
Acetic	Absent		E. R. Long (1921–1922)
	Absent (*M. phlei*)		Stephenson and Whetham (1922)
	Stimulated		Braun and Kondo (1924, 1925)
	Doubtful		Model (1929)
	Doubtful		Merrill (1931)
	Inhibition (0.05 *M*)		Wakabayashi (1933)
		Stimulated	Bernheim (1941)
		Doubtful (*M. phlei*)	Edson and Hunter (1943)
	Stimulated		Schaefer *et al.* (1949)
Benzoic. *See* Salicylic			
Benzoic, *p*-amino	Stimulated		Woods and Fildes (1940, 1941)
	Stimulated	Absent	Zetterberg (1949)
	Inhibition (0.004 *M*)		Dubos (1950b)
	Stimulated (1 mg/ml)	Stimulated (1 mg/ml)	Bernheim *et al.* (1953)
Butyric	Absent		Braun and Kondo (1924, 1925)
	Inhibition (0.5 *M*)		Wakabayashi (1933)
		Stimulated	Bernheim (1941)
	Inhibition (0.0015 *M*)		Dubos (1950b)
N-capric	Absent		Cutinelli (1941)
	Inhibition (0.0001 *M*)		Dubos (1950b)
	Stimulated		Youmans and Youmans (1954)
N-caprylic	Inhibition (0.01 *M*)		Wakabayashi (1933)
	Inhibition (0.0003 *M*)		Dubos (1950b)
	Inhibition (1 mg/ml)	Stimulated	Bernheim *et al.* (1953)
	Stimulated		Youmans and Youmans (1954)
Chaulmoogric	Inhibition		Darzins (1938)
		Inhibition (*M. lacticola*)	Franke and Schillinger (1941)
	Inhibition		Dubois (1944a)
Citric	Stimulated		Proskauer and Beck (1894)
	Absent		Braun and Kondo (1924, 1925)
	Absent		Merrill (1931)
		Absent	Nakamura (1938)
	Stimulated (*M. phlei*)	Absent (*M. phlei*)	Edson and Hunter (1943)

Table 14—*continued*

Compound	Growth	Respiration	Author
	Absent (egg white medium)		Finlayson (1946)
	Absent		Schaefer (1948)
Fumaric	Absent (*M. phlei*)		Edson and Hunter (1943)
	No inhibition (0.05 *M*)		Dubos (1950b)
Formic	Inhibition (0.02 *M*)		Wakabayashi (1933)
		Absent	Nakamura (1938)
		Doubtful	Bernheim (1941)
α-ketoglutaric	Absent (*M. phlei*)		Edson and Hunter (1943)
	No inhibition (0.05 *M*)		Dubos (1950b)
Lactic	Absent		E. R. Long (1921–1922)
	Stimulated (*M. phlei*)		Stephenson and Whetham (1922)
	Doubtful		Braun and Kondo (1924, 1925)
		Stimulated	Loebel *et al.* (1933a)
		Stimulated (*M. phlei*)	Edson and Hunter (1943)
	Absent (egg white medium)		Finlayson (1946)
	Stimulated (Dubos' medium)		Schaefer (1948)
	Inhibition (0.008 *M*)		Dubos (1950b)
Lauric	Inhibition (0.0002 *M*)		Dubos (1950b)
Linoleic	Inhibition		Boissevain (1926)
		Stopped at 1:15,000	Bergström *et al.* (1946)
Linolenic	Inhibition		Boissevain (1926)
		Stopped at 1:30,000	Bergström *et al.* (1946)
Malic	Absent		Braun and Kondo (1924, 1925)
		Absent	Nakamura (1938)
	Absent (*M. phlei*)		Edson and Hunter (1943)
Malonic	Doubtful (1 mg/ml)	Doubtful (1 mg/ml)	Bernheim *et al.* (1953)
Oleic	Stimulated (acne bacillus)		Fleming (1909)
	Inhibition	Inhibition	Boissevain (1926)
	Inhibition (0.001 *M*)		Wakabayashi (1933)
		Decrease 30%	Loebel *et al.* (1933b)
	Inhibition	Inhibition	Cutinelli (1941)
		Inhibition	Bloch (1944)
		Inhibition (*M. lacticola*)	Franke and Schillinger (1944)

Table 14—*continued*

Compound	Growth	Respiration	Author
		Stopped at 1:10,000	Bergström *et al.* (1946)
	Inhibition (0.001 *M*)	Inhibition at 250 μg/ml; stimulation at 100 μg/ml	Gray (1949)
	Inhibition (0.001 *M*)		Dubos *et al.* (1945, 1947, 1950)
	Required by dysgonic strains		Schaefer (1952)
	Inhibition (1 mg/ml)	Inhibition (1 mg/ml)	Bernheim *et al.* (1953)
Oxalic	Inhibition (1 mg/ml)	Inhibition (1 mg/ml)	Bernheim *et al.* (1953)
	Inhibition (0.05 *M*)		Wakabayashi (1933)
Palmitic	Absent		Cutinelli (1941)
	Required by dysgonic strains		Schaefer (1952)
	Inhibition (0.0005 *M*)		Dubos (1950b)
Propionic	Absent		E. R. Long (1921–1922)
	Absent		Braun and Kondo (1924)
	Inhibition (0.5 *M*)		Wakabayashi (1933)
	Inhibition (0.003 *M*)		Dubos (1950b)
	Doubtful (1 mg/ml)	Stimulated (1 mg/ml)	Bernheim *et al.* (1953)
Pyruvic	Absent		E. R. Long (1921–1922)
	Absent		Cutinelli (1941)
		Doubtful (*M. phlei*)	Edson and Hunter (1943)
	Doubtful (Dubos' medium)		Schaefer (1948)
	Stimulated (1 mg/ml)	Stimulated (1 mg/ml)	Bernheim *et al.* (1953)
		Stimulated	Braun (1955)
Salicylic, benzoic		Stimulated	Bernheim (1940, 1941)
		Stimulated (in pathogenic strains)	Lehmann (1946a)
		Stimulated (1 mg/ml)	Bernheim (1948)
	Absent	Stimulated	Andrejew (1951)
	Absent (*M phlei*)	Absent (glucose oxidation) (*M. phlei*)	Darzins (1956)

Table 14—*continued*

Compound	Growth	Respiration	Author
Stearic	Absent		Boissevain (1926)
	Inhibition (0.05 *M*)		Wakabayashi (1933)
	Absent	Stimulated	Cutinelli (1941)
		Stimulated (*M. lacticola*)	Franke and Schillinger (1944)
		Required by dysgonic strains	Schaefer (1952)
	Inhibition (0.0008 *M*)		Dubos (1950b)
Succinic	Absent		E. R. Long (1921–1922)
	Absent		Braun and Kondo (1924, 1925)
		Absent	Nakamura (1938)
	Absent		Cutinelli (1941)
		Doubtful (*M. phlei*)	Edson and Hunter (1943)
	Doubtful (Dubos' medium)		Schaefer (1948)
	No inhibition (0.05 *M*)		Dubos (1950b)
	Stimulated (1 mg/ml)	Stimulated (1 mg/ml)	Bernheim *et al.* (1953)
Tartaric	Absent		Braun and Kondo (1925)
		Absent	Nakamura (1938)
Valeric	Inhibition (0.1 *M*)	Absent	Wakabayashi (1933)
		Absent	Nakamura (1938)
		Stimulated	Bernheim (1941)
		Alcohols	
Ethyl	Stimulated (bacilli of cold-blooded animals)		E. R. Long (1921–1922)
	Absent		Braun and Kondo (1924, 1925)
	Absent		Merrill (1931)
		Absent	Nakamura (1938)
		Absent	Bernheim (1941)
	Absent (egg white medium)		Finlayson (1946)
Methyl	Stimulated (bacilli of cold-blooded animals)		E. R. Long (1921–1922)
	Absent		Braun and Kondo (1924, 1925)
Propyl		Stimulated	Bernheim (1941)
Butyl and *iso*		Stimulated	Bernheim (1941)
Amyl and *iso*	Absent		Braun and Kondo (1924, 1925)
		Stimulated	Bernheim (1941)

Table 14—*continued*

Compound	Growth	Respiration	Author
		Aldehydes	
Heptaldehyde		Stimulated	Bernheim (1941)
Isovaleraldehyde		Stimulated	Bernheim (1941)
Anisaldehyde		Stimulated	Bernheim (1941)
Benzaldehyde		Stimulated	Bernheim (1941)
Furfural		Stimulated	Bernheim (1941)
Citral		Stimulated	Bernheim (1941)
	Chemotherapeutics and Antibiotics		
PAS (*p*-aminosalicylic acid)	Inhibition	Absent	Lehmann (1946a)
	Inhibition (0.019–0.156 mg. per 100 ml.)		Youmans (1946b)
	Inhibition (1 μg/ml)		Vennesland *et al.* (1948)
		Absent	Andrejew (1951)
	Inhibition (0.5 mg/ml)	Stimulated (0.5 mg/ml)	Bernheim *et al.* (1948, 1953)
Sulfonamides	Inhibition		Feldman *et al.* (1940)
	Inhibition		Jensen and Kiaer (1943)
	Absent	Absent	Zetterberg (1949)
Streptomycin	Inhibition *in vitro*		Schatz and Waksman (1944)
	Inhibition *in vivo*, healing effect		Feldman and Hinshaw (1944)
	Inhibition (less than 1 μg/ml)		Youmans and Feldman (1946)
	Inhibition (0.74 μg/ml)		Vennesland *et al.* (1948)
		Absent	Zetterberg (1949)
		Doubtful	Oginsky *et al.* (1950)
		Stimulated	Bernheim (1951)
	Inhibition	Absent	Suter (1952a)
	Synthetic medium *p*H 7.2: stimulation (0.3 μg/ml); inhibition (1.0 μg/ml)		Model and Stcheglova (1955)
	Synthetic medium *p*H 6.2: no action		Model and Stcheglova (1955)
Isonicotinic acid hydrazide	Inhibition (1.6–3.1 μg/ml)		Steenken and Wolinsky (1952)
	Inhibition (0.05 μg/ml)		Suter (1952a)
	No action		Noufflard and Deslandes (1952)
	Bacilli killed (10 μg/ml)		Braunsteiner *et al.* (1953)

"normal" in media containing volatile hydrocarbons as a source of carbon, as well as in liquid media with added kerosene. In the absence of these substances growth did not occur. Saz (1949) investigated pathogenic H37Rv, BCG, and other strains of mycobacteria for their capability of utilizing hydrocarbons. Tubercle bacilli were suspended in a buffer solution and inoculated into Dubos' basal medium without albumin; NH_4NO_3 or $(NH_4)_2SO_4$, as a source of nitrogen, and hydrocarbon, as a source of carbon, were added to the medium. The respiration of the cultures was tested according to the Barcroft-Warburg technique, and changes in the optical density of the cultures were used as a basis for the estimation of the growth. When hydrocarbons of chain length greater than 8 carbon atoms were added to the culture, tubercle bacilli accumulated in the water-hydrocarbon interface. (This phenomenon was known to Courtade and Arnaude and to L. Lange and Nitsche (1909) who utilized it to concentrate tubercle bacilli in sputum-ether or in ligroin interface.) Hydrocarbons of 14, 16, or 18 carbon atoms, saturated or unsaturated, greatly increased the respiration of pathogenic tubercle bacilli. Ligroin, *n*-heptane, and petroleum ether had no effect at all or decreased the oxygen consumption. After four weeks of incubation the growth of mycobacteria with hydrocarbons in the medium stopped, even when asparagine was added as a source of nitrogen. The acidic end products which would result if hydrocarbons were metabolized were sought in vain.

The claims of Braun, Stamatelakis, and Kondo (1924) that the "impurities" of the incubator air may serve as a carbon and nitrogen source to mycobacteria have not been confirmed. Haag (1927) repeated the experiments of these authors with pure chemicals and did not obtain any growth.

Masur (1926) affirmed that tubercle bacilli derive their energy from the oxidation of ammonia and are capable of living on media without a soluble source of carbon. Tubercle bacilli are not known to possess the properties of chemo-autotrophic organisms.

It is necessary to verify once more the data of Söhngen and the data of later investigators of this field. The increased oxygen consumption of mycobacteria in the presence of hydrocarbons does not necessarily indicate the assimilation of hydrocarbons (see p. 112).

The latest survey of petroleum microbiology was made by Beerstecher (1954).

Carbon Dioxide

The first period of discovery. Data on the significance of carbon dioxide in the life of heterotrophic organisms accumulated slowly. Pasteur and Joubert (1877) published the observation that *Bacillus anthracis* is killed in an atmosphere of carbon dioxide. Liborius (1886) found carbon dioxide noxious to aerobic and anaerobic microorganisms; the production of pigments by bacteria ceased in the atmosphere of carbon dioxide. Fränkel (1889) observed that most saprophytic bacteria do not grow in carbon dioxide but some pathogenic species are able to support a high concentration of this substance. The discovery of the destructive action of carbon dioxide on bacteria stimulated attempts to apply carbon dioxide to the conservation or sterilization of foodstuffs and water, and this gas was even advocated as a cure for pulmonary tuberculosis (Weber, 1889).

The second period. The next phase in the history of the investigation of the role of carbon dioxide in heterotrophs began with the observation of Nowak (1908) that the growth of *Brucella abortus,* inoculated in agar, was best not on the surface but about 15 mm. below it, where the oxygen tension is less. Nowak utilized the microaerophily of *B. abortus* to facilitate the cultivation of this microorganism from infected organs. To reduce the partial oxygen tension in the cultures, the plates, seeded with *B. abortus* material, were simultaneously inoculated with the strongly aerobic *Bacillus subtilis.* Nowak took for granted that the stimulation of growth of *B. abortus* in these cultures was due to the diminished oxygen tension produced by the growing *Bacillus subtilis.*

Wherry and Oliver (1916) used this technique to facilitate the cultivation of gonococci. In their attempt to cultivate meningococci, Cohen and Fleming (1918) modified the technique of Nowak. In order to diminish the partial pressure of oxygen, they introduced carbon dioxide into the cultures and observed that the addition of 10 per cent of carbon dioxide to the atmosphere greatly facilitated the growth of microorganisms. The favorable influence of carbon dioxide on the growth of gonococci was confirmed by Herrold in 1920; Th. Smith, in 1924, observed the favorable effect of carbon dioxide on the growth of cultures of *B. abortus.*

The third period. The third phase of the investigation of the carbon dioxide problem began in 1918, when Wherry and Ervin indicated that carbon dioxide itself is the cause of the growth stimulation of tubercle bacilli. The growth of cultures stopped when carbon dioxide was absorbed from the atmosphere by barium hydroxide, although the bacilli remained viable. This discovery shed new light on the stimulation of the growth of *B. abortus,* gonococci, and meningococci by growing *Bacillus subtilis.* The carbon dioxide eliminated by *Bacillus subtilis,* not the reduced tension of oxygen, stimulated the growth of these microorganisms. Corper, Gauss, and Rensch (1921) found that a concentration of approximately 5.5 per cent of carbon dioxide in the atmosphere inhibits the growth of tubercle bacilli, that a concentration of 15 per cent is bactericidal, but that the tubercle bacillus will not grow in the total absence of carbon dioxide. A concentration of 5.5 per cent of carbon dioxide is present normally in the human body and, in the opinion of the authors, is a significant factor in the resistance of the organism to tuberculosis.

Sources of Energy, Growth of Bacillus

According to the investigations of Webb, Boissevain, and Ryder (1924), the growth of tubercle bacilli is fair or vigorous on glycerol broth when the carbon dioxide has been absorbed by a 40 per cent solution of potassium hydroxide, but no growth results under the same conditions on glycerol agar (6 per cent glycerol). In their thorough work on the respiration of tubercle bacilli, Novy and Soule (1925) showed that the tubercle bacillus is capable of growing in high concentrations of carbon dioxide. A concentration of 10 per cent has no inhibiting action on growth. The bacillus can grow in concentrations of carbon dioxide ranging up to 60 per cent, and growth is still possible, though slow, at a concentration of 80 and 90 per cent of carbon dioxide in the atmosphere. The authors concluded from their various experiments with carbon dioxide, that the chief factor interfering with the growth of tubercle bacilli on agar media in the experiments of previous investigators was the alkali used to absorb carbon dioxide which had a dehydrating action on the media.

The conclusions of Novy and Soule were opposed by Rockwell and Highberger (1926). These investigators pointed out that virulent strains of tubercle bacilli and saprophytic mycobacteria (*stercoris*, grass bacilli) are inhibited in their growth when incubated over alkali in closed spaces, but that this inhibition is not caused by the dehydration of media. More efficient dehydrating agents, such as sulfuric acid and calcium chloride, do not prevent the growth of bacilli. The only possible explanation for the absence of growth of mycobacteria on plates exposed to alkali is that carbon dioxide, a factor vital to growth, was lacking. In their further work (1927), these authors recognized that carbon dioxide is necessary for the growth of *Salmonella typhosa*, *Staphylococcus*, *Mucor*, and other microorganisms. They expressed the opinion that microorganisms utilize carbon dioxide as the source of carbon. The fixation of carbon dioxide by the cultures of tubercle bacillus was affirmed by Masur (1926). Rippel and Bortels (1927) indicated indispensability of this substance to the growth of *Aspergillus niger*.

Valley and Rettger (1927) reexamined the carbon dioxide fixation problem in microorganisms of widely different genera. They found that all microorganisms need carbon dioxide for growth. The growth of two strains of tubercle bacilli of human type on glycerol agar and on Lubenau's medium, kept free from carbon dioxide, was scanty or nil. To avoid the error due to the dessication of cultures, Gladstone, Fildes, and Richardson (1935) cultivated a large number of aerobic and anaerobic microorganisms (*Salmonella typhosa, Escherichia coli, Bacillus subtilis*, etc.) in a liquid medium. The growth of cultures through which carbon dioxide–free air was passing was compared with the growth of control cultures gassed with air containing 10 per cent carbon dioxide. The passage of carbon dioxide–free air through the cultures completely inhibited their growth. Carbon dioxide was recognized as a factor essential to the growth of microorganisms. The necessity of carbon dioxide for the growth of tubercle bacilli was confirmed by Schwabacher (1937).

The Japanese investigators Ebina, Nakamura, and Inomata (1938) cultivated pellicles of tubercle bacilli on the liquid medium of Lockemann, in a mixture of gases of different composition. The mixtures of gases were renewed every second and third day, the concentration of oxygen was maintained at 21 per cent, and the *p*H remained constant. The influence of the gases on the growth was estimated by weighing the bacillary mass produced. These workers found that the optimal concentration of carbon dioxide for tubercle bacilli of human and bovine variants is 5 per cent, for the avian type, from 0 to 10 per cent. Carbon dioxide in a small dose stimulated the growth of tubercle bacilli but it was not indispensable.

R. Davies (1940) in reviewing the work done before 1935, said that it was not conclusive as to the role of carbon dioxide in the biology of the tubercle bacillus, because solid media were used, control experiments

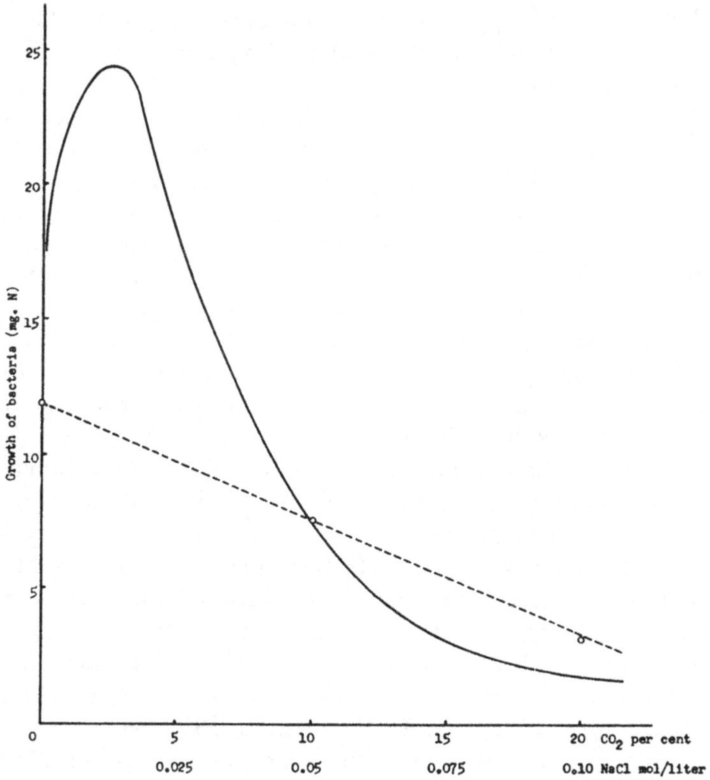

Figure 23. Effect of carbon dioxide and sodium chloride on the growth of tubercle bacilli. Solid line: carbon dioxide. Broken line: sodium chloride. (Davies, 1940.)

were insufficient, and control of the *p*H of the media during growth was not carried out. The first attempts to control these variable factors so as to obtain a precise answer about the effect of carbon dioxide on the growth of tubercle bacilli were made by Ebina, Nakamura, and Inomata (1938), in whose experiments the concentration of oxygen was maintained constant, a liquid medium used, and the *p*H of the medium controlled. Davies studied the influence of 2.5, 5.0, 10.0, and 20.0 per cent of carbon dioxide in the atmosphere on the growth of tubercle bacilli. A medium containing 0.0125 *M* $NaHCO_3$ and 2.5 per cent carbon dioxide gave the optimum growth of strain H37Rv. To exclude a simple salt effect, parallel experiments with sodium chloride were run. The experiments of Davies confirmed the fact that carbon dioxide at a concentration of 2.5 per cent or below has a specific stimulating action on the growth of tubercle bacilli, but inhibits their growth when above this concentration. Analyzing the data of Ebina, Nakamura, and Inomata on the action of carbon dioxide on tubercle bacilli, Davies indicated that, if the growth values found by these experimenters are plotted against the concentration of carbon dioxide, the curve shows that the optimum of carbon dioxide concentration for the growth of human tubercle bacillus is about 2.5 per cent, but not 5 per cent, as stated by the Japanese authors.

Other facts about the role of carbon dioxide in biologic processes have been discovered. In the pathogenic strains of *Bacillus anthracis,* when grown in an atmosphere containing 25 per cent carbon dioxide, the formation of capsules was highly stimulated, although the virulence of bacilli remained unchanged. In nonpathogenic strains carbon dioxide neither provoked the formation of capsules nor the development of pathogenicity (Ivánovics, 1937). Hes (1938) showed that heterotrophic microorganisms do not reduce methylene blue to leucobase in the complete absence of carbon dioxide. For the cell-free maceration extract of yeast cells, the reduction of methylene blue in the absence of carbon dioxide was also suppressed.

The fourth period. The demonstration by H. G. Wood and Werkman (1935, 1936) that carbon dioxide is utilized as a metabolite by heterotrophic propionic acid bacteria marked the beginning of the fourth period. When fermenting glycerol in the atmosphere of carbon dioxide, they fix more carbon dioxide than they produce. In this breakdown of glycerol the succinic acid is formed in quantities approximately equimolar to the amount of carbon dioxide utilized. Little or no succinic acid is formed in the absence of carbon dioxide. This suggests that succinic acid is produced in the carbon dioxide fixation reaction. In this fixation reaction the presence of Mg^{++} is required (Wood and Werkman, 1938). The fermentation of mannitol, adonitol, and glycerol in the atmosphere of carbon dioxide was accompanied by a considerable uptake of carbon dioxide, whereas the fermentation of glucose, arabinose, galactose, xylose entailed but a small uptake of carbon dioxide. Azide, arsenite, and cyanide had no influence on the carbon dioxide fixation. Sodium fluoride and iodacetate inhibited it (Wood and Werkman, 1940).

Redtenbacher, in 1846, and van Niel, in 1928, observed that in the absence of carbon dioxide the propionic acid bacteria convert glycerol quantitatively into propionic acid:

$$\underset{\text{GLYCEROL}}{CH_2OHCHOHCH_2OH} = \underset{\text{PROPIONIC ACID}}{CH_3CH_2COOH} + H_2O$$

Elsden (1938) observed that the washed suspensions of pyruvate fermenting *Escherichia coli,* under increased carbon dioxide concentration, increase the production of succinic acid by about 50 per cent, as compared to the cells which ferment this acid in the air. This observation would support the observations of Wood and Werkman that carbon dioxide is involved in the synthesis of succinic acid, although it is doubtful whether the carbon dioxide fixation in the glycerol fermentation process is going according to the reaction:

$$\underset{\text{GLYCEROL}}{CH_2OHCHOHCH_2OH} + \underset{\text{CARBON DIOXIDE}}{CO_2} \rightarrow \underset{\text{SUCCINIC ACID}}{HOOCCH_2CH_2COOH} + H_2O$$

Wood and Werkman (1936, 1938, 1940) suggested that this fixation is a linkage of carbon dioxide with the 3-carbon keto-acid, pyruvic acid:

$$\underset{\text{PYRUVIC ACID}}{CH_3COCOOH} + \underset{\text{CARBON DIOXIDE}}{CO_2} \rightarrow \underset{\text{OXALACETIC ACID}}{HOOCCH_2COCOOH}$$

The enzyme oxalacetic carboxylase catalyzes reversibly this reaction (Ochoa, 1946).

The fifth period. The fifth period in the investigation of carbon dioxide fixation began when the radioactive isotopes of carbon were made available to research. The isotopes have been used to study the mechanism of the carbon dioxide fixation, the localization of the fixed carbon in the compounds of the cell, the source of energy necessary to reduce carbon dioxide, and, last but not least, the significance of this process for the heterotroph.

Ruben and Kamen (1940) exposed a suspension of fresh yeast cells to the short-lived radioactive carbon dioxide ($C^{11}O_2$). The major part of C^{11} was fixed in COOH groups of the cells. Carson and Ruben (1940) studied the fermentation of glycerol in the presence of $C^{11}O_2$ by the *Propionbacterium pentosaceum.* From the total of carbon dioxide taken up, 72 per cent were found in propionic acid produced from glycerol, 10 per cent were used to form succinic acid, and 17.5 per cent were found in cell extracts of the microorganism. Most of the fixed carbon was located in the carboxyl groups. Liener and Buchanan (1951) reported that growing yeast cells take up rapidly the radioactive $C^{14}O_2$ and that as much as 5 per cent of their total carbon is obtained from the air. At low concentrations of carbon dioxide in the air, the uptake of this substance by cells is proportional to its concentration until the concentration reaches 5 per cent of the air. At this level the quantity of fixed carbon becomes constant. The cells of *Serratia marcescens* in the logarithmic growth phase have a ten times higher fixation rate of C^{14} than in the resting phase. The consumption of carbon dioxide is influenced by the composition of the medium (McLean, Robinson, and Purdie, 1952). Gitterman and Knight (1952) found that the amount of $C^{14}O_2$ fixed by *Penicillium chrysogenum* decreases in the absence of divalent ions Mg^{++}, Fe^{++}, Mn^{++}, Ca^{++}, and that, in the absence of a soluble carbon source (glucose) in the medium, the amount of fixed gas is insignificant. When 0.25 and 0.75 millicurie of radioactive $NaHC^{14}O_3$ were injected intraperitoneally into rats, 50 per cent of the radioactivity was found in the fumarate of the liver. The incorporation of radioactive carbon dioxide in the liver was seven times greater than in the heart of the animals (Hall, Hawthorne, and Marshall, 1953). Utter (1951) using radioactive $C^{14}O_2$ observed that the carbon dioxide fixation was catalyzed by enzyme systems of adenosinetriphosphate and triphosphopyridine nucleotide.

The work of Long, Miles, and Perry (1955) showed that the cultures of tubercle bacilli grown in the atmosphere of C^{14}-labeled carbon dioxide ($C^{14}O_2$) produced proteins of tuberculin containing large quantities of C^{14}. The labeled carbon appeared in soluble polysaccharides and also in the lipids and the bodies of the bacilli.

The studies of the energy balance of carbon fixation by autotrophs and chemo-autotrophs showed that these reactions are endergonic and require an outside source of energy (see p. 78). These sources are known in autotrophs and chemo-autotrophs, but the knowledge as to what the source of energy of carbon dioxide fixation in heterotrophs might be is limited. The mechanism by which energy is supplied in a form capable of reducing carbon dioxide is unknown. (The heat of formation of H_2CO_3 is 167.53 kg.-cal. per gram formula weight.) The question of the source of energy of carbon dioxide fixation by heterotrophs must be regarded as one of the most obscure problems of biology (Utter and Wood, 1951). Some authors consider the fixation of carbon dioxide by heterotrophs as concomitant with the oxidations of inorganic substances (van Niel, 1943).

Lwoff and Monod (1946) expressed the opinion that the fixation of carbon dioxide is necessary to microorganisms because they can synthesize some essential metabolites only by the reaction of carboxylation. The dicarboxylic acids of C_4 and C_5 (glutamic, succinic, aspartic) are such essential metabolites and may act as growth factors. In a normal atmosphere, rich in carbon dioxide, these acids do not have any action as growth factors, but become such in an atmosphere poor in dioxide. They cannot be replaced by monoacids, aminoacids, or glucose. Indirect support of the view that fixed carbon dioxide participates in the synthesis of essential growth intermediates is given by the replacement experiments. If a metabolite synthesized by a cell from carbon dioxide is present in a medium where the cell is growing, the cell will utilize this metabolite, and the carbon dioxide will be dispensable to its growth. Lwoff and Monod (1946) showed that the lack of dicarboxylic acids of C_4-type and the absence of carbon dioxide in the medium were the cause of the standstill of the growth of *Escherichia coli*; the addition of citrate, acetate, lactate, pyruvate, *n*-butyrate, or *n*-valerianate to the culture did not stimulate the growth of *Escherichia coli*; on the other hand, if a mixture of succinate and DL-glutamate at the rate of 1:50,000 was added to the medium, the development of the culture in the absence of carbon dioxide was equal to that of the controls.

Ajl and Werkman (1948) investigated the possibility of replacing carbon dioxide by some intermediate of the Krebs cycle. In *Escherichia coli*, amino acids arginine, proline, aspartic and glutamic acids, dicarboxylic, succinic, fumaric, malic, oxalacetic, and β-ketoglutaric acids and tricarboxylic *cis*-aconitic acid may replace carbon dioxide and provide normal growth of the culture. These compounds are the members of Krebs cycle. Some relative compounds, like alanine, lysine, pyruvic, and citric acids, were not capable of replacing carbon dioxide in this organism. Middlebrook, Cohn, and Schaefer (1954) discovered that biotin is required for the growth of several strains of tubercle bacilli. In these strains, however, biotin can be replaced by carbon dioxide.

Evans and Slotin (1940) were able to observe the assimilation of radioactive carbon dioxide ($C^{11}O_2$) by the tissue of higher animals. Minced pigeon liver formed α-ketoglutarate from pyruvic acid and carbon dioxide. Krebs and Eggleton (1940), on the ground of the observations of Evans and Slotin, agreed that oxalacetate, through successive enzymatic oxidations, reductions and decarboxylation reactions of Krebs cycle is converted into citric acid and α-ketoglutaric acid. Ketoglutaric acid by the addition of amino group leads to amino acid, the glutamic acid. Thus, links between the metabolism of carbohydrates and glycerol, the fixation of carbon dioxide and the formation of amino acids may be established. A fact of general importance is that probably all heterotrophic forms of life take up carbon dioxide from the atmosphere and use it as a source of carbon.

IX

Sources of Nitrogen and Phosphorus

NITROGEN is indispensable to the growth of tubercle bacilli. As tubercle bacilli do not utilize the nitrogen of the air (Proskauer and Beck, 1894), it must be supplied to them in the form of soluble compounds.

The nitrogen content of tubercle bacilli ranges from 7.0 to 7.8 per cent (Bance, 1942) and there is no relation between the level of nitrogen in the bacilli and its concentration in the medium (Henley and LeDuc, 1939). Tubercle bacilli can for a short time proliferate in a medium lacking a source of nitrogen but containing a source of carbon. Such a process of starving mycobacteria was studied by Marschak and Schaefer (1952). When tubercle bacilli were grown in a simple medium, containing an excess of glucose but a limited source of nitrogen (NH_4Cl), the bacilli continued to proliferate, utilizing their own cellular resources of nitrogen, until the nitrogen was depleted to the level where the lysis of the cells started. After fifteen days of starvation, the nitrogen content of the bacilli (strain H37Rv) was reduced to 50 per cent of the original. The dry weight of the bacterial mass increased till the fifteenth day, when its decrease started. In the absence of both nitrogen and carbon sources, the loss of bacterial nitrogen in the same period of time was only 15 per cent. The bacilli did not proliferate and the lysis of the cells was slow.

Nitrogen is drawn by the tubercle bacilli from the medium and incorporated into their bodies. Tiffeneau and Marie (1912) found that after eight weeks of growth, tubercle bacilli had removed, from the synthetic medium of Proskauer and Beck which contains 2 g. of ammonium sulfate per liter as the source of nitrogen, two thirds of the nitrogen contents and produced four grams of bodies. The experiments of E. R. Long (1919) showed that a glycerol-peptone broth containing initially 133 mg. nitrogen per 100 ml., contained only 61 mg. per 100 ml. of nitrogen after tubercle bacilli had been grown on it for four weeks. Out of 1.345 g. of nitrogen contained in a liter of Sauton's medium, 1.185 were utilized or transformed by tubercle bacilli. Of this quantity of nitrogen approximately 0.991 g. were found in bacilli, 0.270 g. recovered from the medium and 80 g. disappeared from the medium in the form of ammonia (Bance, 1942).

Carrel and Baker (1926) found that for the multiplication of tissue cells the amino acids and other dialyzable nitrogenous compounds of the embryonic juice caused no increase in the mass of the tissue, although these substances stimulate the multiplication of the cells. The proteins completely digested by trypsin or pepsin were also unable to support cell proliferation. Tissue cells needed the higher cleavage products of the proteins for growth.

Proskauer and Beck (1894) reported that such simple amino acids as glycine and alanine may serve as the sole source of nitrogen to tubercle bacilli. Contrary to these early findings, Youmans and Youmans (1954b) after testing 25 amino acids for their suitability as nitrogen sources for the growth of tubercle bacilli (strain H37Rv) in three different media, found that only L-asparagine, L-glutamic acid, and DL-aspartic acid stimulated the growth. Few other amino acids, such as L-(—)histidine, L-proline, and DL-alanine, stimulated growth to a lesser degree. Good sources of nitrogen are ammonia compounds and acid amides. Amino nitrogen and nitrogen of the amide group are not utilized by microorganisms with the same ease. The amino group of monobasic amino acids is attacked by the tubercle bacilli and the ammonia is liberated. In the compounds of dibasic amino acids, like asparagine ($CONH_2CH_2CHNH_2COOH$), the amide group connected with the carbonyl ($CONH_2$) is completely deaminized, the amino group ($CHNH_2$) remains almost untouched (Long, 1921–1922). Lieb (1934) made an interesting observation about the assimilation of aspartic acid and its amide, the asparagine, by *Salmonella typhosa.* The amino group of aspartic acid was not touched by *Salmonella,* but after the introduction of the amide group into the molecule, the assimilation was complete. The carbonyl group $=C=O$ has a weakening effect on the intramolecular bonds.

Asparagine, introduced for the culturing of tubercle bacilli by Kühne (1892, 1894) and Proskauer and Beck (1894), was found to be the best source of nitrogen (Henley and LeDuc, 1930, and Andrejew, 1948). When, instead of ordinary L-asparagine, D-asparagine was used in Sauton's medium as a source of nitrogen, the growth of tubercle bacilli was accelerated at the start but in the end the growth on L-asparagine was always more abundant than on D-asparagine (Dello Jojo, 1937).

According to Middlebrook, Cohn, and Schaefer (1954), the growth of tubercle bacilli isolated from patients treated with isoniazid is inhibited by asparagine. The use of glutamate instead of asparagine was suggested for culturing small inocula of these bacilli. The amino acids containing the benzene ring (tyrosine, phenylalanine, tryptophan) are not metabolized by tubercle bacilli. The same is true of purines, pyrimidines, and their derivatives. Creatinine, which contains imino but not amino nitrogen, is not utilized by the tubercle bacilli either (Long, 1921–1922; Campbell, 1925; Finlayson, 1946).

Some sources of nitrogen promote better growth of tubercle bacilli than others: 100 ml. of glycerol-peptone broth yielded 320 mg. dry weight of tubercle bacilli after six weeks of incubation, whereas Sauton's medium produced 1,075 mg., and Long's medium 1,350 mg. of bacilli under the same conditions. When, instead of asparagine, peptone was used as the source of nitrogen in Sauton's medium, the harvest was 655 mg. instead of 1,075 mg; ammonium oxalate as the nitrogen source produced 1,830 mg. of bacilli (Model, 1929).

Ammonium salts of dicarboxylic acids are readily utilized by tubercle bacilli. Tubercle bacilli can grow on a medium containing nitrogen solely in the form of inorganic ammonia compounds, like $(NH_4)_2SO_4$ and NH_4Cl (Proskauer and Beck, 1894). However, the growth is faster and more abundant when additional nitrogen of organic compounds is present in the medium. In the opinion of Long (1921–1922), corroborated by Henley and LeDuc (1939), all nitrogen consumed by tubercle bacilli is, or ought to be, converted to the form of ammonia.

The influence on growth exerted by an unknown substance is clear in a simple mineral solution but it is often vague in a meat infusion or in egg media containing, besides the chief source of nitrogen or carbon, large inestimable quantities of side sources of nitrogen and carbon. The utilization of a nitrogen source is influenced by the source of carbon in the medium. In the liquid medium of Dubos, with glucose as the source of carbon, glutamic acid was the best source of nitrogen for the avian variant of the tubercle bacilli. Ammonium succinate under these conditions was in eighth and asparagine in ninth place. When sodium succinate was the carbon source in the medium, first place was taken by ammonium succinate, asparagine occupying fourth place (Ackart and Murray, 1951).

As was revealed by paper partition chromatography, the strains H37Rv, bovine, and avian, grown on a synthetic medium with asparagine as the source of nitrogen, contained most of the common amino acids in the cell hydrolyzates. The culture filtrates of the medium revealed a decrease in the asparagine concentration of the medium during growth, but an increase in glutamic and aspartic acids and in alanine. The substitution of asparagine with NH_4Cl did not produce any significant variations in the amino acid content of the cell hydrolyzates (Pauletta and Defranceschi, 1952). When the nitrogen level in a medium is sufficiently high for growth, the addition of nitrogen to the medium is not followed by a proportional increase in the output of bacilli. In a media with an insufficient nitrogen content an increase in the nitrogen concentration is followed by a considerable increase in the harvest of the bacilli. In the experiments of Frouin and Guillaumie (1928), a synthetic medium containing 5 g. per liter of asparagine produced 0.424 g. of bacilli, while a medium with 10 g. per liter of asparagine produced 0.613 g. of bacilli from 100 ml. of the medium. When the asparagine concentration in Sauton's medium was increased from 0.1 per cent to 0.8 per cent, the harvest of bacilli increased fivefold (Goyal, 1936). In the cases where the amount of nitrogen present in the media is small but the quantity of carbon is sufficient, nitrogen will be the limiting factor of growth: with 1 per cent of glucose present, the addition of 0.001 mg/ml of nitrogen source (NH_4Cl) was always followed by a rapid rise in the growth rate, which sank to the previous level after the depletion of the nitrogen available (Schaefer, Marshak, and Burckhart, 1949). It is known now that tubercle bacilli, in order to grow, need far less nitrogenous compounds than it was supposed by earlier workers. Schaefer, *et al.* found that 0.001 mg/ml of NH_4Cl is sufficient to support the growth of *M. tuberculosis* in Dubos' medium.

Mycobacteria, as well as other organisms, obtain their energy more easily from the oxidation of carbohydrates than from the decomposition of nitrogenous compounds. Because of this, the rate of liberation of ammonia depends largely on the quantity of carbohydrates present in the medium. When large amounts of carbohydrates are present, they are used up and only a small amount of ammonia is produced. This leads to the saving of ammonia (Kendall, Day, and Walker, 1914) and to the acidification of the medium. In the presence of large quantities of compounds rich in ammonia and of small amounts of carbohydrates in the medium, ammonia is produced in great quantities. It accumulates in the cultures, chiefly during the first weeks of growth. This fact, incidentally, is of consequence to agriculture. Ammonia formation in the soil is largely diminished by fertilization with carbohydrates (Lipman, Blair, and McLean, 1912). The alkalinity of a medium in which tubercle bacilli have been grown is roughly proportional to its ammonia content. The ammonia production in plain meat infusion broth was three times higher than in the cultures containing carbohydrate (Merrill, 1930).

Andrejew (1948) using the Barcroft-Warburg manometric technique, observed that the assimilation by tubercle bacilli of amino acids, as well as of carbohydrates, is not necessarily tied up with the growth of cells. In the absence of easily attackable carbohydrates, amino acids are the source of energy to the tubercle bacillus, although this source is a poor one compared to carbohydrates. In Sauton's medium containing 4 g. of asparagine per liter, tubercle bacilli consumed, in four hours at 38°C., 9.4 cmm. of oxygen per mg. of dry bacilli. Generally, asparagine media produce about 10.0 g. bacilli per gram of nitrogen utilized, but only from 0.30 to 0.38 g. bacilli per gram of glycerol utilized (Henley and LeDuc, 1939). These facts show what significance each of these substances has for the bacilli: nitrogen is chiefly used in growth and plastic activity, glycerol is utilized in respiration and as a source of energy.

The metabolism of radioactive asparagine in the seedlings of lupine (*Lupinus angustifolius*) was compared with the metabolism of radioactive glucose in the same plant. Radioactive asparagine was obtained in seedlings which were permitted to carry on photosynthesis for six days in the presence of three millicuries of $C^{14}O_2$. It was discovered that 55 per cent of the radioactivity of asparagine was located in carboxyl groups of plant cells. Asparagine was utilized mainly for the synthesis of cell substances (Nelson, Drotkov, and Reed, 1953). The tubercle bacillus not only takes up nitrogen from the medium to build up its body, but it also produces nitrogenous or protein substances which are released in the medium. These substances have the nature of tuberculin and are mainly accumulated in the media during the last period of the growth of bacilli.

The increase in the output of tubercle bacilli is chiefly influenced by the concentration of phosphorus compounds in the medium. This dependance of the amount of harvested bacilli on the concentration of KH_2PO_4 in the medium was demonstrated by Frouin and Guillaumie (1928). They found that when 1 g. per liter of KH_2PO_4 was added to the medium, 0.217 g. of dry bacilli were collected; with 5 g. per liter, 0.341 g.; with 10 g. per liter, 0.467 g.; and with 20 g. per liter, 0.1649 g.

Bance (1942) compared the consumption by different strains of mycobacteria of phosphate compounds in Sauton's medium. A BCG strain grown for thirty-five days on this medium containing 0.5 g. KH_2PO_4 per liter, consumed 67.8 per cent of KH_2PO_4. When the growth of the culture ceased, the lowest level of KH_2PO_4 concentration was reached. No considerable differences in phosphate consumption were found in different strains of mycobacteria. The uptake by *M. phlei* of the radioactive isotope of sodium phosphate added to Dubos' medium was parallel to the growth curve of the bacilli (Sternberg and Padoski, 1953).

The distribution of phosphorus in different parts of *M. tuberculosis* was given by Winder and Denneny (1954, 1956) (see Table 15).

Table 15. The Distribution of Phosphorus in *Mycobacterium tuberculosis* in Liquid Medium and on Löwenstein's Medium

	Lipid Phosphorus	Ortho-phosphate	Ribonucleic Acid	Desoxyribo-nucleic Acid	Poly-phosphate
30–80-day-old cultures (liquid medium)	1.2–2.2 *	1.7–4.0 *	1.7–2.8 *	1.2–2.0 *	0–15.0 *
14-day-old culture (Löwenstein's medium)	6%	. . .	29.8%	6.0%	27%

Source: Winder and Denneny (1954, 1956).

* Milligrams of phosphorus per gram of dry weight.

Table 16. Nitrogenous Compounds Stimulating the Growth or Respiration of Tubercle Bacilli

Compound	Growth	Respiration	Author
	Proteins and Related Substances		
Albumin (serum, egg)	Absent		Dorset (1902)
	Stimulated		Buc (1924)
	Absent		Finlayson (1946)
	Absent (coagul.)		Andrejew (1948)
Albumin Fraction V	Stimulated		Dubos and Middlebrook (1947)
	Absent		Sattler and Youmans (1948)
	Stimulated		Schaefer *et al.* (1949)
		Absent	Bretey and Andrejew (1949b)
	Stimulated (H37Rv)		Holmgren and Youmans (1952)
	Absent (H37Ra)		Holmgren and Youmans (1952)
Biuret	Stimulated		Proskauer and Beck (1894)
Blood serum	Stimulated		Koch (1882)
	Stimulated		Roux and Nocard (1887)
	Stimulated		Weber and Taute (1904–1905)
	Stimulated		Buc (1924)
	Stimulated		Kirchner (1932)
	Stimulated		Scholer (1952)
		Stimulated	Loebel *et al.* (1933a)
		Stimulated	Bretey and Andrejew (1949b)
Protamine scombrine	Stimulated		Armand-Delille *et al.* (1913)
	Amino Acids and Related Substances		
DL-alanine	Stimulated		Proskauer and Beck (1894)
	Stimulated		E. R. Long (1919)
	Stimulated		Campbell (1925)
		Doubtful	Nakamura (1938)
	Absent (egg white medium)		Finlayson (1946)
	Stimulated		Braun (1955)
Arginine	Stimulated		Armand-Delille *et al.* (1913)
		Decrease	Andrejew (1948)
L-asparagine	Stimulated		Kühne (1892, 1894)
	Stimulated		Proskauer and Beck (1894)
	Stimulated		Calmette *et al.* (1909)
	Stimulated		E. R. Long (1921–1922)
		Absent	Nakamura (1938)
	Absent (egg white medium)		Finlayson (1946)
		Doubtful	Andrejew (1948)
Betaine	Absent		Proskauer and Beck (1894)
			E. R. Long (1921–1922)

Table 16—*continued*

Compound	Growth	Respiration	Author
Creatinine	Absent		Campbell (1925)
	Absent (egg white medium)		Finlayson (1946)
Glycine	Doubtful		Proskauer and Beck (1894)
	Stimulated		Armand-Delille *et al.* (1913)
	Stimulated		E. R. Long (1919)
	Stimulated ($\frac{1}{10}$ as much as asparagine)		Model (1929)
		Doubtful	Nakamura (1938)
Glycylglycine	Stimulated		Henley and LeDuc (1939)
		Stimulated	Nakamura (1939)
	Stimulated		Braun (1955)
Glutamic acid		Stimulated	Andrejew (1948)
	Stimulated		Ackart and Murray (1951)
	Stimulated		Braun (1955)
Histidine	Stimulated		E. R. Long (1921–1922)
	Stimulated		Campbell (1925)
Leucine	Doubtful		Kühne (1892, 1894)
	Doubtful		Proskauer and Beck (1894)
	Absent		Calmette *et al.* (1909)
	Stimulated		E. R. Long (1921–1922)
Phenylalanine	Absent		E. R. Long (1921–1922)
	Absent		Model (1929)
Sarcosine	Absent		Proskauer and Beck (1894)
		Stimulated	Andrejew (1948)
Taurine	Absent		Proskauer and Beck (1894)
		Absent	Nakamura (1938)
Tryptophan	Absent		E. R. Long (1921–1922)
	Absent		Model (1929)
	Stimulated		D. G. Smith (1947)
	Absent		Benassi and Perisinotto (1952)
Tyrosine	Doubtful		Kühne (1892, 1894)
	Absent		Proskauer and Beck (1894)
	Absent		Calmette *et al.* (1909)
	Absent		E. R. Long (1921–1922)
	Absent		Model (1929)
		Stimulated (apathogenic strains)	Bernheim (1942)
Purines and Related Substances			
Allantoine	Absent		Proskauer and Beck (1894)
Alloxan	Absent		Proskauer and Beck (1894)
Caffeine	Absent		Proskauer and Beck (1894)
Guanine	Absent		Proskauer and Beck (1894)

Table 16—*continued*

Compound	Growth	Respiration	Author
Hippuric acid	Absent		Proskauer and Beck (1894)
Uric acid	Absent		Proskauer and Beck (1894)
	Stimulated (sodium salt in the presence of glycerol)		Braun (1955)
		Amides and Amines	
Acetamide	Stimulated		E. R. Long (1919)
Ethylamine	Stimulated		E. R. Long (1919)
Formamide	Stimulated		Proskauer and Beck (1894)
	Stimulated		E. R. Long (1919)
Glucosamine	Stimulated		Proskauer and Beck (1894)
Hydroxylamine	Absent	Stimulated	Bernheim *et al.* (1953)
Methylamine	Stimulated		E. R. Long (1919)
	Absent	Stimulated	Bernheim *et al.* (1953)
Propionamide	Stimulated		E. R. Long (1919)
	Stimulated		Henley and LeDuc (1939)
Succinamide	Absent		Calmette *et al.* (1909)
		Stimulated	Andrejew (1948)
Urea	Absent		Proskauer and Beck (1894)
	Absent		E. R. Long (1921–1922)
	Doubtful		Henley and LeDuc (1930)
Urethane	Stimulated		E. R. Long (1919)
		Ammonium Salts	
Ammonium acetate	Doubtful		Proskauer and Beck (1894)
	Absent		E. R. Long (1919)
Ammonium aspartate	Stimulated		Henley and LeDuc (1939)
Ammonium butyrate	Absent		Proskauer and Beck (1894)
Ammonium isobutyrate	Absent		Proskauer and Beck (1894)
Ammonium oxybutyrate	Absent		Proskauer and Beck (1894)
Ammonium carbonate	Absent		E. R. Long (1919)
	Absent		Henley and LeDuc (1930)
Ammonium chloride	Stimulated		Proskauer and Beck (1894)
	Stimulated		E. R. Long (1919)
	Stimulated		Schaefer *et al.* (1949)
	Stimulated		Braun (1955)

Table 16—*continued*

Compound	Growth	Respiration	Author
Ammonium citrate	Stimulated		Proskauer and Beck (1894)
	Stimulated		E. R. Long (1922)
	Stimulated		Henley and LeDuc (1939)
	Doubtful		Boquet (1944)
	Absent		Schaefer *et al.* (1949)
Ammonium formate	Absent		Proskauer and Beck (1894)
	Absent		E. R. Long (1919)
Ammonium fumarate	Stimulated		Henley and LeDuc (1930)
	Doubtful		Boquet (1944)
Ammonium glycolate	Absent		E. R. Long (1919)
Ammonium glyoxalate	Absent		E. R. Long (1919)
Ammonium lactate	Stimulated		Proskauer and Beck (1894)
	Absent		E. R. Long (1919)
	Stimulated		Henley and LeDuc (1930)
	Absent (egg white medium)		Finlayson (1946)
		Stimulated (intensity tripled)	Andrejew (1948)
		Stimulated	Edson (1947, 1951)
Ammonium malate	Absent		Proskauer and Beck (1894)
	Stimulated		Henley and LeDuc (1930)
	Stimulated		Boquet (1944)
Ammonium malonate	Stimulated		Proskauer and Beck (1894)
	Stimulated		E. R. Long (1919)
	Stimulated		Boquet (1944)
Ammonium nitrate	Stimulated		Proskauer and Beck (1894)
	Stimulated		Braun and Kondo (1925)
	Stimulated		Henley and LeDuc (1939)
	Doubtful		Boquet (1944)
Ammonium oxalate	Stimulated		Proskauer and Beck (1894)
	Stimulated		E. R. Long (1919)
		Stimulated	Andrejew (1948)
Ammonium phosphate	Stimulated		Proskauer and Beck (1894)
Ammonium propionate	Stimulated		Proskauer and Beck (1894)
	Doubtful		Boquet (1944)

Table 16—*continued*

Compound	Growth	Respiration	Author
Ammonium pyruvate	Absent		E. R. Long (1919)
Ammonium sulfate	Stimulated		Proskauer and Beck (1894)
	Stimulated		Tiffeneau and Marie (1912)
	Stimulated		Henley and LeDuc (1939)
	Stimulated		Boquet (1944)
Ammonium succinate	Absent		Proskauer and Beck (1894)
	Stimulated		E. R. Long (1919)
	Stimulated		Henley and LeDuc (1930)
	Stimulated		Ackart and Murray (1951)
Ammonium tartrate	Stimulated		Proskauer and Beck (1894)
	Stimulated		Model (1929)
	Doubtful		Boquet (1944)
Ammonium valerinate	Absent		Proskauer and Beck (1894)
		Nitrates and Nitrites	
Sodium nitrate	Doubtful		Proskauer and Beck (1894)
Sodium nitrite	Doubtful		Proskauer and Beck (1894)

X

The Mineral Requirements of Tubercle Bacilli

THE good growth of tubercle bacilli on mineral media or on purely vegetable media, such as potatoes and carrots, reversed the conception of the growth requirements of tubercle bacilli, based upon the first successful attempt at tubercle bacilli cultivation on a coagulated serum by Koch. The opinion that the tubercle bacillus is a highly pretentious parasite which, in order to grow, requires complex animal proteins as nutrients, has proved to be erroneous. It was early found that this bacillus lives on relatively simple nitrogen, carbon, and mineral compounds.

The recognition that the tubercle bacillus grows on solutions of relatively simple inorganic compounds led some investigators to oversimplify the biology of the tubercle bacillus. The capability of the tubercle bacillus to synthesize its extremely complicated body substances from simple inorganic compounds indicates the complexity rather than the simplicity of the bacillus. The tubercle bacillus possesses enzymes endowed with powerful general and specific activities, which are located in the heterogenous morphologic elements of the cell.

The growth of a microorganism depends on the presence of the right substance in the right concentration in the medium. A medium made up of chemically and quantitatively known substances will furnish information about the nutrients utilized by a microorganism.

The pioneer work of Raulin (1869) on the cultivation of *Aspergillus niger* in a liquid medium composed of chemically and quantitatively known substances was inspired by Pasteur's successful attempt to cultivate microorganisms on a simple medium, composed of determined substances. Raulin introduced a precise measure, the weight of the produced mycelium, as a means of appraising the influence that different elements in the medium have on the growth. Raulin's method of subtracting the elements one by one from the complete medium and comparing the weights of mycelia obtained from these media with the weights of mycelia obtained from the complete medium, gave precise indications of the physiologic importance of every element in the medium.

H. Martin (1889) cultivated the tubercle bacillus in a medium not containing native protein or protein compounds ("*en milieu purement minéral*"). The medium contained gycerol and sugar as the source of carbon, ammonium tartrate as the source of nitrogen. It also contained potassium phosphate and probably traces of magnesium and iron as a result of the impurity of the chemicals used. The medium was solidified through the addition of agar. The pictures of these cultures attached to the work give evidence of the success of the cultivation.

To determine which nutrients the tubercle bacillus needs, Kühne (1892, 1894) used the subtraction method of Raulin. Omitting one by one from the medium the mineral, nitrogen, and carbon compounds, Kühne observed the changes in the amounts of the bacilli produced, and thus learned which substances are essential to growth. By this method of elimination, Kühne found that the amino acids leucine and tyrosine could be omitted from the medium if asparagine was present in it. Asparagine could supply nitrogen, and glycerol was capable of providing the carbon necessary for growth. The ashes of Liebig's meat extract could be substituted with a mixture of mineral salts containing sodium chloride, magnesium sulfate, soda, potash, phosphoric acid, and lactic acid. These investigations of Kühne had been stimulated by Koch's work toward improvement in the quality of tuberculin.

A further step ahead in the study of the biology of tubercle bacilli was the work of Proskauer and Beck (1894). Their investigations greatly enlarged our knowledge of the exact growth requirements of this bacillus. Proskauer and Beck started at the point where Kühne left off. Sodium chloride was found not to be essential to growth. The partial substitution of magnesium sulfate with magnesium citrate highly stimulated the growth of tubercle bacilli. Ammonium chloride and glucose were found to support the growth, but Proskauer and Beck, like Nocard and Roux, and Kühne did not discover a substitute for glycerol.

These works presented ample evidence that, besides the sources of nitrogen in the form of asparagine or ammonia salts and such sources of carbon as glycerol or glucose, the salts of phosphoric acid, potassium, and magnesium are vital to the growth of tubercle bacilli.

The medium of Proskauer and Beck was reduced to four essential compounds, none of which can be omitted:

Ammonium carbonate	0.35%
Potassium phosphate, primary	0.15
Magnesium sulfate	0.25
Glycerol	1.5

Sources of Energy, Growth of Bacillus

The composition of the synthetic medium given by Proskauer and Beck is the forerunner of all further synthetic liquid media for growing tubercle bacilli. Sauton (1912) gives the following data on the dependence of the growth of tubercle bacilli on the presence of given elements in the medium:

Synthetic Medium	*Weight in Grams of Dry Tubercle Bacilli from 100 ml. of Medium Grown for 20 Days at 38°C.*
Complete	0.95
Without S	0.04
Without Mg	0.01
Without Fe	0.32
Without P	no growth
Without K	no growth

In the experiments of Sauton it was not possible to substitute the elements potassium with nitrogen and phosphorus with arsenic. Three elements, namely potassium, magnesium, and phosphorus, were found to be essential and sufficient to satisfy the mineral requirements for growing tubercle bacilli.

According to Frouin and Guillaumie (1928) the simplest mineral medium for the cultivation of tubercle bacilli has the following components: monopotassium phosphate, 1.0 g.; magnesium sulfate, 1.0 g.; sodium citrate, 1.0 g.; distilled water, 1,000.0 g. The source of carbon was 40.0 g. glycerol, of nitrogen 5.0 g. asparagine. When the concentration of mineral substances in the medium was diminished ten times, the growth of the cultures was less rapid and less abundant. The harvest of bacilli from the liquid medium increased with the increase of mineral salts in the solution; glycerol was a more favorable source of carbon than glucose.

Magnesium is an indispensable element for the growth of tubercle bacilli. Manceaux (1924) in his experiments on the influence of magnesium on the growth of the bovine variant of tubercle bacilli on glycerol potato, observed that when 15 per cent of magnesium sulfate was added to the medium, the growth of the bacilli was scanty. Under these conditions, the tubercle bacillus must resist a very considerable osmotic pressure to prevent the penetration of magnesium ions at a rate that would coagulate the proteins in the interior of the cell of the bacillus. The quantity of magnesium is considerably diminished in the newly developed synthetic media as compared to the synthetic medium of Proskauer and Beck (1894), who used 2.5 g. per liter of this element. Tiffeneau and Marie (1912) obtained good growth with quantities of magnesium sulfate four times smaller, and Dubos and Middlebrook (1947) reduced magnesium in their medium to 0.01 g. per liter. In our liquid medium we found it necessary to increase the amount of magnesium to 0.2 g. per liter.

In the synthetic medium the length of the lag phase of the culture of *Bacterium lactis aerogenes* was considerably increased when the concentration of magnesium ions was reduced (Lodge and Hinshelwood, 1939). The toxicity of nickel, cobalt, cadmium, zinc, and manganese to the cells of *Escherichia coli* and other bacteria was markedly lowered in the presence of magnesium. By the use of isotopes N^{57} and Co^{56} it was found that the presence of magnesium diminishes the amount of nickel and cobalt bound by the cells (Abelson and Aldous, 1950).

XI

Growth Factors and Trace Elements

Inorganic Compounds

THE greatest part of the ingredients of egg media used for the cultivation of tubercle bacilli remains unknown and the preparation of these media stereotyped (van Niel, 1944; Dubos and Noufflard, 1950; Middlebrook, 1950). The basic elements needed for the growth of a cell, carbon, nitrogen, phosphorus, potassium, iron, and others, are supplied by egg yolk, or may be obtained from the added chemicals. From this primary building material the cell manufactures its constituents. Besides these ingredients, derived directly from the foodstuffs or produced from the nutrients by the cell, there are substances, necessary for the growth, which the cell is incapable of manufacturing and which must be introduced into the medium. "The growth factor of a determined organism is the substance which this organism is incapable of synthesizing and in the absence of which the multiplication of the organism is not possible" (Lwoff, 1936–1937). Some strains of *Escherichia coli* utilize nitrates, while others require nitrogen in the form of ammonia. For these latter ammonia is the growth factor. Still others need specific ingredients, such as vitamins or enzymes (van Niel, 1944).

The trace or oligo-elements, also known as catalytic elements, increase the speed of biologic reactions even if present in extremely small amounts. These elements are dispensable to growth, but the presence of the compounds of Zn^{++}, Cu^{++}, Fe^{++}, and some others in the medium highly accelerate the growth. Bertrand and co-workers, in more than a hundred publications, give an account of their investigation of the role of the catalytic elements in the biology of plants and animals (*Bulletin de la Société Chimique de France*).

Iron, Zinc, Magnesium, Copper

The exclusive action of iron as a growth stimulant of tubercle bacilli indicates that this stimulation is of some specific nature and not a general catalytic acceleration of living reactions. Zinc and iron in a 0.005 per cent concentration were recognized by Raulin (1869) as growth stimulants for *Aspergillus niger.* The basal medium of Raulin contained approximately 0.005 per cent of iron and zinc salts. The presence in the medium of Fe^{++} and Zn^{++} salts raised the harvest of mycelium three to five times, as compared with the harvest obtained from the medium without these salts. Raulin also recognized that the action of iron and zinc must be attributed to the metals, for their different anions were without action.

Baudran (1910) was the first to be concerned with the role of iron in the culturing of tubercle bacilli. Starting out with the presupposition that glycerol in the medium is assimilated by tubercle bacilli in the form of glycerophosphate, he introduced into his liquid medium a considerable amount of iron glycerophosphate (0.2 g. in 1,000 ml.) and manganese salt, and observed rapid growth of the cultures. Unfortunately it is not possible to compare the growth stimulation of tubercle bacilli in the experiments of Baudran with that observed later by Sauton, because the bacilli of Baudran were apathogenic for guinea pigs and the weight of bacilli collected from the cultures was not given.

Calmette, Massol, and Breton (1909) introduced the inorganic salt of iron into the composition of their synthetic medium, but did not give an explanation of the function of this compound. The importance of iron for the growth of tubercle bacilli in a synthetic medium was fully demonstrated by Sauton (1912). His complete medium containing 0.005 per cent of iron salt produced, in twenty days of growth, 0.95 g. of dry bacilli; the same medium without iron under the same conditions gave 0.32 g. of dry mass from 100 ml. of the medium. Iron in the medium tripled the harvest. These facts were also asserted in the works of Frouin and Guillaumie (1924b, 1928). These authors recognized that a mass of tubercle bacilli, produced on a synthetic medium with glycerol as the source of carbon, after thirty days of incubation, doubled or tripled in the presence of one part of ferric ammonium citrate added to 100,000 parts of the medium.

The favorable action of iron on the growth of tubercle bacilli does not depend upon the kind of the iron compound added to the medium. The most favorable action of ferric sulfate in glycerinated beef broth was in the range from 0.01 g. to 0.03 g. per 100 ml. of the medium (Henley, 1925). G. B. Reed and Rice (1928) indicated that in the presence of iron in the medium, the growth of tubercle bacilli increased in eight weeks by as much as 20 per cent, but if both citrate and iron salts were added, the increase was more than 100 per cent. This favorable effect was observed in a slightly acidic medium (*p*H 6.5), probably because iron is readily precipitated out of alkaline media. The uptake of iron by tubercle bacilli is very slight; iron in the media after the cultivation usually decreases only by 0.017 to 0.046 mg. per ml.

Not all investigators have found that iron has as favorable an influence on the growth of tubercle bacilli as reported by the above authors. E. R. Long and Seibert (1926) found that the average yield of their cultures containing iron was 0.71 g. per 100 ml., that of those without iron 0.66 g. per 100 ml.

According to Sher and Sweany (1939) iron salts, added in the amount of 7.5 mg. per liter to Long's synthetic medium, more than doubled the yield when the medium was prepared from purified chemicals. When the medium was prepared from chemicals of lower grade purity, no growth enhancement occurred. Iron, when added to egg media or media containing serum, has little or no stimulating effect on the growth of tubercle bacilli. The investigations of Turian (1951) showed that an *M*/60,000 concentration of Fe^{++} in a synthetic medium containing 1 per cent glycerol increased the harvest of *Mycobacterium phlei* by six times. Iron had the same action on the growth of tubercle bacilli. After 21 days of growth 20 ml. of Sauton's medium produced the following amounts of dry bacilli, strain Vallée:

Without iron	57 mg.
M/60,000 Fe^{++} added	331 mg.
M/30,000 Fe^{++} added	350 mg.

According to Turian, the action of iron is specific. There is no other element which has even approximately the same action as iron on the growth of acid-fast bacilli.

The chief reason for the increase in the yield of tubercle bacilli in media containing iron is the increase in the speed of glycerol utilization by the bacilli, although these bacilli, growing at a great speed, contain less lipids than the bacilli grown in the absence of iron (Frouin and Guillaumie, 1924b). Henley (1926) regarded the growth acceleration as a result of a delayed acidification of the medium. This delayed action prolongs the growth time of bacilli and increases their quantity. With the discovery of the histohematin respiration of tubercle bacilli (see p. 83), in which iron is an important element, the whole problem of the growth activation of tubercle bacilli by iron received a different and more complex aspect. The importance of iron in this process is indicated by the fact that in the absence of iron the production of histohematin comes to a halt.

Sauton (1912) found that iron is not essential to the growth of tubercle bacilli. This cannot, however, be affirmed definitely, since in order to stimulate growth of tubercle bacilli, such a small quantity of iron is necessary that hardly any definite conclusions can be drawn from the experiments. An amount of iron sufficient to influence the growth can be introduced into the medium in the form of impurities in the chemicals or it could be dissolved from the glass of the container.

According to Warburg (1914b) the respiration of the liquid prepared from eggs of the sea urchin *Strongylocentratus lividus* increased by 50 to 110 per cent when 0.01 mg. Fe^{++} were added to 1.5 ml. No salts of other metals produced such an effect.

The studies of Pappenheimer and Johnson (1936) showed that the amount of iron necessary for the production of diphtheria toxin was considerably smaller than the quantity of iron found in the form of impurities in the media.

Menkin (1934) reported that ferric chloride (0.25 per cent solution), injected intravenously into tuberculous rabbits, penetrates into the avascular caseous areas of the organs. These claims were not confirmed by Bloch, Gomori, and Sperry-Braude (1948).

Iron (0.4 mg. of $FeSO_4 \cdot 7\ H_2O$) injected repeatedly into mice increased the pathogenicity of nonpathogenic mutants of *Pasteurella pestis* (Jackson and Burrows, 1956).

The findings of Baudran (1910) to the effect that manganese promotes the growth of tubercle bacilli were not substantiated by Calmette (1936). According to the investigations of Frouin and Guillaumie (1928), manganese, copper, and zinc, at concentrations of 0.1 and 0.001 per cent, did not increase the yield of tubercle bacilli. $CuSO_4$ and $ZnSO_4$, in a concentration of 1:0.0000001, in Long's synthetic medium, did not stimulate the growth (Uyei, 1930). Copper sulfate in traces (0.033 mg. per liter) retarded the initial growth of H37Rv strain of tubercle bacilli and, in concentrations greater than 1:3,000, prevented growth altogether (Sher and Sweany, 1939). Edson and Hunter (1943) reported that improvement of the growth of *Mycobacterium phlei* depends on the addition of calcium and iron salts to the synthetic medium. Other elements tested, such as Cu^{++}, Zn^{++}, Mn^{++}, did not improve the growth of this organism.

Recently Dubos and Middlebrook (1947) added copper, zinc and calcium in extreme dilutions to their basal medium. $CaCl_2$ was added in as small an amount as 0.0005 g.; $CuSO_4$ and $ZnSO_4$ in the even smaller amount of 0.0001 g. per 1,000 ml. of the medium (see p. 247). No data were given on the supposed role of these traces of elements in the medium.

Turian (1951), in the range of concentrations between $M/30{,}000$ and $M/240{,}000$, was not able to observe any favorable action of Cu^{++}, Zn^{++}, Mn^{++}, Co^{++}, Ni^{++}, Mo^{++}, and V^{++}, on the growth of acid-fast bacilli. Some metals (Cu^{++}, Zn^{++}, Co^{++}), in a concentration of $M/15{,}000$ were noxious to mycobacteria.

Sulfur, Sodium, Calcium, Barium, Silicon

The influence of sulfur, sodium, calcium, barium, and silicon on the growth of tubercle bacilli was investigated by many researchers.

Not all investigators recognized the necessity of introducing sulfur into the synthetic media for tubercle bacilli. Others found this substance necessary to growth (Model, 1929). Noll, Sorkin, and Erlenmeyer (1950), working with the isotope $^{35}S_4^{11}$, found that tubercle bacilli, grown for nineteen days on Sauton's medium, accumulated from 1.16 to 1.29 μg. of this isotope per mg. of dry bacilli.

The presence of sodium was early recognized as not necessary in a medium for tubercle bacilli (Proskauer and Beck, 1894; Model, 1929); the same was found to be true of calcium and barium (Model, 1929). Sauton (1912) did not see any increase in the harvest of bacilli cultivated on his synthetic medium when calcium compounds were added. The experiments seem to justify the conclusion that the presence of calcium compounds is neither necessary nor desirable (Lockemann, 1919; Long and Seibert, 1926).

The high incidence of tuberculosis among iron and silica workers indicates that some relationship may exist between the inhalation or ingestion of the dusts of these compounds and the increase in growth and virulence of tubercle bacilli, or the decrease of the resistance of the workers to the infection (Vorwald and Delahant, 1938). The experiments of Price (1932) supported the view that silica may enhance the growth of tubercle bacilli.

Compounds of Rare Earths

The compounds of rare earths provide many powerful catalysts widely used in organic synthesis. Frouin (1912) investigated compounds of vanadium, cerium, samarium, and other elements as possible growth catalysts of tubercle bacilli. Becquerel (1913) studied compounds of uranium and thorium with the same goal. These authors observed some activation of the growth of tubercle bacilli when these compounds were added in a concentration of 0.005 per cent to a liquid medium, but the action of these elements cannot be compared with the influence of iron salts on the growth of tubercle bacilli.

Organic Compounds

Egg yolk is the most important substance for growing tubercle bacilli. Some investigators tried to determine which of the components of egg yolk favor the growth of mycobacteria. The early work of Capaldi (1896) showed that the growth of tubercle bacilli is stimulated by "lecithin," ether, and alcohol extract of egg yolk; this discovery was corroborated by Boissevain and Schultz (1938).

Alcohol or ether extract of egg yolk, if added at a rate of 0.3 ml. per cent to the medium, enhances the growth of tubercle bacilli. Finlayson (1946) observed that saprophytic acid-fast bacilli grow moderately well on egg white and on defatted egg yolk media. Human, bovine, and avian types of tubercle bacilli did not grow on these media (Dorset, 1903). The factor stimulating the growth of pathogenic tubercle bacilli on egg yolk was found to be the phosphatide fraction of yolk. Dubos (1949) separated sphingomyelin, a substance with a growth-enhancing effect on tubercle bacilli, from livers and brains of animals. This substance is also present in egg yolk. Eggerth (1950), confirming the findings of Besredka (1913, 1921), showed that autoclaved egg yolk, diluted twenty times with distilled water, supports the growth of tubercle bacilli, if heavily planted. In this medium the growth of 10^{-8} mg. of tubercle bacilli was possible when a phosphate solution, instead of water, was used for diluting. When extracted with acetone, egg yolk does not lose its growth-stimulating properties. However, a further extraction of this material with hot alcohol removes the growth-stimulating properties of the egg yolk.

J. G. Hirsch (1954) attempted to isolate and identify the constituents of egg yolk that stimulate the growth of tubercle bacilli. The growth-stimulating factor was not soluble in water and resisted heating in the autoclave. The substance extracted from egg yolk by organic solvents showed only slight growth stimulation. The growth-stimulating substance in these solutions was identified as cholesterol. The residue obtained after the extraction of egg yolk with organic solvents highly stimulated the growth of tubercle bacilli. The substance responsible for this action was not identified.

Another substance promoting the growth of tubercle bacilli was found in potatoes. Thompson (1929) found that this substance is not a vitamin B–like compound. Extraction of autoclaved potatoes with organic solvents did not remove the active principle from the potato. Extraction of potato residue with 2 per cent trichloracetic acid removed starchy materials from the potato, leaving behind cellulose and protein residue. The active principle was not in the protein but in the nonprotein fraction of the potato. Potato ashes did not stimulate the growth of tubercle bacilli. Potato starch and starches of corn, wheat, and rice all showed the ability to stimulate the growth of small inocula (10^{-6} mg.) of tubercle bacilli. Soluble starch, when added to Long's synthetic medium, has a pronounced stimulating effect on the growth. The presence of 0.02 per cent of soluble starch had the same effect as 0.5 per cent of dextrin (Merck). Glucose, maltose, and inosite slightly stimulated the growth of large inocula (1 mg.), but did not influence the growth if only a small number of bacilli were planted. The findings of Thompson were corroborated by Uyei (1930).

The liver of animals was early recognized as containing substances stimulating the growth of tubercle bacilli. Corper, Fiala, and Kallon (1919) observed that a medium containing liver produced better growth of tubercle bacilli than the medium of Petroff. Liver juice and liver broth were used by many investigators to improve the growth of tubercle bacilli. Böcker (1923) employed these juices to produce submerged growth of tubercle bacilli; Moureau and Gruvel (1926) made a comparative study of the influence of glycerol extracts of liver and other organs on the growth of tubercle bacilli.

Our investigation of this problem (1948) revealed that horse liver is particularly rich in substances stimulating the growth of mycobacteria. The saline extract of organs, after filtration through a Seitz filter, was added to a glycerol agar medium which then was inoculated with a 40-day-old culture of *M. butyricum*.

After 12 to 24 hours of incubation at 37°C. an explosive growth of the *M. butyricum* occurred, whereas controls without liver substance showed only feeble incipient growth. The stimulation is well marked in tubercle bacilli and in Gram-positive bacilli. The growth-stimulating substance, in our experiment, was found not to be vitamin B-complex.

Table 17. Concentration in Organs of Man and Horse of Substances Promoting the Growth of Old *Mycobacterium butyricum* on Glycerol Agar

Organ	Man	Horse
Liver	1:100	1:10,000
Spleen	1:10	1:1,000
Kidney	1:1	1:100
Lung	0	...*
Heart muscle	0	...*
Brain	0	...*
Blood serum	1:1	1:1

* Organs not investigated.

The organs of the guinea pig and the rabbit have growth-stimulating values which are superior in effectiveness to those of man but inferior to those of the horse. Our recent investigations (1957, unpublished) showed that ribonucleic acid (0.2 per cent in a liquid medium) is the most powerful growth stimulant of acid-fast bacilli.

Agar definitely inhibits the growth of tubercle bacilli when added to the synthetic medium in an amount exceeding 0.1 or 0.25 per cent (Drea, 1940). Ordinary commercially prepared agar contains fatty acids which inhibit the growth of microorganisms. These acids are difficult to separate from agar (Ley and Mueller, 1946). The addition of proteins to agar greatly improves the growth of tubercle bacilli. This improvement of the growth of tubercle bacilli is attributed to the protective action of proteins against the bacteriostatic action of fatty acids (Dubos and Davis, 1946, 1947; Darzins, 1956). (See p. 113.)

Hematin, recognized by Hohn in 1931 as stimulating the growth of tubercle bacilli, was found by other investigators to be devoid of such a capacity (Mazzetti, 1932). Hemoglobin is capable of inhibiting the growth of tubercle bacilli (R. Davies, 1939). According to Cohn, Kovitz, Oda, and Middlebrook (1954), growth-supporting substances, such as liver extract, hemin, and serum albumin, have catalase-like activity.

Growth Factors and Trace Elements

The filtrates of old cultures of acid-fast bacilli, added in small amounts to the cultures of tubercle bacilli, favor the growth of the bacilli. The action of these filtrates is increased by heating them to 100°C. but abolished by dry heat at 170°C. The action is not specific (Borrel, Boez, and Coulon, 1923b).

In 1940 Woolley and McCarter, by extracting *Mycobacterium phlei* with boiling water and acetone, obtained a product that stimulates the growth of *M. johnei*, a microorganism that does not grow on plain egg media. The obtained oily material was assumed to have a naphthoquinone structure and to be related to phthiocol and vitamin K, the antihemorrhagic factor. Francis *et al.* (1949) isolated from *M. phlei* a crystalline aluminum derivative which promoted the growth of *M. johnei*, but was not naphthoquinone. In their experiments neither phthiocol nor vitamin K was capable of promoting the growth of *M. johnei*.

Vitamin B-complex is formed by tubercle bacilli. Pope and Smith (1946) found amounts of vitamins in 100 ml. filtrates of H37Rv and Ravenel strains of bacilli grown for six weeks on modified Proskauer-Beck medium, as shown in the accompanying tabulation.

Vitamin	*H37Rv*	*Ravenel*
Biotin	0.002 μg/100 ml	0.001 μg/100 ml
Folic acid	0.015	0.002
Para-aminobenzoic acid	0.020	0.002
Thiamine	0.041	0.014
Riboflavin	0.330	0.060
Pantothenic acid	0.410	0.140
Pyridoxine	0.440	0.090
Inositol	14.170	1.280
Nicotinic acid	37.500	0.740

Seven out of ten tested vitamins, including vitamin C, had no effect on the growth of H37Rv and H37Ra bacilli. Thiamin, inositol, niacin, niacinamide, and coenzyme I were inhibitory in high concentrations to both strains (Holmgren and Youmans, 1952).

Cortisone

Hart and Rees (1950) inoculated 0.0006 mg. dry weight of tubercle bacilli into mice, which had as a result the appearance of nonprogressive tuberculosis in six to twelve weeks. The lesions exacerbated markedly in the mice, which were given daily subcutaneous injections of 0.25 to 0.5 mg. of cortisone during two to three weeks in the stable period of infection.

Spain and Molomut (1950) infected guinea pigs with 0.2 mg. of the H37Rv strain of tubercle bacilli and administered 5 mg. of cortisone acetate to the animals daily. The treated animals developed more extensive, more widely spread and less localized tuberculous lesions than the controls.

Harris and Harris (1950) showed that, in rabbits and guinea pigs sensitized with BCG, cortisone suppresses the dermal reaction to old tuberculin. Four days after the injection of cortisone the skin reaction became positive again.

R. Bloch, Vennesland, and Gurney (1951) administered to tuberculous guinea pigs 5 mg. of cortisone daily. This treatment promoted the development of tuberculous lesions, interfered with the therapeutic effect of the streptomycin therapy of the animals, and, in 50 per cent of the animals, abolished the specific sensitivity to tuberculin.

Uelinger and Siebenmann (1952) found that initial necrosis of the intradermal and corneal tuberculin reaction is not prevented by cortisone, which is only capable of subduing the inflammatory reaction.

The American Trudeau Society (1952) collected data on the action of cortisone or corticotropin on tuberculous infection in man and in experimental animals. Hormone therapy, in 46 cases of active and inactive human tuberculosis out of a total of 81, had a devastating effect on the infected body. Thirty-nine papers published on the effect of cortisone or corticotropin on experimental tuberculosis show striking differences in the results obtained. The type of infection, the dosage of the hormone, and the duration of therapy all influence the results. The hormones may convert the chronic tuberculosis of mice into acute disease. These hormones have no significant effect on tubercle bacilli *in vitro*.

PART THREE

The Isolation and Identification of the Tubercle Bacillus

XII

The Collection of Tuberculous Material

WHEN tubercle bacilli invade an organism previously affected by tuberculosis, they meet with a highly sensitized tissue which reacts to the renewed infection with the death of local tissue or caseation necrosis. This defense mechanism of the organism is a result of the contact between the allergic tissue and the tuberculous antigens and is a by-product of the infection. This defense reaction will, to a great extent, determine the issue of the infection itself. From the moment of the caseation of the tissue on, the organism is combating not only the invasion of tubercle bacilli but also its own dead tissue. The caseated area is from the start a solid, dead, foreign body in the living organ. In this dead tissue the tubercle bacilli are rare until the solid caseum has progressively softened, leaving the fiber-walled cavity filled with liquid and with dead cells. The walls of the cavity contain a few tubercle bacilli but the necrotic internal masses are the breeding medium of tubercle bacilli in the living organism (Koch, 1882; Canetti, 1946, 1955).

The cavity may be connected with the outside atmosphere by a draining bronchus, through which the content of the cavity is discharged. The atmospheric pressure governs the inside of the cavity; the interpleural pressure on the outside is weaker. Because of this, a spontaneous collapse of the cavity is prevented and the tubercle bacilli in the cavity receive the oxygen necessary for their growth.

With caseation and the formation of a cavity, the tuberculous process has definitely gained a hold on the organ; phthisis has developed. A cavity isolated as a foreign body in the organ may last for many years and produce countless generations of bacilli, which may invade new areas of the host or find new victims outside.

The tuberculous infection exists long before the caseation of the tissue has started (closed tuberculosis) but unfortunately in most closed cases the tubercle bacilli are eliminated and may be detected only after the liquefaction of a caseum and cavity formation (open tuberculosis). Rist and Ameuille demonstrated in 1927 that pulmonary tuberculosis may remain closed by three mechanisms: when (a) the localization of the process is strictly interstitial; (b) the outlet of the cavity or the draining bronchus is blocked; (c) the exudate is extremely thick.

Are these closed forms of lung tuberculosis rare? This is still an unanswered question. Cordier indicated in 1927 that from 1 to 2.5 per cent of all cases of lung tuberculosis, mostly among teenagers, are closed. Minimal open tuberculosis may also elude our present-day laboratory and X-ray diagnostic methods. Because of this, there are authors who regard these methods as only supplements to the clinical diagnostic procedures. For Rolland (1952) the laboratory and X-ray procedures presently in use are based on the myth of "*Le Rouge et le Noir*" (red bacilli, black X-ray film), just like the magic of Stendhal's novel. This view embodies a revolt against the oversimplification of, and disregard for, the human and individual side of the disease and also against the inefficiency of diagnostic methods; but when Rolland says, "*Il faut, une fois pour toutes, s'affranchir de la mystique totalitaire de la bactériologie en matière de diagnostique de la tuberculose,*" he gives way to a dangerous attempt to replace science by clinical mysticism.

Tuberculosis has no other cause than the tubercle bacillus discovered by Koch, and there is no tuberculosis without this bacillus. Clinical diagnosis of tuberculosis, by such means as percussion and auscultation, X-ray examination, or tuberculin testing, is presumptive. Definite diagnosis of tuberculosis is established only by the identification of the tubercle bacilli in the pathologic material collected from the patient. Contrary to the opinion of Aronson and Whitney (1930) and some other investigators, there are no healthy carriers of tubercle bacilli. All material containing tubercle bacilli is pathologic, eliminated from the foci of infection. This conclusion is based on the results of the thorough work of Feldman and Baggenstoss (1939) and others.

Feldman and Baggenstoss investigated material cautiously taken from the upper and lower lobes of the lungs and the hilar and tracheobronchial lymph nodes of 50 bodies. In 12 of these bodies no gross or microscopic tuberculous lesions were found, in 38 other cases there were lesions of latent or healed tuberculosis. Three emulsions were prepared from the tissues of each body and injected into 6 guinea pigs. The guinea pigs were inoculated with material taken from the apparently nontuberculous parts of the organs. Only in 2 out of 300 animals inoculated were tubercle bacilli found. In one case the tubercle bacilli were of the bovine type, in the other they were discovered in the guinea pig inoculated with the material taken from the hilar lymph nodes. Pathogenic tubercle bacilli were absent even in the healthy tissue of arrested or latent cases of lung tuberculosis.

Collection of Tuberculous Material

To the physician the discovery of tubercle bacilli eliminated from a patient establishes the diagnosis of open tuberculosis and indicates the further treatment of a patient. To the patient, this discovery complicates and profoundly changes the mental, physical, social, and material aspects of his future life. A physician should announce the discovery of the tubercle bacillus to a patient only when he is sure of the diagnosis and has carefully considered the issue.

A bacteriologist is directly responsible for the diagnosis of tuberculosis, and therefore he must make use of the most refined procedures of extracting tubercle bacilli from their breeding places or trapping them on their way out of the organism, and apply the methods actually recognized as the best for the identification of tubercle bacilli.

The detection of the early tuberculous infection is achieved with the aid of the tuberculin reaction. The tuberculin test is the only fine screen available in the diagnosis of the first tuberculous infection in children. It detects the presence of the infection long before other methods of examination are of any avail (Myers and Harrington, 1934), although the positive tuberculin test does not indicate clinical tuberculosis. Tuberculin testing cannot replace the bacteriologic diagnosis of tuberculosis.

Sputum

Tuberculosis of the lungs is the most frequent form of human tuberculosis and sputum is the pathologic material most important in the detection of the disease.

Only in the upper parts of the respiratory tract does the ciliary movement have a propulsive action on the secreted mucus; the lower part of the respiratory tract is without cilia. The thick secretions in the alveoli are diluted or liquefied by the secretions from the glands of the bronchial mucosa, and moved out by the kinetic energy of the respired air (see reviews by Gordonoff, 1938; and Basch, Holinger, and Poncher, 1941).

"Sputum" is a collective name for all that is evacuated from the mouth with the exception of vomited stomach content or blood (Steigner, 1949). In addition to the pathologic material expectorated from lungs and bronchi, which is "sputum" in the strict sense, the same name "sputum" is applied to saliva and to secretions from nasal, laryngeal, pharyngeal, and mouth cavities.

The results of the investigation of tubercle bacilli are greatly influenced by the material, often of varying bacteriologic value, delivered to the laboratory. Due to this, particular attention must be given to the collection of undiluted and uncontaminated sputum, and ingenious methods have been invented for the extraction of such material from the body.

The secondary infection of the pulmonary tissue in tuberculosis is rare, whereas the secondary infection of the necrotic contents of the cavities is very common. In cases of the latter kind the sputum contains a large quantity of different non-acid-fast microorganisms.

In cases of the tuberculosis of the urinogenital tract, tubercle bacilli are found in urine; in intestinal tuberculosis, or when bacilli are swallowed with sputum, the bacilli are found in the contents of the stomach and in the feces. In cases of tuberculous bacillemia, tubercle bacilli may be found in the blood, urine, feces, and gastric washings (see p. 177).

Diagnostic biopsy (regional lymph node biopsy, aspiration, joint and bone biopsy) is an important procedure for the early separation of tuberculous from nontuberculous infections. The diagnosis should rest on the firm bacteriologic and histologic proof of a tuberculous infection and not on a clinical estimation which is often unreliable (Mills, Owen, and Strach, 1956).

In general, the diagnostic procedures prescribed for sputum are applicable to any other tuberculous material.

A small quantity of sputum, produced in nonactive cases of tuberculosis, may remain in the bronchi or the upper respiratory tract. Often it goes unnoticed by the patient and is expectorated gradually, mixed with saliva or swallowed mainly in the case of children and women. It is possible to extract this pathologic material from the bronchial passages by the introduction of water into the bronchi (bronchial lavage), by catching it up in absorbent cotton in the laryngeal passages (laryngeal swab), or by aspiration from the stomach after it has been swallowed (gastric lavage). All these methods for collecting sputum apply to pathologic material expelled from its place of formation in the lung, but we have no methods for collecting material directly at the site of its formation.

The qualitative investigation of patients' sputum may lead to the discovery of tubercle bacilli. The quantitative estimation of bacilli in sputum provides information about the patient as a potential public health problem and may lead to some suggestions for therapy and prognosis.

Gastric Lavage

The extraction of swallowed poisonous substances from the stomach is an ordinary medical procedure. It was Meunier (1898) who first thought of extracting swallowed sputum from the stomach in the search for tubercle bacilli. The absence of sputum in children directed some investigators, among them Kossel in 1895, to search for bacilli in their feces, until Meunier observed that swallowed sputum containing tubercle bacilli remains for some time in the stomach. The bacilli are not destroyed there and may be found in the morning contents of the fasting stomach. "*C'est dans l'estomac que je conseille d'aller chercher, par un simple lavage, les sécrétions bronchiques dégluties par l'enfant, et c'est dans les crachats ainsi obtenus que je poursuis la recherche du bacille*" (Meunier).

Collection of Tuberculous Material

Meunier (1898) was ahead of his time. Staining and animal inoculation were the only methods of diagnosis for the identification of tubercle bacilli at the disposal of the investigators of those days. Meunier used the staining method to identify acid-fast bacilli. In his brief communication he presented the rather unimpressive results he had obtained. Examining gastric specimens from 17 children and 4 adults, he discovered acid-fast bacilli in three of the specimens. In a second series of 13 observations the method identified one positive case of tuberculosis, which was later verified by autopsy. The publication of Meunier aroused little attention on the part of the physicians of that time.

Thirty years later, Armand-Delille and Vibert (1927), fellow countrymen of Meunier, described Meunier's technique again. Microscopic investigation with added homogenization and concentration of the material revealed acid-fast bacilli in 34 cases out of a total of 110 examined. In later publications, 1936 and 1937, Armand-Delille and his co-workers broadened the application of the method for use with adults and showed its efficacy in detecting different forms of tuberculosis in children. Out of a total of 594 cases of primary tuberculosis or tuberculous reinfection, 57 per cent were positive for tubercle bacilli on gastric lavage.

After these publications and after the introduction of the considerably easier nasal route for the aspiration of liquid, the method was universally recognized as the most reliable for collecting tuberculous material in the absence of expectorated sputum. Of the abundant publications on this subject (Robinson and Dunn (1943) compiled a list of 124, published all over the globe), we will mention only a few.

Stadnichenko, Cohen, and Sweany (1940), inoculating guinea pigs with the gastric specimens from 940 persons whose sputum was negative on direct examination, obtained 249 or 26.5 per cent positive cases. In 1,000 gastric specimens from 738 persons from whom no expectorations had been obtained, Robinson and Dunn (1943) found 303 cases (33 per cent) containing tubercle bacilli. Guinea pigs were tuberculous in 24.4 per cent of the cases and the cultures revealed tubercle bacilli in 22.5 per cent. In 105 patients no tracheobronchial or pulmonary lesions were revealed by X-ray film, but in 21 per cent of these cases tubercle bacilli were detected by gastric lavage.

The chief domain of gastric lavage is the tuberculosis of childhood, as had already been stressed by Meunier and Armand-Delille.

The positivity of gastric specimens for tubercle bacilli declines with advancing age. Langer (1933) showed that one-year-old children with active lung tuberculosis produced 70 per cent positive gastric specimens, two-to-three-year-old children, 62 per cent; but between three and six only 17 per cent of the specimens were positive. Among males under twenty, the specimens were positive in 30 per cent of the cases and in the age group over forty, in 14 per cent of the cases (Robinson and Dunn, 1943). In women these age differences are not so clear-cut because of frequent swallowing of sputum in order to avoid its elimination. Opitz (1933) emphasizes the fact that the normal sedimentation time and the normal blood picture in children do not anticipate the results of culture or animal inoculation of gastric lavage specimens.

According to Cantonnet, Murguía, Cantonnet, and Lieutier (1938), cultures or guinea pig inoculations of 1,563 gastric specimens were positive for tubercle bacilli in children afflicted with hilar shadows in 11 per cent of the cases; with early infiltrates in 81 per cent; with epituberculosis in 32 per cent; with perifocal infiltrations in 28 per cent; with fibrous and ulcerous tuberculosis in 78 per cent; with tuberculosis of the bones and joints in 23 per cent; with tuberculous pneumonia in 100 per cent; and with terminal cases of tuberculosis in 100 per cent.

The discovery of tubercle bacilli in gastric specimens hints at early tuberculous lesions of the lungs, frequently concealed by the diaphragm or the heart. Reaction to tuberculin is generally positive in the presence of tubercle bacilli in the gastric contents. If positive in babies in the first year of life, gastric lavage indicates active tuberculosis.

Sources of tubercle bacilli in gastric contents. The mechanism responsible for the passage of sputum and bronchial secretions from the lungs into stomach may be other than the conscious swallowing of sputum. The contractile muscle fibers form a loose extensive network around the respiratory tubes but disappear in the terminal respiratory bronchioli. Reinberg (1925) and Hudson and Jarre (1929) showed by X-ray photographs that foreign material is expelled from the trachea by peristalsis-like motion without producing a cough. Ulmar and Ornstein (1933) injected iodized oil into the bronchial tree of a patient. After a while X-ray examination revealed that the entire amount of the oil was in the stomach. In no instance did the patient cough. In two other instances the X-ray showed actual spilling over of the iodized oil from the trachea into the esophagus without provoking a cough.

Doubt may arise whether positive gastric specimens always indicate tuberculosis of the person in which the bacilli are discovered. Can transitory tubercle bacilli remain in the gastric contents if swallowed with food?

Debré, Saenz, Broca, and Costil (1936) never discovered tubercle bacilli in gastric contents unaccompanied by tuberculous lesions in the organism. Gad (1937) investigated 23 healthy adult persons and was never able to find tubercle bacilli in their stomach contents. Stadnichenko, Cohen, and Sweany (1940) found that patients with completely healed tuberculosis lesions and nontuberculous diseases uniformly showed no tubercle bacilli in gastric washings.

Besides the pulmonary source another possible origin of tubercle bacilli in gastric contents and feces must be considered. The excretion of tubercle bacilli with bile is intermittent and difficult to determine. Calmette and Guérin (1909) investigated the elimination of tubercle bacilli in the bile of rabbits infected intravenously with bacilli of the bovine type. The rabbits were sacrificed at different times after the infection and their centrifuged bile inoculated into guinea pigs. Bile of animals killed 24 hours, 48 hours, 5 days, and 6 days after the infection did not produce tuberculosis; the bile taken on the third and fourth day after the infection produced tuberculosis in three out of eight guinea pigs inoculated. Perla (1927) infected guinea pigs intraperitoneally with 0.001 mg. of tubercle bacilli and found bacilli in the feces, bile, and urine of the animals. Pezzangora (1936) infected 26 guinea pigs orally with tubercle bacilli and ten days later no tubercle bacilli were found in their duodena. No lesions were left in the digestive tract, but the mesenteric and ileocecal glands of the animals were infected.

An experimental verification of the problem of whether tubercle bacilli found in gastric washings may in some cases have their origin in the blood stream and pass from it into the stomach contents was made by Obrant and Sievers (1950). The esophagi of seven guinea pigs were ligated and 1 mg. of virulent H37Rv strain of tubercle bacilli was injected intravenously into the animals. Four to five hours later the animals were killed and their stomachs opened and irrigated with 10 ml. of saline which was then inoculated on Löwenstein's medium and into guinea pigs. Out of seven guinea pigs investigated four showed tubercle bacilli in their stomach contents. One of four inoculated rabbits had tubercle bacilli in its stomach lavage. Tubercle bacilli injected intravenously produced bacillemia and passed through the wall into the stomach.

Rubinstein (1950) found tubercle bacilli in gastric lavages of rabbits which had been infected intravenously with tubercle bacilli 30 to 60 minutes earlier or subcutaneously 2 hours earlier. Kirchheimer, Hess, Williston, and Youmans (1950) injected intravenously 0.05 mg. of H37Rv strain of tubercle bacilli into mice. After the death of the animals virulent tubercle bacilli were detected in the gastric washings. Feces collected from these animals 7, 14, and 27 days after the injection contained tubercle bacilli. No lesions were found in their digestive tracts. The authors assumed that the sources of the bacilli in the gastric contents and the feces were the pulmonary lesions of the mice.

Löwenstein (1925) published data on the regular presence of tubercle bacilli in the blood stream of some patients affected by diseases regarded as nontuberculous. Kallós and Kallós-Deffner (1932, 1934) collected 250 works by authors of various nationalities, discussing the findings of Löwenstein. With one exception, the authors did not confirm these findings. Without tuberculosis there are no tubercle bacilli in the blood.

Opitz (1930) investigated seven cases of tuberculous meningitis and in all of them found tubercle bacilli in the gastric lavages.

Another source of tubercle bacilli in gastric contents, although a rare one, might be tuberculous lesions of the stomach itself. According to Good (1931), stomach tuberculosis, as discovered by surgery, makes up 0.34 per cent of all tuberculosis cases, according to Kabuki (1942) 0.11 per cent. It is a disease of adults and half of the cases are associated with tuberculosis of other organs.

The sources of error in gastric washings are the attenuated and saprophytic acid-fast bacilli. The cultivation methods make the differentiation between saprophytic and pathogenic mycobacteria possible. In some cases animal inoculation gives a decisive answer (see p. 300).

Action of gastric juice on tubercle bacilli. Gastric juice is not harmless to tubercle bacilli. After the famous experiments of Spallanzani, who lived from 1725 to 1799, showing that digestion is not a process of putrefaction, the problem of the action of the gastric juice on microorganisms became the object of a vast amount of research.

One of the first works dealing with the action of gastric juice on tubercle bacilli grown on glycerol agar was that of Straus and Wurtz (1889). Tubercle bacilli were introduced into gastric juice taken from a dog. After six hours of incubation at 38°C. this culture produced generalized tuberculosis in rabbits and guinea pigs. After eight to twelve hours of incubation, the culture caused only local abscesses, and after twelve to thirty-six hours the culture was harmless to the test animals. Cadéac and Bournay (1893) fed the flesh of tuberculous animals to dogs, and then inoculated rabbits with the contents of the dogs' stomachs and intestines and with their feces. Twelve and twenty-four hours after the infective meals, the presence of pathogenic tubercle bacilli was confirmed in all parts of the digestive tract and in the feces of the dogs.

Fernbach and Rullier (1924) showed that 210 ml. of artificial gastric juice consisting of 0.5 g. pepsin and 10 drops of hydrochloric acid in 70 ml. of water, mixed with 100 ml. of sputum containing five bacilli per field, destroyed these bacilli if heated for three hours at 50°–52°C. and in 37 hours at 15°C. If stained, they retained a small amount of color (Mylius and Sartorius, 1924). Rapid destruction of the viability of tubercle bacilli in gastric juice was observed by Floyd, Novack, and Page (1942), Kramer (1946), and Schwarting (1948). Kramer found that after 10 hours of the action of normal gastric juice at 37°C., sputum began to lose pathogenicity and was innocuous after 21 hours of exposure. Sprick and Towey (1946) divided gastric specimens in three parts, thirty-three specimens each; the first part was cultured immediately, the second was kept for 24 hours at room temperature, and the third one was kept for 48 hours at room temperature. The first part produced 24 positive cultures, the second 15, and the third 7. Kabler and Lundholm (1949) obtained a significantly reduced number of positive cultures from gastric juice stored for 24 hours at 4°C., either undiluted, diluted with distilled or buffered water, or neutralized with sodium bicarbonate.

Tubercle bacilli survive for hours in such feeble solutions of hydrochloric acid as are found in gastric juice (Kramer, 1946). The influence of gastric juice on the tubercle bacilli must be attributed to the joint action of acid and enzymes in the juice. This view is supported by the fact that the action of refrigerated juice on the bacilli is slower. To counteract the action of the juice on bacilli, the neutralization of the juice was proposed. Armstrong (1948) recommended the addition of an equal part of a 25 per cent solution of trisodium phosphate to the gastric juice. The strongly alkaline salt neutralizes the juice and the viability of bacilli is better preserved. Beattie (1949) showed that trisodium phosphate reduces the number of viable tubercle bacilli after a prolonged action on them.

Hylkema and Onvlee (1951) treated one part of a gastric specimen with 3 per cent hydrochloric acid for 30 minutes, the other part with trisodium phosphate at room temperature for 24 hours. The first part produced 100 colonies, the second 39. The addition of trisodium phosphate to the gastric juice might be effective if the specimens are delayed en route to the laboratory but is not otherwise necessary. Kabler and Lundholm (1949), by adding crystalline disodium phosphate to gastric specimens before storage at room temperature, increased the number of positive cultures but slightly. MacVandiviere, Smith, and Sunkes (1952) compared the results of cultivation and animal inoculation of gastric specimens containing few tubercle bacilli, immediately after their collection and 72 hours later. In order to enable the evaluation of the most efficient measures to protect the viability of bacilli in delayed material, the specimens were (1) diluted with water; (2) neutralized with Na_2HPO_4; (3) diluted and neutralized (1.5 ml. of Na_2HPO_4 solution added to the specimens neutralized approximately 45 ml. of $N/10$ HCl). Diluted specimens lost 71.6 per cent, neutralized ones 39.1 per cent, and diluted and neutralized ones 24.3 per cent of their positivity compared to specimens cultivated immediately. The old way – the immediate culturing of gastric specimens – was still the best.

The swallowing of sputum in pulmonary tuberculosis is not without effect on the function of the stomach. It plays an important role in diminishing its motility and secretory activity and leads to delayed and disordered digestion of food (Mohler and Funk, 1916).

Gastric lavage has a diagnostic, prophylactic, therapeutic, and prognostic value. (Cantonnet, Murguía, Cantonnet, and Lieutier, 1938). It is a tool for separating active, open tuberculosis from closed forms of the disease.

Gastric lavage should be adopted as the ultimate standard of negativity for tubercle bacilli and for the purpose of determining the results of therapy.

Bronchial Lavage

The idea of extracting pathologic material in the same way as foreign bodies are extracted from the bronchi is not new. The aspiration of secretions through a tube introduced into anesthetized bronchial passages was attempted, but this method is too complicated to be accepted in routine practice. It was considerably simplified by the Brazilian scientist, de Abreu (1944, 1945, 1947). De Abreu's procedure for collecting sputum from the upper respiratory tract is at present widely used in South America. This method would be useful in many cases, particularly to obtain sputum where there is no direct expectoration or the sputum is scarce.

De Abreu (1947) describes his technique as follows. The patient should be in a sitting position, bending slightly backwards, (gargle position); anesthesia of pillars, uvula, and the pharynx is induced by means of 1 ml. of a 0.5 per cent solution of novotucaine, pantocaine, or chlorhydrate of tetracine. (In 1951–1952, we used in Bahia a 1 per cent solution of cocaine sterilized in an autoclave.) The anesthetic is applied in small portions at the moment of inspiration. After five minutes, when insensitivity is achieved (this must be ascertained) 10 to 20 ml. of saline solution is slowly dropped by a syringe over the tongue into the bronchi at the moment of inspiration. The cough thus provoked expels sputum and saline solution.

De Abreu (1947), after performing 1,100 bronchial lavages (he calls them "pulmonary lavages"), declared his technique reliable. Some authors (Machado Filho, 1945) speak about the possibility of introducing pathogenic microorganisms through the mouth into the lungs and of possible irritation and dispersion of bacilli in the lungs. Up to now such cases are not known (Ibarra, 1948).

A relatively large amount of material has been published, chiefly in the South American countries, on the efficacy of bronchial lavage for the detection of tubercle bacilli. Magarão, Linhares, and Scorzelli (1948) inoculated into two guinea pigs and on Löwenstein's medium gastric and bronchial specimens taken from a large group of patients. The 1,516 bronchial specimens of inactive, residual, or minimal tuberculosis produced 67 or 4.4 per cent positive cases. In the same group of 1,248 patients, gastric lavage was positive in 55 or 4.4 per cent of cases. In cases of active tuberculosis, 393 out of 484 bronchial specimens, or 81.2 per cent, were positive; 352 gastric specimens of this group of patients were positive in 295 cases, or 83.8 per cent.

Burgos (1948), by direct examination and cultivation of 543 bronchial and gastric specimens which were collected simultaneously from 262 tuberculous patients, obtained 35 per cent positive cases by gastric lavage and 28.5 per cent by bronchial lavage. The cultivation in Bahia, Brazil, in the years 1950 and 1951, of material negative on direct examination, collected by bronchial lavage, revealed from 415 specimens, 144 or 34.7 per cent positive for tubercle bacilli. Sputa from 691 patients cultivated at the same time produced 289 or 41.8 per cent positive specimens. In both cases the shaking-precipitation (SP) method and Petragnani's medium were used. The cultivation results of material obtained by bronchial lavage must be considered good, because most of the patients who submitted to bronchial lavage produced little or no sputum at all and their lung lesions were small or minimal compared to most of the patients who produced large quantities of sputum. These results must be attributed to the fact that more concentrated and purer material is obtained through bronchial lavage than is eliminated in sputum. We found no difficulties in the technique and could observe no ill effects on the patients as the result of the intervention.

Laryngeal Swab

The gastric and bronchial lavage procedures have definite limitations in routine use. "The inconvenience for the patient, the complicated technique, time and cost involved, make this method [gastric lavage], although one of our best, unsuitable for serial examination on a large scale" (Nassau, 1941). By contrast, the laryngeal swab procedure is simple. It requires no anesthetic and may be applied at any time and on any patient. Schramek and Hegedüs (1935) call the laryngeal swab "the finest and most reliable method for investigating the sputum for tubercle bacilli."

Children, childish adults, and mentally ill patients are sometimes not cooperative in producing material by means of gastric or bronchial lavage In such cases it is possible to try the laryngeal swab.

The idea of the laryngeal swab first occurred to the Danish physician, Blume (1905, 1906). Observing tuberculosis in patients who did not cough or eliminate sputum, he asked them to cough against glass slides (1905) or extracted sputum from the larynx with the aid of a cotton swab (1906), and thus obtained material for the investigation of tubercle bacilli. This procedure is also often used to collect material for the investigation of diphtheria bacilli in the throats of patients.

To obtain material good for tubercle bacilli investigation, some precautions must be taken. It would not be satisfactory to swab the pharyngeal cavity and to extract mucus or saliva. Rather, a sterile cotton and gauze mop safely twisted on a slightly bent wire is passed behind the epiglottis. The majority of patients start coughing at this moment, discharging sputum particles on the swab. If there is no cough reflex, the patient is asked to cough. The face of the operator must be protected by a mask and by glasses against the infectious particles expelled by the patient. The removed mop is treated with acid or alkalies, and the sediment inoculated on or in media for tubercle bacilli.

The procedure was recommended by Jessen (1927). Behmann (1930) in 20 patients with open tuberculosis, detected tubercle bacilli in 19 cases by one swabbing. In a group of 150 patients he found more positive cases of tuberculosis with the swab procedure than by direct examination of sputum. Grass (1931) found the laryngeal swab procedure useful in dispensary practice. Brucke (1931) suggested the laryngeal swab to detect the dissimulation of open tuberculosis. The procedure was recommended by Bezançon, Braun, and Meyer (1937). In the experiments of Fraenkel (1944), the swab afforded more positive results than the culture of sputum. From 261 samples of laryngeal swab, 54 (20 per cent) revealed tubercle bacilli. Henry (1946) decontaminated material from the swabs and inoculated it into Kirchner's liquid medium. In some institutions the laryngeal swab is used as a basic procedure for collecting tuberculous material. Šula (1948) at the State Institute of Czechoslovakia in Prague, in the years 1944–1947, cultured 16,447 laryngeal swabs and found 2,459 (14.9 per cent) of them positive for tubercle bacilli. According to Šula, the simplicity of the method makes it invaluable in tracking down the sources of infection from among a large number of suspect cases.

Hounslow and Usher (1948) compared the results of tubercle bacilli cultivation of material obtained from tuberculous patients by gastric lavage and by the laryngeal swab method. The results obtained by three consecutive laryngeal swabbings were as good or better than from a simple gastric lavage. A comparative study of the efficiency of the laryngeal swab and that of gastric lavage was carried out on 100 hospital patients and on 101 outpatients by Forbes, Hurford, Smith, and Springett (1948). Two swabs were taken from every patient, decontaminated in 10 per cent sulfuric acid, neutralized with sodium hydroxide, and then rubbed on Löwenstein-Jensen's medium. Gastric specimens were treated with ferrous sulfate solution, 10 per cent sulfuric acid, and 1 per cent hydrogen peroxide. The deposit was inoculated on two tubes of the same medium. One hundred gastric specimens produced 42 positive cultures; 100 specimens from the laryngeal swab, 32. Lowys (1949) obtained results with the laryngeal swab equal to those with gastric lavage. Renoux and Français (1950), in 56 tuberculous patients with directly negative sputum, obtained 19 positive cultures using the laryngeal swab.

Armstrong (1951) cultured 976 gastric lavages and laryngeal swab specimens taken from sanatorium patients. For one lavage, triplicate swabs were taken: one before the lavage, one on the day of the lavage, and one on the day after it. The three consecutive swabs were almost twice as valuable in yielding positive cultures as one gastric lavage. Chaves, Peizer and Widelock (1953) compared the cultivation results of two laryngeal swabs and one gastric washing taken from 1,418 patients by inexperienced personnel in a large number of clinics. The laryngeal material was kept at room temperature for at least 24 hours; the gastric specimens were kept in a refrigerator. The gastric specimens produced 187 cultures and the swab specimens 135.

Laryngeal swab in mentally ill patients. A mentally ill tuberculous patient presents problems of handling, diagnosis, and treatment. Mental debility, tuberculosis, and advanced age are often associated with physical weakness. The elementary rules of hygiene are rejected by a great many such patients. This circumstance favors the spread of tuberculosis among the inmates of mental institutions. From the report of Bettag (1952), chairman of the committee of chest diseases in institutions of the American College of Chest Physicians, presented at the Anoka State Hospital, Anoka, Minnesota, we borrow the figures on distribution of tuberculosis among the inmates of mental institutions. In 1950, 231 institutions for the mentally ill with a population of 511,064, reported 13,911 cases of active tuberculosis, or 2,700 per 100,000 inmates, compared with the 80 cases per 100,000 in the general population of this country.

The rate of death from tuberculosis in the California hospitals for the mentally ill in 1946 was 800 per 100,000. The early detection and isolation of the open tuberculous patients brought down the death rate to 283 per 100,000 in 1953. The tuberculosis death rate of the state at that time was 11.4 per 100,000 (Oechsli, Kupka, and Bush, 1955).

The collection of tuberculous material from mentally ill patients is often a troublesome operation. This is particularly true of the collection of gastric specimens. In many cases sedatives must be administered. There are patients at the Anoka State Hospital on whom, because of their aggressive behavior, gastric lavage was never performed, or performed only a few times in several years. According to the findings of Burns (1945), in the mental institutions of Minnesota it would be extremely difficult to get a specimen of sputum from more than 2 or 3 per cent of these patients. Even if cooperative, most of them would not understand the difference between sputum and saliva.

These circumstances stimulated us (Darzins and Vitols, 1956) to investigate the possibility of the application of the laryngeal swab for collecting material for the investigation of tuberculosis in the mentally ill.

From the 422 mentally ill tuberculous patients at the Anoka State Hospital, 100 male and 100 female patients with recent positive gastric lavage were selected. The cultivation of gastric specimens was done in the laboratory of the state Board of Health, Minneapolis, Minnesota, where the material from Anoka was delivered on the day of its collection. One laryngeal swab was taken from each patient and the cultivation of the swab material was performed at the Anoka hospital laboratory. Out of 200 patients investigated by gastric lavage, 114 or 57 per cent had had, in the years 1952 and 1953, tubercle bacilli in their gastric contents. The results of the cultivation of gastric specimens were regarded as the standard; the results obtained by swab procedure were compared with them.

Most of the 200 patients examined were old inmates of Anoka State Hospital. A total of 2,681 gastric washings, or an average of 13.4 per patient, had been performed on them during the years of their stay at the hospital. In 1,151, or 43 per cent of the cases, these washings had been positive for tubercle bacilli.

The quantity of material obtained by the swab is very small compared with that delivered by gastric washing. The method of concentration by calcium phosphate precipitation was applied to the swab material. (See shaking-precipitation method, Chapter XVI). The treated material was inoculated on two tubes of egg-potato medium and in one tube of our liquid medium (Table 32). The solid medium was incubated for 6 weeks; the liquid medium was investigated after 14 days of incubation.

As Table 18 shows, gastric specimens in our patients were positive in 30.5 per cent of the cases. One swab per patient, concentrated and inoculated on solid and liquid media, revealed 24.5 per cent positive cases of tuberculosis. Gastric lavage and swab procedures produced 38 per cent positive cases. One swab added to one gastric lavage increased the positive results by 7.5 per cent. The value of the liquid media consists in the early results obtained and in the growth-producing pattern of mammalian tubercle bacilli, which renders possible the distinction between pathogenic tubercle bacilli and saprophytic acid-fast bacilli. (See Chapter XXII.)

The gastric lavage gave positive results in 45 mentally ill males and in 31 females. In sane patients gastric specimens are more frequently positive in the female than in the male (J. L. Robinson and Dunn, 1943). This difference probably indicates a characteristic finding about mental patients, where the so-called "esthetic factor," which leads more female than male patients to swallow sputum so as to avoid expectoration, is no longer valid.

Table 18. The Efficacy of the Gastric Lavage and the Laryngeal Swab Methods in Detecting Tubercle Bacilli in 200 Mentally Ill Patients

Method and Medium	Positive for Tubercle Bacilli		Standard Deviation
	No.	%	
Gastric lavage, solid medium	61	30.5	±3.25
Swab (1), solid and liquid media	49	24.5	±3.04
Gastric lavage and swab, solid and liquid media	76	38.0	±3.43
Swab, solid medium	46	23.0	±2.97
Swab, liquid medium	33	16.5	±2.62
Swab, positive in liquid medium only	3	1.5	±0.86

Source: Darzins and Vitols (1956).

XIII

Diagnostic Staining of Tubercle Bacilli

THE early discovery of a simple and highly effective method for staining tubercle bacilli secured for staining a place of great importance among the diagnostic procedures of tuberculosis, a place which it has kept for long years.

The staining method of Koch (1882) required a long time (24 hours), although Koch indicated that by heating the specimen to 40°C. the staining procedure could be shortened to half an hour. Koch's method was not sufficiently sensitive and failed in many instances (Ehrlich, 1913).

Ehrlich (1882), instead of using potassium hydroxide and methylene blue as Koch had, introduced the alkaline aniline oil solution of methylviolet. An important improvement was brought about by Ehrlich's discovery of the resistance of stained tubercle bacilli to the decolorizing action of acids. In his experiments even 33 per cent nitric acid did not decolorize the stained bacilli. The resistance of stained tubercle bacilli to acids was ascribed by Ehrlich to a protective coating of the bacterial cell, the *Hülle*. ("*Wenn nun aber dennoch der Tuberkelbacillus sich durch die Färbung von allen anderen Pilzen unterscheidet, so beruht dies auf dem Vorhandensein einer Hülle, der eigentümliche und spezifische Eigenschaften zukommen*".)

Bienstock (1886) attributed a fatty nature to this hypothetic protective layer. This explanation of the cause of acid-fastness was sanctioned by Ehrlich (1913) when the presence of large quantities of fatty substances was discovered in tubercle bacilli (Hammerschlag, 1891; Kresling, 1901). The fatty layer around the cells of acid-fast bacilli prevents them from being easily stained and, once they are stained, impedes the decolorizing of the bacilli by acids. The idea of the *Hülle* was widely accepted as an easy and plausible explanation for a difficult problem. The idea of a protective fatty layer around the acid-fast bacilli was to play an important role in further experimental and theoretical work in tuberculosis. The term *Schutzhülle* was used by Koch (1897) himself.

Isolation and Identification of Bacillus

In his review of the cytology and microchemistry of the tubercle bacillus, Knaysi (1929) attributed the acceptance of the notion of the *Hülle* to Calmette and some of his co-workers (Darzins, 1926b). This misunderstanding arose from an erroneous interpretation of the term "ectoplasm," which was used by these authors. There must be properties or compounds in the cell which retain the Gram stain, resist alcohol-acid decolorization of the cell, or retain the impregnated silver salts (Darzins, 1926b). These properties of the cell were supposed to be localized in the outer layer of the cell wall. For this layer Zettnow (1899) coined the term "ectoplasm." Churchman (1927) called it the "cortex." This cell layer consists of the cell wall, the cytoplasmic membrane, and probably the outer layer of the cytoplasm. This outer layer contains magnesium ribonucleate (Lamanna and Mallette, 1950), plays an important role in the Gram staining procedure (Bartholomew and Mittwer, 1951), and forms the physiologic unity of the cell. Ectoplasm has nothing in common with the hypothetic *Hülle* (see Eisenberg, 1909; and Gutstein, 1924).

Ehrlich's hypothesis that the alkaline properties of the stain are of importance in staining tubercle bacilli was demonstrated by Ziehl (1882) as not valid in the very year of the discovery of tubercle bacilli. Instead of the alkaline solution of methylviolet, Ziehl used, with results equal to those of Ehrlich, a solution of methylviolet in carbolic acid. The following year (1883) brought the work of Neelsen, an incidental contribution to the problem of tuberculosis with the following important footnote: ". . . I used as staining liquid a ¾ per cent solution of fuchsin in five per cent carbolic acid, with the addition of a bit of alcohol, decolorized in 25 per cent sulfuric acid." The staining method suggested in this footnote to Neelsen's work has resisted the impact of time. The highly stable solution of fuchsin in carbolic acid – which gives to the stained bacilli a brilliant red hue easily recognizable among the debris of pathologic material, uses inexpensive chemicals, is an easy procedure, and produces effective results – secured for the original Ziehl-Neelsen method first place among more than a hundred modifications of staining methods, and on its seventy-fifth anniversary it is still one of the best methods for staining tubercle bacilli.

Osol's Method

The combat against tuberculosis called for a refined method for detecting bacilli in pathologic material containing only a small number of bacilli. In this respect the method of Osol (1927) was an advance over the method of Ziehl-Neelsen. Osol's method is based on the observation that the number of discovered bacilli increases with the increase of the amount of material investigated or with the thickness of the film. In the Ziehl-Neelsen procedure and other techniques the thickness of the film is the limiting factor because the increase of thickness results in an increasing difficulty in decolorizing the slide. Even the strongest decolorizing agents leave red spots in thick preparations. Osol's method has overcome this difficulty and decolorizes completely.

Loll (1922) tried to apply the thick-film technique to the investigation of tubercle bacilli in feces and sputum, counterstaining the preparation with light methylene blue solution. This method attracted little attention on the part of laboratory workers.

According to Carvalho (1932), in order to detect by means of microscopic examination a tubercle bacillus in a thin layer of sputum, the material must contain not less than 100,000 bacilli per ml.; if a thick layer of the material is put on the slide, 10,000 bacilli per ml. are sufficient to allow detection. These circumstances favor Osol's technique. B. Lange (1932) indicated that Osol's principle of thick film is a procedure of concentrating bacilli and that it is understandable that it produces a richer yield than the ordinary film.

The material is spread in a thick layer on a slide. The fixed preparation is stained with carbolfuchsin for 3½ minutes. The stain is heated to the boiling point. The slide is decolorized with a 10 per cent solution of sulfuric acid until the red preparation becomes transparent. The smear is further decolorized with a mixture of five parts of 10 per cent sodium sulfite solution and one part of 96 per cent alcohol. The slide is dried without washing and without counterstaining. The red bacilli can be seen against a bluish or yellowish transparent ground throughout the smear.

As Osol reports, 6,451 sputa investigated in thick smears yielded 988 positive cases of tubercle bacilli (15.32 per cent), whereas the same material in ordinary smears, stained according to the Ziehl-Neelsen method, was positive in 654 cases (10.14 per cent).

The thick smear technique may be combined with the Antiformin concentration procedure (Osol, 1929).

The causes for the superiority of Osol's method to that of Ziehl-Neelsen were investigated by A. Johannson (1938). According to Johannson, the boiling of the material on the slide required by Osol's technique, which is avoided in the Ziehl-Neelsen procedure, stains an additional number of bacilli that the Ziehl-Neelsen technique leaves unstained. The results were particularly superior in cases where the material contained few bacilli. Another important factor responsible for the superiority of Osol's technique is the use of sodium sulfite as a second decolorizing agent. When sodium sulfite is added to the fuchsin solution decolorized with sulfuric, hydrochloric, or nitric acid, the fuchsin solution once more appears red. The tubercle bacilli in the smear, decolorized by acid, regain the red color when treated with sodium sulfite or alkali (ammonia). The decolorized bacilli do not reappear and cannot be seen when the Ziehl-Neelsen technique is employed.

Isolation and Identification of Bacillus

Osol's method was tested by Bartsch (1935), and Joseph (1936), and found superior to Ziehl-Neelsen's. Wissner (1947) recognized Osol's technique to be good for the detection of bacilli in a material containing only a small number of bacilli. Ficker (1940) compared the efficacy of Ziehl-Neelsen's and Osol's methods for revealing tubercle bacilli in smears. The smears of cultures of tubercle bacilli grown on glycerol agar were subjected to staining by both methods and the number of red and blue bacilli in Ziehl-Neelsen's preparations and the number of red bacilli in Osol's preparations were compared (see Table 19).

Table 19. Age of Tubercle Bacilli and Their Red and Blue Count in Five Sputa

Staining Technique	Percentage of Bacilli Stained		Total Bacilli in 5 Sputa
	21 Hours Old	3–4 Days Old	
Ziehl-Neelsen			2,406
Blue	40%	80–90%	
Red	60	20–10	
Osol			5,001
Red	100	100	

Source: Ficker (1940).

The Ziehl-Neelsen technique produced 2,406 bacilli in five sputa investigated, while Osol's technique made visible 5,001 bacilli in the same material.

The Ziehl-Neelsen technique was found to be particularly unfavorable for staining very young and old bacilli in that it reveals too few red bacilli.

Cultivation and inoculation of pathologic material are important diagnostic procedures of tuberculosis which cannot as yet be used in the diagnosis of leprosy. In leprosy the investigator is restricted to microscopy only and all procedures increasing the effectiveness of microscopy are of great importance to him.

Dubois (1944b) compared in 18 cases of leprosy the amount of bacilli on slides stained according to the Ziehl-Neelsen and Osol methods. He counted a total of 1,545 bacilli in 20 fields of a microscope when the Ziehl-Neelsen technique of staining was used, and 2,526 bacilli when Osol's technique was used. Dubois did not attribute the superiority of Osol's technique to the thickness of the smear. In cases of leprosy, only thin smears of nasal mucus could be made. The reappearance of decolorized bacilli after treatment with sulfite was responsible for the superiority of Osol's technique. Osol's technique, however, was not useful in examining histopathologic sections.

Diagnostic Staining of Tubercle Bacilli

Osol's Technique Combined with Dark Ground and Fluorescence Microscopy

Pothmann (1940) used dark ground illumination to investigate tubercle bacilli in pathologic material. The slides were stained according to Ziehl-Neelsen's and Osol's techniques. In dark ground illumination the bacilli in Osol's preparations were more clearly seen than had ever occurred before. In 1,150 microscope fields of 16 preparations, the Ziehl-Neelsen technique and dark ground illumination revealed 3,648 bacilli; the Osol technique 4,383. Fluorescence microscopy was not superior to the dark ground investigation of Osol's preparations.

Egli (1942), on the basis of a report by Pothmann, investigated the usefulness in clinical conditions of dark ground illumination combined with Osol's technique (see Table 20). He compared 310 samples of pathologic material (sputa, gastric washings, urine, etc.). In 15 cases material found negative by the Ziehl-Neelsen technique, but positive by Osol's technique, was cultured and was in all cases found positive for tubercle bacilli. In Osol's preparation, because of a completely decolorized ground and the lack of staining, the brilliant tubercle bacilli stand out clearly against a dark background.

Table 20. Osol's Technique with Dark Ground Microscopy Compared with the Ziehl-Neelsen Method with Dark Ground and Light Microscopy

	Ziehl-Neelsen, Light Microscopy	Ziehl-Neelsen, Dark Ground Microscopy	Osol, Dark Ground Microscopy
Tubercle bacilli positive....	46.6%	68.7%	100%
Counted in one minute......	1.93 bacilli	5.12 bacilli	11.63 bacilli
Slide found positive in......	266 seconds	156 seconds	85 seconds

Source: Egli (1942).

J. König (1951) investigated with a fluorescence microscope the tissue of tuberculous animals and compared the results with the results yielded by the investigation of the same material treated according to Osol's technique and observed with a light microscope. Tissue material was scratched off the surface of a cut, dried on the slide, and stained. Specimens from 56 organs (6 bovine lungs, 15 bovine lymph nodes, 4 chick livers, 2 cat lymph nodes, 3 guinea pig lymph nodes, etc.) were investigated by both methods. In the 6 bovine lung samples, Osol's technique revealed tubercle bacilli in two to ten minutes of investigation. In the fluoresence microscope the same material showed against a violet ground a great quantity of yellow, green, and reddish luminous particles. The observation of these particles with an oil immersion objective did not reveal them as tubercle bacilli. Out of the

15 bovine lymph nodes, 7 showed considerable caseation necrosis. In these cases Osol's technique secured diagnosis in 2 to 15 minutes; fluorescence microscopy did not permit a reliable identification of tubercle bacilli in the material. In cases of productive tuberculous process and the caseation or calcification of the tissue, fluorescence microscopy was not as efficient as Osol's method in detecting tubercle bacilli.

XIV

Fluorescence and Phase Contrast Microscopy as Diagnostic Procedures

HAGEMANN (1938) investigated tubercle bacilli in pathologic material with a fluorescence microscope and compared the results with those obtained with the Ziehl-Neelsen staining method. His results were extremely encouraging. In sputa confirmed by cultivation as tuberculous, the Ziehl-Neelsen staining method revealed 35 per cent of this material as positive, whereas fluoresence microscopy showed 70 per cent as positive; in the case of tuberculous urine, pus, and feces, fluorescence microscopy revealed 200 per cent more positive cases than the Ziehl-Neelsen method.

The publications of Hagemann and the creation by the Reichert Optical Company at Vienna of a simple and inexpensive fluorescence microscope enormously stimulated the expansion of fluorescence microscopy. These events were in turn responsible for the appearance of a great quantity of papers treating the same problem – the comparison of the efficacy of the fluorescence method with the Ziehl-Neelsen staining method in detecting tubercle bacilli in routine work. From the maze of figures contained in these papers it is easy to combine statistics favorable or unfavorable to fluorescence microscopy. Cruickshank (1947) published the statistics of eight authors (see Table 21) revealing the overwhelming superiority of fluorescence microscopy over the Ziehl-Neelsen method. The figures published by eight other authors are also presented in Table 21, which shows, in cases where the investigators based their conclusions on the results of the investigation of a few hundred specimens (Hauduroy and Posternak; Freiman and Mokotoff; and Fribourg-Blanc) that the superiority of the fluorescence method over the Ziehl-Neelsen method was from 2 to 4 per cent; in cases where around a thousand specimens were investigated, the difference between the two methods was statistically insignificant or zero.

Table 21 shows how uncertain conclusions based on unreliable statistical data may be. The results of the 16 studies using the fluorescence method oscillate between 52 per cent superior to those obtained by the Ziehl-

Table 21. Comparison of the Results of Fluorescence Microscopy with Those of the Ziehl-Neelsen Staining Method in Detecting Tubercle Bacilli

Author and Year	No. of Specimens Examined	% of Superiority of Fluorescence Microscopy over Ziehl-Neelsen
Didion (1939)*	702	14.2
Ritterhoff (1945)*	2,918	20.0
Bogen (1941)*	1,000	20.1
Schneider (1940)*	1,100	22.7
Richards *et al.* (1941)*	324	24.3
Lempert (1944)*	300	25.0 (approx.)
Luz and Meding (1940)*	1,000	36.0
Juricic *et al.* (1944)*	5,044	52.0
Dabelstein (1939)	900	0
Hauduroy and Posternak (1941)	115	3.0
Lind and Shaughnessy (1942)	1,221	1.0
Freiman and Mokotoff (1943)	192	2.1
Briggs and Jennison (1947)	500	−1.4†
Bekker (1948)	1,200	0.3
Fribourg-Blanc (1950)	281	4.3
Wilson (1952)	1,098	1.1

* Data from Cruickshank (1947).
† Fluorescence microscopy inferior to Ziehl-Neelsen method.

Neelsen method (Juricic) and 1.4 per cent inferior to the Ziehl-Neelsen method (Briggs and Jennison). The weakness of the fluorescence method cannot be remedied by collecting more statistical data but rather by research in the basic problems involved.

The original method of Hagemann has been modified by some researchers with the intention of eliminating some of its deficiencies. These modifications do not involve the basic technique but chiefly the staining procedure. The most widely known modification of Hagemann's method is that proposed by Herrmann (1938). To shorten the staining time to five minutes, he heated the auramine solution on a slide to the boiling point and decolorized it with 5 per cent acidified ethyl alcohol. To avoid some side fluorescence of the unstained ground, he counterstained the preparation with potassium permanganate and methylene blue solution. Briggs and Jennison (1947) reported that the modification of Herrmann was inferior to the original method because the deep-lying bacilli were covered by the counterstain and their fluorescence was not revealed.

G. C. Hughes (1946) announced an improved fluorochroming method, based on the observation of Graham (1943) that tubercle bacilli stained with a saturated solution of auramine and rhodamine-B have red fluorescence. Acid-fast bacilli when treated with the mixture of these fluorochromes were seen as orange-red rods on a yellow-green ground. Hughes' method is not so simple as the original method of Hagemann; the use of the right type of objective and eyepiece is absolutely essential.

Fluorescence and Phase Contrast Microscopy

The fluorescence technique is apparently of restricted value for the investigation of tubercle bacilli in tissue material. Schallock (1940) says that the elastic fibers and cholesterin showed a fluorescence comparable to that of tubercle bacilli, and the tissue treated with Antiformin or fixed in formalin longer than five days was unsuitable for investigation with a fluorescence microscope (Schallock, 1940; Petrovskaia, 1948). J. König (1951) found the fluorescence method unreliable for detecting tubercle bacilli in tissue material.

The difficulties of the fluorescence method have been summarized by Graham (1943) as follows: "the method is not ready for general use until it has been evaluated by test under the most favorable conditions that can be afforded by the average laboratory." Andrade (1951) compared the acid- and alcohol-fastness, fluorescence, and virulence of *Mycobacterium tuberculosis*, rat leprosy bacilli, and saprophytic mycobacteria. He concluded that there is not a complete correlation between these properties of mycobacteria. Fluorescence is a variable property of mycobacteria and is not sufficient to make a definite diagnosis of tuberculosis. Kölbel (1952) reported that "to take full advantage of the fluorescence method, a careful adjustment of all mutually connected parts, such as the source of light, optical system and filters, must be obtained."

It must be concluded from the reported results that the fluorescence method is influenced by too many factors, most of them still unknown, which makes impossible comparisons between results by different authors, and the method itself less reliable than the staining methods.

Pötschke, Lewandowski, and Mauch (1954) used phase contrast microscopy for the purpose of identifying tubercle bacilli. Their attempts were based on the observation that stained bacteria as well as acid-fast bacilli can be easily seen with the aid of a phase contrast microscope. In this procedure the color of the stained objects is often completely different from what it is in a light microscope. This change in color was not observed in every dye used in bacteriology and cytology but only in some of them. In objects stained with fuchsin and examined in a dark phase contrast microscope, the color intensity of the red region is diminished or the color disappears completely, whereas the blue region remains unaffected. Because of this, the objects stained with fuchsin appear blue while the hue of methylene blue remains unchanged.

To investigate tubercle bacilli, the Ziehl-Neelsen staining technique was used but the counterstaining was omitted. Parallel investigations of tubercle bacilli of 2,028 pathologic specimens (sputa, gastric washings, feces) were made with phase contrast technique and with a light microscope. In 59 cases phase contrast microscopy revealed acid-fast bacilli where the routine method was never alone positive. The use of dry objective of low power increased the positive results.

XV

Cultivation of Tubercle Bacilli

Robert Koch and the Early Pioneers

ROBERT KOCH (1882) was the first to succeed in cultivating tubercle bacilli. He describes this achievement as follows. "The principle involved in cultivating tubercle bacilli is the use of a solid, transparent medium, which even at incubator temperature does not lose its solid consistency . . . Serum of cattle or sheep blood, which is collected as clean as possible, is distributed in test tubes which are closed with a plug of cotton and heated at 58°C. one hour daily for six days. Through this procedure we are able, if not always, at least in most cases, to sterilize the serum. Afterwards the serum is heated at 65°C. for a few hours, until it has coagulated and has become solid. After this treatment the serum has amber color, and is a completely transparent or slightly opalescent, solid, gelatinous mass. When the heating temperature has exceeded 75°C. or when the heating has been extensive, the serum becomes opaque. To obtain a larger surface, the test tubes with the serum are coagulated in an inclined position. . . . The simplest case, when it may be said that the experiment always succeeds, so rare are the exceptions, is when an animal dead of tuberculosis or a tuberculous animal killed for experimental purposes is available. The isolated tuberculous nodules or particles, the size of a millet grain, are rapidly separated from the lung tissue with scissors and immediately brought with a recently heated platinum wire onto the surface of the coagulated serum . . . Then the tubes inoculated with tuberculous material go into the incubating apparatus where they must be kept constantly at a temperature of 37 to 38°C. . . . The cultures originated from the growth of tubercle bacilli become for the first time visible to the naked eye in the second week after the planting, usually after the tenth day, in the form of very small dots and dry looking scales." (P. 224.)

The cultivation of tubercle bacilli on artificial media was successful in the hands of Koch, but, as first described by him, it was a difficult or even impossible task for a less able worker. Cultivation is possible when the material used does not contain contaminating microorganisms. Inoculation into a susceptible animal was, in Koch's time, the only way to separate tubercle bacilli from contaminants and obtain pure material for cultivation on artificial media. Thirty years of hard work were necessary to improve the medium of cultivation, to develop successful methods for the elimination of contaminants, to achieve cultures when the material contains only small quantities of bacilli, and to reach the actual inverse situation in the bacteriologic diagnosis of tuberculosis when it is often quicker, surer, and cheaper to obtain a culture than to obtain a diagnosis by animal inoculation.

Some simplification of the steps leading to the preparation of Koch's medium was achieved by Nocard (1885). Nocard added peptone, sugar, and mineral salts to aseptically collected horse serum before it became gelatinized. On this medium he cultivated avian tubercle bacilli.

Five years after the discovery of tubercle bacilli, Nocard and Roux (1887) made an observation which, from the vantage point of today, stands next in importance to the discovery of the bacillus itself. These authors said that the discovery of the causative agent of tuberculosis did not bring to the study of the disease progress which could possibly be compared to the progress achieved in the study of other infectious diseases after the discovery and cultivation of their causing agents. This, in their opinion, was because of the difficulties of isolation and the poor growth of tubercle bacilli on the medium available, namely coagulated serum. Serum heated at 66° to 68°C. produced a medium on which the growth of tubercle bacilli was weak, and the colonies were not always transplantable. With the intention of preventing the drying of the medium, Nocard and Roux added a small quantity of glycerol to the surface of the coagulated serum. The results were impressive. A ten-day-old culture of tubercle bacilli on serum containing glycerol had far more abundant growth than a one-month-old culture without glycerol. The best results were obtained by adding 6 to 8 per cent glycerol to the serum. Furthermore, Koch had indicated that the growth of tubercle bacilli on ordinary nutrient agar was possible but always poor. But, by adding glycerol to the agar, Nocard and Roux obtained good growth. On ordinary nutrient broth containing 5 per cent glycerol, the tubercle bacilli produced a pellicle within eight to ten days. All attempts to replace glycerol by other substances (glucose, cane sugar) failed.

The growth of bacteria on potato was observed by Esmarch (1887). A year later, another advance in the cultivation of tubercle bacilli was achieved. Pawlowsky (1888) realized the cultivation of tubercle bacilli on potato in sealed test tubes. The potato slices were sterilized in an autoclave and, when heavily inoculated with a pure culture of tubercle bacilli or with tuberculous organs, produced cultures on the twelfth day. Compared with cultures inoculated on coagulated glycerol serum, the growth on potato was more rapid and more abundant. In the early days of the bacteriology of tuberculosis, the potato or the glycerol potato were largely used for the cultivation of tubercle bacilli. The potato as a medium for growing tubercle bacilli has not yet been abandoned; the sulfuric acid method for the isolation of tubercle bacilli from contaminated material (Bossan and Baudy, 1922) is but an elaboration of the glycerol potato method.

Sander (1893) confirmed the findings of Pawlowsky and showed the possibility of cultivating tubercle bacilli on carrots, kohlrabi, and radishes. The growth of tubercle bacilli was poor on these media compared with the growth on potato. In the opinion of Sander, the acidity of the potato medium is favorable to the growth of tubercle bacilli. Schweinitz and Dorset (1896) and Ficker (1900) corroborated the findings of Sander that the growth of tubercle bacilli is facilitated by the acidic reaction of the medium. For the cultivation of tubercle bacilli, Ficker recommended his acid brain medium. Fränkel (1900) did not confirm these findings; according to him the growth of tubercle bacilli is possible and equally good on media within a fairly large range in acidity and alkalinity. N. Hoffmann (1904) found that tubercle bacilli cultivated on glycerol potato for two years had changed in neither morphology nor virulence.

The idea of concentrating tubercle bacilli so as to detect them with greater ease was originated by Biedert (1886). Concentration of bacilli by spontaneous sedimentation was not possible with specimens of high viscosity (sputum, pus, caseous material). To overcome this obstacle, Biedert submitted pathologic material to digestion with sodium hydroxide. In liquefied material the bacilli collected on the bottom of the vessel. At the same time, Philip (1886–1887) recognized the autodigestion and liquefaction of incubated sputum and the increase in number of the bacilli contained in such material.

Coagulated serum, glycerol agar, and potato were the media used by early workers to grow tubercle bacilli, but these workers were hindered in obtaining pure cultures of tubercle bacilli from contaminated pathologic material by rapidly and vigorously proliferating contaminants within the material, which overgrew the cultures.

The one to whom credit must be given for first isolating pure cultures of tubercle bacilli from contaminated material is Hüppe (1887). By seeding contaminated material on a large surface of glucose-serum-agar medium, a medium good for cultivation of tubercle bacilli even in our day (Dubos, 1947), Hüppe obtained isolated colonies of tubercle bacilli.

Kitasato (1892), through successive washings of sputum particles containing tubercle bacilli, tried to free the particles from contaminating microorganisms. When spread over the surface of glycerol agar, tubercle bacilli from washed material produced isolated colonies. Hesse (1899) claimed to have obtained pure cultures of tubercle bacilli from contaminated sputum by inoculating it on alkaline nutrose agar. Römer (1900) verified the results of Hesse and came to the conclusion that not the agar medium, but the mucus or sputum introduced on the surface of the medium causes the multiplication of tubercle bacilli. Fränkel corroborated the findings of Römer. From 20 sputa Fränkel obtained 20 pure cultures of tubercle bacilli on the medium of Hesse. Menzi (1902) states that it is possible to observe the growth of tubercle bacilli on Hesse's medium, but that this medium and procedure are worthless for the practical diagnosis of tuberculosis.

Fränkel (1900) and Ficker (1900) tried to utilize the synthetic medium of Proskauer and Beck as the base for an agar medium for growing tubercle bacilli. The growth of tubercle bacilli on the Proskauer and Beck liquid medium was good; after the addition of agar, it became poor.

The possibility of cultivating tubercle bacilli in pure cultures from contaminated pathologic material was repeatedly confirmed, although it was found to be not a uniformly efficient method but rather to depend on chance. The cultivation of tubercle bacilli remained an academic problem confined to the scientific laboratories without influencing the course of the practical diagnosis of tuberculosis.

The introduction by Dorset (1902, 1903) of the egg medium as a means of culturing tubercle bacilli constituted a great advance in the culturing of tubercle bacilli. The use of fresh egg as a medium for growing microorganisms had been tried by Hüppe as early as 1888. The work of Sclavo (1894) on the possibility of growing the tubercle bacillus in eggs did not provoke any interest on the part of scientists. (*"Il bacillo della tubercolosi dei mammiferi p. es. vi si sviluppa molto bene formando grossi ammassi di batterii."*)

Capaldi (1896) was the first to utilize egg yolk for the cultivation of microorganisms. He added some loops of unheated egg yolk to melted and cooled nutrient agar in the test tubes. This yolk-agar, inoculated with tubercle bacilli, produced colonies as rapidly and of the same size as those produced by coagulated serum. "Lecithin," ether, and alcohol extract of egg yolk, when added to the nutrient agar, also stimulated the growth of tubercle bacilli.

The experiments of Dorset were carried out on (1) whole egg medium, (2) egg yolk medium, and (3) egg white medium. The content of fresh eggs was distributed in tubes and coagulated at 70°C. for two days, four or five hours each day. Dorset observed that the white of egg was alkaline and the yolk acid to phenolphthalein. The tubes with the media were inoculated with the tissue of tuberculous guinea pigs. After seven or eight days, minute colonies were seen on the whole egg medium. Colonies did not appear as rapidly on the egg yolk as on the whole egg medium. There was no growth of tubercle bacilli on egg white. From the organs of nine guinea pigs inoculated with human tuberculous material, pure cultures of tubercle bacilli were obtained on the whole egg medium. The next year, Dorset (1903) obtained, with almost uniform success, pure cultures of tubercle bacilli from seventy-five tuberculous guinea pigs and rabbits.

Then the new solid whole egg medium for growing tubercle bacilli was created. Sterile material for the medium – eggs – was easily obtainable, and the preparation of the medium simple. The cultivation results on Dorset's medium were so uniformly good that this medium, with slight modifications (dilution of the egg mixture, Lubenau, 1907), has lately, in the hands of some workers, proved to be as good as the recently recommended (see p. 257) egg media for the primary cultivation of tubercle bacilli from pathologic material (Topley and Wilson, 1946; Peterson, 1952).

Bezançon and Griffon (1903) incorporated one part of egg yolk in two parts of glycerol agar and obtained a medium on which the tubercle bacilli rapidly produced moist and fatty colonies. Phisalix, in 1903, prepared a medium from egg yolk, potato mash, and glycerol. Agar-egg media did not attract particular attention from investigators until the publication of Herrold (1931); his proposed agar-egg medium is now widely used in laboratories.

As early as 1903, Dorset recognized as the chief cause for the failure of a culture the presence of an insufficient amount of tubercle bacilli in the pathologic material. Concentration of bacilli, proposed by Biedert, was recognized as a solution to this difficulty. No way of consistently obtaining pure cultures of tubercle bacilli from contaminated material has yet been found. The cultivation achievements, added to the basic work of Villemin, Koch, Kühne, Proskauer and Beck, and others, give us the sum of information available on the etiology of tuberculosis, and on the growth conditions and isolation techniques of tubercle bacilli at the turn of the century. A vast number of problems arose in those days, many of which have reached our time unsolved.

Diagnostic Cultivation from Contaminated Material

There are two ways of cultivating tubercle bacilli from contaminated material: (1) the selective elimination or destruction of contaminants in the material to be cultured, and (2) the culturing of contaminated material on selective media that support the growth of tubercle bacilli, but suppress the proliferation of contaminants. Both of these ways were used early.

The idea of selective disinfection of the contaminated material originated from the work of Spengler (1903). Attacking Flügge's method of disinfection with formaldehyde, Spengler announced that tubercle bacilli resist the action of formaldehyde, and that formaldehyde can be used to eliminate the contaminants and to cultivate tubercle bacilli in pure culture.

The formaldehyde method of Spengler was successfully applied by Weber and Taute (1904–1905) to the primary isolation of tubercle bacilli from the livers of tuberculous frogs. The pathologic material was treated for a short time with formaldehyde and then planted on the surface of agar containing malachite green, serum, and glycerol in Petri dishes. Well-separated colonies of acid-fast bacilli appeared in two to three weeks.

The success of Weber and Taute must be attributed to the use of feebly contaminated material from a cold-blooded animal, to the short exposure of the material to formaldehyde, to the use of aniline dye (malachite green) in the medium to prevent the growth of contaminants, and to the addition of serum to glycerol agar. The verification of the formaldehyde procedure by Dworetzky (1904), Jacqué (1904), and others, on contaminated human material (sputum) failed to support the findings of Spengler.

Lannoïse and Girard in 1900, after repeating the experiments of Biedert (1886) with strong alkalies, started to use a commercial alkaline solution of sodium hypochlorite, known as *Eau de Javelle* or *Eau de Labarraque*, for the digestion of sputum and the concentration of tubercle bacilli. To one volume of sputum ten volumes of the solution of hypochlorite were added. The sediment was investigated for tubercle bacilli. No attempts to cultivate the concentrated material were made. Krönig and Paul (1897) attributed the action of hypochlorite on organic substance to the presence of chlorine *in statu nascendi* in the liquid. Andrewes and Orton (1904) recognized hypochlorous acid (HClO) as the active ingredient of hypochlorite. In a 0.05 per cent solution of chlorine more than 90 per cent of this substance exists in the form of hypochlorous and hydrochloric acids (HClO and HCl). The hypochlorous acid is a powerful oxidant. Bleaching powder (calcium hypochlorite – $Ca(ClO)_2$) owes its action to its hypochlorite content. The presence of free alkali in the solution of hypochlorite has an important indirect influence on the disinfectant action of hypochlorite. Bleaching powder was recognized by Andrewes and Orton as the best agent for the digestion of sputa, because "a saturated solution of bleaching powder, containing about 5 per cent of calcium hypochlorite, disintegrates the sponge in one minute into a frothy pulp."

The discovery of egg media for the cultivation of tubercle bacilli and the work of Uhlenhuth and Xylander on Antiformin were the turning point in the solution of the problem of culturing tubercle bacilli directly from contaminated material. In their first communication on Antiformin, Uhlenhuth and Xylander (1908), indicated that Antiformin has a solvent action on all microorganisms except tubercle bacilli, and that they had put this property to good use by applying Antiformin to the direct cultivation of tubercle bacilli from contaminated material. In a further communication,

Uhlenhuth and Xylander (1909) revealed that Antiformin is a solution of 7.5 per cent NaOH and 5.6 per cent sodium hypochlorite, and that it was first used as a disinfectant in the brewing industry.

In contrast to *Eau de Javelle*, Antiformin is stable for a long time, owing to an excess of alkali. After a prolonged exposure to Antiformin, iron, copper, aluminum, and zinc are attacked, and organic products such as hair, wool, silk, and skin disintegrate. Fat is dissolved, but not wax. Sputum is readily dissolved and transformed into a homogeneous liquid. The vegetative forms of microorganisms can be completely dissolved in ten minutes, but not so the spores. Tubercle bacilli, after six hours of action by concentrated Antiformin, were not dead.

These observations suggested the possibility of using Antiformin for direct cultivation of bacilli from contaminated material. This goal was achieved by Uhlenhuth and Kersten in 1909. In their first series of experiments they treated 15 sputa with a 15 per cent solution of Antiformin for one to two hours, then centrifuged the solution, washed the sediment, inoculated it on coagulated serum or glycerol serum, sealed the tubes with paraffin, and incubated them at 37°C. From these 15 sputa 11 produced pure cultures of tubercle bacilli; 4 contained few bacilli. By the means of Antiformin pure cultures of tubercle bacilli were isolated from the spleen of guinea pig and from the putrid liver of chick, and cultures of acid-fast bacilli were obtained from the soil. Notwithstanding these achievements, the authors had reservations about suggesting cultivation as a means of detecting tubercle bacilli. In their opinion, guinea pig inoculation was preferable to culture in cases where few tubercle bacilli were present in the material. Although this was true in the days of Uhlenhuth and Kersten, the situation changed later on; but the conclusion of these two pioneers gave rise to doubts concerning the efficacy of the diagnostic cultivation of tubercle bacilli that have not abated to our day.

After the communications of Uhlenhuth and his co-workers, a stream of publications followed on the use of Antiformin for the direct cultivation of tubercle bacilli. One of the first, confirming the results of Uhlenhuth, was that of Hüne (1909). Impressive results were obtained by Brown and Smith (1910). From directly positive material, 97 per cent provided cultures. From 15 directly negative specimens, 4 cultures were grown. Bacilli from 37 isolated cultures were injected into guinea pigs and all produced tuberculosis. Brown and Smith showed that it is easy to grow tubercle bacilli directly from sputum on the egg medium by means of Antiformin, but that the growth of tubercle bacilli is poor on coagulated blood serum or glycerol agar.

A. S. Griffith (1914), using a 5 per cent Antiformin solution and the egg medium, obtained 27 cultures of tubercle bacilli from the sputa of 29 persons suffering from tuberculosis. He showed that it is not necessary to wash the sediment to free it from Antiformin before it is inoculated on egg media. Of these 27 cultures, 2 were pure cultures of the bovine type of tubercle bacilli. In all, from 115 tuberculous patients, Griffith obtained 115 cultures of tubercle bacilli by means of Antiformin.

Notwithstanding this success in the work toward the cultivation of tubercle bacilli from contaminated material, the Antiformin method did not solve the problem of direct cultivation of tubercle bacilli from contaminated material for the practical diagnosis of tuberculosis (Lippelt, 1939). As Uhlenhuth himself said, after 24 hours of action by Antiformin the spores of contaminants had not been killed. After prolonged incubation they revived and caused the deterioration of egg media.

Petroff (1915a) studied the action of sodium hydroxide on tubercle bacilli and found that tubercle bacilli were not killed if incubated for 24 hours at 37°C. in a solution of 4 per cent sodium hydroxide.

Besides Antiformin and sodium hydroxide, other strong alkalies for the destruction of contaminants have been proposed. Corper and Stoner (1946), showed that trisodium phosphate ($Na_3PO_4 \cdot 12H_2O$), as a 23 per cent solution, slowly destroys the contaminants if they are exposed for 48 hours at room temperature or during 24 hours at 37°C. to the chemical.

Aniline Dyes in the Isolation of Tubercle Bacilli

The antiseptic action of aniline dyes was discovered by Behring (1890). He demonstrated that malachite green was bacteriostatic to *Bacillus anthracis* when one part of the dye was diluted with 40,000 parts of broth, and was equal to the bacteriostatic action of one part of mercuric chloride diluted with 10,000 parts of broth or to that of carbolic acid diluted 500 times.

After these observations general interest in aniline dyes as antiseptic agents was aroused by the publications of Stilling (1890), who claimed that some aniline dyes, like methylviolet (Pyoctanine, Merck), are completely atoxic to living tissue but endowed with great diffusion power and that the antibacterial power of Pyoctanine is nearly equal to that of mercuric chloride. He recommended this dye for the treatment of pyogenic infections. Subsequent experimental works showed a great variation in the toxicity of aniline dyes to living tissues. The antibacterial activity of the dyes in the presence of blood or serum depends on the alkalinity or acidity of medium, the temperature of exposure and other factors.

Beckh and Penzoldt (1890) studied the antibacterial power of dyes, impregnated a solid medium (gelatin) with them, and cultivated microorganisms on this medium. These authors also determined the toxicity of aniline dyes to the rabbit. Malachite green, injected at a rate of 0.1 g. to 1 kg. of the animal, caused paralysis and convulsions; methylene blue was without any toxic action on the organism. Boer (1890) insisted on the necessity of standardizing the conditions for testing the antibacterial power of the substance. A small variation in the composition of the medium may produce great differences in the effect. Boer found that the development of *Bacillus anthracis* was prevented if 1 part of malachite green was added to 120,000 parts of broth and that the bacilli were killed if the concentration of the dye reached the level of 1 part to 5,000. At the same time the respective values for typhoid bacilli were 1 part to 5,000 and 1 part to 500. Boer did not draw any generalizations from these findings.

Weber and Taute (1904–1905) were the first to apply these findings to the cultivation of tubercle bacilli from contaminated material. Their medium consisted of serum-glycerol agar containing 1 part of malachite green to 500 parts of medium.

The studies of Churchman (1912) on the action of aniline dyes on microorganisms considerably clarified the whole problem. His first work, carried out with gentian violet, showed that microorganisms may be divided into two large groups according to their sensitivity to some aniline dyes. If a drop of concentrated aqueous gentian violet solution was added to a broth culture of the Gram-negative *Bacillus prodigiosus* (*Serratia marcescens*) and after one hour transplants from this stained liquid were made on agar, the growth was as luxuriant as with unstained cultures. In the case of Gram-positive *Bacillus subtilis* the results were quite different; the stained culture failed to grow. The same results were obtained when the microorganisms were grown on stained solid media. Parallelism between the action of aniline dyes on growing microorganisms and their Gram staining properties were detected. The growth of Gram-positive organisms was inhibited by the presence of some aniline dyes in the medium, with the exception of acid-fast bacilli, pneumococci, and a few others. The action of dyes on Gram-negative microorganisms was insignificant.

Table 22. Concentrations of Gentian Violet that Inhibit the Growth of Gram-Positive and Gram-Negative Microorganisms

Gram-Positive		Gram-Negative	
Corynebacterium diphtheriae	1:800,000	*Escherichia coli*	1:1,000
Bacillus anthracis	1:650,000	*Proteus vulgaris*	1:1,000
Bacillus subtilis	1:600,000	*Pseudomonas aeruginosa*	1:1,000

Source: Churchman and Siegel (1928).

As can be seen in Table 22, the Gram-positive microorganisms are 600 to 800 times more sensitive to gentian violet than the Gram-negative ones. Eisenberg (1913) discovered that the Gram-positive microorganisms attract India ink, if this liquid is introduced into the medium, and accumulate it around the cells; the Gram-negative ones do not have this property.

Forty-nine basic aniline dyes investigated by Eisenberg all showed bacteriostatic action of varying degrees on Gram-positive bacilli. Out of 41 acidic aniline dyes only 9 had feeble action on these bacilli. The spore-producing bacilli were especially sensitive to the action of the dyes. The cause for this was held to be the greater permeability of the cell membrane of Gram-positive bacilli. These findings were corroborated by Krumwiede and Pratt (1914). In a further study, Churchman (1923) pointed out that the differences in cellular permeability do not explain the whole mechanism of a specific action of basic dyes on Gram-positive bacilli; spores of bacilli are not easily permeable but are easily killed by these dyes. The intravital staining of bacilli does not always lead to their death. It must be assumed that the acidic groups of cell proteins which are of vital importance to the bacilli readily unite with the basic groups of dye.

The action of aniline dyes on Gram-positive bacilli may be divided into four phases: (1) cessation of the mobility of the bacilli; (2) inhibition of their reproduction; (3) suspension of animation; and (4) suspension of sporulation. The action of dyes on bacilli is quantitative; if applied for a sufficiently long time and sufficiently concentrated, the dyes will inhibit the growth of microorganisms or kill them. The action of a dye on microorganisms, as compared to the action of disinfectants, such as mercuric chloride or phenol, is slow (Churchman, 1926; Churchman and Siegel, 1928). The triphenylmethane dyes (brilliant green, malachite green, crystal violet, and gentian violet) have the specific inhibiting action on Gram-positive microorganisms. Acridine and quinoline dyes have practically the same action on Gram-positive and Gram-negative microorganisms. Many factors influence the action of triphenylmethane dyes, such as liquid or solid state, the *p*H of the medium, the presence of carbohydrates or proteins, and the temperature of cultivation. Specific differences in the sensitivity of the strain used may make difficult the determination of pure dye action on microorganisms.

Kligler (1918) states that the higher the concentration of organic nitrogenous compounds in the medium, the lower the effective concentration of the dye. The presence of serum or egg proteins greatly reduces the action of dyes as compared to their action in water solutions. It is also known that the introduction of methyl or ethyl groups in the nucleus of a dye enhances the inhibiting activity of that substance and that the triphenylmethane dyes with primary amino groups are less active than those with tertiary amino groups. According to Dubos in 1929, reduced aniline dyes (methylene blue, gentian violet) are of slight toxicity to microorganisms. Because of this, the organisms that possess a powerful reducing system can stand high concentration of aniline dye in the media.

The investigations of Michaelis (1947) and Kurnick (1950) revealed that triphenylmethane dyes with two methyl-amino groups, such as methyl green, ethyl green, and malachite green, selectively stain polymerized desoxyribonucleic acid and fail to stain depolymerized desoxyribonucleic acid and ribonucleic acid. The dyes with three amino groups, such as crystal violet, victoria blue, and gentian violet, show no such selectivity, but stain both desoxyribonucleic and ribonucleic acids. During the staining process the dye molecule combines with the phosphoric groups of the nucleic acid. The concentration of desoxyribonucleic acid of tubercle bacilli and Gram-positive bacilli in purine and pyrimidine bases (guanine, cytosine, uracil) is considerably higher than in Gram-negative bacteria.

Whether the inhibiting action of triphenylmethane dyes on Gram-positive bacilli is due to one or more specific causes is still an unsolved problem.

First Reliable Procedure for Cultivation from Contaminated Material

Churchman applied his observations that aniline dyes have a different action on tubercle bacilli than on the contaminants to his endeavor to separate tubercle bacilli in pure culture. In one of his experiments he isolated a rapidly growing acid-fast bacillus (tubercle bacillus?) from the contaminating *Bacillus subtilis* by planting a mixture of the bacilli on a medium containing gentian violet. The acid-fast bacillus produced a culture; *Bacillus subtilis* did not grow (1912).

Synthesizing the achievements of Dorset, Uhlenhuth, and Churchman, Petroff (1915a) developed the first practicable method for the isolation in pure cultures of tubercle bacilli from contaminated material. By combining both possibilities, namely destroying nonsporulating contaminants by means of alkali and introducing aniline dye into the egg media so as to prevent the germination of sporulating bacilli, Petroff found a procedure which is the basis of present-day diagnostic methods for the cultivation of tubercle bacilli from contaminated material. Petroff added meat extract to the egg medium of Dorset, and incorporated into it gentian violet at the rate of 1:10,000. To purify the contaminated material, he used a 3 per cent solution of sodium hydroxide, added it in equal parts to the material, and incubated the mixture for 30 minutes at 37°C. The neutralized sediment was inoculated on the gentian violet egg medium. Petroff showed the value of gentian violet in the medium. In an experiment carried out in parallel series, 15 out of the 20 sputa inoculated on the medium without the dye were found to be contaminated, whereas all 20 specimens inoculated on the medium containing gentian violet were free from contamination. Petroff also demonstrated the effectiveness of the method. All of 69 contaminated specimens, 6 of them negative for tubercle bacilli by direct examination, uniformly produced pure cultures of tubercle bacilli.

The use of the egg medium instead of the agar medium, the incorporation of sufficiently diluted dye into the medium, the inoculation of this medium with purified pathologic material, where Gram-negative contaminants were killed and most of Gram-positive ones destroyed or prevented from growing by aniline dye, secured the success of Petroff.

Keilty (1915) was not successful in his first attempt to repeat the work of Petroff. But after improving the technique he succeeded in growing tubercle bacilli in 10 tubes out of a total of 21 inoculated with purified material.

The first analysis of Petroff's procedure was made by Corper, Fiala, and Kallon (1919). These authors investigated the importance of the components of the medium and the necessity of different steps in Petroff's procedure and studied the effectiveness of the method on a comparatively large amount of material. They discovered that the presence of glycerol in a concentration of 1, 2, or 4 per cent in the egg medium did not change the results of cultivation; they also demonstrated that meat juice in the medium is of no importance for the growth of tubercle bacilli. In the hands of these experimenters, 526 microscopically positive sputa yielded 114 (27.3 per cent) pure cultures of tubercle bacilli.

Lurie (1923) compared the Antiformin procedure as used by Griffith with Petroff's method by culturing tubercle bacilli from contaminated material. A solution of 20 per cent Antiformin diluted with equal amount of sputa was digested for 10 minutes at room temperature and the treated material was then inoculated, without having been centrifuged or washed, on Dorset's egg medium. The 34 microscopically positive sputa, after 12 weeks of incubation, produced 2 cultures of tubercle bacilli; the 20 microscopically negative sputa revealed 1 culture. The aliquots of material, treated with 4 per cent NaOH solution, centrifuged, and sowed on Petroff's medium, produced in the same time 14 pure cultures from the positive material and 6 cultures from the negative. Lurie attributed the better results produced by Petroff's technique to the centrifugation of the digested material, to the presence of gentian violet in the medium, and to the use of NaOH solution, which is less noxious than Antiformin, as a decontaminant.

The purpose of aniline dye in the culture media, in the conception of some authors, is to facilitate the early recognition on the colored ground of young, colorless colonies of tubercle bacilli. This view is expressed by Corper and Stoner (1946) as follows: "For those desiring a color background, the color becomes a matter of individual choice covering a wide range from red, green, blue, even black."

From the foregoing one can see that only a definite group of aniline dyes can be used in the media for the cultivation of tubercle bacilli from contaminated material, and that the color of the dye used is of little importance in the procedure.

The work of Petroff remained largely unknown in a Europe devastated and impoverished by World War I. One of the first communications on

Petroff's technique published in Europe was that of Limousin (1921), from the laboratory of Calmette. After his visit to Petroff's laboratory at Saranac Lake, New York, Limousin described Petroff's procedure and the results obtained with Petroff's method of direct cultivation of tubercle bacilli from contaminated material. Limousin's communication was followed by the works of Moreau (1922), Rochaix and Banssillon (1922), and Despeignes (1922) dealing with the direct cultivation of tubercle bacilli from sputum, urine, caseated ganglions, peritoneal liquids, and other materials. These works contributed to the expansion of the use of Petroff's method in Europe.

Acids in the Cultivation of Tubercle Bacilli

Evidence of viable resistance of tubercle bacilli in pathologic material to the action of sulfuric acid was given by the cultivation results of Bossan and Baudy as early as 1922. The credit for the discovery of the possibility of cultivating tubercle bacilli from contaminated material by means of acids was given to Löwenstein (1924) and his co-worker, Sumiyoshi (1924). These authors investigated the use of sulfuric acid for the isolation of tubercle bacilli from contaminated material without mentioning the work done by Bossan and Baudy two years earlier. When one compares the method used and the results obtained by Löwenstein and Sumiyoshi with those of Bossan and Baudy (see Table 23), no differences can be seen and no improvement of the method of Bossan and Baudy can be discerned.

Table 23. Comparison of the Methods and Results of Bossan and Baudy (1922) with Those of Löwenstein (1924) and Sumiyoshi (1924)

	Bossan and Baudy	Löwenstein and Sumiyoshi
Material cultivated	15 sputa	30 sputa
Acid	10% H_2SO_4 (vol.)	10–20% H_2SO_4 (vol.)
Time of treatment	10 minutes	10–60 minutes
Medium	Glycerol potato	Glycerol potato
Time necessary for colonies of tubercle bacilli to appear	13–35 days	14–28 days
No. of pure cultures obtained	13	30

The simplicity, and the reliable results obtained, especially when a strong acid (15 per cent) and material rich in tubercle bacilli were used, contributed to the rapid diffusion of this cultivation method for the routine diagnosis of tuberculosis in laboratories throughout the world. In a few years the cultivation method replaced homogenization, concentration of the material for the direct microscopic examination, and at last, guinea pig inoculation. This diffusion of the diagnostic cultivation of tubercle bacilli through the use of the sulfuric acid method of Bossan and Baudy was considerably enhanced by the publications of Hohn in Germany, Saenz in Uruguay and France, and many others.

In most cases sulfuric acid (in a 6 to 15 per cent solution by volume) is used as a decontaminant, but some workers prefer hydrochloric acid. Corper and Uyei (1930) recommended oxalic acid for this purpose.

Action of Chemicals on Tubercle Bacilli and on Contaminants

There is an abundance of early work on the action of alkalies on tubercle bacilli but this cannot be said of work on the resistance of tubercle bacilli to acids, notwithstanding the fact that the resistance of tubercle bacilli to the decolorizing action of a strong solution of nitric acid was demonstrated by Ehrlich as early as 1882.

The resistance of stained mycobacteria to the decolorizing action of chemicals is different from the viable resistance of these organisms to the action of chemicals. These two phenomena are related, but one is the property of dead, the other of living bacilli. These properties are different in different species of mycobacteria. The *Mycobacterium mölleri*, when stained according to the Ziehl-Neelsen technique, cannot be decolorized by a 2 per cent sodium sulfite solution in 24 hours, and the bacilli are not killed by a 10.5 per cent solution of sulfuric acid within 24 hours. *M. grassbergeri* of the same age and growth condition is killed by a solution of sulfuric acid of the same concentration in five minutes and decolorized by a 2 per cent sodium sulfite solution in three minutes (Darzins, 1932).

Porter (1917) investigated the viable resistance to acids of eleven strains of tubercle bacilli. In his experiments these strains were not killed by *N*/13 sulfuric, acetic, and citric acids in the course of 24 hours, but were destroyed under the same conditions by the *N*/10 solution of these acids. Azzi (1924–1925) investigated the action of a 10 per cent solution of sulfuric acid on tubercle bacilli in the sputum. After 4 to 8 hours of action by the acid it was still possible to cultivate bacilli taken from the material. Warnery (1932) found that the resistance of tubercle bacilli to sulfuric acid increases with the age of the bacilli. A 10 to 12 per cent sulfuric acid solution (by volume) was required to kill a four-day-old culture in 30 minutes; for a five-day-old culture, a 20 to 30 per cent solution; and for a six-day-old culture, a 40 to 50 per cent solution was needed to obtain the same effect in the same time. Gelder (1933) studying the resistance of acid-fast bacilli to a 10 per cent sulfuric acid solution, observed that human tubercle bacilli and saprophytic trumpet bacilli grown under the same conditions survived 24 hours of action; saprophytic *M. smegmatis* and *M. lacticola* were dead after 5 to 15 minutes. *M. phlei* was killed after 40 to 160 minutes of treatment.

Hailer (1938) found great variation in the resistance of different strains of tubercle bacilli to acids. In one series of experiments the bacilli were killed in two to six hours by *N* hydrochloric acid, while other strains resisted twenty-four-hour action of the same dilution of acid. Abel (1939) divided acid-fast bacilli into groups on the basis of their resistance to acids. The pathogenic forms and the acid-fast bacilli from water, turtle, frog, and snake have high resistance to sulfuric acid and Antiformin; the acid-fast bacilli from milk, butter, smegma, and timothy have low resistance to sulfuric acid and Antiformin.

The studies of acid-fast bacilli in their natural surroundings in pathologic material, such as sputum, pus, and exudates, have furnished important information concerning the resistance of these bacilli to acids and alkalies.

Farjot (1933) inoculated 318 guinea pigs with sputum not treated with chemicals: 15.7 per cent of the animals died prematurely, 19.4 per cent were tuberculous. Aliquots of the material, treated for 30 minutes at 37°C. with a 4 per cent solution of sodium hydroxide and inoculated into 780 guinea pigs, were prematurely lethal to 5.9 per cent and rendered 11.2 per cent of the animals tuberculous. Steenken and Smith (1938) observed that acid and alkali digestion affects the growth and acid-fast properties of tubercle bacilli. Hauduroy, Bouvier, and Rosset (1945) inoculated guinea pigs with pathologic material containing tubercle bacilli. One part of the material was treated with a 15 per cent sulfuric acid, another inoculated without any treatment. Of the 28 specimens treated for thirty minutes with acid, 8 (29 per cent) caused tuberculosis in animals. Out of 20 specimens inoculated without prior treatment with acid, 17 (85 per cent) produced tuberculosis. The application of a 15 per cent solution of sulfuric acid in the decontamination procedure killed from 10 to 30 per cent of bacilli (Canetti, 1946).

Spendlove, Cummings, and Patnode (1949) studied the relative toxicity to the tubercle bacilli of the most commonly used decontaminating agents. The action was investigated on the H37Rv strain of tubercle bacilli and on the bacilli in pathologic material. The results obtained with a 4 per cent solution of sodium hydroxide, a 5 per cent solution of sulfuric acid, a 3 per cent solution of hydrochloric acid, Antiformin, trisodium phosphate, and other decontaminants were compared and all found to markedly reduce the number of viable bacilli within the shortest time of action. Sodium hydroxide was relatively less toxic to tubercle bacilli than sulfuric and hydrochloric acid, though approximately 50 per cent of the tubercle bacillus population was killed in 40 minutes of action on the part of these reagents.

Mitscherlich, Reuss, and Gürtürk (1952) at the laboratory of Dr. K. Wagener (Hanover, Germany) investigated the action of different concentrations of sulfuric acid on tubercle bacilli and found that a 6 to 8 per cent solution produces better cultivation and inoculation results than a 10 per cent solution. When a 6 to 8 per cent solution of sulfuric acid was used instead of a 10 per cent, the cultivation results approached those obtained with the SP method (Chapter XVI). In his work of 1952, Reuss made an attempt to show the superiority of the treatment of contaminated material with a 6 to 8 per cent solution of sulfuric acid over a 10 per cent solution or even over the SP method. Omitting the treatment of the phosphate precipitate with citrates, which is an essential part of the SP method, Reuss inoculated the strongly alkaline phosphate precipitate containing free NaOH and Na_3PO_4 directly into a feebly buffered Hohn egg medium. The mistake of regarding the egg media as a potent self-regulating system, which one can inoculate disregarding the *p*H of the inoculum, is still widespread in Europe.

Ficus (1951) in his research for his dissertation, also carried out at the Institute of Veterinary Medicine, Hanover, Germany, under Dr. K. Wagener, found that weak solutions of sulfuric acid have feeble homogenizing effects on sputa and their action on contaminating microorganisms is uncertain. A 10 per cent solution of sulfuric acid was found optimal and far less noxious to tubercle bacilli than a 10 per cent solution of hydrochloric acid. The recent results from the Institute of Hygiene, University of Frankfurt am Main, Germany, under Dr. H. Schlossberger, published by Weigand (1953) affirm the superiority of the 6 per cent sulfuric acid solution over the 10 per cent solution.

The differences in cultivation results obtained from 6, 8, and 10 per cent solutions of sulfuric acid are small and statistically insignificant. (The differences Weigand found between the cultivation results of sputa treated with 6 and 10 per cent sulfuric acid were 2 and 3 per cent.)

Yegian and Budd's (1952) investigation of the toxic effect of sodium hydroxide on tubercle bacilli revealed that the death rate of tubercle bacilli grown in Dubos' liquid medium and exposed to a 3 per cent sodium hydroxide solution is extremely high at the beginning of the action of the chemical. After five minutes of exposure, 50 per cent of the population of the strain H37Rv were dead. After the highly sensitive bacilli had been eliminated, the death rate decreased considerably. The action of sodium hydroxide on tubercle bacilli was comparable to the action of any other disinfectant on microorganisms.

Tubercle bacilli are more sensitive to the action of chemicals than are the spore-producing microorganisms. A great deal of contaminated material treated with the decontaminating chemicals actually in routine use contains living spores of bacilli after the treatment. In one of our experiments (see Table 24) aliquots of five sputa were diluted with equal quantities of 10 per cent sulfuric acid (by volume), 3 per cent sodium hydroxide, and 23 per cent trisodium phosphate. The material treated with acid and hydroxide was incubated at 37°C. for 30 minutes, that with phosphate for 24 hours at 37°C. The sediment of each sample of material was inoculated into three tubes of ordinary broth and upon three tubes of agar slants and incubated for 48 hours. The specimens treated with sulfuric acid produced cultures in one case out of five; those treated with sodium hydroxide and trisodium phosphate in three cases out of five. The growth of the material

Table 24. Results of Incubation for 48 Hours at 37°C. of Broth and Agar Slants Inoculated with Sputa Treated with Sulfuric Acid, Sodium Hydroxide, and Trisodium Phosphate *

	6% H_2SO_4 (vol.)		3% NaOH		23% $Na_3PO_4 \cdot 12\,H_2O$	
Sputum	Broth	Agar	Broth	Agar	Broth	Agar
1	–	–	+++	++	+++	+++
2	–	–	++	+	++	++
3	–	–	–	–	–	–
4	–	–	–	–	–	–
5	++	+	++	++	+++	+++

Source: Darzins, unpublished data, 1950.

* Minus sign indicates no growth. Plus signs indicate the growth rate, in varying degrees.

treated with trisodium phosphate was richer. All cultures grown were sporulating bacilli.

Thus we can corroborate, in regard to sulfuric acid, sodium hydroxide, and trisodium phosphate, the findings of Uhlenhuth and Xylander (1908) for Antiformin, namely, that the spores are not killed by the decontaminating agents. Some authors believe that in the course of the decontamination of the material, the chemicals applied eliminate the secondary microorganisms but the viability of mycobacteria is not affected (Hohn, 1929; Saenz and Costil, 1936; Corper and Cohn, 1942). As the most extreme representative of this view we may mention McNabb (1936), who cultivated tubercle bacilli from material treated with hydrochloric acid only when earlier bacteriologic investigation had indicated the complete destruction of the contaminants.

The difference in action of chemicals on contaminants and on tubercle bacilli is quantitative; actually we do not know any substance which has a specific action on contaminants alone. This is the source of a great deal of our difficulty in the cultivation of tubercle bacilli from contaminated material. Antiformin, sodium hydroxide, sulfuric acid, and other chemicals permit the cultivation of tubercle bacilli from contaminated material rich in bacilli. If the bacilli are few, the cultivation often yields negative results. The importance of bacteriologic diagnosis of tuberculosis actually resides precisely in the discovery of the small quantities of bacilli involved in incipient, slowly progressing, stationary, or healing tuberculosis. In these cases our actual methods of bacteriologic diagnosis of tuberculosis are still insufficient, as they were at the time of Dorset in 1903.

There are only two ways one can nowadays follow when cultivating tubercle bacilli from contaminated material. The first is to decrease the strength and the time of the action of the decontaminant, increasing the percentage of cultures lost by contamination; the second is to increase the strength and the time of action of the decontaminant, decreasing the percentage of positive cultures. The method chosen would have to be a reasonable combination of both possibilities.

Choice of Decontaminant

As shown in the preceding section, the actual decontamination procedures greatly reduce the viability of tubercle bacilli. Penicillin was found not to be efficacious in selectively combating the contaminants. The results of the cultivation methods are only equal but not superior to the results of animal inoculation, probably mainly because of the use of decontaminants that destroy tubercle bacilli in the decontamination procedures.

The team of British investigators (1952) studied under similar conditions the influence of the commonly used decontaminants on tubercle bacilli in contaminated material cultured on Löwenstein-Jensen's medium. To reduce variations to a minimum, twelve laboratories of the British Public Health Service were chosen to participate in the work. The medium was prepared in one central laboratory. It was decided to compare the

Table 25. The Results of Tubercle Bacilli Cultivation from Sputa Treated with Different Decontaminants

Decontaminant	Negative by Direct Microscopy	Positive by Direct Microscopy	Total	Percentage Contaminated
4% sodium hydroxide.				4.0
Number of examinations.	1,243	361	1,604	
Number of positive cultures.	356	311	667	
Percentage of positive cultures. .	28.6%	86.1%	41.6%	
3% sulfuric acid.				4.9
Number of examinations.	1,222	349	1,571	
Number of positive cultures.	267	287	554	
Percentage of positive cultures. . .	21.8%	82.2%	35.3%	
10 or 23% trisodium phosphate.				7.6
Number of examinations.	1,199	347	1,546	
Number of positive cultures.	202	264	466	
Percentage of positive cultures. .	16.8%	76.1%	30.1%	

Source: Team of British investigators (1952).

results yielded by the culturing of aliquots of sputa treated with 3 per cent sulfuric acid, 4 per cent sodium hydroxide, and 10 or 23 per cent trisodium phosphate (dehydrated or crystalline).

The laboratories examined in each stage 52 sputa over a period of six weeks. The figures obtained were subjected to statistical analysis by the other group of workers in order to decide whether differences in the efficacy of decontamination of the material by different chemicals were significant as compared with the random variation in the data of the participating laboratory.

A total of 3,167 sputa were examined; 2,472 sputa were microscopically negative and 695 scantily positive (see Table 25).

The differences among the cultivation results of microscopically positive specimens subjected to three different decontaminants were not statistically significant. All methods employed produced from scantily positive material approximately 80 per cent positive cultures; about 20 per cent of the positive specimens failed to grow on the solid egg media.

The results of the cultivation of microscopically negative series from which the sputa negative by two decontamination methods were excluded (as not containing cultivable bacilli) were different (see Table 26).

Table 26. The Cultivation Results of Microscopically Negative Sputa Treated with Different Decontaminants

Decontaminant	No. of Specimens	No. Positive by Culture	Percentage Positive by Culture
4% sodium hydroxide	394	356	90.3
3% sulfuric acid	340	267	78.6
10% or 23% trisodium phosphate	311	202	65.2

Source: Team of British investigators (1952).

The cultivation of microscopically negative specimens containing scantily cultivable bacilli, when treated with different decontaminants, revealed statistically significant cultivation differences. Sodium hydroxide was the best decontaminant studied; it produced the highest positive results and the lowest contamination rate. Trisodium phosphate produced the lowest positive results and the highest contamination rate.

XVI

The Shaking-Precipitation (SP) Method

THE cultivation results of tubercle bacilli on an artificial medium depend upon (a) the viable properties of the bacilli inoculated; (b) the number of bacilli inoculated; (c) the composition of the medium used.

Both acids and alkalies may be used to eliminate contaminants from pathologic material, and in a material rich in tubercle bacilli the cultivation results will be successful with all these substances. The results will be different if there is a smaller number of bacilli in the material, as in cases where the material has been collected from incipient or healing tuberculosis. The disastrous effect on tubercle bacilli of the chemicals used to decontaminate the pathologic material has never ceased to spur investigators to look for less harmful substances and easier procedures.

The agitation of tuberculous material for the purpose of homogenization was advocated by Biedert (1886), Uhlenhuth and Xylander (1908), Petroff (1915a), and others. Steenken and Smith (1942) proposed the use of a shaking machine, and the American Trudeau Society (1946) recommended the replacement of manpower by machines in laboratory work whenever possible.

The influence of shaking or vibration on microorganisms was an object of study by early authors. Horvath (1878) observed that violent shaking sterilizes the infected liquid and that, in general, motion is detrimental to the life of microorganisms. This conclusion was refuted by Meltzer (1892), who pointed out that motion has on living matter the same effect as any other physical force, like heat, for instance. There is an optimum of heat indispensable to life, but there is also a degree of heat detrimental to it. The same, according to Meltzer, is true of motion. In his experiments *Bacillus ruber* was destroyed after a very long and strong shaking, but a mild shaking was favorable to its growth. The agitation of cultures of microorganisms promotes the growth of aerobic bacilli (*Bacillus anthracis*, Lucet, 1914) and also anaerobic bacilli (tetanus, Bier and Planet, 1937).

Tubercle bacilli ground in a ball mill for two days were still pathogenic for guinea pigs; *Mycobacterium smegmatis* showed the highest resistance of the mycobacteria studied (Willis, 1932).

Curran and Evans (1942) found that suspensions in water of *Escherichia coli*, of spores of *Bacillus megatherium*, and of *Bacillus subtilis* are killed if shaken with sand or glass fragments for five hours. The effect depends upon the size and quantity of the abrasive used, and on the speed and the duration of agitation. Larger and fewer particles are less effective, higher speed has greater germicidal efficiency. After having been shaken with glass beads in a Kahn shaker for 20 minutes at 250 strokes per minute, *Azotobacter*, *Bacillus subtilis*, *Proteus vulgaris*, *Salmonella typhosa*, and *Vibrio comma* were still flagellated (Mallett, Koffler, and Rinker, 1951).

To study the influence of different factors on the results of shaking, Furness (1952) experimented with *Escherichia coli*. The bacteria were suspended in 25 ml. of distilled water and shaken with 25 g. of glass beads from 0.1 to 0.3 mm. in diameter. The agitation with beads had a destructive effect on bacteria which increased with the speed of shaking and decreased with the diminution of the diameter of beads in suspension. The suspension of *Escherichia coli* containing $62{,}300 \times 10^6$ cells per ml. before the shaking, contained 3 to 4 cells per ml. after a three-hour shaking of the suspension with beads at 600 strokes per minute. A complete sterilization of the suspension of *Escherichia coli* by shaking with beads was not obtained. One of the mycobacteria most resistant to disintegration by shaking was *M. smegmatis*. After shaking for sixteen hours with beads in saline solution at a speed of 300–350 strokes per minute, no intact bacilli could be seen in a stained film. The disintegrated organisms were not acid-fast. The culture revealed 10,000 viable organisms per ml. of the treated material (King and Alexander, 1948).

Schaefer, Marshak, and Burkhart (1949) observed that continuously shaken cultures of tubercle bacilli in Dubos' liquid medium (140 oscillations per minute) showed a retarded growth compared to bacilli of cultures that had not been subjected to shaking. This observation was corroborated by Kull and Grimm (1952). A virulent strain of tubercle bacilli, H37Rv, agitated at 240 oscillations per minute, yielded inferior growth in Dubos' medium to a culture not agitated.

The agitation of material with chemicals not only for the purpose of homogenization but also for decontamination is based on our observation that a strong but short agitation of contaminated materials with a weak solution of alkali not only leads to the homogenization of the material but at the same time also eliminates the majority of contaminants, leaving the viability of tubercle bacilli less affected than after a prolonged incubation with strong but not agitated chemicals.

The shaking of tubercle bacilli with acids produces results that are different from the results obtained by shaking with alkalies. After sputum containing few tubercle bacilli per ml. has been agitated in a Kahn shaker for five minutes with 6 per cent (by volume) sulfuric acid, it does not produce a culture. Material containing large quantities of bacilli, when agitated with acid, produces a delayed growth of colonies that are rare in comparison to the abundant growth of the same material agitated with alkalies.

The action of decontaminants in motion on tubercle bacilli in the material is different from their action in static conditions; the tubercle bacilli are resistant to agitated alkali but sensitive to agitated acid. These findings do not support the view of Ehrlich (1882), who ascribed the resistance of stained tubercle bacilli to the decolorizing action of acids and expressed the opinion that the destruction of tubercle bacilli must be expected from alkaline substances. Our investigation showed that the viability of tubercle bacilli is less injured by a short shaking with mixtures of 1 per cent NaOH and 1 per cent of $Na_3PO_4 \cdot 12\ H_2O$ than by shaking with a 3 per cent NaOH solution. The disinfecting action of a mixture of NaOH and Na_3PO_4 on non-acid-fast bacilli is stronger than that of the NaOH solution alone. This can be explained to some extent by the fact that the trisodium phosphate is a wetting agent. The agitated wetting agent damages the surface of non-acid-fast bacilli. After this, the alkali in the solution easily destroys the bacilli. The pathologic material is finely dispersed after the shaking. This process is facilitated by the presence of glass beads in the agitated mixture. Thus, the pathologic material is, in one operation, homogenized and purified of nonsporulating microorganisms.

The inoculation of agitated material on agar and in broth media (not containing aniline dyes) showed that in most cases the material agitated with sulfuric acid does not contain viable microorganisms or the spores of bacilli. The material agitated with 3 per cent sodium hydroxide and with the mixture of sodium hydroxide and sodium phosphate often contains viable spores of microorganisms (Table 27).

The presence of trisodium phosphate in the purifying liquid (purifier) has another advantage. It permits the concentration of bacilli in small volume on the bottom of the container. The cultivation results of tubercle bacilli and the time of the appearance of colonies depend largely upon the quantity of the bacilli inoculated upon the media (Meyn, 1950). The addition of a solution of calcium chloride to the finely dispersed material after shaking produces the flocculation of gelatinous calcium phosphate:

$$2\ Na_3PO_4 + 3\ CaCl_2 = Ca_3\ (PO_4)_2 + 6\ NaCl$$

A short centrifugation projects calcium phosphate, and bacilli in it, onto the bottom of the container.

The precipitation of calcium phosphate for the purpose of concentrating

Table 27. The Influence* of Agitation with Acids and Alkalies on the Viability of Tubercle Bacilli in Sputum after 1, 2, 3, 4, and 5 Weeks of Incubation †

Amount of Bacilli in Sputum	Agitated with 6% H_2SO_4 (by vol.)					Agitated with 3% NaOH					Agitated with 1% NaOH and 1% $Na_3PO_4 \cdot 12\ H_2O$				
	1	2	3	4	5	1	2	3	4	5	1	2	3	4	5
Gaffky 2	−	−	−	−	−	−	−	−	+	++	−	+	+	++	+++
Gaffky 3	−	−	−	−	−	−	−	−	−	+	−	−	+	+	++
Gaffky 4	−	−	−	−	+	−	+	+	++	++	−	++	+++	++	++
Gaffky 5	−	−	−	+	++	+	++	+++	++	++	++	++	++	++	++

Source: Darzins, unpublished data, 1950.

* Minus sign indicates no growth. Plus signs indicate growth, in varying degrees.

† Two ml. of sputum were agitated with 10 ml. of chemicals for five minutes in a Kahn shaker, 275 oscillations per minute, 3 cm. horizontal stroke. The sediment was neutralized, planted on Petragnani's medium, and incubated at 37°C.

tubercle bacilli and other microorganisms was tried by Nunno (1933). To a 10 per cent solution of secondary phosphate, a 10 per cent solution of calcium chloride was added, centrifuged, and the sediment dissolved in acetic acid. The concentration of microorganisms was elucidated by counting them in the Thoma camera. The efficacy of this method of concentrating tubercle bacilli was compared by Beggi and Picasso (1933) with the results of the concentration methods of Ronchese, Angerer, Ylkevitch, and Uhlenhuth. The calcium phosphate concentration of tubercle bacilli was superior to the other methods tested. Zahn (1910) had used the precipitation of calcium hydroxide in sputum digested with sodium hydroxide to collect tubercle bacilli for staining purposes.

The addition of calcium chloride to the sputum after homogenization not only produces flocculation of calcium phosphate but also causes the precipitation of different protein substances of sputum dissolved or in suspension in the liquid. Too abundant a precipitation of these substances was the undoing of all concentration methods and was chiefly responsible for the rejection of these methods for the concentration of tubercle bacilli in sputum for cultivation purposes. In other cases, in order to avoid the heavy precipitation of proteins, the quantity of material used in the concentration was reduced to such a minimum that the bacilli were absent in the sediment (Robinson and Stovall, 1941).

The amount of proteins in sputa varies considerably and there was a time when some prognostic value was attributed to their concentration in sputum. Our study (1951) was conducted to establish the quantity of calcium chloride which will cause not only chemical flocculation of calcium phosphate but will produce a small precipitation of the protein substances of sputum. Such precipitation of protein would be helpful in concentrating bacilli in the liquid. The quantity of calcium phosphate produced from trisodium phosphate and calcium chloride in water solutions was determined. The calcium phosphate produced was washed with hot distilled water, dried over phosphorus pentoxide, and weighed. The quantity of phosphate obtained was in good agreement with the theory. The progressive increase of calcium chloride in the liquid was followed by the linear increase of the weight of formed phosphate.

After this, we investigated the precipitation of proteins from different samples of blood serum, adding increased amounts of a 0.5 per cent solution of calcium chloride to them. In all ten sera of healthy persons studied, the increase of the precipitate was proportionate to the increased quantities of calcium chloride added, until three to four ml. of $CaCl_2$ solution was reached. When four ml. of calcium chloride was added, the sera produced a considerable precipitation, and the straight line of the precipitation increase curve suddenly went up. The critical concentration of calcium chloride was then determined in twenty-five sputa of varying consistency and aspect. The instability of proteins in a sputum solution is considerably greater than that of blood serum. The addition of one ml. of 1 per cent of calcium chloride solution caused some precipitation in all sputa but never led to the heavy precipitation of proteins.

The phosphate formed and the protein precipitate enclose the suspended bacilli, the gelatinous properties of phosphate favoring this process. It is probable that some adsorption of cells to the precipitate also takes place. As early as 1889, Roux and Yersin showed that through the addition of calcium chloride to the solution of diphtheria toxin, the formed precipitate of calcium phosphate removes most of the toxin from the solution. Ungar and Muggleton (1949) observed that aluminum phosphate, cadmium phosphate, and magnesium-ammonium-phosphate precipitate the agglutinable strains of *Haemophilus pertussis*. The adsorption of the organisms takes place the moment the precipitate is formed.

Centrifuging as a Concentration Procedure

Centrifuging of the pathologic material was recommended as a means of concentrating tubercle bacilli. The ordinary laboratory centrifuge with 2,000 to 3,000 rotations per minute is not an efficient instrument for the concentration of tubercle bacilli from pathologic material if used for a short time (Klein, Maltz, Cummings, and Fish, 1952). Prolonged centrifuging (Scartozzi, 1939; Robinson and Stovall, 1941) was recommended. The concentration of tubercle bacilli by means of high-speed centrifuges particularly attracted the attention of researchers. This method was recommended by Davy and Levaditi (1938). The theoretical side of the problem was clarified by Schmidt-Lange (1940).

The sedimentation velocity of a particle heavier than the liquid in which it is floating may be accelerated by centrifuging the liquid. The sedimentation velocity of a round body, as the equation of Stokes shows, is directly proportional to the square of its radius and to the differences between the densities of the body and of the surrounding liquid, and is inversely proportional to the viscosity of the surrounding medium:

$$V = \frac{2\,gr^2\,(d_1 - d_2)}{9\eta}$$

where r is the radius of the sphere, d_1 and d_2 the densities of the sphere and the medium respectively, and η the coefficient of viscosity.

The density of the tubercle bacillus is only slightly greater than that of water. Because of this, after the centrifugation of a dense liquid (purulent sputum), the majority of the bacilli will be found on the top of the centrifuge tube. In the case of viscous liquid (mucous sputum), the bacilli will not be sedimentated. According to Almquist (1898) tubercle bacilli are found at the top of the sodium iodide solution of density 1.4 and 1.5 when centrifuged for 30 minutes at the speed of 8,000 rpm, but they are sedimented when the density of the liquid is 1.2 or 1.3.

The sedimentation velocity of the particle increases with the square of its radius; if the particle is small enough, the given centrifugal force will not precipitate it. The sedimentation of such particles can be achieved by increasing the centrifugal force. The centrifugal force in kilograms produced by a machine may be calculated from the formula:

$$C = \frac{m \cdot v^2}{r}$$

where m is mass in kg., v velocity, in meters per second, r radius. When in the above formula m and r are equal to 1, the centrifugal force increases as the square of the velocity. Thus, when instead of a centrifuge producing 3,000 rotations per minute a machine making 15,000 rotations is used, the increase in centrifugal force will be $15{,}000^2 \div 3{,}000^2$ or 25 times, and particles with a 25 times smaller diameter can be expected in the sediment, or particles with the same diameter will precipitate 25 times more rapidly in a centrifuge with 15,000 rotations than in a centrifuge with 3,000 rotations.

The performance of various rotors may be expressed by the performance index (P) proposed by Pickels in 1951:

$$P = \frac{(\text{rpm})^2}{\log_e R_2 - \log_e R_1}$$

in which R_2 is the maximum radial distance and R_1 is the minimal distance, or the level of liquid in the centrifuge tube.

The practical value of these theoretical considerations was investigated by Kröger and Rosarius (1949). The high-speed centrifuging of pathologic material was found to increase the positive result by 2 per cent compared to the result of ordinary centrifuging. Ahrens and Wanke (1954) investigated the value of high-speed centrifuging in experiments with 1,000 sputa. The direct microscopy of the sediments obtained indicated an increase in the number of bacilli in the specimens centrifuged at high speed but the concentration result predicted by the theory was never reached. (For further information on centrifuging, see Duclaux, 1955).

Calcium Phosphate Precipitation and Concentration by Means of Centrifuging

In our experiments (1951) we compared the efficacy of calcium phosphate precipitation of tubercle bacilli with that of simple centrifuging. The amounts of tubercle bacilli concentrated by calcium phosphate precipitation and from the material subjected to centrifuging without precipitation were compared by direct count of sedimentated bacilli. Twenty different sputa were digested with a purifier ($NaOH + Na_3PO_4$); each sputum was divided into six equal parts and to one of them 1 ml. of a 0.5 per cent $CaCl_2$ solution was added to produce precipitation. All the material was centrifuged in the ordinary laboratory angle centrifuge at 2,000 rpm. After five minutes of centrifuging, a tube with phosphate precipitate and one without it were removed; the other tubes were centrifuged for 15, 30, 45, and 60 minutes; then 0.01 ml. of sediment taken from each tube was mixed with equal parts of egg white, spread over 1 square centimeter of the slide, and stained. Thereupon bacilli in 50 fields of oil immersion were counted.

Figure 24 shows that the quantity of sedimented bacilli after one hour of centrifuging is smaller than the quantity of bacilli sedimentated by the calcium phosphate precipitate after five minutes of centrifuging. The highest rate of sedimentation is reached in the first fifteen minutes of simple

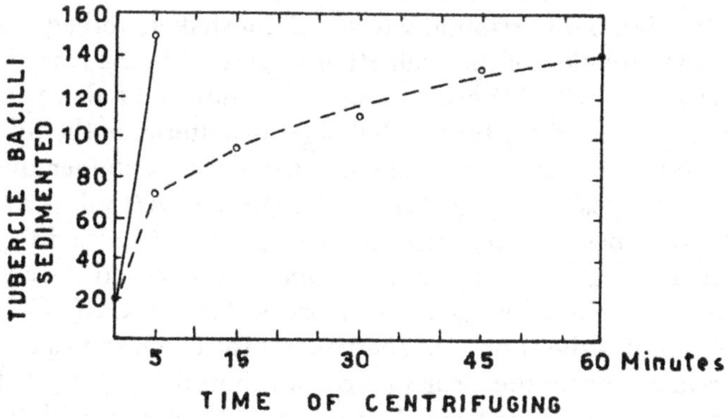

Figure 24. The action of centrifuging and precipitation on the sedimentation of tubercle bacilli. Solid line: centrifuging and precipitation. Broken line: centrifuging without precipitation.

centrifuging; after this the quantity of sedimented bacilli increases slowly. This is in accord with the earlier results of Krzyzanowska (1899) and Davy and Levaditi (1938).

Notwithstanding the small quantities of calcium phosphate formed under the above conditions, it would not be good to spread this mineral substance on the surface of the medium. After drying, it forms a mineral layer that may impede the growth of tubercle bacilli, and, in a liquid medium, may produce a sediment hard to decolorize. Because of this, a solvent was introduced. The phosphates are readily soluble in citric acid and citrates. Calcium salts are little soluble in water. These salts are soluble in citrates because they are dispersed in the liquid and the formation of precipitate is prevented. The formed liquid has all the aspects of a true solution (Gengou, Grégoire, Lagrange, and Thomas, 1950).

To realize the cultivation of a small number of tubercle bacilli, the precise neutralization of the material has to be achieved. The growth of tubercle bacilli is more intensely affected by the *p*H of the medium when a small number of bacilli are planted on the medium than is the case when large amounts of bacilli are inoculated into the media. The use of egg media does not change the situation.

Our SP Technique

About 2 ml. of contaminated material (1 ml. if very purulent) is put into sterile centrifuge tubes with round bottoms containing 10 glass beads 3 mm. in diameter. To the material in the tubes is added 5 ml. of purifier of the following composition: 1 g. NaOH, 1 g. $Na_3PO_4 \cdot 12\ H_2O$ and 100 ml. distilled water (must not be sterilized). The tubes are closed with boiled and dried rubber stoppers and put into a metal box or cylinder, which is secured to prevent the tubes from moving. The container is hermetically closed with a lid, put horizontally into a Kahn shaker, and agitated for five minutes. The direction of the oscillation is parallel to the axis of the tubes. (Any other shaker with 275 oscillations per minute and a three cm. horizontal stroke may be used.) After the shaking, the material in the tubes is finely homogenized. The tubes are removed from the container and 1 m. of precipitant composed of 1 g. $CaCl_2 \cdot 2\ H_2O$ and 100 ml. distilled water (divided into tubes and sterilized in an autoclave) is added to each tube. The tubes are shut with the same stoppers and turned over twice. In a few seconds an abundant gelatinous precipitate of $Ca_3(PO_4)_2$ appears. After five minutes the tubes are centrifuged for five minutes at 2,000 rpm. The tubes are opened, the clear supernatant liquid discharged. To prevent the escape of glass beads from the tube, the stopper is held at the top of the tube. The precipitate on the bottom of the tubes is well shaken with the beads. When opening and shutting the tubes, the infectious liquid is never allowed to escape. To accomplish this, the top of the tube and the rubber stopper must be dried over a flame.

The mineral precipitate on the bottom of each tube is dissolved into solvent (sterilized in an autoclave) of the following composition: 3 g. citric acid, 2.5 g. ammonium citrate, 2 g. sodium citrate, and 100 ml. distilled water.

To neutralize precisely material treated according to the SP method, one small drop of 0.02 per cent bromcresol purple solution sterilized in an autoclave is put into each tube containing sediment. A sufficient amount of solvent must be added to the sediment so as to change the strong blue hue of the sediment into a slightly bluish-gray tint, which would correspond to *p*H 7. The solvent (approximately 0.5 ml.) is aspirated into a 1 ml. sterile pipette and discharged into the precipitate on the bottom of the tube. The liquid is twice aspirated from the bottom of the tube into the pipette, and the material is inoculated, using the same pipette, on the solid or into the liquid medium.

Our Liquid Medium

Our liquid medium consists of three parts, prepared separately and kept in the refrigerator.

The first part is the basal (salt and peptone) solution, the composition of which is shown on Table 32.

The second part is glycerol serum, composed of 50 ml. of bovine serum and 15 ml. of sterile neutral glycerol. The bovine serum comes from blood from the carotid artery of a freshly killed ox, which is collected in a sterile, paraffinated 1 or 2 liter Erlenmeyer flask. To paraffinate the flask we dissolve 1–2 g. of hard paraffin in ether, pour it into the flask, turn it, discard liquid that does not adhere, and dry and aerate the flask for three days. The blood is aseptically collected (we never collect blood that has run over the hair of the animal, but in spite of this and subsequent heating of the serum, it occasionally contains a few live spores of bacilli). The serum is collected and centrifuged, divided among the flasks in 50 ml. portions, and heated in a water bath at 56°C. for one hour. After cooling, the 15 ml. of glycerol are added to each portion. The serum is kept at room temperature for two weeks, and then stored in the refrigerator. It remains clear for months. The occasional surviving spores, after remaining in contact with glycerol for weeks, do not germinate and do not hamper the use of the serum in the medium. The third part consists of a solution of 0.01 g. of malachite green in 100 ml. of distilled water sterilized in an autoclave.

To prepare the medium, 10 ml. of glycerol serum and 1 ml. of malachite green solution are added to 100 ml. of basal solution. This slightly greenish liquid is dispensed into big (2 $\times$ 15 cm.) sterile tubes, 6 to 8 ml. per tube. It is sufficiently buffered to allow the direct inoculation of material treated with a solvent. The final concentration of malachite green in the medium is 1:1,000,000; that of glycerol, 2.3 per cent.

In the course of our four-year-long experiments we did not encounter a case where bovine sera impeded the growth of tubercle bacilli in diluted conditions. We do not use hemolytic sera for the liquid medium. Tubercle bacilli, which may be found in the sera of tuberculous animals (Verge, Davenas, and Dabrigeon, 1952) would be killed by heating the serum and by the prolonged action of glycerol.

The Efficacy of the SP Method

The best way to test the efficacy of a new tubercle bacilli cultivation method for routine use is by comparing the results of cultivation of contaminated pathologic material containing few tubercle bacilli, negative in direct microscopic examination, with the results of cultivation of the same material according to established routine methods. The tested material must be sufficiently abundant and come from different sources. The superiority of a method is proved by (a) superior yields of positive cultures, (b) earlier results, (c) specific appearance of colonies, (d) prevention of contamination, (e) ease of performance, and (g) cheap and easily obtainable chemicals and glassware. A good method involving the use of rare chemicals or complicated procedures will never be adopted by the small laboratories of remote countries where it is most needed.

In order to test the efficacy of the method for cultivation of tubercle bacilli on solid and in liquid media (see Table 28), the sputa and gastric specimens were homogenized and divided into three parts as soon as they

Table 28. The Results of Cultivation of Tubercle Bacilli from Contaminated Pathologic Material by the Routine Procedure and the SP Method on Solid and in Liquid Media

Weeks of Incubation	Positive by Routine Procedure, Petragnani's Medium (455 Specimens) No.	%	Standard Deviation	Positive by SP Method, Petragnani's Medium (210 Specimens) No.	%	Standard Deviation	Positive by SP Method, Liquid Medium (245 Specimens) No.	%	Standard Deviation
1	2	0.4		6	2.8		100	40.8	
2	83	18.2		81	38.6		17	6.9	
3	93	20.4		38	18.1				
4	25	5.5		4	1.9				
5	18	4.0		0	0.0				
Total	221	48.5	±2.35	129	61.4	±2.65	117	47.7	±2.33

Source: Darzins (1951).

arrived at our laboratory. The material, 367 sputa (144 positive by direct examination) and 88 gastric specimens (not examined directly), a total of 455 specimens, were treated according to the routine procedure (3 per cent NaOH for 30 minutes at 37°C., neutralization, centrifuging for 15 minutes, and inoculation on three tubes of Petragnani's medium). After five weeks of incubation this material had produced a total of 48.5 per cent positive cultures. The peak of positivity, 20.4 per cent positive cases, was reached in the third week of incubation. (The same results were arrived at by Hounslow and Usher, 1948.) In the fifth week of cultivation there were 4.0 per cent more positive cases. Our routine procedure after five weeks of cultivation produced 136 positive cultures (94.4 per cent) out of 144 microscopically positive sputa cultivated.

From the same material, 165 sputa (69 directly positive) and 45 gastric specimens – a total of 210 specimens – were treated according to the SP method and each sediment was inoculated on three tubes of Petragnani's medium of the same preparation as in the routine test. After four weeks of incubation there were 61.4 per cent positive cultures. The peak of positivity was reached in the second week (38.6 per cent positive cases), and 69 microscopically positive sputa produced 69 positive cultures (100 per cent).

Also from the same material, 202 sputa (75 directly positive) and 43 gastric specimens – a total of 245 specimens – were treated according to the SP method and each specimen inoculated into two tubes containing a liquid medium. The inoculated tubes were incubated for seven days and then one of them was investigated for tubercle bacilli; if negative, the second tube was incubated one week longer. After the incubation the liquid medium was pipetted off the sediment by means of a sterile 10 ml. pipette. With the same pipette about 0.5 ml. of the sediment was spread over half the surface of an ordinary slide, dried cautiously over a flame, boiled for one minute with Ziehl's fuchsin (Ficker, 1940), decolorized in acid alcohol, and stained for 15 seconds in a half-saturated aqueous solution of picric acid. The stained slides were observed with the weak lens of a microscope, binocular if possible. In cases of tuberculosis, stained serpentine or cordlike colonies of pathogenic tubercle bacilli were seen (see p. 295).

After two weeks of cultivation, the material treated according to the SP method and inoculated into a liquid medium yielded 117 positive cultures out of 245 specimens (47.7 per cent); 100 or 40.8 per cent were positive in the first week of cultivation. The peak of positivity was reached in the first week of incubation. Out of 75 microscopically positive samples of material inoculated into a liquid medium, 75 (100 per cent) were positive in the first week of incubation.

In the cultivation of gastric specimens, the SP method and the solid

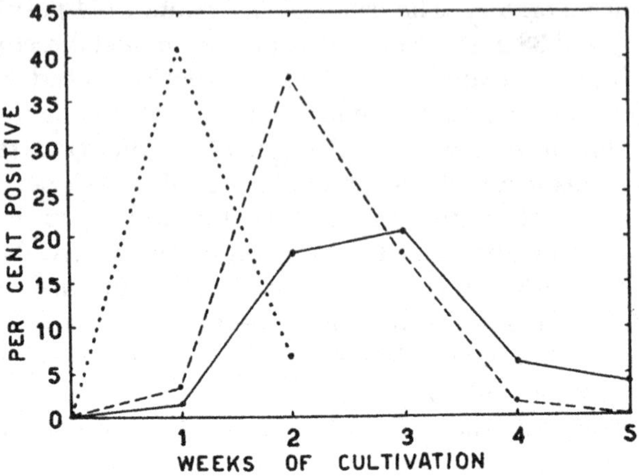

Figure 25. The results of cultivation of contaminated material according to the SP-method and the routine method. Dotted line: SP-method and liquid medium. Broken line: SP-method and Petragnani's medium. Solid line: routine method and Petragnani's medium.

egg medium were more efficient than the routine procedure or the liquid medium alone. The SP method, applied to gastric specimens on Petragnani's medium, produced, in four weeks, 42.2 per cent positive cultures. By the routine procedure, 29.5 per cent positive cases were obtained on Petragnani's medium from the same material. The SP method and the liquid medium produced, in two weeks, 25.6 per cent positive cases. The dying tubercle bacilli in gastric juice need a long revival time to produce a culture.

These statistically significant cultivation differences between the SP and routine methods encouraged us to introduce the SP method into the bacteriologic laboratory of the Brazilian Institute for Tuberculosis Research as the routine procedure for the diagnostic cultivation of tubercle bacilli from contaminated material. In two years 1950–1951, 1,606 samples of pathologic material were cultivated according to the SP method. Sputa were delivered to the laboratory in sterilized flasks, gastric and bronchial washings were done in the laboratory. All sputa were microscopically screened for acid-fast bacilli and only negative material was cultivated. Three tubes of Petragnani's medium were inoculated with each type of material.

As Table 29 shows, the gastric specimens produced the lowest rate of positive cultures. The gastric washings of twenty tuberculous patients were divided into two parts, the first part was cultivated according to the SP method, the other one was inoculated into guinea pigs (one or two guinea pigs were used for each specimen). After five weeks of cultivation,

Table 29. The Results of Routine Cultivation of Contaminated Pathologic Material According to the SP Method

Material	Total	Positive No.	Positive %	Standard Deviation
Sputa	691	289	41.8	±1.87
Gastric lavage	475	117	24.6	±1.98
Bronchial lavage	415	144	34.7	±2.34
Pleural effusions	25	15	...	...

eleven positive cultures were obtained. In three months of observation seven animals were tuberculous.

It was important to estimate the degree of contamination of cultures inoculated with the material treated according to the SP method. Our routine method produced 6 per cent contaminated tubes out of 4,818. The same number of tubes, inoculated with material treated according to the SP method, produced 348, or 7.2 per cent contaminated tubes.

Experience of Other Investigators with the SP Method

Reports of examinations of the SP method by other investigators are beginning to appear. Weidmann (1952), working under the direction of Professor H. Schlossberger at the Institute of Hygiene, University of Frankfurt am Main, Germany, divided 91 sputa, 58 of them containing tubercle bacilli, into three parts. The first part was treated with a 6 per cent solution of sulfuric acid, neutralized, centrifuged for 10 minutes, and inoculated on one tube of Petragnani's medium. The other two parts were treated according to the SP method and each specimen inoculated on one tube of Petragnani's medium and into two tubes of our liquid medium.

Table 30 shows that the material treated according to the SP method and inoculated on Petragnani's medium produced 78 per cent positive cultures and the majority of positive cases were revealed in two to three weeks of cultivation. The material treated according to the routine method (sulfuric acid) produced 73.6 per cent positive cases and most of the positive results were observed in five weeks of cultivation. The material treated according to the SP method and inoculated into our liquid medium revealed, after two weeks of cultivation, 72.5 per cent positive cases, practically the same result as obtained by routine treatment of material with sulfuric acid and eight-week-long incubation on Petragnani's medium (73.6 per cent).

The assumption that liquid media are easily contaminated is not true for our liquid medium when it is inoculated with material treated according to the SP method. Weidmann showed that the rate of contamination of our liquid medium was below that of Petragnani's medium.

Isolation and Identification of Bacillus

The chief reason for the loss of inoculated tubes of solid medium through contamination was, in the case of Weidmann, the fact that a small number of tubes was used for each sample, each inoculated with a large amount of material. Notwithstanding this limitation, the work of Weidmann shows the superiority of the SP method over the routine method and the efficacy of a liquid medium in routine work.

Another trial of our method was made by Mitscherlich, Reuss, and Gürtürk (1952) in the laboratory of Professor K. Wagener in Hanover, Germany. The study was conducted to compare the efficacy of our SP method with that of the standard German procedure of Hohn. The divided material was treated with a 10 per cent solution of sulfuric acid and according to the SP method, and inoculated on Hohn's egg medium. Each specimen, treated according to Hohn's and according to our method, was also inoculated into two guinea pigs. The first study was performed with 27 microscopically positive sputa (see Table 31).

Table 30. The Results of Cultivation of Tubercle Bacilli from Contaminated Material * by the Routine Procedure and the SP Method on Solid and in Liquid Media

	6% Sulfuric Acid, Petragnani's Medium		SP Method, Petragnani's Medium		SP Method, Liquid Medium	
Weeks of Incubation	No. Positive	%	No. Positive	%	No. Positive	%
1					55	
2			3		11	
3	1		24			
4	19		25			
5	26		9			
6	12		5			
7	6		4			
8	3		1			
Total	67	73.6	71	78.0	66	72.5

Source: Weidmann (1952).
* Total of 91 sputa, 58 (63.7 per cent) directly positive.

Table 31. Efficacy of the SP Method and the Standard German Method (Hohn) in Detecting Tubercle Bacilli in 27 Microscopically Positive Specimens

Method	By Cultivation	By Inoculation	By Cultivation and Inoculation
Hohn, 10 per cent sulfuric acid (by volume)	4	14	15
SP	14	26	26
Both	15	26	26

Source: Mitscherlich, Reuss, and Gürtürk (1952).

Table 32. Liquid Media for the Cultivation of Mycobacteria

	Synthetic				Semisynthetic	
Ingredients	Proskauer and Beck (1894)	Sauton (1912)	Long and Seibert (1926)	Kirchner (1932)	Dubos and Middlebrook (1947) *	Darzins (1951) †
KH_2PO_4	5.0 g.	0.5 g.	3.0 g.	4.0 g.	1.0 g.	1.0 g.
$Na_2HPO_4 \cdot 12\ H_2O$				3.0 g.	6.3 g.	5.0 g.
$MgSO_4 \cdot 7\ H_2O$	0.6 g.	0.5 g.	1.0 g.	0.6 g.	0.01 g.	0.2 g.
Citrate	2.5 g. (magnesium)	2.0 g. (citric acid)	5.0 g. (ammonium)	2.5 g. (sodium)		1.0 g. (sodium)
Ferric ammonium citrate		0.05 g.	0.05 g.		0.005–0.05 g.	0.02 g.
Glycerol	15.0 g.	60.0 g.	50.0 g.	20.0 g.		
Glucose					5.0 g.	
Asparagine	5.0 g.	4.0 g.	5.0 g.	5.0 g.	1.0–2.0 g.	2.0 g.
Serum, bovine or human				100.0 g.		
Bovine serum + 30% glycerol						100.0 g.
Albumin (Fraction V)					5.0 g.	
Peptone (Difco, Witte)						5.0 g.
Enzymatic digest of casein					1.0–2.0 g.	
$CaCl_2$					0.0005 g.	
$ZnSO_4$					0.0001 g.	
$CuSO_4$					0.0005 g.	
Na_2CO_3			3.0 g.			
NaCl			2.0 g.			
Tween 80					0.5–0.2 ml.	
Malachite green						0.001 g.
Distilled water	1,000 ml.	1,000 ml.	1,000 ml.	1,000 ml.	1,000 ml.	1,000 ml.
*p*H of medium		7.4	7.0	7.0	6.5–6.8	7.0

* For dispersed growth.
† For primary cultivation from pathologic material.

Out of 27 samples investigated, the culture of the material by Hohn's method revealed tubercle bacilli in 4 samples, by animal inoculation in 14 samples; the SP method found tubercle bacilli by culture in 14 samples and by animal inoculation in 26 samples. This difference in positivity was due to the greater number and the higher viability of the tubercle bacilli in the material treated according to the SP method. The authors concluded that the SP method is highly superior to Hohn's sulfuric acid procedure.

In the United States the SP method was tried out by M. E. Clark (1952) in the laboratories of the Department of Health of the state of New York.

The Brazilian investigators, Chaves and Magarão (1954), working at the Laboratorio Central, Rio de Janeiro, compared the cultivation results of contaminated tuberculous material treated with trisodium phosphate according to Corper and Stoner, and according to the SP method. The treated material was planted upon slants of an egg-potato medium. In 103 parallel tests the SP method produced approximately four times more positive cultures than the trisodium phosphate technique (19.4 per cent and 4.8 per cent positive respectively). The colonies on the medium inoculated with the material treated according to the SP method appeared in two to three weeks. The contamination rate of this material was 2.17 per cent of tubes inoculated. Each of the cultures obtained by means of the SP method was inoculated into two guinea pigs. All but one animal became tuberculous. The authors conclude that the superiority of the SP method over that of the trisodium phosphate technique was the result of three factors: (1) low concentration of chemicals in the purifier, (2) short action of chemicals on the bacilli, and (3) concentration of bacilli in small volume by the phosphate precipitate.

XVII

Submerged Growth

EXPERIENCE derived from the preparation of tuberculin has taught that pellicles that have sunk to the bottom of the vessel will not produce a culture. It was deduced from these observations that tubercle bacilli are only able to grow on the surface of a liquid medium.

The adequate aeration of the surface of liquid media inoculated with pellicles of tubercle bacilli has always been of concern to investigators, and the death of submerged cultures was attributed to the asphyxia of the bacilli, although the first culture of tubercle bacilli in a liquid medium, which was accomplished by Nocard and Roux (1887) was submerged on the bottom of the vessel. Hüppe wrote in 1887: "The growth of tubercle bacilli, gonorrhoecocci and bacilli of glanders under similar conditions is better in a liquid blood serum than on a coagulated one." Contrary to this observation, Spengler (1903) declared that submerged cultures of tubercle bacilli die without exception. As a consequence the cultivation of tubercle bacilli in the depth of a liquid was regarded as an erroneous procedure. The luxurious growth phenomena on the surface prevented the investigators from visualizing the events in the depths.

Diffusion through the surface is the only way in which oxygen can be supplied to tubercle bacilli growing on the bottom of liquid media. The solubility of a mixture of gases in water is governed by Dalton's law of partial pressures. Under identical conditions, the solubility of gas in liquid is a constant physical property of each gas. Water exposed to air of 760 mm. pressure dissolves at 0°C. with 10.29 ml. of oxygen per liter, 20°C. with 6.57 ml. of oxygen per liter, and at 30°C. with 5.57 ml. of oxygen per liter. A liquid exposed to air will always contain oxygen; in deep layers, oxygen is found in small quantities because of its slow diffusion rate. At incubator temperature or at that of the human body, the solubility of gases in a liquid is considerably reduced. A thin paraffin or oil film on the surface of the liquid may be a considerable factor in preventing the penetration of gas into it.

Isolation and Identification of Bacillus

The direct polarographic estimation of the oxygen content of a liquid was first carried out by Petering and Daniels (1938), and then applied by Wise (1951) to determine the aeration of culture media. The polarographic estimation of gas requires but a few minutes. When the culture is adequately aerated, the aerobic metabolism of the microorganism is independent of the rate of aeration. In insufficiently aerated cultures, oxygen is available only at the rate at which it is dissolved in the medium. In submerged cultures aerated by passing air bubbles through the liquid, a limited number of microorganisms can profit from the aeration, namely the ones that have direct contact with the bubbles.

There is a great difference between the amount of oxygen required by tubercle bacilli growing on the surface of a solid or a liquid medium, and that required by bacilli growing submerged in the media. The cultures on the surface need a considerable supply of oxygen; when oxygen is cut off, death occurs. Submerged growth takes place at the expense of the oxygen dissolved in the liquid; it is good at considerable depths (8 cm.) and is not impeded by the sealing of the tubes (Herrmann, 1949). These growth conditions are more similar to the conditions existing in an infected body than the growth conditions on large surfaces of media. The injurious action of noxious substances, such as oleic acid, is stronger on the growth of tubercle bacilli in the depth of the medium than on the surface (Scholer, 1952).

Larson, Cantwell, and Hartzell (1919) performed the following experiment. Some tubes containing broth were inoculated with a culture of *Bacillus subtilis.* The inoculated medium was covered with a layer of sterile oil. After 48 hours of incubation a heavy pellicle had formed beneath the oil layer.

We repeated the experiment of Larson *et al.* with tubercle bacilli. Ten ml. of our liquid medium, dispensed in Erlenmeyer flasks of 50 ml. capacity, was freshly sterilized and then inoculated with pellicles of the H37Rv strain of bacilli, and covered with a 1 cm.-thick layer of sterile paraffin oil. The control flasks contained distilled water instead of a nutrient medium. At the moment of contact between the oil and the bacilli the pellicle was broken and spread over the whole interface of the oil and medium. After three months of incubation at 37°C. the pellicles had disappeared from the surface of the medium, but on the bottom of the flasks abundant clumps of yellowish culture had formed, consisting of acid-fast, highly granular bacilli. These bacilli, after 18 months of growth under the oil, produced cultures on egg media and were pathogenic to guinea pigs. In the control flasks, containing distilled water, the pellicles remained spread over the water's surface and no growth resulted.

These experiments showed that aerobic organisms, such as *Bacillus subtilis* and *Mycobacterium tuberculosis,* need small quantities of oxygen for their growth, and that under restricted oxygen supply the growth of tubercle bacilli is greatly retarded but their viability and pathogenicity is preserved for a long time even at 37°C.

The depletion of oxygen in liquid media may change the growth pattern of tubercle bacilli. In these cases the regular growth curve would change to the linear growth type (see p. 96).

The experiments of Buc (1924, 1928) confirmed the findings of Nocard and Roux (1887) that a simple glycerol broth or mineral solution is not sufficient to induce a luxuriant growth of tubercle bacilli. The addition of protein substances to the medium was found necessary. Buc's medium was composed of egg white or peptone solution, phosphate, glycerol (5 per cent), or glucose (1 or 2 per cent). The pellicles of tubercle bacilli, when brought to the bottom of this medium, produced colonies. The supernatant liquid remained clear. Uncontaminated tuberculous pleural liquid, and the blood or the organs of a tuberculous guinea pig inoculated aseptically into this medium, produced white colonies of tubercle bacilli on the bottom of the tube in ten days to three weeks. Agitation of the vessel favored the growth of the colonies.

The work of Buc aroused considerable interest among his fellow investigators. The good growth of tubercle bacilli in Buc's solution was confirmed by Bezançon (1924). Out of 27 uncontaminated pleural liquids inoculated into Buc's medium, Nedelkovitch (1933) obtained 24 cultures of tubercle bacilli. The same material on Hohn's egg medium produced 16 cultures. Axen (1933) inoculated 97 pleural fluids into a liquid medium containing 1 per cent glucose and obtained 26 cultures of tubercle bacilli. Passini (1934) added glycerol and asparagine to the spinal fluids of persons known to have tuberculous meningitis and obtained cultures of tubercle bacilli in 50 per cent of the cases.

A further development of the liquid media for submerged cultivation of tubercle bacilli was made by Kirchner (1932), who showed that a liquid medium consisting of a modified Proskauer and Beck's mineral, asparagine, and glycerol solution containing 10 per cent human serum was effective for the cultivation of tubercle bacilli even from contaminated material. (For the composition of Kirchner's medium see Table 32.) Kirchner obtained, out of 86 microscopically positive sputa treated with sulfuric acid, 31 cultures on the egg medium and 13 in the liquid medium. If the medium was inoculated with abundant bacilli, the colonies appeared within 6 to 10 days. Kirchner did not recommend the use of his medium instead of egg media for the diagnostic cultivation of tubercle bacilli, but suggested that the liquid medium should be used concurrently with the egg media. Agnello (1935) incubated 10 microscopically positive pleural liquids but did not observe the multiplication of tubercle bacilli in them. The addition of saline solution or 5 to 10 per cent glycerol to the pleural liquids did not improve the results of incubation. The dilution of pleural liquids with Kirchner's medium produced abundant depth and surface growth of tubercle bacilli.

Šula (1948) used the liquid medium for routine diagnostic cultivation of tubercle bacilli from contaminated material. His medium was by and large the same as Kirchner's; however, he used, instead of animal serum, human ascitic liquid, which Kirchner had rejected as not suitable for this purpose. To combat the growth of contaminants, Šula added 1 part of malachite green to the 500,000 parts of the medium. For decontamination of the material, hydrochloric acid was used, and an exact neutralization of the medium was found to be important. Šula compared the cultivation results of 2,562 directly negative specimens in liquid medium, upon Löwenstein's medium, and in guinea pig inoculation. The liquid medium produced 446 or 18.2 per cent positive results; the egg medium 401 or 16.6 per cent; and guinea pig inoculation 381 or 16.2 per cent. The growth of tubercle bacilli from 116 samples of bovine material was nearly as good in the liquid medium as on Löwenstein's medium (75.9 and 84 per cent positive cases respectively). The cultivation method was superior to animal inoculation, but the cultivation in liquid medium of material containing few bacilli was not always satisfactory. In the liquid medium, 4 per cent of the material was lost through contamination.

Göbel (1948) showed some of the deficiencies of Kirchner's medium for the direct cultivation of tubercle bacilli from contaminated material. The growth of tubercle bacilli in 29 different liquid media was highly influenced by the *p*H changes of the medium. The growth of two human and two bovine strains in these liquid media was optimal between *p*H 6.6 and *p*H 6.9 and much reduced when the *p*H reached 6.4 or was over 7.5. Göbel suggested that in order to be able to inoculate into a liquid medium material that had not been exactly neutralized and to avoid at the same time the *p*H changes of the medium, the buffer capacities of the medium should be increased by augmenting the phosphate concentration of the medium to 10 g. or even 15 g. per liter. The increase of the serum concentration in the medium above 10 per cent was not followed by an increase in growth. The concentration of malachite green used in the media was 1:50,000. According to Göbel, in routine work the effectiveness of the liquid media was lower than that of Hohn's egg medium, but sometimes the liquid media added up to 21 per cent additional positive cases to those of the egg media. Liquid media were more effective for growing bovine than human strains of tubercle bacilli. Of eight bovine cultures isolated, six were obtained in liquid media.

Pothmann (1949) obtained 25 cultures of tubercle bacilli from 600 contaminated specimens treated with sulfuric acid and inoculated into Kirchner's liquid medium, as modified by Göbel. On the egg medium, the same material produced 40 cultures. The liquid medium was not capable of replacing the egg media for diagnostic cultivation of tubercle bacilli.

The study of liquid media by Herrmann (1949) revealed that Kirchner's medium is relatively deficient in nitrogen compounds. Herrmann increased the amount of secondary sodium phosphate, diminished the amount of acid potassium phosphate, and added ammonium chloride to the medium as the complementary source of nitrogen. The modified medium permitted good growth of both the human and the bovine types of tubercle bacilli.

Unholtz (1950) treated contaminated material with 10 per cent sulfuric acid, and inoculated it into Kirchner's medium containing malachite green 1:100,000. Colonies could be seen on the bottom of the medium within four to six days. The liquid medium added 17 per cent more positive cultures to the cultures obtained on Hohn's medium. Meyn (1950) compared the cultivation results of bovine and avian material in the liquid medium of Herrmann, with the results obtained on Petragnani's medium. The contaminated material was treated with sulfuric acid. From 74 bovine specimens in a liquid medium without glycerol, 70 were positive for tubercle bacilli; on Petragnani's medium without glycerol, 48 were positive. Avian tuberculous material also produced more positive cultures in liquid medium than on Petragnani's medium (63 and 48 respectively). Meyn emphasizes the fact that the cultivation results and the time of appearance of colonies depend largely on the quantity of bacilli inoculated in or on the media. A liquid medium was found superior to a solid medium for the purpose of cultivating animal tuberculous material.

Künzel (1950) tested the liquid medium of Šula, but used human serum in the medium instead of the ascitic liquid. The specimens were treated with sulfuric acid and inoculated in liquid and upon Petragnani's media. The simultaneous use of solid and liquid media gave better results than cultivation on a single medium. Kröger (1950) came to the same conclusions. The simultaneous use of Herrmann's liquid medium and of Hohn's solid medium increased the positive results by 50 per cent.

The results obtained during recent years in the field of diagnostic cultivation of tubercle bacilli from contaminated material in liquid media embody an indisputable advance over the results obtained by Buc, but they do not solve the problem. The use of harmful sulfuric acid for the decontamination of material, the difficulties of precise neutralization of treated material, uncertainties in reading results—as well as scientific prejudices—have prevented these innovations from gaining the importance they deserve in the diagnostic cultivation of tubercle bacilli.

Cultivation on Slides (Pryce Technique)

Pryce (1941) indicated a relatively simple technique for the submerged cultivation of tubercle bacilli in a liquid medium. The pathologic material to be investigated was spread over a slide, dried and decontaminated in diluted acid, and washed. The slide was transferred into a vessel containing hemolyzed blood. After a week of incubation, the slide was withdrawn from the vessel, stained, and examined with the low-power lens of a microscope for micro-colonies of tubercle bacilli. Out of 14 microscopically negative sputa from tuberculous patients, 13 produced positive cultures. Liquid sputa were not good for cultivation.

In an analogous procedure, Gelder (1933) and Saleck dried and decontaminated sputa on slides and cultured the material on solid egg media.

The possibilities of the use of the slide technique in different areas of research, as well as its practical application in the bacteriology of tuberculosis, are being widely investigated.

Rosenberg (1943) found the slide method simple and inexpensive. Improvements in the method were proposed by Muller (1944). He used the method to study the action of sulfonamides on tubercle bacilli. Bergström, Theorell, and Davide (1946) used this technique to study the effect of fatty acids on the growth of tubercle bacilli. An estimation of the efficacy of the method as compared to routine methods was given by Berry and Lowry (1949, 1950). Kirchner's liquid medium instead of blood was used. The slides were decontaminated in a 6 per cent solution of sulfuric acid. Out of 51 microscopically negative sputa the slide cultures were positive in 19 cases. Routine cultivation on Petragnani's medium, preceded by treatment of the material with a 4 per cent solution of sodium hydroxide, produced 44 cultures of tubercle bacilli. The average time of incubation of egg media was 37 days; for the slide, 3.5 days. Cummings, Drummond, and Schwartz (1950) arrived at similar results. They used Dubos' liquid medium for the slide culture. Out of 176 directly positive sputa the routine method on egg medium revealed 19.3 per cent more positive cases than the slide method. In cases where the sputum contained small numbers of tubercle bacilli the slide cultures often showed no growth. The main advantage of the slide method consists in the short incubation time. When it is necessary to cultivate many samples, the method is time-consuming. The high percentage of contaminated cultures is also disturbing.

Oeding (1951) cultivated pathologic material on a slide and on Löwenstein's medium. His results are comparable to those obtained by earlier workers. The slide method has been repeatedly recommended in cases where a quick answer is needed (Vaccaro and Alonso, 1951). Königstein, Cheng, Königstein, and Suen (1951) used this method to determine the resistance of tubercle bacilli to antibiotics. The method was also applied to the study of problems of the chemotherapy of tuberculosis (Iland, 1946; Bernard and Kreis, 1949; Dissmann and Iglauer, 1950; Bonfiglioli, Cetrángolo, and Acuña, 1950; Badoux, 1951; Illemann-Larsen, 1953).

Reed (1953) investigated the growth of tubercle bacilli on the slides in different liquid media and compared these results with those obtained from the cultivation of the same material on the Herrold egg-agar medium after the material had been decontaminated with trisodium phosphate. The contaminated sputa were decontaminated on the slides for seven minutes in a 6 per cent solution of sulfuric acid and incubated in Kirchner's medium containing fresh human serum. Good growth was obtained in blood solution but the cellular debris greatly interfered with the microscopic examination of the slides. The cultures were observed for 6 or 14 days, and out of 114 specimens positive by direct examination, 80 were found positive by the slide and routine methods. In a group of 132 specimens negative by direct examination, 28 were positive by both methods, while 4 were positive by slide culture alone. Dehydrated beef serum, when used instead of fresh, produced poor growth.

The Chinese investigators Kuei-Chk'ing, Shih-Hsuan, and Tsung-Yu (1955) compared the efficiency of the various liquid media used in the Pryce method for growing tubercle bacilli. Dubos' medium, human blood, serum, and ascites media were investigated. Human plasma from a blood bank was found superior to human blood. The best medium was that of Kirchner-Youmans enriched with 30–50 per cent of ascitic fluid. Malachite green in a concentration of 0.0002 per cent was not deleterious to the bacilli.

XVIII

Dispersed Growth

S. ARLOING (1898) like all other workers of his time, met with little success in his attempts to obtain a homogeneous suspension of human tubercle bacilli grown on solid media. The occasional observation of the presence of diffuse growth in the liquid on the bottom of potato slants inoculated with tubercle bacilli gave S. Arloing the idea of creating a homogeneous culture of tubercle bacilli and of using such a culture instead of a suspension of tubercle bacilli. To facilitate the dispersed growth of bacilli in the liquid, the culture in glycerol broth was agitated daily. Growth throughout the broth started in three days and the culture consisted of acid-fast bacilli and mobile organisms which had the appearance of micrococci. This homogeneous culture was not pathogenic to mammals, but it was toxic to chickens, frogs, and fish (F. Arloing, 1910).

Although its lack of pathogenicity, the appearance of mobile organisms, and its toxicity to cold-blooded animals indicate that Arloing's diffuse culture was apparently contaminated by a mobile organism, the idea of homogeneous cultures of tubercle bacilli exerted a great fascination upon investigators. Bossan and Roset (1923), instead of agitating the containers, agitated and aerated the liquid medium by blowing a constant stream of air bubbles through it. Under these conditions, human, bovine, and avian types of tubercle bacilli grew throughout the liquid in the form of a homogeneous culture. Aeration of the culture with a stream of finely pulverized air bubbles did not produce homogeneous growth. On the contrary, constant agitation of the culture by means of voluminous air bubbles was necessary.

The early investigations of W. P. Larson and co-workers (1919, 1921, 1922, 1923) considerably illuminated the relations existing between the form of the growth of tubercle bacilli in a liquid medium and the nature of the medium's surface. The works of Larson foreshadowed the understanding of, and ultimate success in, dispersed cultivation of tubercle bacilli in liquid media. The density of the pellicle of bacteria growing on the surface of a liquid medium is greater than that of the medium. The pellicle is supported on the surface by the surface tension of the liquid. Pellicle-forming bacteria, such as *Mycobacterium tuberculosis,* will grow throughout the liquid medium if the surface tension of the ordinary broth is lowered from 59 dynes, to 40–45 dynes. Through the addition of soap to the glycerol broth, the surface tension can be lowered to 44 dynes, enabling tubercle bacilli to grow dispersed in the medium. These cultures were apathogenic to the animals. The addition of bile, used by Calmette and Guérin to develop BCG culture, to glycerol broth leads to the growth of bacilli beneath the surface of the medium. Larson and Larson (1922) observed that factors other than surface tension may enter into the phenomenon of dispersed growth of bacteria, since not all bacteria form pellicles when grown on a liquid medium of the same surface tension. W. P. Larson (1921–1922) states: "It may be assumed that when the pellicle-growing bacteria are properly wetted they no longer grow upon the surface of the medium but throughout the body of the broth or even at the bottom of the flask." If pellicle formation is due to the incomplete wetting of the cells, then there must be differences in the surface wetting properties of various bacteria. Larson assumes that "the amount and possible disposition of the fats of the cell might account for the differences in the behavior of bacteria grown under identical conditions." Cultures of *Escherichia coli, Bacillus megatherium,* and *Staphylococcus* grown on a 3 per cent glycerol medium increased in fat content to the extent that some of them finally reached the fat level of tubercle bacilli (*Escherichia coli,* 19.19 per cent, *Staphylococcus,* 29.9 per cent, and *Bacillus megatherium,* 33.8 per cent). These organisms did not turn acid-fast after growing on glycerol media nor did they ferment the glycerol, but all of them, contrary to their ordinary growth form, produced pellicles on glycerol broth. The absence of the wetting of the cells' surfaces because of increased fat content of these organisms may provide an answer to this phenomenon.

The experiments of Mudd and Mudd (1927) further demonstrated the dependency of the mode of growth of tubercle bacilli in liquid media upon the wetting properties of their surfaces. Tubercle bacilli in saline solution produce an unstable suspension; if brought in contact with oil, bacilli pass spontaneously through the water-oil interface into the oil. The clumps of tubercle bacilli in a saline suspension, after coming in contact with oil, are dispersed explosively by the tension along the interface. After the bacilli have entered the oil, they do not return to the water phase. Tubercle bacilli extracted with alcohol, although still acid-fast, are highly stable in the water-oil interface, like non-acid-fast bacteria. These phenomena are due to the fact that the surface of mycobacteria is water repellent; however, mycobacteria can be wetted by oil. In alcohol, the water-repellent property of the surface is lost. Some substance of fatty nature, soluble in alcohol, has been removed from the cells of mycobacteria. These observations were confirmed by Reed and Rice (1931).

Lecithin, the phosphatide extracted by alcohol or ether from egg yolk, if added to the liquid medium, not only promotes the growth of mycobacteria, but makes the organisms grow throughout the medium. Water and acetone extracts of egg yolk are inactive in this respect (Capaldi, 1896; Boissevain and Schultz, 1938). The action of lecithin is not specific; the suspension of kephalin has the same effect on the growth of tubercle bacilli (Boissevain and Schultz, 1938).

Besredka (1913, 1921) and Besredka and Jupille (1913) showed that egg yolk diluted with distilled water at the rate of 1:20, clarified with sodium hydroxide, and sterilized in an autoclave produces a transparent medium. It does not contain meat extract, peptone, or glycerol, but is suitable for producing a dispersed growth of tubercle bacilli. If the inoculum is sufficiently large, growth appears throughout the liquid in four days and bacilli start to settle down on the bottom of the vessel in the form of fine white filaments. In 15 days, the bottom is covered with a white layer of the culture. If slightly shaken, the deposit breaks up and is dispersed in the liquid in the form of a fine dust. The liquid contains tuberculin.

The work of Besredka on the cultivation of tubercle bacilli in liquid egg yolk medium opened a serviceable way for obtaining dispersed cultures but did not add much to elucidate this form of growth of tubercle bacilli. There was no lack of attempts to use the medium of Besredka for practical purposes. One of the first who confirmed the efficacy of Besredka's medium for growing tubercle bacilli was Böcker (1922, 1923). He states that the growth of tubercle bacilli is good in this medium when it has been inoculated with particles of tubercle bacilli "as small as half a pinhead." Prunell (1926) tried to use Besredka's medium for the cultivation of tubercle bacilli from spinal fluid in cases of tuberculous meningitis. Thirty out of 31 noncontaminated specimens, 14 directly positive, inoculated in this medium and incubated for six to eight days, produced cultures of tubercle bacilli.

Poiré and Arzeno-Carranza (1926), in a comparative study of the efficacy of different media, found that the medium of Besredka was good for the isolation of tubercle bacilli from contaminated material. In their experiment, the cultures appeared in 8 days.

Wolters and Dehmel (1930) added malachite green (1:10,000) to Besredka's medium and utilized it for the cultivation of tubercle bacilli from contaminated material treated with 10 per cent hydrochloric acid, and for the differentiation of the types of tubercle bacilli.

van Riemsdijk (1932) cultivated contaminated material, treated with 6 per cent sulfuric acid, in Besredka's medium. The tubercle bacilli showed a slow and difficult growth. Carvalho (1932) found the efficacy of Besredka's medium, when the material contained small quantities of tubercle bacilli, to be inferior to that of solid media. Jensen, Bindslev, and Holm (1935) in their inhalation experiments, used the dispersed growth of tubercle bacilli in Besredka's medium to produce a uniform spray. van Deinse (1937) used Besredka's medium for the conservation of the bovine strain of tubercle bacilli. B. Lange (1939) suggested the use of Besredka's egg yolk medium to culture tubercle bacilli for the early diagnosis of tuberculous meningitis.

Insufficient basic knowledge about the growth conditions of tubercle bacilli in liquids led to a gradual loss of interest on the part of scientists in Besredka's medium and in the dispersed growth of tubercle bacilli in general. The recent work of Dubos and co-workers has promoted new interest in these media.

Dubos' Media

Dubos (1945) published the observation that synthetic, nonionic wetting agents or detergents, known in industry as "Tweens" (registered trademark of the Atlas Powder Company, Wilmington, Delaware), enhance the growth of tubercle bacilli and render it submerged and dispersed. Tween 80, the polyoxyethylene derivative of sorbitan esters of oleic acid, was found to be most favorable for dispersed growth and least toxic to tubercle bacilli. The action of Tweens on the growth of tubercle bacilli depends on the nature of the ester of the fatty acid in the compound. The esters of lauric and palmitic acids impede the growth of tubercle bacilli, whereas the esters of oleic acid do not. Dispersed growth of tubercle bacilli is also produced by the polyethers of phenol, known as Tritons.

Tween 80 is not a chemical individual but a mixture of closely related substances. Different lots of Tween may vary in their properties. Tween 80 is a viscous yellowish liquid, water-soluble in all concentrations. The solutions support sterilization in an autoclave. It possesses both lipophilic and hydrophilic properties. The hydrophilic character of Tween is caused by the free hydroxyl and oxyethylene groups, while the lipophilic properties are found in the long-chain fatty acid of the compound. When adsorbed on the hydrophobic surface of the tubercle bacillus, Tween renders the organism hydrophilic and water-dispersible. Because of this, Tween 80, when added to a liquid synthetic medium in concentrations ranging from 0.01 to 0.05 per cent, produces a diffuse growth of tubercle bacilli (Dubos, 1945; Dubos and Davis, 1946; Dubos and Middlebrook, 1947).

The unsaturated fatty acids, particularly oleic acid and its salts (soaps), are toxic to tubercle bacilli. According to Dubos (1946), one part of oleic acid, added in the proportion of 10:100,000,000 parts of the medium, inhibits the growth of small inocula (10^{-7}mg.) of tubercle bacilli. (In another publication, Davis and Dubos (1946b) say that the inhibiting action of oleic acid was calculated as one part of the acid per one million parts of medium.)

According to Davis and Dubos (1946b), Tween 80 contains 0.6 per cent of unesterified oleic acid; according to Dubos, Davis, Middlebrook, and Pierce (1946), Tween 80 contains 0.3 per cent of unesterified oleic acid. The detoxification of fatty acids can be achieved in two ways: (1) through their esterification, and (2) by the addition of the serum albumin to their solutions. When one of the two procedures has been carried out, the growth of tubercle bacilli becomes possible in a medium containing 0.01 per cent oleic acid (Dubos and co-workers). Proteins have free $-COOH$ and $-NH_2$ groups. These groups account for the amphoteric character of proteins and for their ability to neutralize acids and bases.

According to Dubos and Middlebrook (1947), many samples of blood serum contain substances that inhibit the growth of small inocula of tubercle bacilli. Fractionated and desiccated serum albumin can be used instead of blood serum (commercially available Fraction V, or albumin prepared from blood serum through separation of globulins by acidification and heating, Armour Laboratories, Chicago, Illinois). Purified albumin added in the quantity of 0.5 per cent to the liquid synthetic medium binds fatty acids, soaps, phenols, and heavy metals, and protects inoculated tubercle bacilli against the noxious effect of oleic acid released in the medium by unpurified Tween 80. Rendered nontoxic, the unsaturated long-chain fatty acids and Tween 80 acquire the opposite quality: they enhance the growth of tubercle bacilli. The addition of serum albumin (Commercial Fraction V) to the synthetic liquid medium further promotes the growth of tubercle bacilli, so that inocula as small as 10^{-8} mg., produce visible cultures in 10 to 14 days. The growth enhancement of tubercle bacilli by Tween 80 was observed by Dubos (1946) in an avian strain of tubercle bacilli and deduced by him from the experiments of Loebel, Shorr, and Richardson (1933a), who observed the stimulation of the respiration of tubercle bacilli by added fatty acids (see p. 99).

The communications of Dubos and co-workers promised to solve some of the most urgent problems of present-day tuberculosis bacteriology: (a) the detection of bacilli in the early period of the disease and the rapid growth of the bacilli; (b) obtaining cultures from specimens containing a small number of bacilli; (c) the standardization of the suspensions of tubercle bacilli.

At length the composition of the Tween-albumin medium underwent changes. First, Dubos proposed the use of the synthetic medium of Long with added Tween 60 and purified serum albumin. The source of nitrogen in this medium was asparagine, and possibly albumin; the source of carbon was glycerol and glucose (Medium I in Table 33). Furthermore, Tween 80 was recognized as a growth-promoting substance and glucose and glycerol were found noxious to the growth of small inocula of tubercle bacilli. Because of this, glycerol, glucose, and blood serum were omitted from Kirchner's synthetic medium used at that time by Dubos and Davis (1946). As the source of nitrogen, asparagine, albumin, or enzymatic digest of casein was introduced; the source of carbon was undefined (Medium II in Table 33). The growth of tubercle bacilli in this medium was doubtful. Considerably different from the previous media of Dubos, was the medium of 1947 (IV in Table 33). To this medium were added a source of nitrogen in the form of asparagine, digested casein, or albumin, and a source of carbon in the form of glucose or glycerol.

An agar-albumin-oleate medium was also created. Oleate was introduced as the supposed promoter of the growth of tubercle bacilli (Medium V, Table 33).

The investigations and findings of Dubos and co-workers on the liquid media and the dispersed growth of tubercle bacilli aroused a great deal of interest among scientists. A considerable part of Dubos' experiments and theories was re-examined by other researchers.

Table 33. Dubos' Media *

Medium	Source of Nitrogen	Source of Carbon	References
I. Long's synthetic medium, Tween 60, purified serum albumin	Asparagine, albumin	Glucose or glycerol	Dubos (1945)
II. Kirchner's synthetic medium without glycerol, glucose, or blood serum; with Tween 80, albumin, asparagine, or hydrolyzate of casein.	Asparagine, hydrolyzed casein, albumin	Unknown; growth doubtful	Dubos and Davis (1946)
III. Medium II with ferric ammonium citrate	Asparagine, hydrolyzed casein, albumin	Unknown; growth doubtful	Dubos, Davis, Middlebrook, and Pierce (1946)
IV. Medium II with $MgSO_4$, ferric ammonium citrate, $CaCl_2$, $ZnSO_4$, $CuSO_4$, asparagine, enzymatic digest of casein, glucose, or glycerol	Asparagine, hydrolyzed casein, albumin	Glucose or glycerol	Dubos and Middlebrook (1947)
V. Solid agar medium: liquid medium IV, with sodium oleate, albumin, penicillin; without Tween 80, agar 1.5%	Asparagine, hydrolyzed casein, albumin	Glucose or glycerol	Dubos and Middlebrook (1947)

* For the composition of Dubos' liquid albumin-Tween medium, see Table 32.

Serum albumin, oleate, Tween 80, and trace elements in Dubos' media. As early as 1887, Nocard and Roux made the observation that egg albumin enhances the growth of tubercle bacilli. Dorset (1902), from his studies on egg media, concluded that coagulated egg albumin does not support the growth of tubercle bacilli. Buc (1924) added egg albumin to improve the growth of tubercle bacilli in his liquid medium.

The investigations of Bainbridge (1911) showed that crystalline egg albumin, coagulable protein (globulin and albumin) of horse serum, and alkali albumin prepared from egg albumin were not utilized by *Escherichia coli*, *Salmonella*, *Staphylococcus*, and other microorganisms, because they are not able to break down the protein molecule. The addition of glucose did not improve the growth. Even *Pseudomonas aeruginosa* and *Proteus* grew feebly on this medium. The presence of very minute amounts of nitrogenous food in the protein was sufficient to promote growth. These experiments were repeated and confirmed by Sperry and Rettger (1915), who showed that even very vigorous anaerobic putrefactive microorganisms, such as *Bacillus putrificus* and *Clostridium oedematis maligni*, are unable to attack and decompose proteins if there is no peptone or other nitrogenous foodstuff present to start their life.

The causes for the variations in the response of a body under tuberculosis infection were sought in the properties of blood or its components. Among the blood components, the proteins were those that attracted most attention. Kirchner (1932b) studied the influence of 32 tuberculous and 20 nontuberculous sera on the growth of tubercle bacilli, using the serum itself as a medium. A synthetic liquid medium, with serum added at the rate of 3 to 10 per cent, was found to be an excellent medium for tubercle bacilli. It was possible to detect the bactericidal action of the sera on tubercle bacilli when undiluted sera were used. The bactericidal property disappeared when the sera were diluted. These findings of Kirchner were confirmed by Kallós and Nathan (1932). Lurie (1923) reported that in an undiluted serum from tuberculous animals tubercle bacilli did not develop well. Carvalho and Vidal (1936) did not detect any influence of the presence of blood in liquid media upon the growth of tubercle bacilli.

Evans and Hanks (1939) found that the presence of blood in solid media interferes with the growth of tubercle bacilli but, if diluted in a liquid medium, blood permits the growth of a small number of bacilli. Boissevain (1940) reported that the addition of human, guinea pig, rabbit, sheep, or horse serum enhanced the growth of tubercle bacilli in a synthetic medium. The separation of albumin from globulin fraction had no effect on growth or inhibited it. Davis and Dubos (1946b) confirmed these findings and showed that all other albumins and globulins, such as gelatin, protamin, milk albumin, and egg albumin – with the exception of serum albumin – have no effect on the growth of tubercle bacilli.

Besides the assertion of the role of albumin as an oleic acid–detoxicating agent, other theories on the function of this substance in media for growing tubercle bacilli were proposed. Dubos (1945) and Davis and Dubos (1946b) stated that "albumin alone facilitates the initiation of growth of small inocula (10^{-7} mg.) of tubercle bacilli in synthetic liquid media, but does not increase very markedly the total amount of growth produced." Furthermore, Davis and Dubos (1946a) say, "the mode of action of the albumin does not appear to be nutritive. Although the growth promoting factor is nondialyzable, a solution of albumin, suspended in the medium in a cellophane bag, promotes growth. Since there is no contact between the protein and the bacteria, it is clear that the albumin must exert its effect by interaction with dialyzable constituents of the medium." In another publication, the following statement can be found: "In addition to its protective effect, bovine plasma Fraction V (serum albumin) exerts on the growth of tubercle bacilli an enhancing effect which is not exerted by highly purified preparations of crystalline albumin. This effect is not due to the albumin protein but to a heat stable component of serum, apparently soluble in alcohol, which has not yet been identified" (Dubos and Middlebrook, 1947).

Schaefer, Marshak, and Burkhart (1949), from their study of the growth of the strain H37Rv of tubercle bacilli in Dubos' liquid medium containing 0.02 per cent Tween 80, concluded that this substance acts not only as a dispersing agent, but also as an accelerator of growth. Their estimation of the amount of growth was made by visual observation of the amounts of cultures on the bottoms of the tubes after centrifugation. Albumin was found to be the source of carbon and nitrogen for the tubercle bacilli studied. In the absence of albumin, growth did not occur.

With the aid of shaking method, we investigated in 1955 the oxidation of glucose in *Mycobacterium phlei* and the protective action of human blood serum against the noxious action of oleate in this oxidation. The glucose solution was shaken in 500 ml. flasks containing 200 glass beads (3 mm. in diameter) in a Kahn shaker making 275 3-cm. strokes a minute. The first series of control flasks were shaken with 15 ml. glucose solution and 300 mg. *M. phlei* culture (wet weight) 72 hours old; the second series of flasks contained the same amount of glucose solution and *M. phlei*, and 5 per cent oleate solution prepared according to Dubos and Middlebrook (1947); the third series of flasks were shaken with the same amounts of mycobacteria, glucose, and oleate as the second series but also contained 5 per cent human blood serum. The dilutions of glucose were made equal, and the amounts of glucose in the flasks before the shaking and after one, two, and three hours of shaking were determined by means of the Somogyi method, modified by N. Nelson (1944). The readings were made in the Evelyn photoelectrometer.

As Figure 26 shows, the amount of oxidized glucose in the first three hours of shaking, when plotted against time, assumes the course of a nearly straight line, indicating that the oxidation has proceeded with undiminished force. The oxidation of glucose in the presence of oleate was insignificant; the addition of serum to the oleate solution restored the oxidation almost fully.

Some other findings of Dubos and co-workers were subjected to experimental analysis by Sattler and Youmans (1948). The growth rates of H37Rv strain of tubercle bacilli cultured in the modified synthetic medium of Proskauer and Beck, and of the same strain grown in Dubos' medium, were estimated by the amount of their nitrogen content. Both media contained 0.05 per cent Tween 80. Bovine albumin (Fraction V), when added in the rate of 0.2 per cent to both media containing purified or unpurified Tween 80, did not enhance the growth of tubercle bacilli. (In later investigations, Holmgren and Youmans (1952), by means of a method using small inocula, recognized some growth stimulation of the pathogenic strain H37Rv by albumin Fraction V.) After the first five days of incubation a decrease in the growth rate of tubercle bacilli was noted in both Proskauer and Beck's and Dubos' media even though large inocula were used. Probably the albumin protected only the early growth of tubercle bacilli against

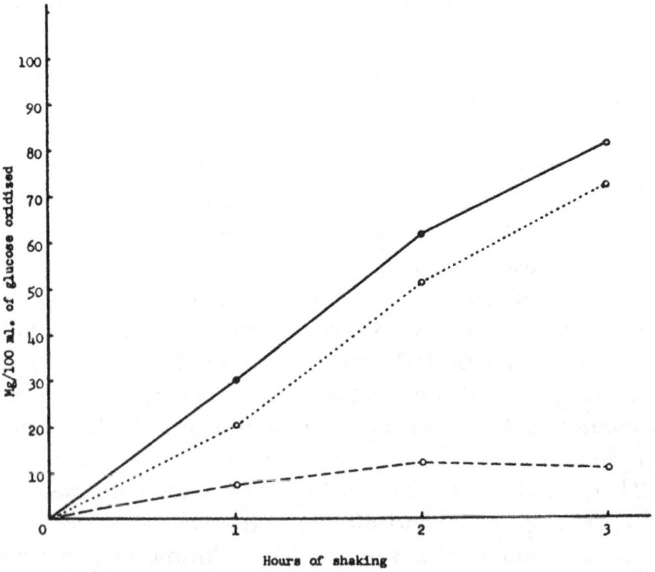

Figure 26. Oxidation of glucose by *Mycobacterium phlei* in shaking experiment, showing the protective action of human blood serum against the noxious action of oleate. Solid line: glucose alone, control. Broken line: glucose and oleate. Dotted line: glucose, oleate, and serum.

the inhibitory effect of Tween 80. The absence of glycerol or glucose in the media resulted in a marked reduction in the growth rate of tubercle bacilli. The albumin Fraction V and Tween 80 in the synthetic media failed to increase either the rate of growth or the total yield of tubercle bacilli.

Bretey and Andrejew (1949a, b), using Warburg's technique, studied the influence of different components of Dubos' liquid medium on the respiration of tubercle bacilli. The addition of bovine serum to the medium increased the respiration rate of tubercle bacilli by 30 per cent; the addition of Fraction V in the same conditions did not have any influence on the respiration of the bacilli.

Zetterberg (1949), in cultivation experiments on tubercle bacilli in Kirchner's liquid medium containing 25 per cent bovine serum, obtained the same growth rate as in the original Dubos' liquid medium. Scholer (1952), in a thorough study, investigated the role of albumin Fraction V, Tween 80, and oleate in Dubos' liquid medium. Scholer used the method of Youmans to determine the growth rate of small numbers of tubercle bacilli. The human laboratory strain H37Rv and freshly isolated strains of tubercle bacilli were used. Out of seven bovine sera used instead of Fraction V, five showed the generation time of 14 hours, recognized by Youmans as optimal for tubercle bacilli growing in a liquid medium. The added oleate never enhanced the growth of strain H37Rv, and often impeded it. Fraction V and oleate in the medium produced scarcely any improvement of growth. The human sera in Kirchner's medium with added Tween were superior to Fraction V for dispersed growth of tubercle bacilli (Reed, 1953).

Millberger, Bartmann, and Zander (1954) found that the addition to the medium of whole serum led to better growth of tubercle bacilli than the addition of albumin (prepared in Behringwerke, Germany) or of Fraction V prepared by the authors. The action of Tween 80 as a growth-promoting and dispersing agent depends largely on the individual properties of the strain of tubercle bacilli.

By adding agar, albumin, and oleic acid to the basal medium, Dubos obtained transparent solid agar medium which could be used in Petri dishes for the surface inoculation of pathologic material. In the absence of iron and oleate the colonies of tubercle bacilli on such a medium remains small (Dubos, 1947). The toxic effects of agar (Drea, 1940) and of oleic acid on the growth of tubercle bacilli were supposed to be neutralized by serum albumin present in the medium. The growth of small inocula of tubercle bacilli on this oleate-albumin-agar medium becomes visible in 10 days or earlier (Dubos and Middlebrook, 1947).

Kürsteiner (1950) used, without any loss in the efficacy of the medium, bovine serum instead of albumin Fraction V in Dubos' agar medium. Scholer (1952) compared the growth of tubercle bacilli in Dubos' agar medium containing 0.5 per cent Fraction V and 0.05 per cent oleate with the growth results in the medium without oleate and containing, instead of Fraction V, 10 per cent serum. Scholer concluded that the presence of Fraction V in the medium facilitated the growth of small inocula (10^{-8} mg.) of tubercle bacilli, but that bovine serum, in an agar medium in the absence of oleate, produces more rapid growth of small inocula of tubercle bacilli than the oleate-albumin-agar medium of Dubos. Horse sera were inferior to bovine sera in promoting the growth of tubercle bacilli.

Serum-agar or serum-glycerol-agar media without any additional substances were early used with success for the cultivation of tubercle bacilli. Even the first cultivation of tubercle bacilli from contaminated material was realized on serum-glycerol agar (Hüppe, 1887) (see page 196). Important early observations about the role of bovine serum in the agar media for the cultivation of mycobacteria were made by Weber and Taute (1904–1905). These authors cultured frog tubercle bacilli from frog liver treated with formaldehyde by planting the treated material on bovine serum–glycerol agar (see p. 199). When serum was absent from the agar, the primary isolation of the bacilli from the material treated with formaldehyde could not be made; the bacilli did not grow on glycerol agar without serum. Weber and Taute concluded that bovine serum neutralizes the traces of formaldehyde which remain in the treated material and inhibit the growth of bacilli.

Powelson and McCarter (1944) found that Dorset's synthetic medium with 1 per cent agar and 0.5 per cent human serum albumin was as good for growing tubercle bacilli as Corper's egg medium. Herrmann (1949), through the addition of 1.5 per cent agar to the modified synthetic Kirchner's medium containing serum without oleic acid or Tween 80, obtained a solid medium highly efficient for the culture of tubercle bacilli.

Byham (1950) compared the efficacy of the egg media of Dorset and Petroff with that of Middlebrook's agar medium not containing oleic acid. The agar medium was about twice as efficacious as the egg medium for the primary cultivation of tubercle bacilli from contaminated material.

Tween 80 influences the permeability of acid-fast bacilli very profoundly. Added to Ziehl-Neelsen's carbolfuchsin, acid-fast bacilli are stained in three minutes without heating (Aubert, 1950). This observation was corroborated by Desbordes, Fournier, and Guyotjeannin (1952).

The hemoglobin-reducing capacity of tubercle bacilli cultivated on egg, Sauton's, or potato media is practically zero. Saprophytic bacilli, on the other hand, reduce the hemoglobin rapidly. Tubercle bacilli growing in Dubos' liquid medium containing Tween 80 undergo a considerable increase in their capacity for hemoglobin reduction (Lévy, 1951). The pathogenic bacilli grown in the presence of large amounts of Tween 80 decolorized methylene blue just as did saprophytic mycobacteria.

The action of Tween 80 on the virulence of tubercle bacilli was investigated by Bloch and Noll (1953). The decrease in virulence was slight when the concentration of Tween 80 was between 0.05 and 1 per cent, but considerable in cultures with 2.1 per cent.

All Tweens, at concentrations of 0.5 to 0.05 per cent, are definitely toxic to animal cells in tissue cultures (Morton, Morgan, and Parker, 1950). Some polyoxyethylene esters inhibit the growth of the apathogenic strain of mycobacteria but do not influence the pathogenic H37Rv strain (Rees and Hart, 1952).

Compounds of calcium, zinc, and copper were introduced into the medium of Dubos and co-workers in extreme dilutions (0.0005 g. $CaCl_2$, 0.0001 g. $ZnSO_4$, and 0.0001 g. $CuSO_4$ in 1000 ml.). There are no data or explanations available about the necessity of this step (concerning trace elements, see p. 160).

Dubos' liquid medium in diagnostic cultivation. Dubos and Middlebrook (1947) indicated that the albumin-Tween liquid medium may be used for early diagnostic cultivation of tubercle bacilli from contaminated pathologic material.

The verification of these data, which are of practical significance, was started by Foley (1946, 1947). Foley treated contaminated material with 3 per cent hydrochloric acid and, after centrifugation and neutralization, the sediment was inoculated into Dubos' liquid medium and into guinea pigs. Fifty-seven microscopically positive specimens inoculated in guinea pigs produced, after 8 to 12 weeks of observation, fifty-four positive cases of tuberculosis (94.6 per cent). Cultures were positive in fifty cases (87.7 per cent). Forty-four of these cultures in liquid medium were positive in 14 days or less. Brun and Viallier (1949) inoculated eighty-seven specimens of contaminated material, treated with 15 per cent sulphuric acid, into Dubos' liquid medium. Fifty-seven cultures were obtained in 6 to 10 days. In cases where the material contained few bacilli, the growth of the cultures stopped 3 weeks after inoculation, probably because some growth factor in the medium had been exhausted. The same phenomenon was observed by Sattler and Youmans (1948), Gernez-Rieux, Sevin, and Spy (1948), and Gernez-Rieux, Sevin, and Chenet (1949). Beattie (1949) found that the inoculation of contaminated material into liquid Dubos' medium is possible only after the decontamination of the material. This hardship, the technical difficulties of the preparation of the Dubos medium, and the necessity of investigating the stained smears taken from the liquid would prevent the adoption of this medium in public health laboratories. Brodhage (1950) observed that the use of malachite green in Dubos' albumin-Tween medium to prevent the growth of contaminators was not possible; the medium with added malachite green became brown and not suitable for the growth of tubercle bacilli. The infected material must be decontaminated before inoculation into the medium.

Gernez-Rieux, Sevin, and Spy (1948) and Gernez-Rieux, Sevin, and Chenet (1949) investigated the possibility of utilizing Dubos' liquid medium for direct cultivation of tubercle bacilli from noncontaminated, microscopically negative material (pleural effusions, spinal liquids). The initial growth of tubercle bacilli in Dubos' medium started well but then the growth ceased, likely because of the presence of some inhibiting substance in, or the absence of some growth factor from, the medium. The results obtained from the cultivation of 765 noncontaminated pathologic specimens were superposable over the results obtained on solid media. The frequent failures of the liquid medium were due to contamination. H. König (1948) used Dubos' liquid medium for early diagnosis of tuberculous meningitis. Out of seven specimens of spinal fluid, microscopically negative to tubercle bacilli, inoculated directly into this medium, four produced cultures in 6 to 14 days. The same material revealed, in 3 to 6 weeks, two positive cases on Löwenstein's medium.

The attempts made by Valtis, van Deinse, and Solomidès (1948) to cultivate tubercle bacilli from aseptically obtained fragments of ganglions and spleens of three tuberculous guinea pigs, inoculated without any treatment into Dubos' medium, failed completely. The same material inoculated on Löwenstein's medium produced abundant cultures of tubercle bacilli.

Penicillin as a decontaminant in Dubos' media. Goldie (1947b) cultured pathologic material treated with sodium carbonate in Dubos' albumin-Tween medium. To combat the contaminants, 0.5 to 2 units of sodium penicillin per ml. were added to the medium. The contamination of the medium by Gram-negative bacteria and molds was "quite abundant," but did not obscure the presence of tubercle bacilli. Mollov, Hill, and Oshinsky (1950) cultivated 1,560 contaminated specimens in Dubos' liquid medium containing 10 units of penicillin per ml.

The use of penicillin in media for tubercle bacilli cultivation so as to prevent the growth of contaminants is largely based on the early publications of the Oxford workers, Abraham, Chain, Fletcher, Florey, Gardner, Heatley, and Jennings (1941), who showed that the addition of penicillin, in an amount 1,000 times greater than that necessary to inhibit the growth of the *Staphylococcus* used as the test microorganism, does not stop the growth of tubercle bacilli. As was pointed out by Iland (1946), these experiments were performed with heavily infected glycerol broth, the highest concentration of penicillin was approximately 40 units per ml. of medium, and the drug of those days was neither pure nor accurately standardized.

M. I. Smith and Emmart (1944) studied the action of penicillin, penatin, and extracts of the culture medium of *Penicillium cyclopium* and *P. notatum*, prepared in their laboratory, on the development of tuberculous infection of chick embryo membrane, on guinea pigs, and on the growth of bacilli in glycerol broth inoculated with 1 mg. of bacilli. They found that 50 to 3,000 units of penicillin (Florey) per 100 ml. of glycerol broth in no way inhibited the growth of tubercle bacilli. Friedmann (1945) obtained rapid growth of tubercle bacilli in a chick embryo tissue in the presence of 20 units per ml. of penicillin.

Ungar and Muggleton (1946) observed that the growth of tubercle bacilli is stimulated by the addition of 1 to 5 units of penicillin per ml. of the medium. Woodruff and Foster (1945) studied the destruction of penicillin by penicillinase of different microorganisms. The enzyme penicillinase catalyses the reaction:

$$\text{penicillin} + H_2O = \text{penicilloic acid}$$

To 800 units of penicillin per ml. of the medium, fully developed cultures were added and, after two hours of incubation at 37°C., residual penicillin was determined. *Mycobacterium tuberculosis* was found to be one of the most powerful destroyers of penicillin. A seven-day-old culture incubated for two hours with 800 units per ml. of penicillin destroyed all penicillin; at the same time in the cultures of *Pseudomonas aeruginosa* 800 units per ml. of penicillin remained, and in the cultures of *Escherichia coli*, 670 units per ml.

Iland (1946) used the Pryce slide method to study the sensitivity of tubercle bacilli to penicillin in strongly positive sputa. Slides were treated with 10 per cent sulfuric acid and incubated in a liquid medium for seven to eight days. A recently isolated pathogenic strain was inhibited by penicillin when the inocula were small enough. When the inocula were too large or the dose of penicillin added too small, the penicillin was destroyed and growth occurred. The avirulent strain R607 grew so readily and destroyed penicillin so effectively that even 0.00001 mg. of tubercle bacilli would grow in the presence of 500 units of penicillin per ml. of the medium. Because of this, the strain was recognized as insensitive to penicillin. The errors in the determination of the sensitivity of mycobacteria to penicillin are due to (a) the large inoculum (0.1–1.0 mg.) and (b) the use of a laboratory strain of tubercle bacilli. The effect of penicillin on recently isolated strains depends on the size of the inoculum; an old laboratory strain may be a very active destroyer of penicillin.

Solotorovsky, Bugie, and Frost (1948) studied the action of penicillin on recently isolated and on old laboratory strains of tubercle bacilli of different concentrations grown in Dubos' medium. The 14-day-old undiluted cultures of recently isolated human strains were inhibited by 80 to 200 units of penicillin per ml.; the same cultures, diluted tenfold, were inhibited by 20 to 150 units, the culture diluted a hundredfold was inhibited by 1 to 60 units; and the culture diluted a thousandfold was inhibited at the concentration of 20 units or less of penicillin per ml. of medium. Espersen (1949) observed, in glass-covered cultures in serum-Tween agar, that the action of penicillin is bacteriostatic and bacteriolytic and that this action can be demonstrated in a medium containing as little as 5 units of penicillin per ml.

Fallin, Patnode, and Hudgins (1952) studied the influence of penicillin on scanty tubercle bacilli in pooled sputum (one to three bacilli in 50 oil immersion fields), and found that 100 to 400 units of penicillin per ml. exert a definite toxic effect on small numbers of tubercle bacilli in sputum. Penicillin significantly reduced the number of viable tubercle bacilli in direct proportion to the concentration of the drug added. Soltys (1952) observed the inhibition of the growth of an avian strain of tubercle bacilli in Dubos' medium in the presence of 50 ml. of penicillin per ml. Mammalian strains of tubercle bacilli were inhibited in the presence of 500 units of penicillin per ml.; *Mycobacterium phlei* and BCG strain were the least sensitive to penicillin.

Kirby and Dubos (1947) in their study on the action of penicillin on tubercle bacilli, concluded that "small inocula of tubercle bacilli are highly susceptible to concentrations of penicillin as low as one unit per cc. in the albumin-Tween medium."

Dubos' agar medium in diagnostic cultivation. Smith, Humiston, Creger, and Kirby (1949) compared the results of cultivation of 1,300 pathologic specimens on Dubos' albumin-oleate agar with the results obtained from the cultivation of the same specimens on egg-potato media. The contaminated material was treated with 4 per cent sodium hydroxide and shaken in a shaking machine, then 100 units of penicillin were added per ml. of the medium. The agar medium produced 134 positive cultures; the egg-potato medium 120. The cultures appeared on the agar medium ten days earlier than on the egg medium.

Kürsteiner (1950) tried, in a thorough work, to evaluate the different properties of Dubos' oleate-albumin-agar medium. He concluded that penicillin added to the medium in an amount as high as 40 units per ml. does not interfere with the growth of tubercle bacilli and that the Fraction V of bovine albumin can be replaced with whole bovine serum. For greater protection of the medium against contamination, he added malachite green in the concentration of 1:300,000. All attempts to inoculate this medium composed of serum, oleate, penicillin, malachite green, and agar directly with material not decontaminated were unsuccessful. Two hundred twenty specimens were inoculated after decontamination with hydrochloric acid or sodium hydroxide onto this medium in Petri dishes. In four to five weeks 34 positive cultures (15.5 per cent) were obtained. The same material inoculated into guinea pigs produced 35 cases of tuberculosis (15.9 per cent).

Molloy, Miner, and Berry (1951) cultivated on Dubos' agar medium and on Löwenstein's medium, aliquots of 395 decontaminated specimens of routine material (200 gastric washings, 46 sputa, etc.) and inoculated them into guinea pigs. Each Petri dish contained 20 ml. of agar medium and 1,000 units of penicillin. Plates were read until the end of the sixth week and animals were observed for six weeks. Dubos' medium was positive in 44 cases (11 per cent); Löwenstein's medium in 30 (7.6 per cent); guinea pig inoculation in 31 cases (7.8 per cent). No explanation for the breakdown of animal inoculation was given.

Armstrong (1950) compared the results of cultivation of 1,891 samples of sputum and gastric specimens on Petragnani's medium and on Dubos' oleate-albumin-agar medium. The material was treated with Na_3PO_4 solution. Observation of cultures was carried on for eight weeks. Agar medium tubes were subjected to microscopic examination each week and smears from colonies were made. The two media were found to be roughly equal in sensitivity. Dubos' agar medium was superior to the Petragnani medium in regard to speed of growth; 58 per cent of the positive cultures appeared within the first two weeks of cultivation, but the sediment on the surface of the medium made gross identification of colonies impossible. Each culture that yielded acid-fast bacilli had to be identified by the inoculation of Petragnani's medium. Dubos' agar medium was found to have no advantage for culturing sputum and lavage material except insofar as positive cultures appear earlier on it than on Petragnani's medium.

Abbott (1951) claims that the major cause for the failure of the bacteriologic diagnosis of tuberculosis is the contamination of media, and that this hazard might be partly eliminated by the introduction of penicillin. To one or two ml. of material, partly decontaminated with 4 per cent sodium hydroxide, Abbott added 200 units of crystalline penicillin and inoculated treated material on three or four tubes of Löwenstein-Jensen's egg medium. On the preliminary tests of 925 specimens, the contamination of cultures decreased approximately 50 per cent from his 1950 results. (In 1950, Abbott's rate of contaminated cultures had been 41.8 per cent; in 1951, when penicillin was used, it dropped to 20.6 per cent.) The rate of growth of tubercle bacilli was not affected by the penicillin. In the second series of 9,477 sputa, the growth of tubercle bacilli on the medium containing penicillin was slower than on the medium without penicillin. In 265 specimens treated with 200 units of penicillin, the contamination rate for staphylococci was reduced from 47 to 2 cases, for Gram-positive bacilli from 25 to 5, but the contamination rate from Gram-negative coliform organisms remained unaffected.

Melvin, Klein, Jones, and Cummings (1951) cultivated 1,500 pathologic specimens. Because of the polymorphous and atypical growth of tubercle bacilli on oleate-albumin media it was difficult to identify the colonies of tubercle bacilli on the basis of their morphology. Frequently tubercle bacilli grew in smooth dewdrop-like colonies.

Medlar, Bernstein, and Reeves (1951) cultivated as routine work, 2,157 contaminated specimens in three different egg media and on Dubos' and Herrold's agar media. Dubos' albumin-oleate-agar medium containing 50 units of penicillin per ml. produced 94.8 per cent, and the egg medium 98.3 per cent positive cultures from microscopically positive specimens. Microscopically negative specimens revealed on egg mediums 36.6 per cent, and on Dubos' medium 29.3 per cent positive cases. On albumin-oleate-agar medium, no recognizable colony formation was observed prior to the fourth or fifth week of incubation. Microscopic examination was necessary for the identification of colonies on agar media. The greatest variation in the colony growth of tubercle bacilli was observed on Dubos' and Herrold's agar media.

New facts about the growth of acid-fast bacilli on agar media were brought forth by the study of Ross and Landry (1952). By culturing 204 sputa on Löwenstein's medium, these workers obtained 52 cultures of tubercle bacilli. The stained preparations from cultures of the same material on Dubos' albumin-oleate-agar medium showed 62 strains considered to be tubercle bacilli by one technician, but 9 of them were regarded as doubtful by another. All 62 strains of acid-fast bacilli grown on Dubos' medium were transferred to Löwenstein's medium, where 44 of them showed typical growth, but 18 failed to grow. These 18 strains from Dubos' medium were inoculated into guinea pigs. Four of the inoculated animals developed tuberculosis; 14 were reported as negative. So Dubos' medium produced *in toto* 48 cultures of tubercle bacilli. The origin and nature of 14 apathogenic acid-fast strains (7 per cent) obtained on Dubos' medium remains unknown.

From the analysis of the foregoing works it must be concluded that albumin or Fraction V can be replaced by bovine serum in Dubos' albumin-oleate-agar medium (Kürsteiner, 1950; Scholer, 1951, 1952). Up to the present there is no proof of oleic acid or oleate assimilation by tubercle bacilli. The growth of tubercle bacilli of some recently isolated strains was stimulated by oleic acid when small inocula were used; to other strains (H37Rv) oleic acid was toxic (Scholer, 1952).

In Dubos' agar medium it is possible to eliminate oleic acid as nonessential for the growth of tubercle bacilli. Thus the medium of Dubos is transformed into a serum-agar medium which had been shown by many earlier authors to be efficient for the cultivation of tubercle bacilli (Hüppe, 1887; Powelson and McCarter, 1944; Herrmann, 1949; Byham, 1950).

Penicillin has little influence on the growth of the heavily inoculated cultures of tubercle bacilli (Smith and Emmart, 1944; Iland, 1946). It is toxic for small inocula of tubercle bacilli; freshly isolated strains are more sensitive to it than old laboratory strains (Iland, 1946; Solotorovsky, Bugie, and Frost, 1948; Fallin, Patnode, and Hudgins, 1952). The tubercle bacillus is a powerful destroyer of penicillin and this may simulate the insensitivity of the strain to the antibiotic (Woodruff and Foster, 1945; Iland, 1946).

The application of Dubos' albumin-oleate-penicillin-agar medium in diagnostic cultivation of tubercle bacilli from contaminated material in routine work has, by now, been sufficiently tested to permit the comparison of results with those yielded by egg media. Most investigators observed earlier development of tubercle bacilli colonies on agar-serum-albumin media than on the egg media. One of the causes for this must be the soft, colloid consistency of the former. A 2 per cent agar medium contains 98 per cent water; coagulated egg yolk contains only 50 per cent water. The agar medium is transparent, allows the count of the colonies, and often the observation of cord formation also. The claims for the superiority of this medium over egg media, advanced on the basis of laboratory experiments (Dubos, 1947; Lagergren and Frisk, 1950; Zuckermann and Rantz, 1951), were not confirmed in large-scale diagnostic cultivation of tubercle bacilli from contaminated material. Dubos' medium did not produce results statistically superior to those obtained with egg media (J. W. Smith, Humiston, Creger, and Kirby, 1949; Medlar, Bernstein, and Reeves, 1951; Armstrong, 1950; Abbott, 1950, 1951). The disadvantage of Dubos' agar medium lies in the use of ingredients that, in many countries, are rare and expensive (Fraction V, penicillin), the uncharacteristic growth of tubercle bacilli on agar media (if the growth on egg media is accepted as characteristic), and the difficulty of recognizing colonies among the debris of inoculated material (Armstrong, 1950).

Because of the lack of criteria for absolute truth, man assesses an unknown value by comparing it with a known one, the arbitrary "norm" or "standard." This standard in the routine cultivation of tubercle bacilli can at the present only be the well-known egg media, contrary to the opinion of Dubos and Noufflard (1950): "*On ne saurait prendre comme critère du 'type' l'apparence des colonies de bacille de Koch sur le jaune d'oeuf coagulé.*" Notwithstanding its empiricism ("*l'empirisme total des milieu à l'oeuf,*" Dubos and Noufflard, 1950) and the "uncontrolled complexity of the egg media" (Middlebrook, 1950), there are, at the present moment, no other media and methods which could be substituted for these media and methods in routine diagnostic work.

Further advance will be only possible when more basic knowledge has been gained about the growth and specific resistance factors of tubercle bacilli, but the accumulation of scientific facts, as the foregoing has shown, has been difficult and slow in this field.

Although Dubos' media did not solve the problem of early cultivation of tubercle bacilli and the cultivation of a small number of tubercle bacilli from contaminated material, the liquid albumin-Tween medium of Dubos rendered outstanding service to many branches of tuberculosis research.

Dubos' liquid medium in research. The growth of tubercle bacilli in Dubos' liquid medium takes place mostly in the form of separated cells, in small heaps of cells (Hauduroy and Rosset, 1947), or in "units" (Fenner, 1951), if albumin but not whole serum is used in the medium (Scholer, 1952). Such dispersion of mycobacteria cells, which is practically equal to the suspension of single cells, could not be achieved with the aid of old methods of trituration, filtration, or centrifugation of a bacterial suspension prepared from a solid medium. This achievement diminishes the important dilution error in the quantitative problems of research on mycobacteria and renders the results obtained by different investigators statistically comparable.

D. G. Smith (1947); Wolinsky and Steenken (1947); Youmans and Youmans (1949); Schaefer, Marshak, and Burkhart (1949); and Hurwitz and Silverman (1950) used the wetting agent Tween 80 to produce dispersed growth of tubercle bacilli and to estimate their growth rate and generation time. Some authors, such as D. G. Smith (1947), studied the influence of streptomycin on the dispersed growth of tubercle bacilli; Schraufstätter (1950) used Kirchner's medium with added Tween to obtain precise inocula of tubercle bacilli and to study the action of bacteriostatic agents on the organisms. Ström and Rudbäck (1949) labeled the growing tubercle bacilli with radioactive phosphorus by adding radioactive Na_2HPO_4 to Dubos' medium. Bacilli were inoculated into animals and their distribution in organs was determined by an investigation of the radioactivity of tissue. Fisher, Kirchheimer, and Hess (1951) reported that tubercle bacilli of the H37Rv strain have, in Dubos' liquid medium, a linear growth curve, like the cultures with a constantly renewed supply of nutrients. Marshak and Schaefer (1952) used Dubos' liquid medium to study the growth of tubercle bacilli in a medium rich in carbon but poor in nitrogen sources.

XIX

Efficacy of Microscopic Examination, Culture, and Animal Inoculation

Microscopic Examination

A TREMENDOUS amount of work was devoted to the problem of direct microscopic examination and culturing or animal inoculation as a means of revealing the presence of tubercle bacilli in pathologic material. The avalanche of publications about this problem has brought very few new data, but it keeps on rolling.

The microscopic examination of pathologic material was for a long time, and in many countries still is, the limit beyond which it is impossible to go in detecting tubercle bacilli. The history of the cultivation of tubercle bacilli shows that for many years the cultivation of tubercle bacilli was the exclusive privilege of tuberculosis research laboratories. The works of Dorset, Bossan and Baudy, Uhlenhuth, Churchman, Petroff, and others, brought this procedure to such perfection that it became more reliable for detecting tubercle bacilli than direct microscopy or even the inoculation of animals with the material.

The problem of how strong the concentration of tubercle bacilli in the pathologic material must be in order for the bacilli to be detected by direct examination was investigated by Carvalho (1932). He used sputa artificially infected with known quantities of tubercle bacilli. This work revealed that tubercle bacilli stained according to the Ziehl-Neelsen technique can be consistently detected by an ordinary five-to-ten-minute microscopic examination of the thin film when the number of the bacilli is about 100,000 per ml.

A smear on an ordinary slide usually takes 0.01 ml. of sputum, which will cover about 600 sq. mm. As the field of an oil immersion objective magnifying 1,000 diameters has an area of about $\frac{1}{125}$ sq. mm., there would be approximately 75,000 such fields on the slide. A worker can cover 100 fields, or $\frac{1}{750}$ of the total area of a slide, in 5 to 10 minutes. When 0.01 ml.

of sputum is put on the slide and 1/150 of this amount is investigated, 1/75,000 ml. of the material is examined, and therefore 100,000 bacilli per ml. would be the smallest amount necessary to assure the detection of one bacillus by microscopic examination in the given time. The investigation results of thick smears, however, are considerably better (see p. 187).

The recent results of microscopic examination and cultivation of large numbers of specimens uniformly showed the superiority of cultivation over microscopic examination.

A discrepancy between the results obtained by the direct microscopy of the pathologic material and by culturing or the inoculation of this material into animals may be caused by the reduced viability of the bacilli (see p. 211).

Table 34 shows that the methods of cultivating tubercle bacilli from contaminated material produce approximately three times more positive results than the direct microscopic examination of the material. "Without the culture it is impossible to affirm that a given material does not contain tubercle bacilli" (Meyer, Galland, and Kobrinsky, 1951).

Notwithstanding these results, the microscopic examination of material still has valuable application in some fields. According to Freiman and Pinner (1949), this method is an important tool for classifying the patients entering a sanatorium. From the total of 611 specimens from patients examined by Freiman and Pinner, 65.8 per cent were positive by microscopic examination, while the rest of them were found positive by culture. Microscopic examination of material should be performed when a prompt answer is needed (Cummings, 1949–1950). The microscopic examination of sputum indicates the degree of danger for the contact persons, and suggests the policy to be adopted about the patient's employment. However, in order to secure diagnosis, microscopic examination must, in every obscure case, be supplemented by the cultivation of the material. There are no facts substantiating the view expressed by Maassen and Dietz

Table 34. The Efficacy of Microscopic Examination and Cultivation in Detecting Tubercle Bacilli

Author and Year	Number of Specimens Examined	Decontaminant	Positive by Microscopic Examination	Positive by Culture
Cancela Freijo (1946)	2,706	H_2SO_4	8.1%	23.4%
Levin, Brandon, and McMillen (1950)	10,280	Na_3PO_4	6.8	15.1
Holm (1950)	92,759	NaOH, H_2SO_4	7.7	20.1
A. Meyer, Galland, and Kobrinsky (1951)	1,433	NaOH	Negative	25.0
Gifford, McKinley, and Hunter (1951)	3,380	NaOH, Na_3PO_4	12.9	24.0

(1954) that direct microscopy may substitute for cultivation in detecting tubercle bacilli.

The statement of Friis, Lester, and Rasmussen (1955) that the results obtained by culture are poor compared with those obtained by microscopy, contradict the data published by these authors, and probably is caused by some error: 194,641 sputum specimens produced 23,945 cultures of tubercle bacilli, but only 8,495 specimens were positive by microscopy.

C. R. Smith (1951) performed a microscopic examination of 707 specimens of gastric contents; 25 per cent of the cases found positive by this examination were not confirmed by the culture method. This demonstrates that microscopic examination should not be carried out on stomach contents. MacVandiviere, Smith, and Sunkes (1952) reported that for only 2 out of 696 (0.28 per cent) gastric lavage specimens studied by them was the microscopic examination of the material of some value. They consider this procedure absolutely unnecessary. Contrary to this, the French authors Joussaume, Mornand, and Yalcin (1952) hold the microscopic examination of the gastric contents in high esteem. In the opinion of these authors, this examination is an easy procedure and ten slides stained according to Ziehl-Neelsen's technique have more value for the detection of tubercle bacilli in gastric contents than one culture or animal inoculation of the material.

Egg Media

The properties of a good medium for the cultivation of tubercle bacilli were indicated above (see p. 198).

The publications of Dorset (1902, 1903) and Petroff (1915a) on the use of egg media for the diagnostic cultivation of tubercle bacilli stimulated a flow of formulas and suggestions for the preparation of better media and modifications of culturing procedures. The authors of these suggestions sincerely believed that they had found something basically new and that their discoveries placed their medium or procedure above all others (Löwenstein, 1931).

In formulating the recently developed media, researchers have tended to synthesize the growth-favoring qualities of the egg and the potato and to reject ingredients unfavorable to growth, such as meat juice. In some cases, peptone was rejected as a growth-inhibiting factor, egg white was partially abandoned, distilled water replaced by a solution of salts, and chemically inconstant gentian violet was replaced by malachite green or some other dye. One of the first media created as a result of this trend is that of Petragnani, the modification (1926) of which is still widely used. Whole egg, milk, potato flour, peptone, glycerol, and distilled water are its chief ingredients. The addition of a solution of malachite green to this medium greatly improved the protection of the medium against the surviving contaminants in inoculated material and rendered the cultivation results better and more reliable. Most of the ingredients of Petragnani's medium are used in the medium of Löwenstein (1930), the peptone having been replaced by asparagine, the distilled water by a solution of salts. The modification of Löwenstein's medium by Jensen (1932) has recently been found by some workers to be more useful for the cultivation of tubercle bacilli than the original version.

The preparation of the egg media is not complicated, but the basic ingredient of these media, fresh eggs, is not easily obtainable.

The importance of fresh eggs for the cultivation of tubercle bacilli was emphasized by Corper and Cohn (1933). The influence of stale eggs on the growth of tubercle bacilli I demonstrated in the following experiment (1951): Twelve eggs, 24 hours old, were divided into two lots. One lot was put in the refrigerator, the other kept in the incubator at 37°C. After five days two sets of Petragnani's medium were prepared from each lot and the tubes of both series were inoculated with aliquots of microscopically positive sputa. After five weeks of incubation abundant cultures of tubercle bacilli appeared on the medium prepared from the refrigerated eggs. The medium from the incubated eggs showed no growth. In tropical and subtropical countries the temperature for many months is over 30°C. and the eggs on the market rarely come from refrigerators. To avoid grave errors in cultivation results it is of importance for every tuberculosis laboratory to secure its supply of fresh eggs from a reliable farm.

These observations are confirmed by the recent findings of Hudgins and Patnode (1952). These investigators showed that the use of eggs more than 2 or 3 days old in media for the primary cultivation of tubercle bacilli leads to a statistically significant reduction of the sensitivity of the medium and to a decrease in the size of the colonies. The inhibiting action of stale eggs on the growth of tubercle bacilli is attributed to the development of fatty acids in the egg yolk. Bad cultivation results were yielded when dry egg powder was used in the media.

The Efficacy of Different Egg Media

A comparative study of the efficacy of different media is possible only when the material inoculated, the treatment of the material, and the cultivation conditions are comparable in some respect. There are two ways of comparing the efficacy of the media: (1) by the inoculation of a small number of bacilli from diluted cultures into the media and the observation of the number and size of the early colonies, and (2) the inoculation of the media with aliquot samples of pathologic material containing small numbers of cultivable bacilli. Objections have been raised against the first method, principally on the grounds of the impossibility of dispersing tubercle bacilli in water. The error of small number (see p. 318) is unavoidable in these experiments and the viability of the bacilli in the culture is extremely variable. Every colony consists of individuals of different ages and many of them at the moment of the dilution of the colony are already dead. When laboratory strains are used, bacilli accustomed to artificial media are inoculated into the media, and their start of growth will be different from that of bacilli taken from pathologic material. The action of chemicals, which destroys contaminating organisms in pathologic material and reduces the viability of the bacilli is eliminated in the experiments with cultures.

Table 35 shows the results produced by the most commonly used egg media, namely the Petragnani medium, the Löwenstein-Jensen medium, and the egg yolk–potato medium. The Petragnani medium yielded approximately 15 per cent positive results (Gifford, McKinley, and Hunter); the Löwenstein-Jensen medium produced 15 to 21 per cent positive cultures (Holm and Lester; Levin, Brandon, and McMillen; Gifford, McKinley, and Hunter; Smith), the egg yolk–potato medium was positive in 17 per cent of the cases (C. R. Smith). The pathologic material positive for tubercle bacilli produced cultures and was positive in guinea pig inoculation in 80 to 90 per cent of the cases, but failed to demonstrate the presence of tubercle bacilli in 10 to 20 per cent (Abbott).

Medlar, Bernstein, and Reeves (1951) comparing the cultivation results of 447 microscopically positive and 1,710 microscopically negative specimens of sputa cultivated on Löwenstein-Jensen's and Petragnani's media and on the agar media of Herrold and Dubos, found that both egg media appeared to be approximately equally capable of stimulating the growth of tubercle bacilli; on the other hand, Herrold's agar medium was insufficient for growth, and the identification of the colonies of tubercle bacilli was difficult on Dubos' agar medium.

Melvin, Klein, Jones, and Cummings (1951) studied the efficacy of six media for the primary cultivation of tubercle bacilli. The number of colonies that appeared on the slants, the time of their first appearance, and the morphologic characteristics of the colonies were compared with the results of cultivation of the same material on the Löwenstein-Jensen medium. A total of 7,362 specimens of sputa was employed in the study. The Löwenstein-Jensen medium yielded 95.5 per cent, Petragnani's medium 92 per cent, and Dubos' agar medium 89.9 per cent positive cultures. The average number of days needed for the bacilli to produce visible colonies was 23.1 on Löwenstein-Jensen's and 23.4 on Dubos' medium. The identification of colonies was difficult on Dubos' agar medium.

These data, obtained by study of a relatively large amount of tuberculous material cultivated under comparable conditions, indicate that the different egg media in use at present are essentially of the same value for the primary cultivation of tubercle bacilli from contaminated material.

Table 35. The Results of Cultivation of Pathologic Material on Some Egg Media Compared with the Results Yielded by the Inoculation of the Same Material into Guinea Pigs

Author and Year	No. of Specimens Examined	Decontaminant	Positive				Efficacy Index * (E)
			Petragnani's Medium	Löwenstein or Löwenstein-Jensen's Medium	Egg Yolk–Potato Medium	By Guinea Pig Inoculation	
Holm and Lester (1942)	20,090	H_2SO_4		16.9%		14.5%	1.2
Beller (1942)	212	HCl	77.8%			72.2	1.1
Robinson and Dunn (1943)	209	NaOH		22.5		24.4	0.9
Šula (1948)	2,562	HCl		16.6		16.2	1.0
Levin, Brandon, and McMillen (1950)	10,014	Na_3PO_4		15.1			
Abbott (1950)							
Sanatorium specimens	1,260	NaOH, Na_3PO_4		89.4		87.1	1.0
Field specimens	299	NaOH, Na_3PO_4		73.2		79.2	0.9
Gifford, McKinley, and Hunter (1951)	3,380	NaOH, Na_3PO_4	14.4	16.2			
C. R. Smith (1951)	1,999	NaOH		21.2	16.9%		

$$^* \frac{\text{Cultivation results}}{\text{Inoculation results}}$$

Microscopic Examination, Culture, Inoculation

The great range in cultivation and inoculation results shown in Table 35 (from 15.1 to 89.4 per cent positive) is the result of the different amounts of viable bacilli in the material examined. Comparison of these results is possible when the results of guinea pig inoculation are taken as a standard and the cultivation results compared with it. The indices of efficacy

$$E = \frac{\text{cultivation results}}{\text{inoculation results}}$$

of the six investigators, who used various egg media and decontaminants, were almost equal to 1 – indicating that the cultivation results are equal to the inoculation results.

Differences of 1 to 5 per cent in results are statistically insignificant and do not indicate the superiority of one medium over another. Such differences are random variations caused by some unknown factors in the preparation of the media or in the distribution of bacilli in the material, but not by the influence of some essential ingredient in the medium. The improvement of cultivation results may be expected from the methods such as the shaking-precipitation method that use less harmful decontamination procedures and allow the concentration of bacilli only sparsely present in the material, or from repeated examination of the material.

The inoculation of the guinea pig as a diagnostic procedure is losing ground to the cultivation methods. Once regarded as the most sensitive and reliable procedure, inoculation of guinea pigs can no longer be considered superior to the diagnostic cultivation of tubercle bacilli on the egg media. Revolutionary discoveries, such as the discovery of the action of glycerol on the growth of tubercle bacilli, may lead to the successful cultivation of every viable tubercle bacillus in a pathologic material and to the virtual elimination of guinea pig inoculation as a diagnostic procedure. The agar media, recently taken out of the historical storehouse, show no promise of being the promulgators of a new era.

Improvement of Cultivation Results

Repeated examination. Constant improvement in cultivation results of tubercle bacilli was achieved without new media or new decontamination procedures, by preparing the media carefully, by performing each step in the experiment carefully, and by preventing the desiccation of the media during incubation.

Meyer, Galland, and Kobrinsky (1951) increased their cultivation results as follows: in 1944, 887 specimens produced 118 cultures, i.e., 13 per cent were positive; in 1950, 891 specimens produced 196 cultures, i.e., 22 per cent were positive.

The specimens described in Table 36 came to the laboratory from the dispensary of the Brazilian Institute for Tuberculosis Research; during

Table 36. Cultivation Results at the Brazilian Institute for Tuberculosis Research

Year	No. of Specimens	No. Positive	% Positive
1948	251	27	10.8
1949	520	152	29.2
1950	1,062	441	41.5

these 3 years there were no appreciable changes in attendance at the dispensary. The considerable increase in positive results in 1950 was due to the introduction in that year of the shaking-precipitation method as a routine cultivation procedure.

The efficacy of the cultivation methods, as well as that of microscopic examination, is increased by obtaining and examining material repeatedly. Repeated examination is important because of intermittent excretion of tubercle bacilli by the patient. Strandgaard (1950) showed that 52 out of 404 patients examined (12.9 per cent) excreted bacilli irregularly. Such elimination of the bacilli was observed in cases of early tuberculosis as well as in cases of chronic cavernous phthisis.

Burgos (1948) performed gastric lavages repeatedly on his tuberculous patients with the following results: 1 gastric lavage was positive in 23.8 per cent of patients, 2 in 38.6 per cent, 6 in 91.0 per cent, and 8 in 100 per cent.

Freiman and Pinner (1949) found that the direct examination and cultivation of sputum specimens from 611 patients were positive in 51.5 per cent of the cases on the first examination, in 14.2 per cent more on the second examination, and in 16.7 per cent more on the third examination.

Daddi and Nuti (1949) examined 326 tuberculous patients with sputum negative on the first microscopic examination, and found 52.7 per cent of them positive after the fifth consecutive day of examinations; the positivity rose to 73.4 per cent after nine days of examination.

Most radical in this direction was C. R. Smith (1949), who examined by cultivation and partly by animal inoculation ⅔ to ⅘ of all sputum expectorated by 648 patients for three months. During a period of ten years, positive bacteriologic results were obtained in 97.4 per cent clinically active cases of pulmonary tuberculosis and in 94.6 per cent of cases of clinically active minimal tuberculosis.

Specimens from a group of 330 tuberculous patients, 35 per cent of whom had no radiologic evidence of tuberculosis, produced cultures of tubercle bacilli; 70 per cent of the patients examined yielded cultures of tubercle bacilli as a result of the first examination but 10 per cent of the patients were found positive for tubercle bacilli after ten and up to thirty cultures had been performed (Hay, 1956).

Microscopic Examination, Culture, Inoculation

The Clinical and Laboratory Subcommittee of the American Trudeau Society indicated (1952) that the criteria for the absence of tubercle bacilli in sputum in patients under antimicrobial therapy can be based on the results of repeated investigations of the material collected on the patients after the lapse of two or three months following discontinuation of therapy due to the revival of tubercle bacilli.

Tubercle bacilli of human origin under the action of pyrazinamide and isoniazid disappeared from the organs of mice insofar as could be detected by microscopy, culture, or guinea pig subinoculation. Ninety days after the discontinuation of the treatment, tubercle bacilli could be cultured from approximately one third of infected animals (McCune, Tompsett, and McDermott, 1956).

XX

Quantitative Aspects of Tubercle Bacilli in Sputum

THE idea of a classification and prognosis of tuberculosis on the basis of the number and the morphology of bacilli in sputum provoked extensive works and discussions in the early days of tuberculosis bacteriology, and the scale of classification of Gaffky (1884) particularly attracted the attention of physicians. The following years were poor in results pointing toward a cure for active tuberculosis, so that physicians gradually abandoned Gaffky's classifications as worthless for the estimation of the results of the treatment and the prognosis. An easy way of dealing with the problem was adopted. In the presence of few or thousands of tubercle bacilli in the field of sputum film, the case was labeled as "open" tuberculosis; in the absence of bacilli, there was no tuberculosis or the case was "closed."

Cruickshank (1952) tried to apply the most recent discoveries of tuberculosis bacteriology and clinics to the creation of a scale of classification based on the number of bacilli in the sputum. His scale (Table 37) was built on the assumption that the direct microscopic examination of sputum film stained according to the Ziehl-Neelsen technique will reveal the presence of bacilli when their number is between 100,000 and 10,000 per ml., and that 6,900 bacilli will be the "equipoint" – the limit at which there will be an equal chance to find or to miss the organisms. Fluorescence microscopy, in the opinion of Cruickshank, can reveal bacilli in the "transition zone" (Table 37), where the Ziehl-Neelsen technique produces negative results, and the culture will be found positive. The third division of the scale is taken up by sputa negative both by Ziehl-Neelsen and by fluorescence microscopy, but positive in the cultures. These are sputa containing between 10^4 and 10^1 bacilli per ml. The sputa with 1 bacilli per ml. would produce negative cultivation results. In Cruickshank's scale each division contains ten times fewer bacilli than the preceding one.

According to Cruickshank, the divisions of the scale have a definite

Table 37. Cruickshank's Scale

	Bacilli per ml.	
Ziehl-Neelsen film positive		
+ + + +	10^9	1,000,000,000
+ + +	10^8	100,000,000
+ +	10^7	10,000,000
+	10^6	1,000,000
(+)	10^5	100,000
Ziehl-Neelsen film negative —		
Fluorescence microscopy (+)		
Transition zone		
Culture positive		
100–1,000 colonies	10^4	10,000
10–100 colonies	10^3	1,000
1–10 colonies	10^2	100
0–1 colonies	10^1	10
Culture negative	10^0	1

Source: Adapted from Cruickshank (1952).

clinical and prognostic significance for the patient, for the understanding of his condition as a potential problem of public health, and for the classification of sanatorium inmates. Generally, incipient and healing cases of tuberculosis produce small quantities of sputum containing few bacilli. The decrease in number of bacilli in the sputum would indicate the progress of healing, while the conversion of sputum from positive to negative indicates recovery.

The changes in the quantity of tubercle bacilli in the sputum of a patient under treatment may follow different patterns.

1. *Complete conversion.* The bacilli diminish progressively and finally disappear from the sputum.

2. *Protracted conversion.* After their first disappearance from the sputum, the bacilli reappear, but finally disappear completely.

3. *Improvement.* The number of bacilli diminishes in the sputum but they never disappear completely.

4. *Failure.* The bacillary count remains unchanged. The treatment has failed.

5. *Reversion.* After the disappearance of bacilli from the sputum, they reappear after a while and increase in number.

The aims of quantitative sputum bacteriology will be fulfilled when it becomes possible to demonstrate the direct relationship between the quantity of bacilli in the sputum and the clinical condition of the patient and the course of his disease under treatment. There are cases with such a direct relationship, but in many cases these correlations still have not been sufficiently understood.

The Significance of the Discovery of Tubercle Bacilli in Treated Patients

After treatment or intervention, the decisive question in every tuberculosis case is whether tubercle bacilli have disappeared from the patient's body or not. This question is answered by bacteriology. Until the elimination of the bacilli has ceased, the patient is not healed and prognosis is not good, as seen from the statistics of Poulsen and Andersen (1934); Bogen and Bennett (1939); Leston, Gómez, and Cetrángolo (1950); and Takaro, Clagett, Hodgson, and Carr (1952).

Poulsen and Andersen (1934) investigated by gastric lavage 622 children with vague symptoms and negative X-ray findings but positive tuberculin reaction, and found 199 of them positive and 423 negative for tubercle bacilli. The rate of mortality of these children is shown in the accompanying tabulation.

Age	*Tubercle Bacilli*	*Mortality*
0–4 years	Positive	25.3%
4–10 years	Positive	22.9
0–4 years	Negative	8.5
4–10 years	Negative	5.5

Table 38 shows the relation of the quantity of bacilli eliminated in sputum to the annual death rate of the patients in Olive View Sanatorium, California.

Leston, Gómez, and Cetrángolo (1950) published the results of their observations gathered in the course of ten years, on 115 tuberculous patients with artificial pneumothorax and on 170 patients on whom thoracoplasty had been performed. When the bacilloscopy of sputa was negative, the material was cultivated and guinea pig inoculation was performed; when sputum was not expectorated, gastric lavage was done. To detect intermittent elimination of bacilli four inoculations of negative material were performed at different times. The results are shown in Table 39.

All these publications reveal the importance of the discovery of tubercle bacilli in pathologic material for the prognosis of treated patients. In no instance was healing achieved if expectorations contained tubercle bacilli after artificial pneumothorax or thoracoplasty had been performed.

Contagiousness of Pulmonary Tuberculosis

There is a direct relation between the infectiousness of persons with open tuberculosis and the amount of bacilli in their sputa. Many factors – such as the number of persons living together, the carelessness with which the tuberculous person coughs or spits, the age of the healthy persons of contact, and the length of contact – influence the outcome of the contact

Table 38. The Relation of the Number of Tubercle Bacilli in Sputum to the Annual Death Rate at Olive View Sanatorium

Sputum	No. of Cases	Annual Death Rate
Never positive	3,655	4.1%
Negative on discharge	1,981	6.0
Positive on discharge		
To culture or to guinea pig inoculation only	82	7.7
Scanty to smear or positive on concentration only	1,238	27.7
Few on smear	1,688	34.1
Numerous on smear	1,008	48.6

Source: Bogen and Bennett (1939).

Table 39. Conversion of Sputum and the Therapeutic Results of Pneumothorax and Thoracoplasty

Sputum	No. of Patients	Years of Observation 0–2	2–5	10	Percentage
Pneumothorax					
Positive, 40 cases					
Dead	24	16	8	...	60.0
Stationary	6	1	5	...	15.0
Amelioration	10	5	5	...	25.0
Negative, 23 cases					
Dead	1	...	1	...	4.3
Stationary	1	...	1	...	4.3
Amelioration	8	2	6	...	34.8
Healing probable	2	...	2	...	8.7
Healing sure	11	4	7	...	47.8
Thoracoplasty					
Positive, 62 cases					
Dead	33	12	19	2	53.2
Stationary	17	2	13	2	27.4
Amelioration	12	1	11	...	19.4
Negative, 32 cases					
Dead	2	...	2	...	6.1
Stationary	1	...	1	...	3.1
Amelioration	10	...	9	1	31.3
Healing probable	19	...	16	3	59.4

Source: Leston, Gómez, and Cetrángolo (1950).

between a healthy person and an open tuberculous person (see the discussion of tuberculosis in mental institutions, p. 183).

We are ignorant as to the stage at which a tuberculous person becomes noninfectious. Some investigators have tried to answer this question. McPhedran and Opie (1935) of the dispensary of the Henry Phipps Institute, Philadelphia, showed that in children from open tuberculous families the rate of reactors to tuberculin in the 10–14 age group reaches 87.5 per cent. In the tuberculous families whose members have no bacilli in their sputum, 54.7 per cent of the children reacted to tuberculin, approximately the same percentage as in the healthy families (53.1 per cent). Shaw and Wynn-Williams (1954) tried to link the degree of risk of infection with the various amounts of bacilli in the sputa. The work was carried out in Bedfordshire, England, from 1948 to 1952 on children under five years of age. The tuberculin conversion reaction from negative to positive (old tuberculin jelly, 1:100) was taken as the criterion of infection. Of 374 children who had contacted tuberculous patients positive on microscopic examination, 244 were reactors (65.2 per cent); 228 contacts with patients negative on microscopic examination but positive on culture produced 61 reactors (26.8 per cent); whereas contacts with tuberculous persons with negative sputum produced 17.6 per cent reactors. The control group, in which no contacts with tuberculous persons were known to have occurred, showed 22.1 per cent reactors.

Hertzberg (1957) investigated in Norway the risk of infection with tuberculosis in 0–4-year-old-children. In households of persons who had tubercle bacilli detectable by direct microscopy of their sputum, 58.2 of 100 investigated children were tuberculin-positive; when the bacilli in surrounding persons were detectable by culture of sputum only, the rate of infection was 31.3 per cent; when the bacilli were found in gastric washings, 14.8 per cent of children were tuberculin-positive. Of clinically identical cases of tuberculosis, those associated with cough were considerably more infectious than the cases without cough.

The rate of reactors to tuberculin was highest in the group that came into contact with persons whose sputum was positive for tubercle bacilli on microscopic examination. The rates of infection in all other groups were close to the rate of the control group. Only persons positive for tubercle bacilli on microscopic examination must be regarded as dangerous to contact persons. The importance of these conclusions lies in the evaluation of the degree of danger inherent in contact with tuberculous persons in social life, and in the employment policy for tuberculous persons.

Contagiousness of Persons with Tubercle Bacilli in Gastric Contents

As we have seen, the number and virulence of tubercle bacilli in the gastric juice undergo a considerable reduction in the intestines. Compared to their number in gastric contents, only a fraction of virulent bacilli may be found in the feces. Frequently in cases of minimal tuberculosis with few bacilli in the gastric lavage, no bacilli are found in the feces. Considerations and practical experience divide clinicians and pediatricians into two opposing groups: Opitz (1928, 1930); Nalbant (1934); Wallgren (1936); and Lesne, Dreyfus-See, and Saenz (1938) consider persons with bacilli in the gastric contents, chiefly children, as a menace to their associates, and recommend their separation from the healthy persons. Priesel (1932), Zederbauer (1935), Brügger (1941), and Bluhm (1947) profess that the danger from children with positive gastric lavage is minimal or nonexistent and do not dictate special measures for their isolation (for bibliography see Bluhm, 1947).

The bacteriologic discovery of tubercle bacilli in feces is far from perfect, as the elimination of the bacilli is intermittent. A man's notion of hygiene and his conscientiousness in carrying out the rules imposed on him are the result of his education and social milieu. The child of an educated family with tubercle bacilli in his gastric lavage, living in good material conditions, would be no menace to his surroundings. But another child with tubercle bacilli in his gastric lavage who comes into daily contact with many other children in a one-room family apartment, in an overcrowded school, or in an orphanage, may be a great menace to healthy children and must be isolated from them.

PART FOUR

The Types and Pathogenicity of the Tubercle Bacillus

XXI

Do Fixed Types of Tubercle Bacilli Exist?

THE identity of human and bovine tuberculosis was assumed by the early investigators, even before the tubercle bacillus itself was discovered. Villemin's (1865, 1868) classical experiments on the transmission of the human and bovine tuberculous virus to animals led him to this conclusion. His observations were confirmed by Chauveau's (1868), Klebs' (1870), and Gerlach's (1870) successful attempts at infecting animals with tuberculosis by feeding them with tuberculous material of human and bovine origin. Koch (1882) held that *Perlsucht* (the pearly disease of cattle) is identical to human tuberculosis and, consequently, transmissible to humans. The identity of tubercle bacilli derived from different sources was not questioned until Th. Smith (1898), in a comparative study of the pathogenicity of seven cultures obtained from sputum and from bovine material, demonstrated the differences in virulence of bacilli from these different sources. Smith found that the bacilli from sputum were incapable of infecting cattle, whereas he held that bovine bacilli, because of their higher virulence were capable of infecting humans.

Pathogenicity is the disease-producing property of microorganisms. Virulence expresses the degree of pathogenicity of bacilli. At present, only tubercle bacilli lethal to experimental animals are regarded as pathogenic or fully virulent. Even if bacilli should cause morbid lesions in an organism without killing the animal, they will be labeled nonpathogenic. By inference, only the bacilli lethal to experimental animals are actually regarded as dangerous to human beings.

Trends in the Studies of the Pathogenicity of Tubercle Bacilli during the Half-Century after Th. Smith

After the publications of Th. Smith, Koch and Schütz began extensive investigations of the virulence of tubercle bacilli of different origins. Koch (1912a) communicated the results of his first series of investigations to the

International Tuberculosis Congress at London in 1901. His views may be summarized as a break with his original unitarian concept and the recognition of the plurality of tubercle bacilli types. These ideas were further developed by Koch and presented in a more definite form at the International Tuberculosis Congress at Washington in 1908.

To designate differences in origin and virulence of tubercle bacilli, Koch accepted the term "type" proposed by Kossel but emphasized that to him this term is no better than the word "variant" or any other name. The biologic differences implied by these words did not interest Koch.

Koch's convictions that bovine tuberculosis is different from human tuberculosis, and that it "does not seem advisable to take any measures against bovine tuberculosis," were most striking, because they were diametrically opposed to the opinions which he had held before the work of Th. Smith.

Koch defended his new views with extreme tenacity. At a special meeting of the International Tuberculosis Congress at Washington in 1908, he rejected the evidence of the British Tuberculosis Commission on the existence of types of intermediate and unstable pathogenicity as well as the arguments of Calmette, Fibiger, Ravenel, Dorset, and others who defended the possibility of the evolution of types.

The Washington International Tuberculosis Congress split the tuberculosis workers into two unequal groups: the great majority followed Koch and accepted the existence of different constant types of tubercle bacilli, responsible for tuberculosis in humans, bovines, and birds. This was the beginning of the reign of the dogma of types in tuberculosis bacteriology. The scientists of the opposite camp, who regarded the types, varieties, and intermediate forms as links between the evolving forms, remained a small minority.

The seemingly high practical importance of the types of tubercle bacilli stimulated work on this problem. The presence of the "bovine type" of tubercle bacilli in humans was early discovered by Ravenel (1902), Th. Smith (1904–1905), Griffith (1914), and others. It was taken for granted that the persons afflicted with the bovine type of tubercle bacilli had directly or indirectly acquired the infection from cattle. Research projects toward the classification of tubercle bacilli according to their types were started all over the world. Great national tuberculosis commissions (German, British, and American) were created for the study of tuberculosis and especially for the investigation of the role of bovines in spreading tuberculosis to humans.

Differences in Virulence

The most important difference between the human and bovine types of bacilli was found in their virulence. The British Tuberculosis Commission found that rabbits inoculated intravenously with 0.01 or 0.1 mg. of bacilli of bovine type died from generalized tuberculosis within five weeks; when infected with bacilli of human type the majority of the animals stayed alive for three months, although some died within twenty days. To these findings Griffith added observations that the intravenous inoculation of 1 or 0.1 mg. of bacilli of the human type sometimes produced in rabbits an acute and rapidly fatal tuberculosis indistinguishable from that caused by the bacilli of bovine origin.

Cultural Differences

A promising cultural method of differentiating between the variants of tubercle bacilli was indicated by Th. Smith (1904–1905). It was based on the differences in the degree of utilization of glycerol by the human and the bovine types of bacilli. The acidity or alkalinity changes of the medium during the growth of the bacilli was supposed to differentiate the types. "The curve of the bovine type of bacilli tends only toward the alkaline level, while that of the human type tends at first toward the alkaline level and then retreats again toward greater acidity" (Th. Smith). Of the two strains of tubercle bacilli isolated by Th. Smith from the mesenteric lymph nodes of children, one showed the bovine, the other the human curve of growth. The aspirations of Th. Smith were early frustrated by the work of Griffith, who showed that the difference between the alkalinity and acidity curves of bacilli of human and bovine types produced in glycerol broth are only quantitative and not qualitative in nature and cannot serve to differentiate the various types of bacilli. ("The glycerin broth test does not bring out distinct bio-chemical differences in the action of bovine and human tubercle bacillus on glycerin broth.") Th. Smith's (1910) defense of his views was vigorous but did not contribute any new facts and thus could not refute the findings of Griffith. Further work in the direction indicated by Th. Smith – that is, toward the determination of differences in the utilization of glycerol as a source of carbon by bacilli of human and bovine types – was done by the British Tuberculosis Commission. The amount of growth and the appearance of colonies on media containing glycerol was found to be different in the cases of bacilli of human and of bovine types. The growth of bacilli of human type on glycerol media was found to be profuse or *eugonic*, that of bacilli of bovine type restrained or *dysgonic*. A light yellowish pigmentation was recognized as characteristic of the colonies of bacilli of human type. No morphologic differences were found between the bacilli of the two types.

The differences between the bacilli of human and bovine type were summarized by Jensen (1949), as shown in Table 40.

The subtle differences between the human and the bovine types of bacilli sometimes are simplified as far as in Bergey's (1948) *Manual*:

Table 40. The Differences in Pathogenicity between Colonies of the Human and the Bovine Types of Tubercle Bacilli Grown on Löwenstein's Medium and Inoculated into Rabbits and Guinea Pigs

Type	Growth and Morphology on Löwenstein's Medium	Rabbit Inoculated Intravenously: .01 mg.	Rabbit Inoculated Intravenously: 1 mg.	Guinea Pig Inoculated Intraperitoneally
Human	Eugonic, pigmented	No tuberculosis	Few regressive tubercles in lungs and kidneys	10^{-4}–10^{-6} mg. produce generalized tuberculosis
Bovine	Dysgonic, not pigmented	Generalized tuberculosis	Acute generalized tuberculosis	10^{-6} mg. produce generalized tuberculosis

Source: Jensen (1949).

"*Mycobacterium tuberculosis var. hominis* produces tuberculosis in man, monkey, dog and parrot. Experimentally, it is highly pathogenic for guinea pigs but not for rabbits, cats, goats, oxen or domestic fowls" (p. 878).

Human Infections Caused by the Tubercle Bacilli of Bovine Type

The statistics indicating the high rate of bovine tuberculosis among the rural population, especially in children in localities with high incidence of tuberculosis in cattle, seemingly support the view that the bovine type of bacilli are acquired from tuberculous cattle.

Price's (1932), study of the incidence of human and bovine tuberculous infection in children and adults living in the same region of Canada revealed 14.1 per cent of bovine infection in 286 tuberculous children and only 3.5 per cent in 168 tuberculous adults. The bacilli of bovine type were found in 22.2 per cent of the 877 cases of tuberculosis in children (up to 16 years) but only in 2.2 per cent of the 1,330 cases of tuberculosis of adults (Rich, 1951).

The facile explanation for this "very curious phenomenon" (Rich, 1951) offered by the supporters of the theory of stable types of bacilli is generally to the effect that children are more frequently exposed to bovine infection than adults, because milk is the chief food of children, and that the resistance of adults to tuberculous infection is greater than that of children. These hypotheses are insufficient to explain why the bacillus of bovine type disappears from the human body and why the bacillus of human type takes its place when the infected child develops into a tuberculous adult. The theory of the superinfection with bacilli of human type cannot explain this phenomenon; consequently, it is necessary to seek a different answer to the problem.

Types of Tubercle Bacilli in Cases of Extrapulmonary and Pulmonary Tuberculosis

The percentage of the bovine type of bacilli in cases of extrapulmonary tuberculosis is high, as shown in Table 41.

Contrary to the appearance of a high percentage of the bovine type of bacilli in cases of extrapulmonary tuberculosis, the incidence of the bovine type of bacilli in the cases of pulmonary tuberculosis is low. Griffith and Munro (1943) found 1.5 per cent of the bovine type of bacilli among patients with pulmonary tuberculosis in England and 5.8 per cent in Scotland, although there was no evidence that these differences had a connection with the differences in the spread of tuberculosis in cattle in England and Scotland. Out of 241 cases of pulmonary tuberculosis caused by the bovine type of bacilli, in only 70 cases did the autopsy suggest the possibility of the infection's having occurred through the alimentary tract, and only 2.5 per cent of the infected persons had ever worked with cattle. The percentage of the bovine type of bacilli in cases of pulmonary tuberculosis in Hanover, Germany, was 1.9 per cent (Wagener, 1950–1951).

Table 41. Percentage of the Bovine Type of Tubercle Bacilli in Cases of Extrapulmonary Tuberculosis

Localization	England and Wales *	Germany †
Cervical glands	46.5	49.4
Meninges	27.1	
Bones and joints	10.8	13.8
Abdomen, genitourinary system	12.8	16.3

* Data from Wilson (1950).
† Data from Goeters (1950–1951).

The Intermediate Strains

The present situation in tubercle bacilli classification resembles the situation that existed in biology before Darwin — before it was found that the intermediate, atypical, or labile species of the plant and animal kingdom could not be forced into the artificial classification schemes of the time. Later these "rebel" species were to provide the theory of evolution with important links between seemingly unrelated forms, and indicate the course of their evolution.

Tubercle bacilli that could be classified as neither human nor bovine were early discovered by the British Tuberculosis Commission. Griffith, a member of this commission, showed that tubercle bacilli cultured from cases of lupus were seemingly of the bovine type but of low virulence for calves, rabbits, monkeys, and guinea pigs. He further found that the bacilli from lupus may show the characteristics of the human type but yet be of lower virulence for the monkey and the guinea pig than the ordinary bacilli of human type. These cultures are not mixtures of both types of bacilli. Griffith designated these strains as intermediate in virulence between the true bovine and human types. These findings of Griffith were confirmed by Kirchner (1922) and Rabinowitsch-Kempner (1927).

Griffith (1932) summarized his findings on 188 strains of acid-fast bacilli isolated from cases of lupus in the following manner:

Strain	*Human*	*Dysgonic Human*	*Bovine*	*Eugonic Bovine*
Standard virulence	32	2	31	0
Attenuated virulence	59	2	61	1

Jensen and Frimodt-Möller (1936a) found in a total of 35 lupus strains 30 attenuated or atypical strains. Beller (1942) investigated 203 cases of lupus. Bacilli from these cases subcutaneously inoculated in the amount of 0.01 mg. into rabbits, produced in only 7 animals some lesions of the internal organs. Beller concluded that the inoculation of tubercle bacilli from skin lesions into animals is an unsuitable method for differentiating these strains of tubercle bacilli. According to this author, only cultural methods can show the type differences of these bacilli.

The problem of whether these organisms are related to the acid-fast bacilli recently isolated from skin lesions contracted in swimming pools (*Mycobacterium ulcerans*, MacCallum, Tolhurst, Buckle, and Sissons, 1948; *M. balnei*, Linell and Nordén, 1954) remains to be investigated.

The later investigators who attempted to differentiate types by means of animal inoculation found a considerable number of intermediate, atypical, or labile bacilli among the human and bovine strains.

Table 42. Results of Attempts to Differentiate Types of Tubercle Bacilli

Author and Year	Human	Bovine	Intermediate or Atypical	Percentage
Rabinowitsch (1909)	27	4	5	
Jensen and Frimodt-Möller (1936a)	2,545	391	7	0.24
Arena and Cetrángolo (1946)	186	13	27	11.9
Grumbach (1949)	157		33	21.0
Mitscherlich (1952)		9	3	

Changes in Virulence

By repeated passage of tubercle bacilli of the human type through calves, Ravenel (1902) succeeded in increasing their virulence so much that the bacilli produced progressive tuberculosis in a calf. The British Tuberculosis Commission recognized virulence as a transitory property of tubercle bacilli. This conclusion was based on the following findings:

(1) two strains of tubercle bacilli isolated from the horse grew like bacilli of bovine type but were less virulent for the calf and the rabbit than the ordinary bacilli of bovine type, and by passage through animals the virulence of these bacilli was increased to the level of fully virulent bacilli of bovine type; (2) two bovine strains of attenuated virulence isolated from cases of lupus after two passages through calves acquired the virulence of fully pathogenic bacilli of bovine variant; (3) two strains isolated from two cases of lupus showed the cultural characteristics of bacilli of human type but were of feeble virulence for a monkey. After the passage through the monkey the virulence of the strain reached in 139 days the level of fully virulent bacilli of human type. From these observations the British Tuberculosis Commission concluded that "if it were to be held that virulence is a fixed quality, it would be necessary, in order to classify the lupus bacilli, to recognize several new types of tubercle bacilli."

Borrel, Boez, and Coulon (1923a) investigated strains of tubercle bacilli which had lost a great deal of their pathogenicity to the guinea pig after being cultured for some time on glycerol potato. These strains (H1036, Marmorek, etc.), when inoculated subcutaneously into a guinea pig at the rate of 10 mg., killed the animal after 249 days. A second animal, inoculated with material taken from the first, died within 135 days; the third animal, inoculated with material from the second animal, died within 82 days, and the fourth, inoculated with material from the third animal, died from generalized tuberculosis within 62 days. It was not possible to change the pathogenicity by transferring the strain B.B. through the guinea pigs.

Jensen and Frimodt-Möller (1936b) described seven strains of tubercle bacilli, all of low virulence for rabbits, as bacilli of human type. In all seven cases the authors were able to cultivate bacilli of the bovine type from rabbits inoculated with these strains. They concluded that the appearance of the bovine type of bacilli was the result of the transformation of the original human type of bacilli into the bovine type within the rabbit organism. Particularly interesting is the history of strain 1832 as reported by Jensen and Frimodt-Möller (1936b). This strain of human type was cultured from urine and grew dysgonic, being virulent for guinea pigs and only slightly virulent for rabbits and calves. The passage of this strain through a rabbit produced a typical bovine type of bacilli. This transformation of the human type into a bovine one was performed seven times. Strain 1832 was not a mixture of bovine and human type of bacilli.

Pinner (1935) by means of passages through guinea pigs succeeded in transforming two strains of nonpathogenic acid-fast bacilli, isolated from tuberculous patients, into bacilli producing typical tuberculosis in guinea pigs. Smithburn (1939) restored the virulence of attenuated bovine and human types of bacilli by serial transfer of these strains to rabbits and by serial brain-to-brain passages through guinea pigs.

Larmola (1947) cultured strains of acid-fast bacilli of low virulence from the sewage tank of a tuberculosis sanatorium. Some of these strains recovered their virulence after passage through guinea pigs. Apparently not all attenuated strains can be restored to their former virulence by the presently known methods. Willis (1933) did not succeed in restoring the virulence of the R1 strain by making it traverse 900 guinea pigs, during a period of ten years. According to Uhlenhuth and Seiffert (1930) the recrudescence of the virulence of an attenuated strain occurs sporadically and cannot be forced upon the strain in any known way.

The pathogenicity differences among the various types of tubercle bacilli are restricted to a few animal species (rabbit, calf). The differentiation of types cannot be made in guinea pigs. In mice both types of bacilli produce similar lesions. In dogs there are no pathogenicity differences between the human and bovine type of bacilli (Francis, 1956). In humans, tuberculosis caused by the bacilli of human or bovine type has the same course.

The experiments of Lurie and Zappasodi (1955) have indicated how easily the resistance of rabbits to the human type of tubercle bacilli can be changed. In the experiments with the susceptible race C of rabbits, 47 tubercle bacilli had to be inhaled by the animals to produce a single tubercle in the lungs, whereas in the resistant race III, it took 648 bacilli to obtain the same result. After cortisone had been administered in therapeutic doses to the rabbits, three to four times more tubercles were generated in the lungs of the hormone-treated animals than in the lungs of animals that had not been treated.

Mixed Infections

The British Tuberculosis Commission, while studying the various types of tubercle bacilli derived from cases of human pulmonary tuberculosis, discovered cultures consisting of a mixture of both the human and bovine types of bacilli. Griffith (1919–1920) summarized these findings and indicated that out of 1,068 cases studied, 5 were mixtures of bovine and human types of bacilli. According to Griffith, two explanations for the origin of these mixed infections are possible: (1) transformation, within the human body, of one type of bacilli into another; and (2) the later association of another type of bacilli with the already existing infection.

The facts that led to the correct answer to this question accumulated at a slow pace. The possibility of the transformation of the primary type of bacilli was admitted by Rabinowitsch-Kempner (1927). Important data were contributed to the elucidation of this transformation by Jensen (1949). In 17 cases of lung tuberculosis, caused by the bovine type, the course of the disease and the change of the type of bacilli were studied during a period of one to four years. In nine cases the initially pure bovine infection was transformed into a mixed infection of bacilli of bovine and human variants. The strains derived from mixed infections were labile and atypical. It was shown that out of 28 colonies obtained by Jensen and his associates from mixed infections, 20 had full virulence of bacilli of human type, but 8 were of attenuated virulence.

Tubercle Bacilli of Human Type in Domestic Animals

Important information about the pathogenicity of tubercle bacilli of the human type was provided by the studies of tuberculosis in domestic animals, often living in close contact with tuberculous human beings.

Nocard (1898) investigated a case of horse tuberculosis. The bacilli cultured could not be classified as mammalian although they also deviated from the standard avian type of bacilli. F. Griffith (1928) investigated material from eight cases of tuberculosis in horses. Three of the strains cultured from this material exhibited the virulence of the bovine type of bacilli but the other five strains were of low virulence for the rabbit. Notwithstanding these results, Griffith concluded that the horse "undoubtedly derives its infection from the ox," and that the bovine type of bacilli becomes modified in the organism of the horse. Influenced by the doctrine of types, Griffith did not question the possibility of a human source of infection.

Stableforth (1929) investigated material from 16 tuberculous dogs and in 10 of these cases found the human type of tubercle bacilli as a causing agent. In four of these cases definite association of the dogs with tuberculous persons was established. From a tuberculous parrot bacilli of human variant were cultured. The bacilli of human type are also known to be the cause of tuberculosis in pigs.

Cases of infection of bovines with tubercle bacilli of human type are known, although rarely observed. The early experiments of Ravenel (1902) showed that a typical tuberculosis infection can be produced in young cattle by the repeated inoculation with large doses of tubercle bacilli of human origin. Feldman and Moses (1941) isolated from the lung lesions and bronchial lymph nodes of an adult cow tubercle bacilli with the cultural and pathogenic properties of the human type. In the same publication, Feldman and Moses also summarized the earlier discoveries about the infection of bovines with tubercle bacilli of human type.

Cattle can become sensitized to tuberculin as a consequence of contact with open tuberculous persons. McKinstry and Blampied (1955) described six instances of the appearance of reactors in an otherwise tuberculin-negative herd. This led to the discovery of open pulmonary tuberculosis in five persons who were in contact with the cattle.

The discovery of the bovine type of tubercle bacilli in humans and the infectiousness of the human type of bacilli to animals established beyond any doubt the intercommunicability of the disease.

The Ultimate Attempts at Typing Tubercle Bacilli

A great amount of work and large sums of money have been spent on the typing of tubercle bacilli during the half-century that has elapsed since the investigation of Th. Smith. It could be expected at least that definite methods for the differentiation of types and the standard characteristics of the types would be established. The steady flow of new publications dealing with the problem of the differentiation of types indicates that this goal has not yet been achieved. Gervois (1937) composed a list of no fewer than 221 works dealing with the differentiation of types all over the world before 1937, when the projects of the great national tuberculosis commissions were concluded. Since 1937, a considerable number of additional works have appeared. The impossibility of classifying the mammalian tubercle bacilli into two types, either by culture methods or by means of animal inoculations, was clearly recognized by the latest investigators of the problem.

Grumbach (1949a), in a total of 157 human strains studied, found 33 strains (21 per cent) impossible to classify into the two types. Wagener (1950–1951) in his investigation of 160 strains of tubercle bacilli, found 33 that could not be classified on the basis of their cultural characteristics. Wagener and Mitscherlich (1951) in order to differentiate the types, tried to revive the method of Th. Smith – distinguishing the human and bovine types of bacilli by their different rates of utilization of glycerol. The titration method was not applied to determine the *p*H changes in the medium, but, instead, an indicator (bromcresol purple) was added to the medium and changes in color observed. Ninety-nine mammalian strains investigated revealed that the bovine strains BCG and Vallée had become intermediate between human and bovine types. Animal inoculation confirmed these findings. The strains K221 and Kalo, originally classified as bovine, could neither by culture nor by animal inoculation be differentiated from the bacilli of human type. Mitscherlich (1952) emphasized the difficulty of typing freshly isolated tubercle bacilli by means of animal inoculations (Koch had put all the emphasis on the use of freshly isolated bacilli for the determination of their types). The lungs of rabbits subcutaneously infected with bacilli of bovine type were regularly affected, but similar lesions were also found in 24 per cent of the rabbits inoculated with bacilli of human variant. According to Mitscherlich, the extension and number of lung lesions in infected rabbits has only a restricted value for the differentiation of types of tubercle bacilli.

Thiel (1956) found that tubercle bacilli of bovine type often cause generalized tuberculosis in wild mice but that bacilli of human type sometimes also produce similar lesions in these mice. The size of the tuberculous lesions in wild mice could not be used as a criterion in differentiating tubercle bacilli of bovine and human types.

Altevogt and Kuckhern (1955) made one more attempt to differentiate the types of strains of tubercle bacilli grown for 3 to 4 years in the laboratory. Neither by animal inoculation nor by the use of bromcresol purple–glycerol or other media, was it possible to determine the type of these bacilli. The authors agreed with Wagener and Mitscherlich that through cultivation on artificial media the bovine type of bacilli does acquire the properties of the human type.

The investigations of Heidelberger and co-workers revealed that there are no serological differences between polysaccharides of different types of tubercle bacilli. Polysaccharides extracted from human type H37 were built up mostly of D-arabinose and D-mannose. None of these polysaccharides appeared to be type-specific (Heidelberger and Menzel, 1937). The horse serum prepared with the polysaccharides from human type gave definite precipitin reaction with the polysaccharides extracted from the bovine type of bacilli (Menzel and Heidelberger, 1939).

Agglutination tests (Furth, 1926) and the reaction to tuberculin protein (Seibert and Morley, 1933) did not reveal any differences between the types. The studies of Schaefer (1940) on the serologic differentiation of bovine and human types of bacilli, confirmed the findings of earlier authors that lipid and polysaccharide antigens are present in pathogenic and nonpathogenic acid-fast bacilli and that these antigens cannot be used as a criterion for the differentiation of bacilli of bovine, human, and avian types. In the filtrates of the bovine type of bacilli, Schaefer discovered an antigen of protein nature. The protein antigen was identified in complement fixation reaction, by the use of filtrates from the cultures and serum of rabbits prepared by the injection of bacilli killed by heat and enrobed in paraffin oil. Only the smooth colonies of the bovine type of bacilli contained protein antigen. This antigen was not discovered in the ten strains of human type investigated, but it was also not found in the BCG and TB-18 Uhlenhuth strains of bacilli, both of attenuated virulence and of bovine origin.

In his further work, Schaefer (1947) simplified the technique for the demonstration of the presence of protein antigen in tubercle bacilli. Instead of complement fixation reaction, the reaction of precipitation was applied to demonstrate the presence of the antigen. This technique was identical to the ring precipitation technique of Ascoli as it is used to demonstrate the heat-stable antigen of Anthrax bacilli. Schaefer prepared his antigen from the tubercle bacilli of smooth colonies by boiling the bacilli in $N/5$ hydrochloric acid. This antigen, in the reaction with specific rabbit serum, showed that "in the case of human, avian or saprophytic acid-fast bacilli the ring precipitation appeared considerably later and was considerably weaker than in the case of bovine bacilli." On the basis of these findings, it must be concluded that the protein antigen, just like the lipid and polysaccharide antigens, is also present in acid-fast bacilli of different origin and pathogenicity and that the serologic differences between the types of acid-fast bacilli are quantitative and not qualitative.

Tubercle bacilli of high virulence are found in bovines. These bacilli are pathogenic to humans, but the assumption that all bacilli of high virulence found in humans have been acquired from bovine sources has not been substantiated in spite of a half-century of efforts. Hedvall (1941) in a systematic study of bovine tuberculosis in man in southern Sweden, could find some connection between the infected persons and tuberculous cows or infected milk in only 12 cases out of 67. Francis (1947) indicated that the spread of bovine tuberculosis in humans is not simply related to the incidence of tuberculosis in cattle. Bovine tuberculosis in man does not differ in any of its forms from human tuberculosis, being on the contrary indistinguishable from the latter in its appearance and development. Nor is any aid obtained in this respect from tuberculin tests (Hedvall, 1941).

We do not know the causes for the high percentage of tubercle bacilli of high virulence (bovine type) in the cases of nonpulmonary tuberculosis and in infantile tuberculosis, just as we do not know why these bacilli are rarely the cause of pulmonary tuberculosis in humans, and moreover why the tubercle bacilli from cases of lupus are of low virulence.

We do not know an outside source for the bacilli of intermediate or attenuated virulence. If these strains were found in some animal, we would not hesitate to incriminate the animal as the source of tubercle bacilli of human skin afflictions. This is precisely what is being done when bacilli of high virulence are found in the cases of tuberculosis of human joints or lymphatic nodes.

Pneumococci were classified in serologically well-defined types, more distinct than those of tubercle bacilli. Some of these types are pathogenic, others apathogenic to animals. These types were regarded as stable and unchangeable until F. Griffith (1928) and Dawson and Sia (1931) showed that the types of pneumococci can be transformed by means of *in vitro* and *in vivo* methods (see p. 52). Braun (1947) observed that a tumor-inducing principle is required to transform normal cells into crown-gall tumor cells. Klein and Klein (1953) showed that avirulent crown-gall bacteria (*Agrobacterium tumefaciens* and other species) were transformed permanently into virulent, tumor-inducing bacteria when grown in the presence of desoxyribonucleic acid from virulent crown-gall bacteria.

The opinion of the British Tuberculosis Commission, expressed in its final report in 1911, that "man's liability to infection from animals remains, of necessity, purely a matter of inference," still stands unshaken.

Conclusions. Fifty years' work toward the typing of tubercle bacilli has shown the inconstancy of the types, and in a great many cases the impossibility of differentiating them. The unity of the various clinical manifestations of tuberculosis indicated by Laënnec in 1804, the transmissibility of human and bovine tuberculosis to animals discovered by Villemin (1865, 1868), the identity of cause of human and bovine tuberculosis discovered by Koch (1882), and the intercommunicability of the disease—all these facts are not compatible with the opinion of Th. Smith and the final views of Koch on the constancy of the types of tubercle bacilli. The assumption of Park and Krumwiede (1910) that the "culture and rabbit give us all the information needed for the differentiation of type," cannot be upheld. A return to the early unitary concept is necessary.

We used the expressions "type" or "variant" in the above discussion, not because constant types or variants of tubercle bacilli do exist in nature, but to indicate their relative virulence and frequency of distribution in animals and humans. The bacilli of "bovine type" are those with high virulence to experimental animals and more frequent in bovines than in humans; the bacilli of the "human type" are bacilli less virulent to experimental animals than the bovine ones and more common in humans than in bovines.

Mode of Origin of the Strains of Different Virulence

Ravenel said as early as 1902, that "it is certain that the various types of tubercle bacilli known to us sprung from a stock common to them all, and that they have acquired their racial peculiarities by residence in different animals." In opposition to this theory of adaptation as the cause for the development of new types of tubercle bacilli is the theory of mutation of bacilli, which was greatly in favor when children vaccinated with BCG vaccine developed tuberculosis.*

Petroff and Steenken (1930) published the observation that acid-fast bacilli can be dissociated in apathogenic "R" and pathogenic "S" forms. These authors claimed that four strains of BCG produced colonies that caused progressive tuberculosis in animals.

Dysgonic tubercle bacilli cultured from human cases of tuberculosis produced in subcultures eugonic and dysgonic colonies. Typical bovine cultures after six to eight months of cultivation on Löwenstein's medium yielded a few eugonic secondary colonies emanating from primarily dysgonic bovine colonies. Out of thirteen cases of dissociated bovine strains, five had eugonic variants with a virulence identical with those of the dysgonic primary strains, whereas six eugonic cultures were of more or less attenuated virulence to guinea pigs and rabbits. Two of the eugonic bovine dissociants were nonpathogenic to guinea pigs and rabbits and similar to the BCG strain in every respect. The change in virulence resulting from dissociation proved to be unstable. The possible reversion of the BCG strain from nonpathogenic to pathogenic must be admitted, although such reversion may happen rarely (Frimodt-Möller, 1939).

* Concerning the catastrophe of Lübeck, 1929–1930, see the report of the state investigation commission, *Arbeiten aus dem Reichgesundheitsamte*, 1935, vol. 69.

Types and Pathogenicity of Tubercle Bacillus

The observations of Petroff, Steenken, Frimodt-Möller, and others provoked a controversy that has not yet been settled. The new data on the pathogenicity of BCG indicate the necessity for further work on the pathogenicity of seemingly nonlethal strains of mycobacteria (see p. 303).

The knowledge of the origin and development of new races of organisms was advanced by the studies of the action of X-rays on *Neurospora*, by the investigation of the development of streptomycin-resistant strains of bacteria, and by the discoveries of sexuality in bacteria (see p. 70). In any case, there is no doubt that, at present, experimental science is in possession of tools capable of influencing directly the hereditary substance of the organisms.

XXII

Methods of Determining Virulence

In vivo Methods

UNDER the influence of the hypothesis of the stability of types, the study of the basic property of tubercle bacilli — their virulence — was overshadowed by the conventional typing of bacilli as a means of determining the presumed sources of infection. It is evident that the degree of pathogenicity or virulence of bacilli must play a decisive role in an attempt to determine the types of bacilli. To cause the disease, tubercle bacilli must establish and multiply in the host, although the rate of multiplication alone does not explain the degree of their virulence. The slowly evolving tuberculous lesions of a resistant animal (mouse) may be stuffed with bacilli, whereas the rapidly progressing lesions of a susceptible species (guinea pig, man) may contain only few bacilli. The virulence of bacilli is determined by the relationship between the host and the parasite. This relationship is influenced by many variables, such as (1) the racial and individual resistance of the animal, (2) individual properties of the strain used, (3) the route of the infection, and (4) the nutrition conditions of the animal. The virulence of the bacilli will probably be known when these variables have been determined, although in species susceptible to tuberculosis the course of the infection is largely determined by the size of the infective dose.

To the early investigators of the virulence of tubercle bacilli, only one procedure, animal inoculation, was available. Vagedes (1898) working under the guidance of Koch, used the eye chamber of rabbits to follow up the development of lesions. The differences in the extent of lesions were regarded as indications of differences in the virulence of the various strains. Vagedes recognized that the extent of lesions, or the virulence of the strain, depends upon the amount of bacilli injected and the species of animal used in the experiment.

Krompecher and Zimmermann (1903) injected 0.25 to 10.0 mg. of human tubercle bacilli intravenously into rabbits and did not see any differences in the virulence of the strains investigated. A different approach to the problem was chosen by Fränkel and Baumann (1906). To compare the virulence of different strains these investigators tried to determine the smallest amount of bacilli that produces tuberculosis in animals. Because of great fluctuation in the resistance of the rabbit to tuberculous infection, guinea pigs were used in the experiments. All 37 strains studied showed approximately the same degree of virulence. Fränkel's and Baumann's conception of virulence as the minimal infective amount of bacilli (*Dosis minima inficiens*) was abandoned after it was established that one virulent bacillus, isolated by means of a micromanipulator from the suspension of bacilli, is capable of producing tuberculosis in susceptible animals (Levinthal, 1927; Wámosher and Stöcklin, 1927; Bretey, 1944).

Calmette, Boquet, and Nègre (1923) showed that individual resistance or the factor of "terrain" does not influence the course of experimental tuberculosis in rabbits and guinea pigs of the same age and race. The course of the disease was inversely proportional to the amount of bacilli inoculated (fewer bacilli, prolonged disease; more bacilli, shortened disease). B. Lange (1930, 1932), from his experiments on the inoculation of guinea pigs with varying amounts of bacilli, concluded that the virulence of the tubercle bacilli, as manifested by the course of the disease, is the function of the amount of bacilli inoculated.

Doerr and Gold (1932), using the micromanipulator technique, inoculated thirty guinea pigs with 1 bacillus; three of these animals developed tuberculosis. The animals inoculated with 10 bacilli all developed tuberculosis, and no influence of the virulence of the bacilli on the course of the disease could be seen. Rather, the course of the disease was determined by the amount of bacilli inoculated. The minimal infective amount of bacilli overshadowed all the differences in virulence, if any. According to Doerr and Gold, the course of human tuberculosis too is not determined by virulence but by the amount of bacilli causing the primary infection.

Fust (1938) also observed that the course of the disease depends upon the quantity of bacilli inoculated. A dose of 10^{-4} to 10^{-7} mg. of bacilli led to rapidly progressing generalized tuberculosis, whereas an injection of 10^{-8} mg. resulted in two out of four guinea pigs inoculated, in nonprogressive tuberculosis of the lymphatic nodes. The increase of the infective dose above the critical minimal level has no enhancing effect on the course of the disease (Svedberg, 1951).

Stewart (1951), Stewart and Tamargo-Sanchez (1952) investigated the possibility of determining the gradations in virulence of recently isolated human strains of tubercle bacilli. The strains were subcultured in Dubos' Tween-albumin medium, plated to obtain the viable count of bacilli, and injected intracerebrally at the rate of 0.05 ml. into mice. The virulence of the H37Rv strain was accepted as an arbitrary standard of virulence, with which the virulence of other strains was compared. When the mean 50 per cent mortality time was plotted against the number of bacillary units injected, a linear relationship was found to exist within the inoculum range of 400,000 to 1,320,000 bacillary units. Out of the 37 strains tested, 22 showed equal or higher virulence than H37Rv; of 15 subvirulent strains, 13 were obtained from sources other than sputum (abscesses, urine). Two strains of BCG were slightly virulent: they caused occasional deaths of mice in 50 days. The BCG strains were more virulent than the H37Ra strain. No correlation between the virulence of the strain and the severity of the disease could be found. A large dose of slightly virulent tubercle bacilli produced lesions similar to those caused by a small dose of virulent bacilli. The size of the inoculum was the dominant factor in determining the outcome of the infection.

In addition to subcutaneous, intravenous, intraperitoneal, and intracerebral ways of infecting experimental animals, percutaneous and intracutaneous ways were used to differentiate the virulence of tubercle bacilli. Tomarkin and Peschič (1912) found that out of 52 guinea pigs infected by rubbing the human strain of the bacilli into the shaved, intact skin, 7 developed tuberculosis, whereas all 26 animals treated in the same way with the bovine strain of bacilli became tuberculous. No local skin lesions developed in either case.

B. Lange (1930) also used this procedure to infect guinea pigs. Richmond and Cummings (1950) and Kite, Patnode and Read (1952) found the percutaneous method of infection valuable in their studies of the virulence of tubercle bacilli. Toda (1930) inoculated rabbits intracutaneously with 10^{-5} mg. of tubercle bacilli and observed the differences in the lesions produced by the bovine and human strains. Three inoculations were performed in one animal. Lester (1939) applied the method of intracutaneous inoculation of guinea pigs to differentiate between the pathogenic and saprophytic bacilli.

Conclusions. The inoculation of animals with acid-fast bacilli leads to the recognition of two groups of microorganisms. The smaller group consists of bacilli capable of causing the death of the inoculated animal. This group is recognized as pathogenic. The larger group is made up of bacilli which do not cause the death of the animal, although some bacilli in this group may bring about morbid lesions. This group is recognized by many investigators of our day as nonpathogenic. According to their conception, the pathogenicity is identical to the lethal properties of the bacilli.

The search for criterion of pathogenicity led Pinner (1935) to "assign the term pathogenic only to those microorganisms that cause progressive disease." It is obvious that the term "progressive disease" means nothing else than the lethal outcome of the inoculation. The confusion which arises from the use of animal inoculation to differentiate between pathogenic and nonpathogenic acid-fast bacilli was analyzed by Pinner, who said that "if any demonstrable tissue alterations be called disease, and accordingly any organism that causes them is considered pathogenic, then, there are no apathogenic acid-fast organisms."

The insufficiency of animal inoculation as a means of differentiating gradations of virulence – other than lethal and nonlethal – brought on the search for other ways of recognizing the differences in virulence of acid-fast bacilli.

In vitro Methods

The inoculation of animals with acid-fast bacilli revealed differences between lethal and saprophytic acid-fast bacilli but failed to reveal any gradations in the virulence of attenuated or intermediate strains, to establish quantitative methods for testing virulence, or to lead to the discovery of the cause of the pathogenicity of tubercle bacilli.

In vitro methods made it possible to recognize the following differences between pathogenic, nonpathogenic, and saprophytic strains of mycobacteria.

Chemical differences. The early works on the chemical composition of tubercle bacilli (Hammerschlag, 1891; Kresling, 1901; and others) were followed by extensive works devoted chiefly to the investigation of the composition of lipids extracted from bacilli.

The lipids of tubercle bacilli can be divided into two groups according to their solubility in boiling acetone. The acetone-soluble fraction of lipids of pathogenic bacilli contains 65 to 85 per cent mycolic acid; the insoluble fraction consists of lipopolysaccharides. The lethal (H37Rv) strains contain 7.6 per cent lipopolysaccharides, the nonlethal, attenuated H37Ra strain contains 0.56 per cent of lipopolysaccharides. The lipopolysaccharide retains the neutral red stain of Dubos and Middlebrook (Asselineau and Lederer, 1950). Seibert, Long, and Morley (1933) found that pathogenic strains of mycobacteria, when extracted with ether and chloroform, yielded larger amounts of lipids than the nonpathogenic strains. These differences were chiefly due to the different amounts of wax extracted by chloroform.

The acetone-soluble fats containing phthioic acid were studied in detail by Sabin and associates. According to these researchers, the extracts produce tuberculoid structures in experimental animals. The formation of giant cells is stimulated by some methylated long-chain fatty acids. The α-ramified acids are active in this respect, whereas the β-acids are not (Gerstl and Tennant, 1943). (See diagram on p. 291.)

Choucroun (1943) obtained toxic paraffin oil extract from dead tubercle bacilli. The toxic substance was precipitable from the oil and 2 μg. of the precipitate were lethal to the guinea pigs. The substance proved to be acid-fast, free of nitrogen and phosphorus. Hydrolysis of this substance yielded sugars and compounds related to mycolic acid.

According to Philpot and Wells (1952), the petroleum ether extracts of live pathogenic tubercle bacilli have no toxic effect when injected into mice or guinea pigs.

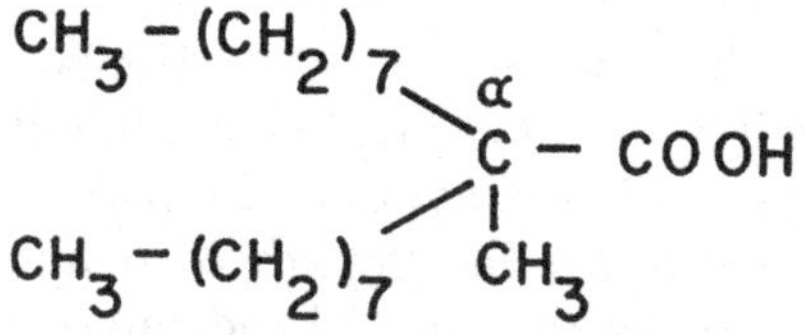

α-BRANCHED FATTY ACID

Attempts to differentiate the bovine, human, and avian types of bacilli by the fractionation of their lipids and the identification of the fractions by means of chromatography and infrared spectroscopy were made by Kubica, Randall, and Smith (1955). The experiments were based on the assumption that microorganisms differing biologically should also differ chemically. A component with an absorption band at 6.63 μ was found in the three strains of the bovine type but was absent in nine strains of the human type of bacilli. These components were recognized as the long-chain fatty acids and their esters. The amounts of these substances varied in the bacilli, indicating that these differences between the tubercle bacilli are of quantitative nature.

The chemical disintegration of tubercle bacilli produced some toxic fractions of tubercle bacilli; and some of these substances, when injected into susceptible animals, caused tuberculoid structures but failed to establish the cause of pathogenicity. The chemical methods have not elucidated the cause of another most striking property of pathogenic tubercle bacilli, i.e., their ability to cause caseation necrosis of the tissue.

Biologic differences. As was emphasized by Hanks and Grady, 1953, in the scale of acid-fast bacilli, ranging from saprophytic to fully pathogenic ones, the organisms gradually lose their ability to utilize ordinary nutrients, become less and less able to grow on artificial media, and finally are transformed into parasites on living cells. Saprophytic organisms, when inoculated into a living organism, may increase in number for a short time, but their multiplication is restricted mostly to the site of inoculation. Pathogenic tubercle bacilli, inoculated into the peritoneal cavity of guinea pigs, multiply freely outside the cells in the liquid of the cavity; this property is not possessed by the saprophytic bacilli (Woodruff and Kelly, 1940).

According to Syverton, Werder, Friedman, Roth, Graham, and Mira (1952), cortisone and X-rays when employed in combination for the preparation of test animals, alter the animals' resistance to enhance the pathogenicity of a variety of infectious agents, such as poliomyelitis virus, streptococcus, *Mycobacterium tuberculosis* var. *hominis*, and others.

Bernheim (1940), with the aid of the Warburg manometric technique, observed the increase of oxygen uptake in tubercle bacilli when salicylate or benzoate was added to the medium. Lehmann (1946b) observed increased oxygen uptake in the presence of salicylate or benzoate in pathogenic strains of bacilli only (see p. 106). Heplar, Clifton, Raffel, and Futrelle (1954), using the Warburg technique, found that some nonpathogenic strains respire at a higher rate than the pathogenic strains. At a low oxygen tension (1 per cent), the growth of nonpathogenic strains was inhibited to a greater extent than that of the pathogenic ones. Heplar and associates held this property responsible for the failure of nonpathogenic strains to multiply in live tissues, where the oxygen tension is low.

The Italian investigators Cattaneo, Morellini, Ortali, and Penso (1950) showed that among the mycobacteria exists a considerable difference in sensitivity to *para*-aminosalicylic acid. In the liquid medium of Dubos, saprophytic mycobacteria grew in the presence of 1,000 micrograms of PAS; the pathogenic tubercle bacilli did not develop in the presence of 1 microgram of this substance. The avian type of tubercle bacilli grew like the saprophytic bacilli. However, exceptions to this rule are known.

Oxidation-reduction potentials. The oxidation-reduction potentials of mycobacteria were investigated in pathogenic and nonpathogenic strains. Aksjanzew (1933) found that these potentials oscillated between +360 and +16 millivolts. No differences were found in the reducing capabilities of pathogenic and nonpathogenic strains. By means of the Thunberg technique, Bloch (1950) observed the reduction of methylene blue by saprophytic mycobacteria but not by pathogenic strains. F. Wilson, Kalish, and Fish (1952) studied the reduction (decolorization) of phenol-indophenol, sodium benzenoneindophenol, and other dyes by pathogenic (H37Rv), attenuated (H37Ra, BCG), and saprophytic strains of mycobacteria. The enzyme dehydrogenase causes the reduction of the dyes. In all pathogenic strains studied, when the dehydrogenases were lacking, the dyes were not decolorized. The reduction potentials were found to be in the range of —0.28 to —0.29 volt. All nonpathogenic and saprophytic strains, except BCG and H37Ra, decolorized these dyes. The latter strains, derived from pathogenic bacilli, behaved like pathogenic strains.

The cytochemical test. Dubos and Middlebrook (1948b) proposed the cytochemical test as a means of differentiating pathogenic from nonpathogenic mycobacteria. The bacilli were washed in 50 per cent methanol and suspended in an alkaline buffer solution (1 per cent barbiturate). To this alkaline solution was added a small amount of aqueous solution of neutral red. The pathogenic strains of bacilli absorbed the dye and became red. In saprophytic strains the fixation of the dye does not occur, and the organisms remain yellow like the ambient liquid. Hauduroy and Posternak-Gallia (1949) confirmed the findings of Dubos and Middlebrook. In their experiments on 67 pathogenic strains, all acquired a red hue, whereas the 67 saprophytic strains studied remained yellow. Other investigators of the problem did not find close accord between the neutral red binding ability and the pathogenicity of mycobacteria.

Richmond and Cummings (1950) investigated in a cytochemical test the behavior of 14 strains of mycobacteria. These strains showed equal virulence in the animal tests, while there was a varying degree of staining in the cytochemical test. The cytochemical test was found to be not directly related to the virulence of the bacilli. Viallier and Tigaud (1952) investigated 25 strains of mycobacteria by means of the cytochemical test and by guinea pig inoculations. They did not find any concordance between the results yielded by the cytochemical test and the virulence of bacilli to guinea pigs.

Catalase activity. According to Cohn, Kovitz, Oda, and Middlebrook (1954), in most cases pathogenic tubercle bacilli isolated from patients who have not been previously treated with isoniazid manifest catalase activity *in vitro*. Most of the strains resistant to 10 μg/ml isoniazid and of reduced pathogenicity were catalase-negative. Cohn and co-workers attributed the attenuation of pathogenicity of these bacilli to their deficiency in catalase activity. These findings were supported by Neumayr, Morse, and Morse (1955).

Stief and Hall (1956) found that out of 22 catalase-negative strains resistant to 1 μg. of isoniazid, 12 were pathogenic to guinea pigs and 10 were nonpathogenic or of doubtful pathogenicity.

Schierholz and Jeder (1956) point out that in *Brucella abortus* catalase activity can be correlated with pathogenicity if the speed of the decomposition of peroxide is known. This speed depends on the temperature of the suspension and is directly related to the concentration of cells in the suspension. However, the estimation of catalase activity in many instances is impossible when the concentration of peroxide is higher than 0.1 mol/liter, because concentrations of peroxide higher than this destroy the catalase. All this is based on the assumption that catalases vary only quantitatively – not qualitatively – in various substances. Such data on catalase activity in mycobacteria are not known.

The investigations at the Anoka laboratory revealed (our unpublished data, 1957) that it is doubtful whether the peroxide splitting property of mycobacteria is caused by the presence of catalase in the cells. As in the case of glucose oxidation in mycobacteria in shaking experiments (see page 243), it may be the result of catalytic action of the cell surface. Saprophytic acid-fast bacilli show high catalase activity.

Generation time. The generation time of lethal H37Rv and attenuated

H37Ra bacilli in Proskauer and Beck's medium was found to be approximately 24 hours. The growth of the H37Rv strain was stimulated by the addition of blood serum to the basal medium, so that the generation time was cut down to approximately 14 hours.

Bacteriophages. The bacteriophages which produce lysis of saprophytic acid-fast bacilli have been isolated by Gardner and Weiser (1947). Froman, Will, and Bogen (1954) and Froman, Will, Bogen, and Black (1957) obtained from soil bacteriophages active against *Mycobacterium tuberculosis,* as well as phages active against saprophytic mycobacteria. The phages were propagated on susceptible, saprophytic acid-fast hosts, and concentrated by differential centrifugation. The phages exhibited the typical head-tail morphology. Grouping of 69 strains of mammalian and avian tubercle bacilli and 329 strains of saprophytic acid-fast bacilli according to their resistance or susceptibility to bacteriophage lysis was attempted. The susceptibility of mycobacteria to phage lysis varied. Mammalian tubercle bacilli showed susceptibility to one phage.

Morphologic differences of colonies. Koch (1884) described the early colonies of tubercle bacilli in the following terms: "They appear as very elaborate spindle-shaped formations, in most cases bent in an S or a similar form," and published a drawing of these colonies. This S-form, or serpentine growth pattern, or cord formation of tubercle bacilli, was well known to investigators. The mode of formation of these cords was described by Miehe (1909): "the tubercle bacilli grow by sliding one over the other, thus showing considerable plasticity and forming very compact characteristic growth units."

The relation between the serpentine growth pattern and the pathogenicity of tubercle bacilli was first indicated by Middlebrook, Dubos, and

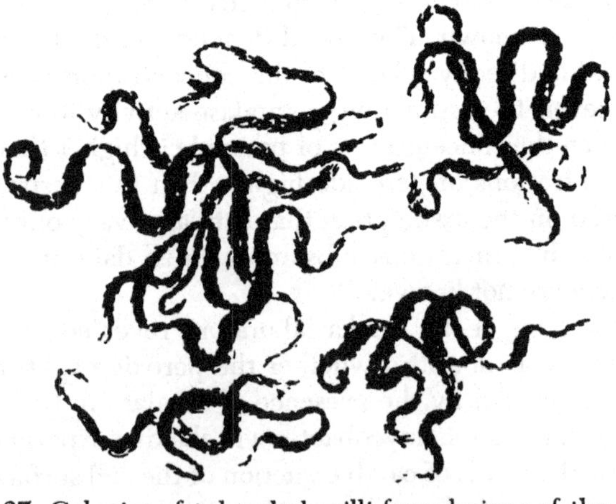

Figure 27. Colonies of tubercle bacilli from lesions of the human kidney, × 700 (Koch, 1884).

Pierce (1947). They found the serpentine growth pattern characteristic of pathogenic mammalian strains; the saprophytic bacilli, avian bacilli, and bacilli of cold-blooded animals did not show the oriented pattern of growth; rather their growth was unorganized or dispersed.

The findings of Middlebrook and associates were confirmed by Roth (1949), who indicated that after the transversal division, the ends of the newly formed bacilli do not separate from one another but, as the growth proceeds, slide one over the other and form cord-like structures. In the case of the saprophytic strains, the bacilli do separate one from another after the division. Obviously, the surface of the bacilli in each case is different. In the pathogenic strains the surface is adhesive to the newly formed bacilli and thus prevents their separation. H. Bloch (1950) also found a close relation between the cord formation and the pathogenic properties of bacilli.

Yegian and Kurung (1952) confirmed the correlation between the cord formation and the pathogenicity of bacilli. The attenuated strains showed a slight degree of cord formation. The findings of Brieger and Glauert (1952) that avian bacilli grown in chick embryo extract produce cords, have not been confirmed yet. Engbaek (1952), on the basis of direct observation of the growth of tubercle bacilli in an agar medium, has confirmed the formation of cords by pathogenic and the attenuated BCG bacilli. These confirmatory findings favoring the observation of Middlebrook and associates were opposed by Richmond and Cummings (1950), who said that "only two of the acid-fast bacilli showed true serpentine growth, and those were saprophytes." Similar observations were made by Bassermann (1954) and others.

The true and false cords of mycobacteria. Although the cord formation was first observed in bacilli grown on solid media, only the liquid medium permits its full development. In tuberculous organs, the cords are found in lesions surrounded by liquids, such as urine or exudate (see Fig. 27.) Cords are lacking in infected tissue. Our liquid medium (see Table 33) is favorable to the formation of cords. In this medium pathogenic bacilli grown for 14 days and then stained according to Ziehl-Neelsen and counterstained with a solution of picric acid when observed with a low-power lens, show bright red cords against a uniformly yellow background. These cords are extremely compact structures with a smooth surface. The separate bacilli in the true cord are difficult to see with an oil-immersion objective. This is the most characteristic feature of the true cord of the lethal mammalian tubercle bacilli (see Figs. 28 and 29).

Disregard for these structural differences between the true and false cords has led even some recent investigators (Goldman and Goldman, 1956; Aitoff, 1956) to misinterpret the observed cell formations of saprophytic acid-fast bacilli.

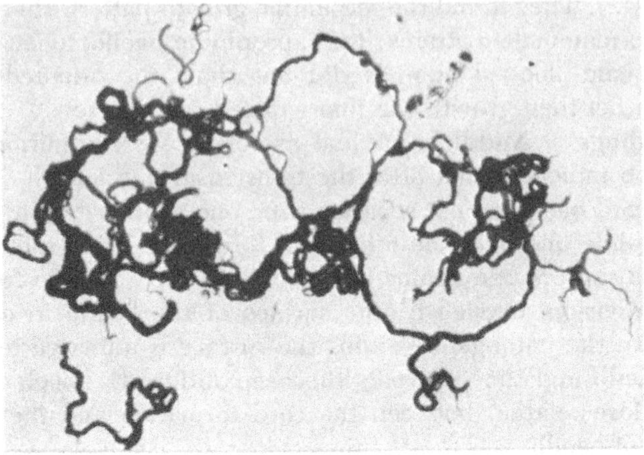

Figure 28. Cords of lethal tubercle bacilli, × 126.

The decreasing virulence of bacilli is reflected in changes in the structure of the cord. The diminishing virulence entails the loosening of the cord structure. Bacilli detach themselves from the surface of the cord, and sometimes the whole formation looks like a brush. The oil-immersion objective of a microscope is capable at this stage of detecting the separate bacilli even in the axis of such a formation. With the progressive loss of virulence, and the breakup of the formation, the bacilli increasingly separate from one another until at last only disconnected bacilli, as seen in saprophytic strains (Fig. 30), are left, sometimes still arrayed in heaps or in one line (false cords, Fig. 31).

The Cord Substance

A parallel array of bacilli in a cord may be the result of some substance located on the surface of the cells that prevents their separation. Such a substance, of lipid nature, was extracted from the cords by treatment with petroleum ether (Bloch, 1950). Saprophytic strains did not yield this substance. The attenuated strains (BCG) contained small quantities of it. The extracted pathogenic bacilli were not dead, their ability to grow on artificial media was not reduced, but they became totally or partly apathogenic to mice. The extracted substance was found to be toxic to mice. The mice injected with this substance three or four times died in 10 to 14 days emaciated and showing hemorrhage in the lungs. Bloch compared the role of this substance in the pathogenesis of tuberculosis to the function of the polysaccharide capsule in pneumococcus infection. The loss of the capsule results in the loss of the pathogenicity of the pneumococcus. The naked microorganisms are readily phagocytized by polymorphonuclear leucocytes.

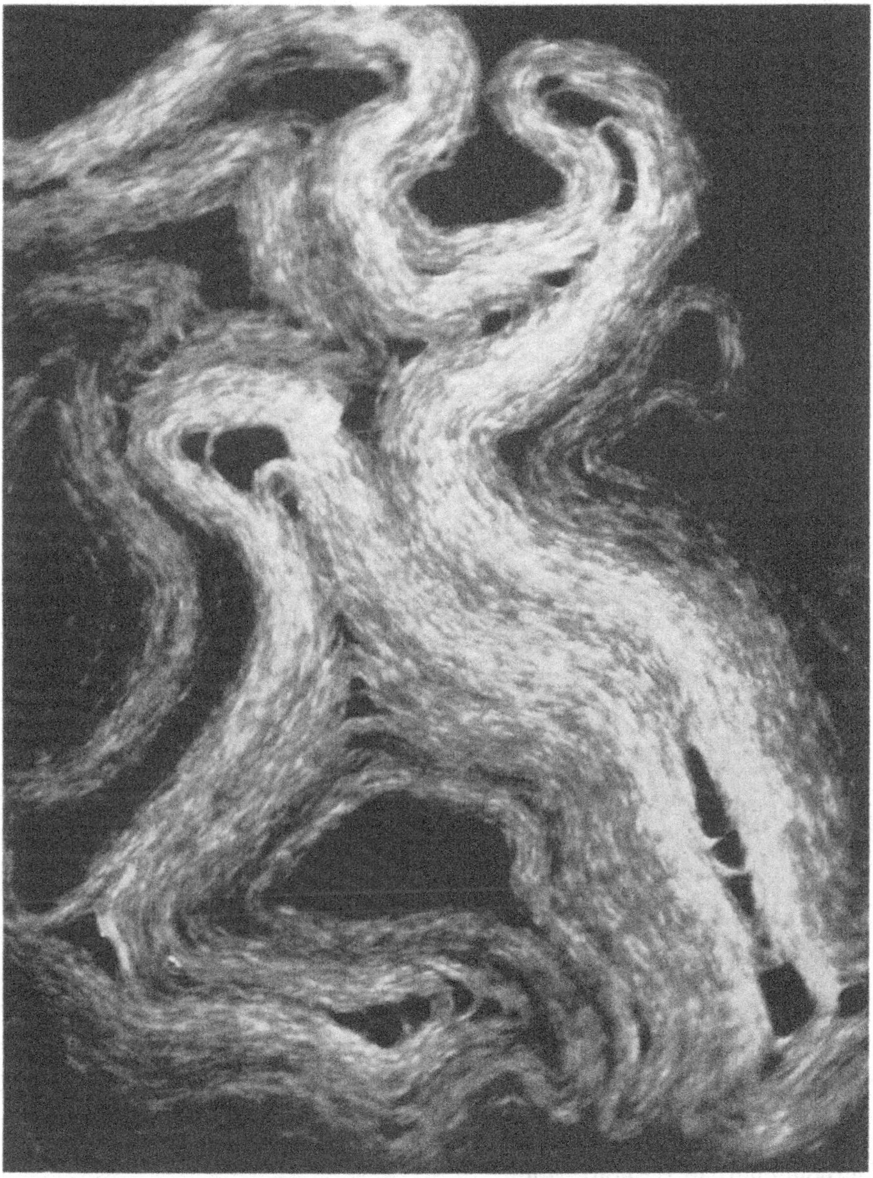

Figure 29. Cord structure of pathogenic tubercle bacilli, × 1,100 (Kölbel, 1954).

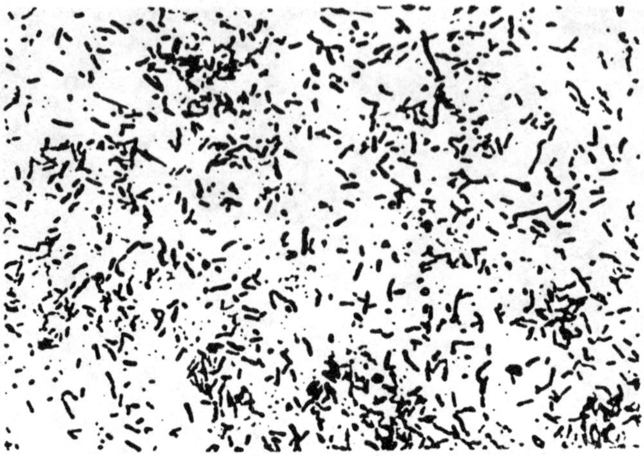

Figure 30. Saprophytic acid-fast bacilli, dispersed growth, × 480.

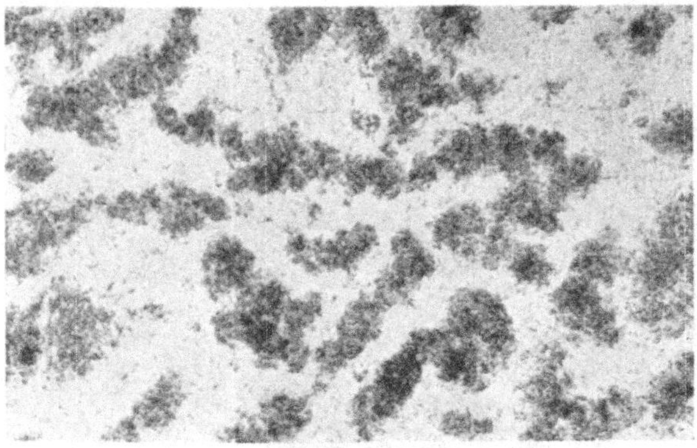

Figure 31. False cords of nonlethal acid-fast bacilli, × 126.

The cord substance of tubercle bacilli is, to some extent, analogous in its pathogenicity to the virulence (Vi) antigen of typhoid bacilli. The higher virulence of freshly cultured typhoid bacilli than that of old laboratory strains was attributed to the presence of superficially located Vi antigen in fresh bacilli. The discovery of Vi antigen in nonpathogenic *Escherichia coli* showed that Vi antigen alone does not account for the pathogenicity of typhoid bacilli.

The cord substance inhibited the migration of leucocytes. The inhibition of leucocyte migration *in vitro* was found to be caused by the pathogenic tubercle bacilli but not by the nonpathogenic ones (Allgöwer and Bloch, 1949). The crude cord substance was partly purified (Sorkin, Erlenmeyer, and Bloch, 1952). When heated in acetone, the crude substance yielded about 1 per cent insoluble residue which showed characteristic toxicity.

This residue was soluble in petroleum ether, chloroform, and ether, but insoluble in methanol, ethanol, and water. Further purification and separation of the components of the cord substance were obtained by extracting young human and bovine bacilli with chloroform. The crude extract was fractionated by chromatography on silica gel. For the identification of the microquantities of the separated fractions infrared spectroscopy was used. The fraction C contained the cord substance. The infrared spectra of cord substance of five strains of tubercle bacilli were identical. Strong hydrolysis of the cord substance liberated a reducing compound identified as glucose. The rest of the fraction C consisted of esters of low melting point. The cord substance was recognized as glucolipid of molecular weight of approximately 1570, containing 83 per cent mycolic acid and 9 per cent glucose in ester linkage. The composition of the residual substance remained unknown (Noll and Bloch, 1955).

Asselineau and Lederer (1955) confirmed the findings of Noll and Bloch and added some additional information about the chemistry of the cord substance. According to Asselineau and Lederer, the cord factor of the strain H37Rv is a wax with the melting point 42°–44°C., and has the total formula

$$C_{95}H_{189}O_9N \pm 5CH_2 \pm O$$

This compound is made up of mycolic acid ($C_{87}H_{174}O_4 \pm 5CH_2$) and of carbohydrate containing some unknown compound of nitrogen ($C_8H_{17}O_6N$).

The interpretation of some biologic properties of the cord substance as toxic or instrumental in the genesis of tuberculosis, suggested by Bloch and his co-workers, was subjected to criticism.

The migration of leucocytes is influenced by the contact between leucocytes and various bacteria (*Salmonella typhosa, Pseudomonas aeruginosa, Neisseria intracellularis*) and their soluble products (Martin and Chaudhuri, 1952). The migratory ability of leucocytes is not influenced by the presence of tubercle bacilli in their bodies, as was revealed by the electron micrographs of Bassermann (1954) (Fig. 32), but, under the influence of tuberculin, the leucocytes undergo cytolysis (Witte, 1950).

These findings do not warrant any changes in the use of the migratory ability of leucocytes as a specific diagnostic tool. The findings of Bloch and associates on the specific role of cord substance in tuberculosis were not confirmed by Philpot and Wells (1952). These investigators extracted live and heat-killed tubercle bacilli with organic solvents (petroleum ether, ether, chloroform). The extracts were fractionated according to their solubility in the admixtures of solvents and subjected to chromatographic analysis. The petroleum ether extract of live bacilli was found to have no toxicity for mice and guinea pigs. Eleven intraperitoneal injections of 0.1 mg.

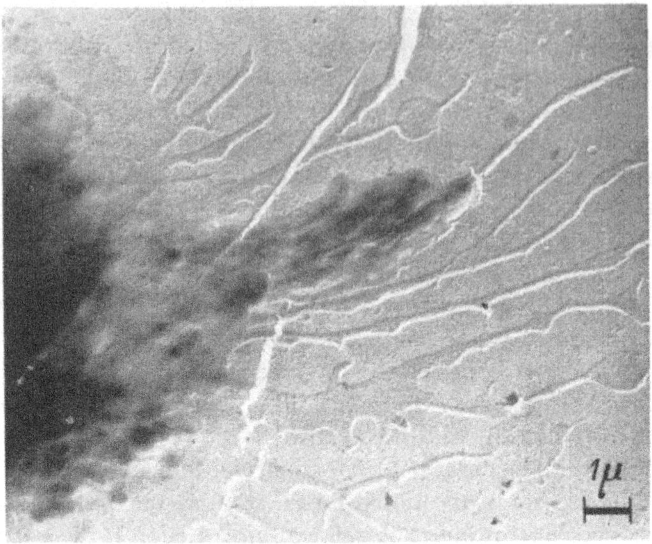

Figure 32. Electron micrograph of tubercle bacilli in the leucocyte, platinum-palladium shadowed, × 4,700 (Bassermann, 1954).

of cord substance were given to the susceptible strain of mice (C57, used also by Bloch) without any harmful effect.

Cord Formation as a Diagnostic Tool

The formation of true cords is the property of pathogenic mammalian tubercle bacilli. It would be theoretically and practically important to know to what extent the disappearance of the pathogenicity of tubercle bacilli to guinea pig is reflected in the structure of cords. If the partial or total loss of pathogenicity of tubercle bacilli may be detected in cords, it might be possible to use the *in vitro* method instead of animal inoculation to differentiate attenuated or pathogenic mycobacteria from nonpathogenic or saprophytic ones.

An investigation of this problem was carried out in two Minnesota laboratories (Darzins and Fahr, 1956). At the laboratory of the state Department of Health, Minneapolis (referred to as the Minneapolis laboratory), cultures of acid-fast bacilli were isolated from the pathologic material and the pathogenicity of each culture was tested by inoculation into two guinea pigs. These cultures were sent to the laboratory of the Anoka State Hospital, Anoka, Minnesota (referred to as the Anoka laboratory), where their pathogenicity *in vitro* on the basis of their cord formations was tested. The personnel of the Anoka laboratory was not informed about the results of the animal inoculation at this time.

Methods of Determining Virulence

The cultivation was done in our liquid medium (see Table 33). After 14 days of incubation at 37°C., the deposits in the tubes were stained and investigated for cords. A total of 245 cultures was tested by animal inoculation and by cord formation; 192 of these cultures were designated as M strains; 40 strains as C; 8 strains as N, and 5 strains as R. The M strains produced typical cords and were classified as lethal. These strains caused tuberculosis in guinea pigs. The C strains produced yellow pigment and abundant, early, dispersed growth with formation of heavy pellicles on the surface of the medium. Cords were not formed. The C strains were classified as saprophytic. These strains did not kill guinea pigs or cause morbid lesions in the animals.

The growth of N strains was relatively slow, without pigment formation, and resembled the growth of pathogenic strains. These strains had been isolated from patients and, since they were not lethal to guinea pigs, classified as nonpathogenic. The N strains showed, in the liquid medium, some cord formation and one of them (N-5), because of such a formation, was classified as pathogenic. This N-5 strain produced considerable caseation of the lymphatic nodes in guinea pigs, but the animals were alive after three months of observation. The other N strains were recognized as attenuated, although it was presumed that they had originated from the lethal strains.

The R strains uniformly produced cords and were classified as lethal. These strains had been isolated from the sputa and gastric washings of tuberculous patients, and all were resistant to 10 micrograms of isoniazid. Two of these strains were lethal when inoculated subcutaneously into guinea pigs; the three others were not lethal to guinea pigs. These strains, inoculated intravenously into mice, were lethal.

Conclusions. The pathogenicity of 245 strains of mycobacteria was tested by means of guinea pig and mouse inoculation. In the Anoka laboratory the same strains were tested for their cord-forming ability in our liquid medium (see Table 43). Both methods recognized 192 lethal and 40

Table 43. The Results of Tests for the Pathogenicity of 245 Cultures of Mycobacteria by Cord Formation (Anoka Laboratory) and Animal Inoculation (Minneapolis Laboratory)

Strain	No. of Cultures	Cord Formation	Tuberculosis in Animals
M	192	Present	Present
C	40	Absent	Absent
N	8	Absent in 7; present in 1	Absent
R	5	Present	Present *

Source: Darzins and Fahr (1956).
* 2 cases in guinea pigs, 3 in mice.

saprophytic strains with equal efficiency. These two groups of mycobacteria represented 94.3 per cent of the strains tested.

The remaining material consisted of eight N strains showing rudimentary cord formation. These strains were not lethal to guinea pigs but caused a number of morbid lesions in them. The origin of these strains from the lethal ones was presumed. Five isoniazid-resistant R strains formed true cords. They were classified as lethal. Two of these strains were lethal to guinea pigs; when injected intravenously, the other three strains were lethal to mice.

Cord Formation in Nonlethal Strains of Mycobacteria

The nonlethal strains BCG, H37Ra, and N-5 form cords. (Micrographs of BCG serpentine growth pattern were published by Kölbel, 1951; Engbaek, 1952; of H37Ra by Hart and Rees, 1954.) Tubercle bacilli which have acquired resistance to antibiotics and chemotherapeutics have not lost their cord-forming ability (Yegian and Kurung, 1952; Patnode, Dail, and Hudgins, 1955; our R strains). Dubos (1950a) posed the question of how to reconcile the fact that BCG and H37Ra strains form cords while these strains are not pathogenic.

The confusion which at the present time still surrounds the question of the pathogenicity of tubercle bacilli is illustrated by the studies of Yegian and Budd (1953). To these authors "the ability to produce progressive disease in guinea pig was the criterion for pathogenicity." At the same time, "the cord-forming tendency of each strain was also studied and proved to be a reliable measure of virulence." Some strains studied by Yegian and Budd formed cords and were grossly indistinguishable from tubercle bacilli. When inoculated into guinea pigs, these strains did not cause progressive disease. The question arises as to which should be the criterion of pathogenicity: the results of guinea pig inoculation or the cord-forming ability of the strains. Yegian and Budd decided to call these strains nonpathogenic, and to ignore their cord-forming ability, because they did not kill the guinea pigs.

This difficulty in reconciling the results yielded by guinea pig inoculation and the cord-forming ability of the strains arises from the acceptance of lethal properties of a strain to the experimental animal as criterion of pathogenicity. Only a fully virulent strain is lethal (our M strains, see Table 43); the partial loss of virulence, such as was observed in attenuated strains (BCG, H37Ra, and our N strains), results in the definite or temporary loss of lethality, although the strain is not apathogenic. BCG is a strain derived from pathogenic bacilli. Inoculated into animals, this strain will produce varying amounts of specific lesions with giant cells, epitheloid cells, and caseation necrosis; in the appropriate medium this strain will form cords. These findings were well known, but nevertheless the BCG strain was regarded as nonpathogenic to animals and humans because it was not lethal.

According to Friedmann and Russel (1953), cord formation was a prominent feature of BCG and H37Ra strains grown in media containing embryonic tissue. The culture of BCG-313 strain (Pasteur Institute, No. 891, series 2) produced tuberculosis in two out of five guinea pigs inoculated. (See also the findings of Hauduroy, p. 360.) The results of the investigation of the pathogenicity and the cord-forming ability of the nonlethal H37Ra strain by Hart and Rees (1954) are of the same order. These authors called the strain H37Ra avirulent. The addition of 0.001 per cent of wetting agent Triton A20′ to the liquid medium increased the cord-forming ability of the strain, but the pathogenicity of the strain for mice was not increased. Hart and Rees said that "at the peak the cords were usually less packed, less serpentine, and more branched, than those of H37Rv." One has to deal here with the cords of an attenuated mycobacterium, which, like other strains derived from pathogenic bacilli, have retained some rest-pathogenicity. This was confirmed by Hart and Rees: in the animals inoculated with the H37Ra bacilli the pin-point pulmonary lesions were seen when the animals were killed 40 days later, except for one group, where definite lesions were present.

The publications of Meyer and Jensen (1954) and Oeding, Hesselberg, Thrap-Meyer, and Waaler (1954) revealed that under some undetermined conditions, BCG may produce tuberculosis in humans. These Scandinavian investigators described two fatal cases of tuberculosis in men following BCG vaccination. According to the Polish investigator Verzhbovskaia (1955) 2 per cent of children vaccinated intracutaneously with the BCG vaccine developed lymphadenitis followed by suppuration of the lymph nodes.

Borch Jørgensen and Horwitz (1956) collected data of 100 persons, mostly children, vaccinated intradermally with BCG in whom 150 specific tuberculous lesions developed. The lesions consisted in scrofuloderm surrounding the site of inoculation, regional and universal adenitis, local and universal tuberculide, and lupus vulgaris. The specific nature of some of the lesions was verified bacteriologically.

van Deinse (1956), head of BCG department of the Pasteur Institute, Paris, is of the opinion that the recorded cases of death and of lupus-like infections after BCG vaccination may be caused by some unknown BCG-related *Mycobacterium.*

Between the fully virulent (lethal) strains of mycobacteria and the totally nonpathogenic (saprophytic) ones lies the spectrum of virulence. Tubercle bacilli lose their lethal properties with relative ease but conserve with considerable tenacity their rest-pathogenicity and cord-forming ability. The decrease of pathogenicity in bacilli is reflected on the structure of their cords.

Tubercle Bacilli in the Lesions of Patients Treated with Antibiotics or Chemotherapeutics

Discrepancies have been observed between the results arrived at by investigating pathologic material positive for tubercle bacilli by microscopy and the results obtained by the culturing or animal inoculation of the same material. Aronson and Whitney (1930) were unable to infect guinea pigs with 12 different samples of tuberculous material in which acid-fast bacilli were seen by direct microscopy. Canetti (1946), in two samples of material taken from patients not treated with antibiotics and chemotherapeutics, counted 960 and 250,000 acid-fast bacilli, respectively. When planted on egg media, the material did not produce any growth. According to Canetti, the bacilli in the cultured samples were dead, and their death and autolysis in the tissues contributed to the development of lesions and produced specific tuberculous conditions in the organism. These data are in agreement with the findings in animals. Rolle and Mayer (1953) investigated material taken from the lungs of 14 aging cows. In nine cases acid-fast bacilli were seen by microscopic examination of the material. Guinea pigs inoculated with this material showed no signs of tuberculosis after 54 weeks of observation.

With regard to material obtained from patients treated with antibiotics and chemotherapeutics, the situation is still more complicated, mainly because of the poor growth and low virulence of the bacilli. Beck and Yegian (1952) cultured and inoculated into guinea pigs 50 specimens of material from the resected lungs of 28 tuberculous patients treated with streptomycin and PAS. Of 17 specimens, in 16 the presence of acid-fast bacilli was demonstrated by microscopic examination. When cultured, this material yielded 4 cultures of tubercle bacilli. Medlar, Bernstein, and Steward (1952) investigated 209 specimens of resected lung tissues from 72 tuberculous patients treated with streptomycin and PAS. Of these, the contents of 35 open cavities produced cultures in 29 cases, contents of 58 filled in cavities yielded cultures in 14 instances, and, out of specimens of contents of 122 solid necrotic lesions, only 9 were positive by culture. In all cases in which the tubercle bacilli were cultured from closed lesions, the number of colonies obtained was a small fraction of the number of bacilli seen in the material by direct microscopy.

Granville, Jenkins, Cooley, DeBakey, Whitcomb, and Halpert (1953) found by direct microscopy acid-fast bacilli in material obtained from nine patients treated with streptomycin and PAS. The same material produced five positive cultures. Hall and Gleason (1953) investigated 130 pulmonary specimens resected from 119 patients after chemotherapy. Microscopically acid-fast bacilli were discovered in 72 per cent of nodular lesions and in 92 per cent in lesions with cavities. The culturing of the material, however, produced growth of acid-fast bacilli in 5 per cent of the nodular lesions and in 58 per cent of the lesions with cavities. Guinea pig inoculations revealed tuberculosis in 10 per cent of the nodular lesions and in 39 per cent of the lesions with cavities.

Kaufmann, Wanner, and Amsler (1954) investigated 68 lesions from the resected lungs of 41 patients who for three months had been under treatment. The cavities, filled with air, produced cultures in ⅔ of the cases, whereas only ¼ of the solid lesions yielded cultures.

A panel discussion at the annual meeting of the American National Tuberculosis Association at Los Angeles in 1953 was devoted to the problem of whether acid-fast bacilli visible by direct microscopy in tuberculous lesions of patients treated with streptomycin, PAS, or isoniazid, but not cultivable on artificial media and not lethal to guinea pigs, are dead or alive. Six hospitals reported 515 resections of tuberculous lesions; bacteriologic investigations were made in 661 apparently closed lesions. These closed lesions were in 346 cases positive for acid-fast bacilli by microscopy, but only 85 of them yielded tubercle bacilli by culture or guinea pig inoculations. The conclusions drawn from these discussions were that there is no proof that the bacilli in tuberculous lesions of patients under chemotherapeutic or antibiotic treatment are dead; all that has been demonstrated is that there are large amounts of acid-fast bacilli in the lesions of these patients which neither grow on the media presently in use nor produce tuberculosis in guinea pigs.

Wier, Storey, Walrath, Weiser, and Tempel (1955) drew attention to the frequent occurrence in patients treated with antibiotics and chemotherapeutics of microscopically positive sputum specimens which are negative by culture. Out of 8,447 sputa from 494 patients, 351 showed acid-fast bacilli by microscopy (4.2 per cent), but these sputa were negative by culture. The highest incidence of noncultivable bacilli was at the beginning of the treatment. According to Bogen (1955), these findings indicate that, under the above circumstances, acid-fast bacilli found in sputum, even when negative by culture, should be regarded as tubercle bacilli.

Some strains of tubercle bacilli rapidly lose their pathogenicity under the influence of streptomycin or isoniazid treatment, while other strains retain their pathogenicity. A nonpathogenic streptomycin-dependent strain derived from the pathogenic H37Rv strain was observed by Yegian and Kurung (1952); Karlson and Ikemi (1952) obtained an isoniazid-resistant H37Rv strain by culturing bacilli on media containing 2.5 and 10 micrograms of isoniazid per ml. The strain was not pathogenic to guinea pigs. Steenken and Wolinsky (1953) obtained from patients treated for 120 and

179 days with isoniazid 14 strains of acid-fast bacilli. These strains were nonpathogenic to guinea pigs; 9 strains obtained from seven other patients under isoniazid treatment had conserved their pathogenicity for guinea pigs. The tubercle bacilli isolated from patients under isoniazid treatment show progressive loss of virulence. This loss is not correlated with the degree of isoniazid resistance obtained, or with the length of the treatment of the patients (Steenken and Wolinsky, 1953). Peizer, Widelock, and Klein (1953) arrived at findings identical with those of Steenken and Wolinsky.

Isoniazid-resistant bacilli rapidly revert to sensitivity when they have come into contact with the drug during only one subculture; after they have been in contact more than once, the bacilli retain their resistance during many passages through drug-free media (Barnett, Bushby, and Mitchison, 1953).

Tubercle bacilli (strain H37Rv) resistant to 10 μg. per ml. of isoniazid produced characteristic lesions in guinea pigs which were seen in animals killed 21 days after the infection. Lesions could not be found, or they were limited to the site of inoculation, in animals killed 88 days after the infection. The lesions produced by resistant bacilli regressed in guinea pigs. The action of isoniazid-resistant bacilli injected into mice, however, was different. All infected animals died of progressive tuberculosis, and there were no differences between the survival rate of mice infected with tubercle bacilli sensitive to isoniazid and those infected with bacilli resistant to isoniazid (Karlson and Ikemi, 1954). The observations of Karlson and Ikemi were confirmed by Gernez-Rieux, Jacquet, and Fabre (1954).

Noufflard (1955) found that out of four strains resistant to isoniazid, three produced generalized infection in mice, although less severe than the infection brought about by the fully virulent strains. The isoniazid-resistant strains were a mixture of bacilli sensitive and resistant to isoniazid. The thirteen strains of tubercle bacilli resistant to isoniazid investigated by Patnode, Dail, and Hudgins (1955) were found to be less virulent for guinea pigs than the strain H37Rv. The findings of Karlson and other investigators are in agreement with the earlier observations of Branch (1933) on the greater susceptibility of mice in comparison to guinea pigs to the attenuated strains of tubercle bacilli or to the chromogenic bacilli isolated from tuberculous patients.

In the lesions of guinea pigs and mice, inoculated with the mixtures of isoniazid-resistant and isoniazid-sensitive bacilli, only pathogenic, isoniazid-sensitive bacilli were found (Widelock, Peizer, and Klein, 1955). Obviously, nonpathogenic, isoniazid-resistant bacilli had been used for the animal inoculations. The results might have been different if the animals had been inoculated with mixtures containing isoniazid-resistant bacilli pathogenic to the animals.

The tuberculosis of mice caused by isoniazid-resistant strains was accessible to streptomycin therapy (J. Hirsch, 1952).

The erroneous interpretation that tubercle bacilli which have lost their pathogenicity under the action of antibiotics or chemotherapeutics are harmless must be avoided (Steenken and Wolinsky, 1953). The virulence of isoniazid-resistant bacilli does change from one species of animals to another. We do not know the degree of virulence of these bacilli to humans (Noufflard, 1955).

Chromogenic Acid-Fast Bacilli from Human Sources

The production of either yellow or orange or pink carotenoid pigment, besides nonpathogenicity to experimental animals and the absence of cord formation, is the chief characteristic of saprophytic acid-fast bacilli. The decrease in virulence of pathogenic, acid-fast mammalian strains is generally accompanied by the increased pigmentation of the cultures. The highly virulent bovine strains are colorless; the less virulent human strains are of yellow hue. Our cultures of H37Rv strain, grown for 18 months under paraffin in liquid medium, are bright yellow.

Chromogenic acid-fast bacilli are widely distributed in nature. They are constant inhabitants of soil, dust, water, and sewage. These bacilli are also found in human pathologic material.

The possibility of increasing the virulence of acid-fast saprophytic bacilli to the level of pathogenic ones has been proclaimed feasible by some investigators (Kolle, Schlossberger, and Pfannenstiel, 1921). These claims were not supported by further investigation of the problem (Strauss, 1922; Calmette, 1924; Willis, 1933).

Recent works have revealed the difficulty of classifying these organisms and of interpreting their etiologic significance in human pathology. Schwabacher (1933) cultured chromogenic bacilli from six blood cultures of tuberculous patients, tuberculous rabbits, and three normal rabbits as well as from other material. These strains were nonpathogenic for rabbits, guinea pigs, and mice. No classification of the bacilli was possible. (A review of the earlier works in this field is given by Schwabacher, 1933).

Pinner (1935) studied 15 strains of chromogenic acid-fast bacilli cultured from the sputa, gastric washings, urine, and blood of patients. The colonies of these strains were lemon-yellow to dark orange in color and always smooth. When 10 mg. of these bacilli were injected subcutaneously into guinea pigs or intravenously into rabbits, a few white nodules, 0.5 to 2.0 mm. in diameter, were occasionally found in the liver, spleen, and lungs of the animals. Histologically, these lesions consisted of granulomatous tissue, containing some epitheloid and giant cells. Caseation was absent.

Histologically the process resembled suppuration. The infected animals reacted typically to injections of old tuberculin (1:10).

Lester (1939) discovered in 26,343 specimens of human material 130 strains of acid-fast saprophytic bacilli. Of these, 58 per cent came from gastric specimens, 18 per cent from urine, and 10 per cent from sputum; 55 strains had bright orange colonies.

Laporte (1940) reported three cases of subcutaneous abscesses which developed following the injection of nonsterile remedies. The causative agents, acid-fast bacilli, were cultured from the pus. The bacilli grew on ordinary agar at 20°C. and were not pathogenic to experimental animals. Baldwin (1942) cultured from the sputum of a patient a chromogenic nonpathogenic acid-fast bacillus. Hauduroy (1950), in his review of saprophytic acid-fast bacilli (the French *bacilles paratuberculeux*), admits that some of these bacilli have been the causative agents in human disease. Spanedda (1951) isolated ten strains of nonpathogenic mycobacteria from the feces, urine, and sputum of tuberculous patients.

The investigation of 620 strains of acid-fast bacilli cultured in Bahia, Brazil, from sputa and gastric and bronchial washings by Silveira, Darzins, and Ventura de Matos (1951) revealed 15 strains nonpathogenic to guinea pigs (2.5 per cent approximately). Part of these strains were chromogenic, and they did not produce cords in a liquid medium. A partial explanation for the high percentage of these strains in Bahia lies in the fact that the giant frog (*gia*) used as food by the population is always tuberculous. The infection is caused by the chromogenic acid-fast bacillus *Mycobacterium giae* (Darzins, 1952). The water of pits habitated by *gias* is heavily infected with an acid-fast bacillus similar to that found in the *gias*. This water is consumed untreated by a considerable part of the population of Bahia.

Tarshis and Frisch (1952) studied 26 strains of chromogenic acid-fast bacilli cultured from sputa, gastric washings, and lung abscesses of tuberculous patients or persons suspected of being tuberculous. The intraperitoneal inoculation of enormous amounts (25 mg.) of these bacilli was fatal to guinea pigs, but the smaller inocula showed no virulence. The lesions produced by these organisms were of the same nature as described by Pinner (1935).

Lominski and Harper (1953) cultured the chromogenic organism from the sputum and lung lesions of a patient. This bacillus was nonpathogenic for guinea pigs, rabbits, and chickens, but highly virulent for mice. Two carefully studied cases of human infection by chromogenic acid-fast bacilli were reported by Buhler and Pollak (1953). The bacilli were recovered on several occasions from the sputum and the pus of two patients. The same bacilli were cultured in the first case from the excised lung tissue and on the other occasion from the autopsy material. Pathogenicity of these bacilli to guinea pigs was negligible, and in mice a generalized disease developed in some instances following the injection of the bacilli. These strains, in Proskauer and Beck's liquid medium, produced yellow homogeneous or granular cultures. No cord formation was reported.

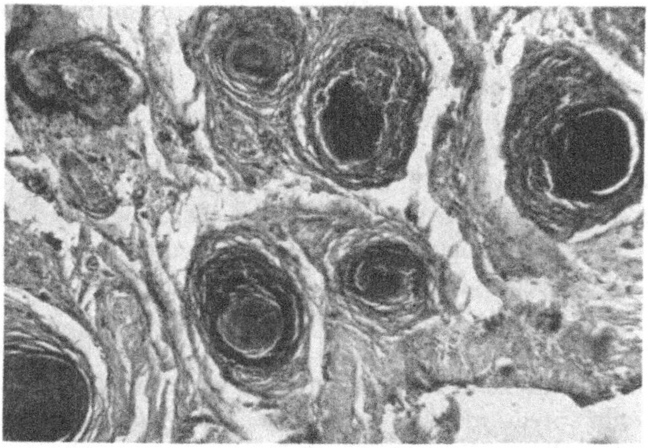

Figure 33. Tuberculosis in gia liver, eosin-hematoxin stain, × 215 (Darzins, 1952).

Timpe and Runyon (1954) collected chromogenic acid-fast bacilli from 120 persons, some of them suffering from pulmonary diseases. Inoculated (1 mg.) into guinea pigs, these strains caused transient swelling of regional lymph nodes, but did not produce lesions of internal organs. In mice, some of these organisms caused fatal infection. Lesions were found in lungs, spleen, and liver. No cord formation has been observed in these strains. Timpe and Runyon made a tentative classification of these organisms on the basis of the appearance of their colonies. The forty strains of chromogenic acid-fast bacilli of human provenance investigated by Darzins and Fahr (1956), showed no cord formation in a liquid medium. In guinea pigs, these strains did not produce progressive lesions. These organisms were classified as saprophytic (see p. 301).

Wood, Buhler, and Pollak (1956) reported about 15 more patients infected with the "yellow" acid-fast bacillus. Five patients died of the disease. In most cases the "yellow" bacillus was resistant to high concentrations of isoniazid, but susceptible to streptomycin. Mantoux tests (0.0001 mg. of purified PPD tuberculin) were performed on eleven patients. The reaction was positive in seven but negative in two instances.

Weed, McDonald, and Needham (1956) published data collected during ten years on 19 patients of the Mayo Clinic suffering from a wide variety of closed lesions containing acid-fast bacilli. Among those patients were 8 children not over five years of age with swellings of cervical or submaxillary glands. The tuberculin test was positive in most cases. The histologic examination of the material taken from the lesions revealed caseous tuberculosis. Acid-fast bacilli were cultured in all 19 cases. The bacilli grew readily at 30°C., the colonies were pale or bright yellow in color. The bacilli were nonpathogenic to guinea pigs, although many of the inoculated animals became sensitized to old tuberculin. The cord-forming ability of these strains was not thoroughly investigated.

Weed and co-workers described the case of a student who had suffered for ten years from heavy granulomatous lesions in the forehead, ribs, scapula, and tibia. The lesions contained nonpathogenic acid-fast bacilli. This infection resembles that of another student, described by Norwegian investigators, who was afflicted with widely disseminated lesions of similar character. These lesions allegedly developed after BCG vaccination (see p. 303).

Weed and co-workers do not claim that the acid-fast bacilli found in the lesions of these patients were the cause of these lesions. Rather they assume that the bacilli spread to these areas from some unknown focus by hematogenous or lymphogenous routes.

Florence (1956) reported on 23 cases of pulmonary disease in which sputa, gastric contents, or other material taken from the patients yielded chromogenic acid-fast bacilli by culture. In 15 patients, originally presumed to be tuberculous, the cultures produced only acid-fast chromogenic organisms before chemotherapy was started. In some of these cases chromogenic acid-fast bacilli were cultured from resected lung tissues and from the pus of cervical lymph nodes. Tuberculin reaction was positive in these patients. The cultures of these bacilli became chromogenic at room temperature. The bacilli injected into guinea pigs caused local abscesses or regional lymphadenopathy but not generalized disease. None of these bacilli showed cord formation. According to Florence these organisms are potential pathogens for humans and may produce a lung disease similar to tuberculosis.

The critical specific dose of tuberculin for identifying tuberculous infection is 0.0001 mg. of standardized tuberculin (PPD or its equivalent). This dose of tuberculin was given to 10,000 nursing school students from different schools who had lived all their lifetimes in widely separated areas of the United States. Those who failed to react to the first dose were administered a second dose of 0.005 mg. of tuberculin. In southern states (New Mexico, Missouri, Virginia) twice as many persons reacted to the second dose of tuberculin as to the first. In contrast to the first-dose reactors the proportion of second-dose reactors was higher in rural than in urban areas.

This pattern of tuberculin sensitivity suggests the existence of a local widespread nonspecific sensitivity to tuberculin in the population of the South of the United States (Palmer, Ferebee, and Petersen, 1950).

Conclusions. The chromogenic acid-fast bacilli found in the human body may be true saprophytic organisms introduced into it from the outside. These bacilli are not pathogenic to guinea pigs and do not produce cords in a liquid medium. This group of organisms apparently does not contain the causative agent of human tuberculosis, but these bacilli may associate with pre-existing nontuberculous lesions and cause grave diagnostic errors. The other group of acid-fast bacilli, pigmented or not, originate from the tubercle bacilli. These bacilli have lost their lethality and partly their virulence during their inhabitation of the human body, mostly as the result of antibiotic and chemotherapeutic treatment, or during their growth on artificial media. This group of bacilli will not produce progressive lesions in guinea pigs, but some of them may be virulent to mice. They will produce fractions of true cords in liquid media, indicating their residual virulence. The organisms of this group, including the BCG and our N-5 bacilli, may be the cause of primary infections, although their role in human pathology is still controversial. Without cultivation in liquid medium and the study of their cord-forming ability, these two groups of acid-fast bacilli, both found in the human body and nonlethal to guinea pigs, cannot at the present be differentiated.

Pathogenicity Factor of Tubercle Bacilli

As the foregoing shows, there have been many attempts to identify the factor or substance that causes the pathogenicity of tubercle bacilli and by which the pathogenic bacilli differ from the saprophytic acid-fast bacilli. Most of these attempts were devoted to the study of fatty or lipid substances extracted from the bacilli and to the search for the specific pathogenicity factor among these compounds.

Although there were substances found among the extracted fats which do produce in the tissue of susceptible animals some tuberculoid structures, none of these substances known at present can be regarded as the specific pathogenicity factor of tubercle bacilli. The same must be said of the cord substance of tubercle bacilli. Pathogenic tubercle bacilli, when grown in dispersed form in the presence of wetting agents (egg yolk, Tweens), do not lose their virulence (Besredka, 1913; Dubos, 1945). These considerations led some investigators to deny the existence of any specific pathogenicity factor in tubercle bacilli. There are also authors, such as Middlebrook (1945), who defend the existence of such a factor.

The problem of the pathogenicity factor of tubercle bacilli will be narrowed by finding the relation between the amount of bacilli inoculated and the duration of the disease produced. If an increased amount of bacilli should kill the animals early and a decreased amount prolong the duration of the disease, the increase in the amount of bacilli will be identical to the increased virulence, and the decrease in the amount of bacilli will be equal to the decreased or attenuated virulence. Thus, a direct relation between the amount of bacilli and their virulence would be established.

An early investigator of the pathogenicity of tubercle bacilli, Vagedes (1898), indicated the existence of relations between the dose of bacilli inoculated and the duration of the disease. Later investigators, such as Calmette, Boquet, and Nègre (1923), Lange (1930), Doerr and Gold (1932), Fust (1938), and Stewart (1951), came to identical conclusions.

Youmans and Youmans (1951) determined the effect of the size of the infecting dose of tubercle bacilli on the survival time of mice and confirmed the earlier findings; namely, that the survival time of mice infected intravenously with virulent tubercle bacilli is inversely proportional to the number of bacilli injected. When the size of the inoculum reaches 7.8 mg. of the H37Rv strain of bacilli (wet weight), the mice die immediately. This effect of large doses suggests the presence of some specific toxic factor in tubercle bacilli.

Boquet and Bretey (1950), repeating the experiments performed by Calmette, Boquet, and Nègre (1923), came to the conclusion that the differences in the speed of development of tuberculosis caused by the inoculation of different amounts of bacilli depend on the speed with which bacilli are dispersed into the organism from the point of inoculation. The amount of bacilli inoculated determines the speed with which they break through the local defense mechanism of the organism. In guinea pigs inoculated subcutaneously with 1 mg. of tubercle bacilli the bacilli were found in the blood stream within 30 to 45 minutes after the infection; a dose 1,000 times smaller produced generalized infection between the ninth and the fourteenth days.

The local-defense theory of Boquet and Bretey does not explain the cause of pathogenicity. Why is it that the pathogenic bacilli can break through the local defense and the saprophytic ones cannot? The data of Boquet and Bretey support the findings of earlier authors and those of Calmette, Boquet, and Nègre (1923) that the course of the disease produced by the inoculation of tubercle bacilli is the function of the amount of bacilli inoculated. According to Boquet and Bretey, 1 mg. of bacilli, strain Vallée, inoculated intracutaneously into guinea pigs, killed them within two months; 10^{-2} mg. of bacilli were lethal in three to four months; 10^{-4} mg. in four to five months; and 10^{-6} mg. in four to six months.

The uniform results arrived at by the investigators point to some pathogenicity factor in the cells of tubercle bacilli. This substance seemingly opens the way through which bacilli can enter the organism. The presence of such a pathogenicity factor is indicated by the preponderance of the quantity of bacilli inoculated over all other agents and circumstances involved in the course of the infection. The parallel with the action of a poison is striking. In both cases the quantity dominates the picture of the disease. When nonliving poison is inoculated in a sublethal amount, the recovery of the organism occurs. When living tubercle bacilli are inoculated in a sublethal dose, the amount of toxin, or the "pathogenicity factor," introduced with them into the organism is not sufficient to permit their immediate dispersion. Time is necessary to allow the increase of this factor in locally multiplying bacilli to reach the level that permits the bacilli to invade the organism. Thus, the course of the disease is inversely related to the amount of bacilli inoculated.

Tubercle bacilli substances causing allergy account for the development of tuberculous conditions in chronic cases of tuberculosis but they do not explain the rapid death of animals or human beings infected with a large dose of tubercle bacilli. To explain an early death from a tuberculous infection, it is not necessary to accept the notion that tubercle bacilli produce a soluble exotoxin as do tetanus or diphtheria bacilli. The cases of anthrax and gas gangrene infections may illustrate the point. To explain death in cases of anthrax infections, investigators since Davaine, in 1850, have unsuccessfully tried to find toxic products in anthrax bacilli or in their cultures. Just recently, Smith and Keppie (1955) found that anthrax toxin is produced in the organism and can be found only *in vivo* in the plasma of infected animals. The clostridia of gas gangrene (*Cl. septicum*, *Cl. oedematiens*, and others) produce formidable soluble toxins in cultures, but toxins cannot be found in infected organisms (Macfarlane, 1955).

The inability of bacilli to establish themselves and to proliferate in the host may be caused by the inability of bacilli to obtain specific nutrients in the host. Purine-requiring mutants of *Klebsiella pneumoniae* are nonpathogenic when inoculated into the peritoneal cavities of mice. The addition of purines (adenine, guanine, xanthine) to the inoculum results in the death of mice (Garber, Hackett, and Franklin, 1952).

At present we do not know the pathogenicity factor of tubercle bacilli or the mode of its action. The large-scale and painstaking work done with the fatty substances of tubercle bacilli in search of this factor has dominated this field of research. The pathogenicity factor is probably some substance of nucleic acid nature.

The role of nucleic acids in the pathogenicity of bacteriophages was established by Hershey and Chase (1952–1953). When bacteriophages infect a bacterial cell, the nucleic acid component of the bacteriophage enters the cell and causes intracellular multiplication of bacteriophages. The protein component of the bacteriophage remains outside the infected cell.

The reconstitution experiments of Fraenkel-Conrat and Williams indicated that nucleic acid plays a role in the pathogenicity of tobacco mosaic virus (see p. 53).

Only the discovery of the pathogenicity factor will offer the possibility of an exact assay of the pathogenicity of mycobacteria.

PART FIVE

Experimenting with the Tubercle Bacillus

XXIII

Problems in Experimenting with Tubercle Bacilli

EXPERIMENTS with tubercle bacilli bring up some problems which are common to general microbiology and others that are restricted to the bacteriology of mycobacteria.

Experiment, observation, and reasoning, which were recognized by Francis Bacon and Claude Bernard as the only sources of human knowledge, has its limitations because our senses and the procedures we employ to collect scientific data (weighing, diluting, injecting, etc.) are imperfect and subject to variations which lead to errors. To overcome this, a large number of average data are often collected. These created averages do not exist in nature (Claude Bernard). In an account of an experiment, it is better to give the total result and to indicate the size of possible deviation or the standard error of the data. This gives information about the degree of accuracy of the method used and the certainty of the conclusions drawn from the facts revealed by it. Statistical methods, mostly mathematical, provide an answer to many of these questions. The tests of significance of observed data and the calculation of χ^2, as devised by Pearson in 1900, supply objective measures which permit the determination of whether the observed variation is due to chance or to the technique employed.

The examination of data is facilitated by the construction of diagrams. Ordinarily, the number of things measured (population) is put on the abscissa, and the frequency on the ordinate. If the distribution is normal, the greatest frequency is in the center and the diagram has the shape of a regular bell. Departures from the normal distribution will distort the bell's form. In other cases some variable (population) is plotted against some invariable factor (time). Instead of numbers their logarithms may be used. More instructive results are obtained when one variable phenomenon is plotted against another variable. In such cases a scatter diagram is obtained which tells us whether a close connection exists between the variables.

Experimenting with Tubercle Bacilli

The distribution of variables may not be uniform if the variable is found not in all but only in some values or samples. If one microorganism is in a sample of 100 ml. and we withdraw 1 ml. from the sample, our microorganism may be in the 1 ml. withdrawn or in the remaining 99 ml. The chances are 99 out of 100 or $^{99}/_{100}$ or 0.99 that our organism will not be in the withdrawn ml. In general, if V represents the number of volumes in the sample, X the number of microorganisms in the sample, and 1 volume is withdrawn, the probability that this volume will not contain the microorganisms is given by the formula (McGrady, 1915):

$$\left(\frac{V-1}{V}\right)^{X}$$

In bacteriologic work, when small numbers or highly diluted suspensions of microorganisms are handled, the nonuniform or random distribution of particles makes the result subject to the operation of chance. The frequencies with which the value is given is known as the Poisson series of probabilities or the law of small numbers. In the bacteriology of tuberculosis, when efforts are concentrated on the discovery of small numbers of bacilli, the law of small numbers illuminates some obscure facts observed in experiments. Examples of such order are given by Berg (1941) (see Table 45). B. Lange (1926) injected 86 guinea pigs with doses of tubercle bacilli ranging from one ten-millionth to one billionth mg. Seven of the animals became tuberculous from a dose containing 0.2 of a bacillus, three from 0.1, and one from 0.01.

Table 45. The Distribution of Small Numbers of Tubercle Bacilli in Equal Doses According to the Poisson Series of Probabilities

Number of Bacilli in One Unit Volume	Mean Number of Bacilli in One Unit Volume Calculated from Actual Count and Dilutions							
	0.1	0.5	1	2	3	4	5	10
				Probabilities				
0	0.90	0.61	0.37	0.14	0.05	0.02	0.01	
1	0.09	0.30	0.37	0.27	0.15	0.07	0.03	
2	0.005	0.08	0.18	0.27	0.22	0.15	0.08	
3		0.01	0.06	0.18	0.22	0.20	0.14	0.01

Source: Berg (1941).

To explain these results we need not admit the existence of some "virus" or infective fragments of tubercle bacilli. These results are understandable if the distribution of bacilli in a suspension is examined statistically. Even in the absence of any agglutination, the distribution of small numbers of bacilli in a liquid medium is not uniform.

If a liter of a concentrated suspension of bacilli is diluted so as to contain 3 bacilli per ml., every ml. taken from the final dilution – theory and practice agree – will not contain 3 bacilli. A probable distribution of bacilli is given in Table 45. The column headed 3 states that probably 0.05 of one liter or 50 ml. will contain 0 bacilli, and 0.15 of one liter or 150 ml. will contain 1 bacillus. In higher dilutions, where the number of bacilli is smaller in the separate unit, the probability of having 0 bacilli in a single unit is higher. If, for example, we aspire in a syringe 10 ml. of suspension with a probable 3 bacilli per ml., and inject the suspension into guinea pigs at the rate of 1 ml. to each, the guinea pigs will receive 0 to 9 bacilli each.

The number of colonies grown on a solid medium seeded with a highly diluted suspension of bacilli does not correspond to the numbers estimated theoretically. B. Lange (1930) seeded 10^{-7} and 10^{-8} mg. of tubercle bacilli on slants of solid medium; in each case only one colony developed on the slants. In another experiment, tubes inoculated with 10^{-6} mg. bacilli produced 26 colonies, those planted with 10^{-7} mg., on which 2 to 3 colonies were expected, remained sterile.

Frimodt-Möller (1939) inoculated 72 tubes of media with dilutions of tubercle bacilli presumably containing 1 bacillus per ml. After incubation, 43 tubes were sterile, 23 tubes contained 1 colony each, 4 tubes 2 colonies, and 2 tubes 3 colonies. The mean number of colonies was $^{37}/_{72} = 0.514$ colonies per tube. The column headed "0.5" in Table 45 indicates that there should be $0.61 \times 72 = 43.9$ sterile tubes (actually there were 43). These 43 doses did not contain bacilli and would not produce tuberculosis if injected into guinea pigs. The actual distribution of bacilli was in agreement with the theory.

Theoretically, it is not possible to seed media or to inoculate animals with equal numbers of bacilli even in the absence of agglutination in the suspension when the numbers of the bacilli are small.

In studies of virulence, in the estimation of the action of antibiotics and chemotherapeutic agents, and in many other problems, the determination of the density of the bacterial population in the culture or the suspension is an everyday problem of primary importance. Fisher, Thornton, and Mackenzie (1922) pointed out that the results of the estimation of viable bacilli by the plating method would be of the highest possible accuracy when (1) each plate would offer the same facilities for development; (2) the development of any organism would be independent of other organisms present; (3) every bacillus would produce only one colony; (4) each plate would have an equal chance of receiving planted organisms. The fulfillment of the first and fourth conditions depends upon the degree of perfection of the technique employed; the fulfillment of the second and third conditions depends on the nature of the organisms studied.

The variation in the distribution of organisms in diluted suspensions on parallel plates is due to the chance distribution and will vary in the same manner as the samples in the Poisson series. The total error involved in estimating a bacterial population by the plating method is the result of two different sources of deviation: (a) the distribution or sampling error, and (b) the dilution error (Jennison and Wadsworth, 1940). The distribution

$$\text{Total Error} = \pm \sqrt{(\text{Percentage distribution error})^2 + (\text{Percentage dilution error})^2}$$

error is due to variation in the number of colonies on replicate plates, the dilution is produced by the dilution of the suspension and by pipetting. The dilution error increases with higher dilutions, the distribution error does not. To minimize the distribution error, the plates must not be overcrowded with colonies, and a sufficient number of replicate plates (3–5) must enter into the count.

Besides the dilution error, the common practice of seeding media or of inoculating animals with a quantity of bacilli determined by weight is followed by errors resulting from differences in the amount of moisture in the media and also from the fact that, even in the logarithmic phase of growth, the cultures contain a considerable quantity of dead bacilli.

The estimation of the number of bacilli per mg. of culture, i.e., the total count, may be performed in the counting chambers (Petroff-Hausser, Helber); the proportion of living organisms – the viable count – is revealed by the quantity of colonies developed on a solid medium. Quantitative experiments on tubercle bacilli must be based on the estimation of viable bacilli in the material. The dosage of bacilli based on the weight or the total count is not a reliable procedure (B. Lange, 1926; Kirchner and Li, 1932). According to G. S. Wilson and Schwabacher (1937), cultures of 4 avian strains of tubercle bacilli contained, in different phases of growth, from 41.4 to 80.3 per cent, 12 bovine strains from 0.2 to 15.4 per cent, and 4 human strains from 1.1 to 8.7 per cent viable bacilli.

The inoculation of tubercle bacilli into susceptible animals does not give a reliable answer as to the viability of the bacilli. Bretey (1944) found that of 9 guinea pigs inoculated with 1 bacilli from a virulent human strain of tubercle bacilli isolated with the aid of a micromanipulator, only 5 animals contracted tuberculosis.

Dubos (1945), by introducing wetting agents, opened the way to the production of dispersed cultures of tubercle bacilli (see Chapter XVIII). The dispersed cultures provide an easier and more precise way of quantitatively estimating a bacillary mass and the amount of living bacilli in it than the earlier methods of weighing, trituration, and centrifuging.

Cells growing in a liquid medium containing wetting agent Tween 80 produce a uniform turbidity. The degree of turbidity or optical density of the liquid depends on the quantity or weight of the cells suspended in it.

This makes it possible to express in terms of turbidity readings the mass of bacilli produced. The amount of bacilli in a culture can be estimated in terms of weight by comparing the turbidity of the culture with the turbidity produced by a known weight of bacilli (D. G. Smith, 1947); the weight of bacilli may be determined by filtering them out of the medium (Wolinsky and Steenken, 1947), or by separating them by centrifuging the medium (Hurwitz and Silverman, 1950). The weight of the bacillary mass obtained at different growth phases or under the influence of chemotherapeutic agents or antibiotics may be plotted against the turbidimetric readings of the photometer or against the time and growth curves of the culture obtained. By the same token, the viable count of bacilli, if the colony counts are made on solid media, can be correlated with the turbidimetric readings. Unfortunately, when these methods are used the weight of the harvested bacilli cannot be determined with precision; traces of the medium remain in the bacterial mass; the determined optical densities are proportional to a number of bacteria of the same size; under the influence of antibiotics (penicillin) the optical density is the measure of the volume or mass rather than of the number of bacteria (Treffers, 1945–1946).

Kaplan, Traum, and Bankowski (1948) estimated the amount of mycobacteria present in a suspension producing radioactive bacilli by growing them on Sauton's medium containing radioactive Na_2HPO_4. The weight of the bacilli in suspension was determined by the radioactivity of the suspension; the concentration of the suspension was correlated with its turbidity.

Fenner (1951) compared the total count of tubercle bacilli of Tween-albumin liquid medium in a Petroff-Hausser chamber with the viable count of colonies developed on the surface of the transparent agar medium. The colony count showed that the ratio of the viable count to the total count was high and that most of the organisms in the liquid medium were viable. This method provides an easy way to estimate the viable tubercle bacilli and makes it possible to express the doses of bacilli in terms of the number of viable bacilli instead of expressing it inaccurately in terms of weight or volume.

Yegian and Budd (1951) used the same procedure as Fenner, but inoculated by the pour-plate technique into a solid agar medium 10^{-7} mg. of H37Rv strain of tubercle bacilli cultivated in Tween-albumin liquid medium. As shown by the earlier experiments of Buc, Lange, Second, and Chatelain (see p. 89), tubercle bacilli inoculated into agar develop colonies mainly in the subsurface of the agar. In the experiments of Yegian and Budd, the number of colonies grown in the subsurface exceeded considerably the number of colonies grown on the surface of the plates.

XXIV

Estimating the Antituberculous Activity of a New Drug

CAREFULLY collected and critically selected data will produce lasting achievement. The investigation of a new drug must always be started with the study of the action of this drug *in vitro*. The results obtained may give important indications about the mode of its action as well as save time and work. However, the actions of drugs *in vitro* and *in vivo* rarely run parallel. Generally, the action of a drug is the result of its concentration. High concentrations have bactericidal or bacteriolytic, low ones bacteriostatic, action.

The chemotherapeutic or serotherapeutic action of an unknown compound must be compared with the action of a known standard substance in standard conditions (Prigge, 1940). Without such a standard, improvement or advance in research is hardly to be expected. The discovery of penicillin by the Oxford workers illustrates this rule.

According to the principles laid down by Ehrlich, the standard penicillin was prepared. A determined but arbitrary quantity of this brand of penicillin, which under standard conditions showed uniform activity, was chosen as an arbitrary unit of penicillin (Oxford unit). The activities of antibiotics produced by different strains of *Penicillium* were compared with the activity of this unit.

The rules which govern the testing of antituberculous substances have been fixed by Feldman and Hinshaw (1945). A satisfactory chemotherapeutic agent (1) should be supported by animals and should not bring about disturbances of their health; (2) should favorably influence the course of experimental tuberculosis of animals; (3) should produce the favorable effect within a reasonable period of time.

The animals used in testing antituberculous drugs are guinea pigs, mice, rabbits, and occasionally hamsters. Important factors in chemotherapeutic testing are good care, good food, and the good health of the animals. The death of animals from causes other than tuberculosis is a serious obstacle to the success of an experiment. It may reduce the animal population to a level which would no longer secure trustworthy results. To avoid this and to accelerate the work, the animals are treated for a definite period and then killed (guinea pigs 6–8 weeks, mice 4 weeks).

The animals must be inoculated with doses of tubercle bacilli of known virulence, such as the Saranac Lake laboratory strain H37Rv. The choice of the appropriate infective dose is of importance. When the animals are infected with too small a dose or when the bacilli inoculated are of low virulence, the control animals may show no signs of infection, and the results of the experiment may be inconclusive. When the infective dose is too big, the course of the disease may be greatly accelerated, the influence of the treatment annihilated. The sensitivity to tuberculosis of the animal species used in the experiment must also be taken into consideration.

The quantitative administration of the test substance to animals can be made by means of the stomach tube. The uptake of the drug mixed with food cannot be regarded as quantitative. The absorption and the changes undergone by the drug in the digestive tract would remain unknown. The parenteral route of introduction is preferable. The action of the drug introduced parenterally may be different from that obtained by stomachal application. In general, the drug introduced through the digestive tract shows only a fraction of the activity it reveals when it is introduced through the parenteral route.

The administration of a therapeutic agent may be started some days before, simultaneously with, or some time after the infective inoculation. It should be administered at regular intervals. The gross examination of the organs of animals who died or were killed must be followed by a histologic examination.

A drug that shows some promise as an antituberculous agent must be subjected to rigorous screening in animals that were infected some weeks before therapy was started and show a positive tuberculin test.

The greatest obstacle to the elucidation of the antituberculous activity of a substance is the absence of an impartial standard whereby an effective substance could be definitely distinguished from a noneffective one (Feldman and Hinshaw, 1945). The sum of conclusions derived from (1) the survival time of treated animals as compared to untreated ones, (2) the loss of weight by untreated animals, (3) the amount and character of tuberculous lesions in the organs of treated animals as compared to those in untreated ones, and (4) the quantity of bacilli present in the lesions, will indicate the therapeutic value of the compound studied.

Besides animal inoculation, another *in vivo* method, the treatment of infected chorioallantoic membrane of chick embryo, may be used to estimate the antituberculous activity of a drug. This method cannot replace the animal experiment but it may be of use in the preliminary screening of a promising compound (see Chapter XXIX).

The difficulty of evaluating *in vitro* the activity of a relatively simple antituberculous drug and of estimating the influence of secondary factors on the outcome is illustrated by the results obtained by various authors investigating the action of isonicotinic acid hydrazide on tubercle bacilli.

Steenken and Wolinsky (1953) studied the action of Rimifon and Marsilid on the growth and viability of H37Rv strain of tubercle bacilli cultivated in Tween 80–albumin liquid medium. Marsilid (1-isonicotinyl, 2-isopropyl hydrazine dihydrochloride) brought about the complete inhibition of growth in a concentration of 1.6 to 3.1 μg. per ml., and reduced, in 24 hours, the count of viable bacilli from 200,000 to 15,000 per ml.

Middlebrook (1952), also using the Tween-albumin liquid medium and bovine strain Vallée instead of H37Rv, found that the presence of 0.1 μg. per ml. of isonicotinic acid hydrazide in a 24-hour-old culture diminished by approximately twenty times the viable count of the bacilli.

Suter (1952a) found that 0.05 μg. per ml. of isonicotinic acid hydrazide completely inhibits the growth of tubercle bacilli in Tween-albumin liquid medium.

Braunsteiner, Mlczoch, and Zischka (1953) investigated the action of Rimifon on tubercle bacilli cultivated in Tween-albumin medium containing 10 μg. of the drug per ml. After 24 hours of contact the tubercle bacilli were no longer cultivable.

While the works of the foregoing investigators confirm the bacteriostatic and bactericidal action on tubercle bacilli of isonicotinic acid hydrazide at different concentrations, different conclusions were reached by the French authors, Noufflard and Deslandes (1952) who worked with a Dubos' liquid albumin medium not containing Tween 80. These investigators did not observe any bactericidal action of the drug on the H37Rv strain of tubercle bacilli. After one month of contact with 13.7μg. of the drug per ml., the viable count of bacilli did not show any decrease when cultivated on Löwenstein's egg medium. Noufflard and Deslandes attributed the difference between their results and those obtained by American investigators to the presence of Tween 80 in the media of the latter authors. The cultivation of bacilli on an egg medium instead of the less favorable Tween 80–albumin medium may have influenced the results.

Goulding, King, Knox, and Robson (1952) observed the inactivation of isoniazid in Dubos' Tween 80–albumin medium not inoculated with tubercle bacilli but incubated at 37°C.

Pansy, Koerber, Stander, and Donovick (1953) studied the constituents of Dubos' Tween-albumin medium to detect the component causing the inactivation of isoniazid. The activity of the solutions was tested against the BCG strain of bacilli in a modified Kirchner's medium. The minimal growth-inhibiting concentrations of isoniazid were determined. The inactivation of isoniazid took place only in the solutions containing ferric ammonium citrate and accompanied by the phosphates. Ferric ammonium citrate without phosphate produced no inactivation of isoniazid. The inactivation took place at *p*H 8.3, but not between *p*H 4.9 and *p*H 7.0.

It is doubtful if the ferric ion is the only cause of the inactivation of isoniazid in Dubos' medium, because the *p*H of Dubos' medium is 6.8.

Brieger, Cosslett, and Glauert (1953) studied, by means of an electron microscope, the action of isonicotinic acid hydrazide on tubercle bacilli in a concentration of 10 μg.; the drug had hardly any visible effect on the bacilli.

Of particular difficulty is the collection and the proper analysis of data derived from observation and experiments on human beings. The manifold physiologic and pathologic manifestations of race, age, sex, nutritional conditions, individual resistance or susceptibility, earlier infections, and many other factors will intervene and break the uniformity of data collected from these experiments or observations. Because of this, clinical studies must be preceded by extensive animal experiments. To evaluate the result of an experiment or to appraise a new drug, the course of the pathologic process in a sufficiently large number of spontaneously afflicted, untreated individuals should be known. How many cases must be observed to collect trustworthy data does not depend so much upon the number of observed cases, as upon the homogeneity of the material. When we deal with human beings, statistically pure material can rarely be collected. The chief cause of an event is accompanied by one or more supplementary causes. When a tuberculous patient is subjected to hospital care, undergoes pneumothorax therapy, and receives gold injections, the favorable outcome of the treatment cannot be ascribed to the chemotherapeutic effect of gold (Martini, 1940).

When the results of observations or experiments on animals or human beings are recorded in numbers, the rules of statistics must be applied. Errors of judgment may creep in if seemingly related phenomena are accepted as having a common cause. (*Post hoc non est propter hoc.*) The emotional approach of an investigator to a problem is another source of error. To prevent this, control experiments with the injection of saline or water instead of the drug are conducted.

Some problems will inevitably require experimentation on human beings. The rules guiding the investigator in this field were formulated 2,000 years ago by Hippocrates and have lost none of their meaning but gained in force through the centuries. The supreme law in experimenting with human beings — *Nil nocere* — was recently called to the attention of investigators by the French Academy of Medicine (Académie Nationale de Médecine, 1952): "Experiments on human beings are not only allowed but they are the duty of the physician when: (1) the new experimental methods of therapy or surgery are applied to the patient in the interest of his health in cases when the existent methods have not secured diagnosis or have not produced recovery; (2) when the experiments proper have other goals than the healing of a determined patient, for example the solution of important problems (such as those of epidemiology) which it would be impossible to solve in other ways. Such experimentation should be only practiced on informed volunteers completely free to accept or to refuse, and performed by a highly qualified person capable of reducing the possible risk involved in the experiment to a minimum."

In the trials of new drugs clear answers can be obtained in a relatively short time if clinicians who have previously worked independently each within his hospital center are willing to merge their individualities and take part in group investigations, accepting only patients approved by an independent team, conforming to an agreed plan of treatment, and submitting results to analysis by an outside investigator (Daniels, 1950).

The results achieved in cooperative clinical research in tuberculosis were stressed by Hinshaw (1953). The solution of the problem of the clinical value of streptomycin in the therapy of tuberculosis was possible only through an extensive series of cooperative investigations performed, in the United States by Veterans' Administration hospitals and the American Trudeau Society, and in England by the British Medical Research Council. That attempt at cooperative research was so successful that investigators in other fields should seriously consider the use of cooperative research work, Hinshaw asserted.

A complex problem can be solved more rapidly when systematically attacked by the members of a team than when it is attacked by a single worker, but the results will either be a mosaic of opinions or will perforce be reduced to a common level to conform with the results of the majority or of the leader of the team. The submission of individuality and creative reasoning (as the chief sources of scientific achievement) to a nonpersonal team opinion is not accepted by many workers. In teamwork there is also the danger of the "influence error" (Martini, 1933). The problems of teamwork in research are treated by Bush and Hattery (1953).

XXV

The Guinea Pig in Experimental Tuberculosis

THE guinea pig is the animal most sensitive to infection with tubercle bacilli. It is universally used to detect tuberculous infection, to screen the pathogenicity of acid-fast bacilli, and to test the efficiency of antituberculous drugs.

A guinea pig infected with pathogenic tubercle bacilli develops exudative, progressive, and lethal tuberculosis which resembles but slightly the pathology of the torpid cavernous phthisis of human beings. These peculiarities of guinea pig tuberculosis forced investigators to look for animals whose tuberculosis is more similar to that of men (mice, rabbits, hamsters).

In tuberculosis experiments young and healthy guinea pigs not under 300 g. of weight are generally used. Before the experiment the animals must be tested with an intradermal injection of standardized tuberculin. (When old tuberculin is used, 0.1 ml. of 1:100 dilution is injected.) Only nonreactors can be accepted for tuberculosis experiments. The chosen animals, a week before the experiment, are segregated in uniform units composed of a sufficiently large number of individuals (10–20 or more) to provide data reliable not only experimentally, but also statistically. In each unit only one unknown factor is tested. It is of importance to select a sufficiently large number of control animals so as to establish the role of the tested component of infection with the greatest accuracy possible.

The development and progress of a tuberculous infection depends on the virulence of the bacilli, the quantity of bacilli injected, and, to a lesser degree, on the way of infection. Bacilli of known virulence, such as the human strain H37Rv, the bovine strains Ravenel, Vallée, and others, must be used in the experiment. For example, 0.1 mg. of H37Rv strain inoculated subcutaneously into a guinea pig produces rapidly progressing disease; 0.001 mg. produces a long-term infection of slow progress (Feldman and Hinshaw, 1945).

Feldman and Hinshaw (1945), who discovered the healing effect of streptomycin in guinea pig tuberculosis, developed a procedure for recording tuberculous lesions in the guinea pig (see also Karlson and Feldman, 1949). The various organs of the guinea pig are schematically represented on the record card of the animal by means of a large rubber stamp (5 x 10 cm.) (Fig. 34). At the necropsy the approximate size and form of the tuberculous lesions in the organs are sketched on the card. The record cards are easily comparable and demonstrate the gross differences in pathologic changes of organs more clearly than descriptions.

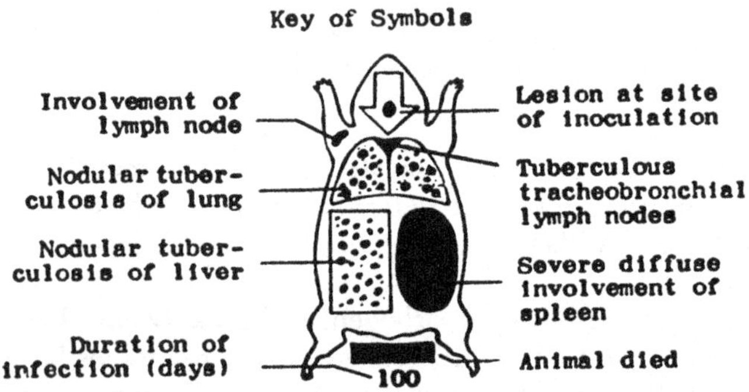

Figure 34. Schematic representation of tuberculous lesions in sites of predilection of an experimentally infected guinea pig (Feldman and Hinshaw, 1945).

In order to follow the course of infection, some importance has been put on the continuous control of body temperature and body weight of the animals. Long experience has shown that these two tedious procedures provide little useful information.

The problem of the sensitivity of the skin of infected animals to tuberculin attracted the interest of a large number of workers. The rules governing the time of appearance of this sensitivity, relation to the amount of the infective dose, the course of this sensitivity during the disease, and its diagnostic value were established.

The active principle of tuberculin is a heat-stable protein. The claims of Paraf and Desbordes (1945) that the active substance of tuberculin is α-α-disubstituted fatty acid have not been confirmed (see the review by Seibert, 1950).

The studies of Römer (1909, 1910) revealed the direct relation between the appearance of the sensitivity of the skin of the infected animals to tuberculin and the amount of bacilli inoculated. Debré, Paraf, and Dautrebande (1920) found that the development of the sensitivity of the skin of guinea pigs to old tuberculin diluted 1:100 coincides with the development of local lesions at the site of the inoculation of bacilli. The duration of the antiallergic period is inversely proportional to the amount of bacilli injected. Parish and Okell (1929) studied this problem in fifteen guinea pigs infected with a large dose (0.5 mg.) of tubercle bacilli and tested them weekly with standard tuberculin. Ten guinea pigs, one week after the infection, gave definite positive reaction with tuberculin diluted 1:50 and 1:100. One week later seven of these animals were sensitive to tuberculin diluted 1:1,000 and 1:4,000. The development of tuberculin sensitivity varied considerably in individual guinea pigs. A guinea pig may be insensitive to tuberculin one week but sensitive seven days later. On the whole, the guinea pig is far less sensitive to tuberculin than man.

Uhlenhuth and Seiffert (1932) studied the sensitivity to tuberculin of guinea pigs infected with tubercle bacilli of different virulence. The animals infected 5 to 6 weeks earlier with tubercle bacilli of high virulence were killed by 0.1 ml. of tuberculin injected intraperitoneally; 0.0002 ml. of tuberculin injected intracutaneously provoked strong local reaction in them. Animals infected with strains of low virulence showed little pathologic change in organs; 0.005 to 0.02 ml. of tuberculin was needed to obtain positive skin reaction. In guinea pigs infected with BCG, 0.1 to 0.05 ml. of tuberculin was needed to obtain positive skin reaction, and 1 to 1.5 ml. of tuberculin to cause death. These latter doses were not harmful to animals not infected.

Boquet and Bretey (1933, 1934) confirmed the fact that the duration of the insensitivity of the skin (the antiallergic period) of an infected guinea pig is variable and depends on the route of infection and the doses of inoculated bacilli (see Table 46 and Fig. 35).

Table 46. The Relation between the Amount of Injected Tubercle Bacilli (Strain Vallée) and the Duration of the Antiallergic Period in Guinea Pigs

Amount of Bacilli	Duration of the Antiallergic Period
0.0001 mg.	12–14 days
0.001	10–12
0.1	10–12
1.0	5

Source: Boquet and Bretey (1934).

After the antiallergic period ends the skin sensitivity increases rapidly. Guinea pigs inoculated with 0.001 mg. of virulent bovine bacilli (Vallée) reacted on the eighth day to 0.05 or 0.01 ml. of old tuberculin; between the eighth and the thirtieth day after the infection the animals reacted to 0.0004 ml. of tuberculin. A dose of 0.01 ml. at that time produced necrosis of the skin. The skin sensitivity to tuberculin increased progressively till the

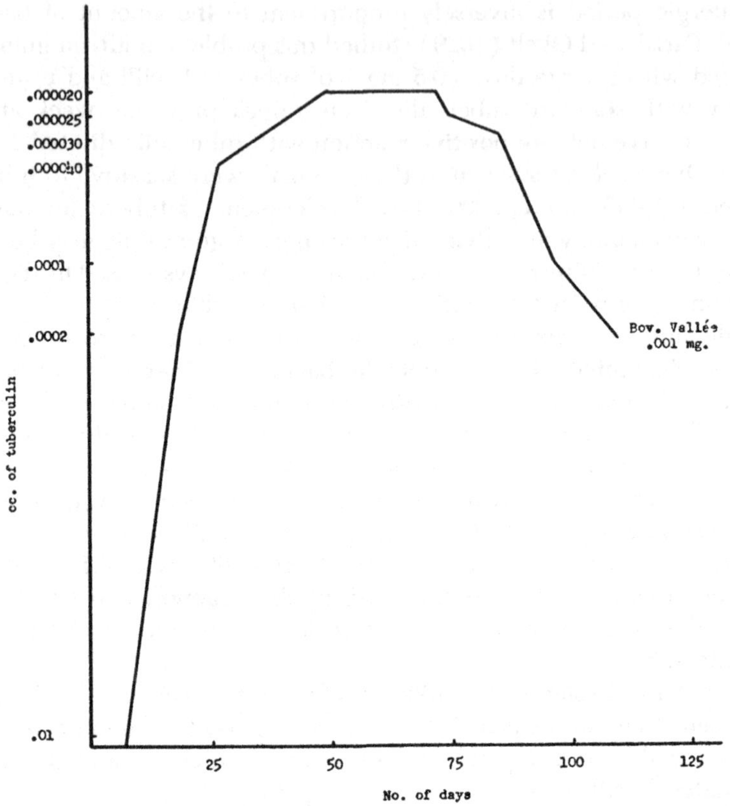

Figure 35. Development of skin sensitivity to tuberculin of guinea pig infected with 0.001 mg. tubercle bacilli of bovine type (Boquet and Bretey, 1934).

thirtieth day; the necrotic reaction had the same course. After a short period of stability the skin sensitivity declined rapidly.

The skin sensitivity induced with dead bacilli is less intense than that created with living ones. Tubercle bacilli killed by heat and enveloped in hard paraffin (melting point 45°C.) produce in guinea pigs an extremely strong and prolonged skin reaction (Coulaud, 1934). Repeated injections of bacilli into the animal decrease the sensitivity of the skin to tuberculin (Kourilsky and Coulaud, 1952). The great variability of the reaction of the skin to tuberculin was particularly stressed by Seibert and Morley (1933). In their experiments the proteins of bovine bacilli produced a more intense reaction than those of human bacilli. The proteins of avian and grass bacilli produced a weak skin reaction. The seasonal fluctuation of the intensity of skin reactions in tuberculous animals was observed by von Engel (1933).

Some authors, impressed by the high coincidence of positive tuberculin reaction and tuberculous lesions in the organs, advocated the use of tuberculin reaction as a diagnostic procedure. Müller (1920) recommended it as an easy means of recognizing early tuberculosis in guinea pigs inoculated with pathologic material for diagnostic purposes. Müller regarded the positive tuberculin reaction as sufficient to confirm a diagnosis of tuberculosis, even the autopsy of the animals being, in his opinion, superfluous. These ideas were recently shared by Tison (1951). According to him, the diagnosis of tuberculosis in guinea pigs can be made in 20 to 30 days. The diagnosis is secured when 0.1 ml. of old tuberculin, diluted 1:10, produces necrotic lesions in the skin of the animal.

Pinner (1935) studied 15 strains of nonlethal chromogenic acid-fast bacilli. The animals infected with these bacilli reacted typically to old tuberculin diluted 1:10. Fernbach and Rullier (1941) observed that 5 ml. of old tuberculin were inactivated when incubated with 50 mg. of glutathione. Harris and Harris (1950) showed that in rabbits and guinea pigs sensitized with BCG, 34 mg. of cortisone, injected daily for 3½ days, suppressed the skin sensitivity to old tuberculin diluted 1:10. Guinea pigs sensitized by injections of 2 mg. BCG, and grossly but not completely deficient in ascorbic acid, developed a high skin sensitivity to tuberculin. This sensitivity was diminished or abolished by the addition of ascorbic acid (20 mg. daily) to the food of the animals. The skin sensitivity to tuberculin was not diminished when ascorbic acid was provided by feeding raw cabbage to the animals. The factor in the cabbage that opposes the desensitizing action of ascorbic acid also inhibits the desensitizing action of ascorbic acid added to the diet of the sensitized animals. A single injection of cortisone (5 mg. per kg.) diminishes the sensitivity of the skin to tuberculin in guinea pigs on a cabbage diet (D. Long, Miles, and Perry, 1951). Tuberculin sensitivity in guinea pigs is depressed by a single subcutaneous injection of 10 to 100 mg. of non-ionic, surface-active polyoxyethylene ether (detergents D2, D14). The action of these ethers is independent of dietary factors (Hart and Long, 1952). (See p. 310.)

The sensitivity of the skin to tuberculin does not in itself permit a diagnosis of tuberculosis (Lippelt, 1939). To take a transitory positive skin sensitivity of an inoculated animal as sufficient evidence of tuberculosis is an oversimplification of tuberculosis diagnosis that may lead to errors of grave consequence. Only the presence of the characteristic acid-fast bacilli and specific anatomic lesions of organs can justify a diagnosis of tuberculosis in animals. The positive skin reaction of an animal to tuberculin may indicate tuberculosis and should be followed by the autopsy of the animal to confirm or disconfirm the diagnosis.

Rubbo and Pierson (1953) suggested a rapid and inexpensive method of large-scale screening of antituberculous substances in guinea pigs. The method consists in inducing four tuberculous ulcers on the shaven back of guinea pigs (Fig. 36). The activity of the drug was estimated by measuring

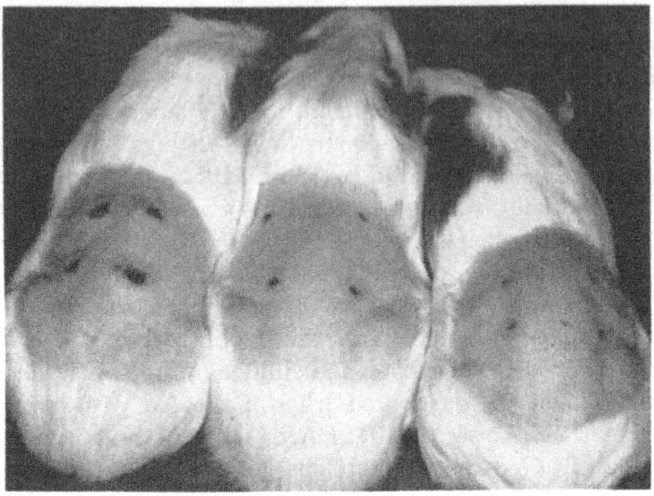

Figure 36. The effect of chemotherapy in experimentally induced skin lesions in guinea pig. Left to right: untreated; treated with 30 mg. streptomycin per kg. for 28 days; treated with 30 mg. isoniazid per kg. for 28 days. (Rubbo and Pierson, 1953.)

the shrinkage of the ulcers in treated animals compared with the ulcers of untreated ones. The age of the animals is an important factor in the procedure. In young animals of less than 400 g., the ulcers tend to be irregular in shape and size. To perform the measurement, the back of the animal is swabbed with alcohol and shaved once weekly, the operator being protected against infection. This method seems to be rapid but more dangerous than other methods, since the open ulcers tend to disseminate tubercle bacilli.

XXVI

The Rabbit in Experimental Tuberculosis

Inhalation Tuberculosis in the Rabbit

RABBITS are used for the differentiation of human and bovine types of tubercle bacilli and in the study of the problems of the pathogenesis and therapy of tuberculosis. Lurie (1949b) showed that rabbits uniformly develop ulcerative chronic pulmonary phthisis when exposed to the inhalation of controlled numbers of virulent bovine tubercle bacilli. Tubercle bacilli multiply in the walls of the lung cavities, and the tuberculous process in the animal closely resembles human chronic pulmonary tuberculosis. The testing of chemotherapeutic substances under these experimental conditions may be of importance in the evaluation of new antituberculous drugs.

In the experiments of Lurie, an aerosol of almost separated tubercle bacilli was produced by atomizing a suspension in a Wells centrifuge (see p. 390). The fine aerosol of bacilli, visible only by Tyndall effect, was carried into a chamber in which the rabbits were exposed to it. The estimation of the quantity of bacilli in the aerosol was made possible by passing a predetermined quantity of aerosol into a broth which was then cultured, and in which the count of viable bacilli was made. When the concentration of living bacilli in the air respired, the duration of exposure, and the respiring volume were known, it was possible to calculate the number of bacilli inhaled by the animals.

A general formula for the determination of tidal air of resting and fasting animals was given by Kleiber (1944). It was assumed that animals, like humans, take up 5 per cent of oxygen from the respired air, and that thus for each 20 liters of air inhaled, 1 liter of oxygen is consumed. The oxygen consumption in warm-blooded animals from rat to steer in the space of 24 hours can be estimated from the basal heat production as being equal to $72 \times W^{0.75}$ calories, where W is the body weight in kilograms.

One liter of oxygen consumed by a fasting animal is equivalent to 4.7

kilocalories of heat; the oxygen consumption would be $72/4.7 \times W^{0.75}$ liters of oxygen per day, or $306 \times W^{0.75}$ liters of air daily.

Kleiber determined by means of the above formula the tidal air of groups of 10 resting and fasting albino Swiss mice at a temperature of 30°C. as being 7.0 ml. per minute.

The tidal air of a 3.5 kg. *Rhesus* monkey under deep pentobarbital anesthesia was found to be 546 ml. per minute; according to the formula the amount should have been 543 ml. per minute.

The difficulty presented by the use of inhalation as a standard procedure to produce lung tuberculosis lies in the impossibility of estimating the natural resistance of rabbits to inhalation tuberculosis and the high death rate of bacilli in aerosol. As was pointed out by Lurie, the naturally resistant rabbits of race III required as many as 1,000 tubercle bacilli units to generate a single microscopic tubercle, but in the susceptible FC strain, 50 units of bacilli produced caseous tubercles. In resistant animals human tubercle bacilli often did not produce any infection.

The survival of sprayed microorganisms in the clouds of aerosol is greatly influenced by the construction of the atomizer and the nature of the diluent used. The number of viable organisms is considerably reduced during the spraying process. From the aerosol cloud of *Serratia marcescens* suspended in distilled water, 0.9 per cent viable bacteria were recovered; from the bacilli suspended in gelatin solution, 14.1 per cent remained alive (Rosebury, 1947).

The Ear Chamber as a Site of Continuous *in vivo* Observation

The classical object of study of such processes as blood circulation, wandering cells, and inflammation has been the transparent tail of the tadpole or the web of the frog's foot. From these studies a considerable amount of basic knowledge of physiology and pathology was gained. In mammals, there are very few transparent tissues which can be adapted to direct microscopic observation. The omentum and the mesentery provide some possibilities, but the time of observation is greatly limited by the inflammation which soon sets in because of the exposure of these internal parts of the body to outside conditions.

Ziegler (1875) had the idea of introducing under the skin or between the muscles of rabbits a chamber made from two cover-glasses fastened together. By periodically removing the chamber from the body, he was able to follow the changes of the tissue in the chamber.

Maximow (1902), in his studies on the origin of inflammatory connective tissue carried out in the laboratory of Ziegler, further developed this glass chamber method. His chambers were made of coverslips fused together at their edges or of sterile celloidin. The chambers were introduced into the intermusculary connective tissue of rabbits, dogs, and pigeons. At a suitable moment they were extracted from the animals, and Maximow was able to keep the tissue in the chamber alive and observe it for 1½ hours on the warm stage of a microscope.

The problem was approached from a different angle by Sandison (1924, 1928), who developed a chamber consisting of two mica slides which was not introduced deeply into the animal tissue, but was sewed into the ear of a rabbit. The tissue, connected with the mother substance and containing blood vessels, was put into the chamber or was allowed to grow into the chamber, thus making continuing observation possible.

Maximow was able to preserve the tissue in his chamber for 1½ hours in a living state, whereas Sandison's technique permitted him to keep the tissue alive for many weeks and rendered it accessible to direct microscopic examination. Later on Sandison improved his technique by using fragments of celluloid photographic film instead of mica slides. Sandison's chamber made it possible to see under the microscope individual cells, growing and moving, and offered possibilities of study equal or superior to those of tissue cultures.

The ear chamber method of Sandison was modified by Ebert, Ashern, and Bloch (1948), and applied to the study of the development of tuberculous infection in the rabbit ear. The chamber consisted of a transparent, round lucite base with a central table rising 2 mm. above the base. The skin was removed from the cartilage, and the table was covered with the mica coverslip leaving a film of tissue 40 to 50 μ thick on the table. Within 14 to 28 days the covered area was vascularized from the surrounding cartilage. This chamber permits microscopic observation by means of oil immersion objectives, and a record of findings can be made by means of motion pictures.

The tissue in the chamber was infected with 0.001 to 0.003 ml. of suspension of bovine Ravenel strain of tubercle bacilli grown in Dubos' liquid medium. The early reaction of the tissue to infection could not be distinguished from the reaction to trauma. Slight dilatation of vessels and stasis of cells could be observed in the first seven days. Between the tenth and the twenty-fourth day the changes were revolutionary and progressive. Dilatation of vessels, infiltration of white cells into the tissue, increase of exudate, and appearance of some giant cells were observed. Thrombosis of blood vessels proceeded until the area was avascular and necrotic and the tissue on the table contained numerous tubercle bacilli. At that time the animals developed positive tuberculin reaction. In the tissue adjacent to the central table, tubercles consisting of central necrotic parts surrounded by epitheloid and giant cells were formed.

A plastic chamber may be implanted in the peritoneal cavity of the animal to study the humoral factors in tuberculosis (Tsuji and Ito, 1955)

Experimenting with Tubercle Bacilli

The Cornea of the Rabbit

Koch (1882) found that the cornea of animals can only occasionally be infected with tubercle bacilli. It was easy to infect rabbits through the eye chamber. In his fifth, sixth, seventh, and eighth series of experiments, he inoculated 14 rabbits in the eye chamber. All of them developed heavy iritis, the cornea was cloudy, and the lungs showed widely disseminated tuberculosis.

Extensive studies of experimental tuberculosis of rabbit's eye infected with avian tubercle bacilli were made as early as 1893 by Kostenitsch and Wolkow. In their first series of experiments, the tubercle bacilli were rubbed in the scarified center of the cornea of 10 rabbits. In the first day of infection, hyperemia of the eye was observed. A considerable amount of polynuclear leucocytes appeared and the ulceration of cornea followed. Epitheloid cells were formed from the fixed tissue cells. In twenty-four days the infection stopped, and healing started.

Friedrich and Nösske (1899) and Daels (1907) observed that a considerable number of rabbits infected by the intracardial or intravenous way with a heavy suspension of tubercle bacilli developed ocular tuberculosis.

Manfredi and Frisco (1903) inoculated tubercle bacilli into the eye chambers of rabbits and observed a direct relation between the dose of bacilli inoculated and the course of infection. Large amounts of bacilli produced generalized tuberculosis, the minimal dose of 10^{-4} mg. produced a local, rapidly healing infection.

Many problems of the pathology and immunity of tuberculosis were studied in the infected eye. E. Long, Holley, and Vorwald (1933) and E. Long and Holley (1933) studied the cellular reaction and the origin of cells taking part in the formation of tubercles in the nonvascular cornea. The polymorphonuclear leucocytes of tuberculous lesions, and the large monocytes which subsequently replaced them in the cornea as in the vascularized organs, were found to be of vascular origin. In the corneas of rabbits, guinea pigs, and cats inoculated with human strain H37 of tubercle bacilli, the cellular response started around the blood vessels of the limbus. The elements of the tubercle, such as epitheloid cells, were also derived from the vascular elements.

Angevine and Huntington (1941) used the incidence of eye tuberculosis in rabbits to estimate the vaccination effect of tubercle bacilli killed by heat. The incidence of eye tuberculosis in immunized rabbits was less than in unvaccinated controls (27.2 and 49.1 per cent respectively). In 18 nonimmunized rabbits out of 28, eye tuberculosis developed within 164 days; in immunized rabbits at that time, tuberculosis of the eye was observed in 4 out of 37 animals.

In rabbits inoculated with 0.00001 mg. of bovine culture (40–200 bacilli) ocular tuberculosis was observed not earlier than three months after infection. The incidence of ocular tuberculosis was closely parallel to the number of tuberculosis lesions in the lungs. (See Fig. 37 for distribution of tubercles in eye.)

Robson (1944) produced experimental ulcers in the eyes of rabbits to study the action of antituberculous substances on the lesions. Bovine and human strains of bacilli were injected in the amount of 0.001 ml. into the anesthetized cornea. Bovine strains, after a week of latency, produced infiltrations made up of small nodules which increased in size and, three weeks after the inoculation, broke down, producing caseating ulcers. Robson showed that for the testing of chemotherapeutic substances it is important to produce equal lesions with the minimum of inoculum.

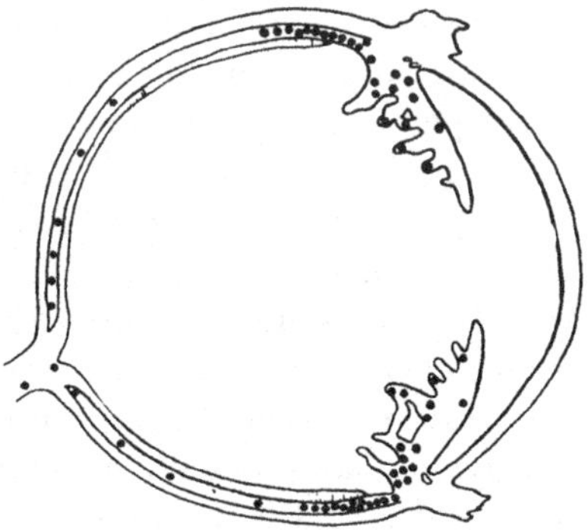

Figure 37. Distribution of tubercles in different parts of the eye of a rabbit inoculated intravenously with 0.00001 mg. bovine type of tubercle bacilli (Angevine and Huntington, 1941).

Gardiner, Rees, and Robson (1949) indicated that most of the screening procedures of therapeutic substances *in vivo* are laborious and time-consuming. The corneas of rabbits infected with tubercle bacilli have advantages over other *in vivo* methods for the testing of therapeutic substances. The comparative development of the lesions can be easily followed, since the lesion of one eye can be treated, the lesion of the other eye left untreated. In thirty days this method indicates whether the drug is active against tuberculous infection.

In the experiments of Gardiner *et al.* the eyes of a mature rabbit were inoculated with approximately 300 bovine tubercle bacilli contained in 0.03 ml. of liquid. This inoculum consistently produced progressive corneal lesions and about 50 per cent of all lesions appeared between the twelfth and the fourteenth day after the inoculation. Minute white nodules appeared in the needle track, increased in size rapidly, and caseation occurred in the centers of the lesions. Approximately 30 days later the lesions broke down and tuberculous ulcers, surrounded by spreading blood vessels, appeared.

The therapy was started with intravitrous injection of 10,000 μg. of streptomycin into the right eye, the left eye of the animals remaining untreated for control purposes. One out of seven eyes treated did not develop the lesion in 94 days. Six untreated eyes developed lesions after a prolonged latent period, but only one of these progressed.

When the standard inoculum was used, consistent lesions of the eye were produced, which enabled the investigators to evaluate the antituberculous activities of the drugs and produced results comparable with those obtained in other *in vivo* screening tests.

Rees and Robson (1949) observed considerable increase of therapeutic effect on early corneal tuberculosis of rabbit when para-aminosalicylic acid was added to streptomycin.

Bunn and Drobeck (1951) and Adair, Drobeck, and Bunn (1951) used the anterior chamber of the rabbit's eye to evaluate the antituberculous activities of drugs. The rabbits inoculated in the anterior chamber with human H37Rv strain of bacilli grown in Tween-albumin liquid medium, developed chronic, destructive, but nonfatal phthisis.

Minimal eye lesions were produced in 23 out of 47 eyes inoculated into anterior chamber with 0.002 mg. (dry weight) of bacilli. Mild diffuse iritis developed and was followed by the increased vascularity of the eye. The fluid in the anterior chamber became cloudy, but in ten to fourteen days it was clear again, and in thirty days the normal appearance of the eyes was restored. When a large dose of bacilli was injected (0.02–0.04 mg.) progressive tuberculosis developed in 8 out of 11 eyes inoculated. The increased caseation destroyed the eye. The final outcome of untreated eye tuberculosis in rabbits depends almost exclusively upon the amount of tubercle bacilli injected.

Streptomycin, when applied 24–96 hours after the infection, failed to influence the course of tuberculosis in rabbit eyes. When given 24 hours before the infection, streptomycin favorably influenced the disease. The action of PAS, terramycin, and other drugs on the course of ocular tuberculosis was also studied.

The speed of the tuberculous process and the easily accessible observation of it made the eye method particularly useful for the study of tuberculosis therapy.

Steenken, Wolinsky, Bristol, and Costigan (1953) proposed using the rabbit in evaluating antituberculous drugs by serial chest roentgenograms. The method permitted them to follow up visually the development of miliary tuberculosis, caseous pneumonia, or cavitary disease, and to study the action of antituberculous drugs on the process.

A rabbit was infected by the injection into the marginal ear vein of 0.01 mg. (dry weight) of bovine Ravenel strain of tubercle bacilli. To minimize radiation hazards the X-ray apparatus was equipped with a steel cone; 400 milliamperes and 46 to 50 kilovolts were used to obtain roentgenograms. A chest roentgenogram was obtained for each animal prior to the infection and, after the infection, at intervals of two or four weeks. Treatment was not started until the roentgenograms revealed widespread miliary lung tuberculosis. The first lesions of the lungs were usually noted two or three weeks after the infection.*

* For information on physiologic experiments on rabbit see H. M. Kaplan, *The rabbit in experimental physiology* (Scholar's Library, New York, 1956).

XXVII

The Mouse in Experimental Tuberculosis

Ways of Infection and Peculiarities of Mouse Tuberculosis

THE susceptibility of the white mouse and the field mouse (*Arvicola arvalis*) to infection with the tubercle bacillus was demonstrated by Koch (1884). Tubercle bacilli, injected subcutaneously or intraperitoneally into mice, produced a slowly progressing infection. Koch concluded that the mouse possesses high resistance to tuberculosis. This view was to be shared by most later workers in this field.

Straus (1895) reports his successful attempts to infect mice with tubercle bacilli. Römer (1903) was the first to use large numbers of white mice in a comparative study of the biology of tubercle bacilli, although mice at that time were regarded as refractory to tuberculous infection. Römer was the first to infect mice intravenously. Even the injection of 0.01 g. of tubercle bacilli produced slowly progressing tuberculosis in the mice, leading to an enormous accumulation of bacilli in the organs. Römer explained this phenomenon as the result of the insensitivity of the mice to the poison (tuberculin) of the tubercle bacilli. A tuberculous mouse can support the injection of 0.5 ml. of tuberculin, an amount representing the tenfold minimal lethal dose for a tuberculous man.

The pathogenicity of tubercle bacilli from different sources to mice and rats was studied by Fränkel and Baumann (1906). Subcutaneous and intraperitoneal inoculation showed that the mouse is considerably more susceptible to infection with tubercle bacilli than had been thought earlier. These investigators confirmed the complete absence of the toxicity of tubercle bacilli to the mouse. The mouse and the rat were found to be animals not suitable for virulence studies of tubercle bacilli.

Marmorek (1906) approached the problem of the pathogenicity of tubercle bacilli from an angle which has received particular attention from investigators during recent years. He indicated that it is difficult or even impossible to estimate the virulence of tubercle bacilli from the death rate of a highly susceptible animal, such as the guinea pig, in which the infection is rapidly progressing and always fatal, and cannot be compared with the torpid tuberculous process in human beings. The development of tuberculous lesions in an animal relatively resistant to tuberculosis, such as the mouse, can furnish information useful in studies of human tuberculosis.

Trommsdorff (1909) used the intravenous way to infect the mouse with tubercle bacilli. Bacilli suspended in 1–2 ml. of liquid were injected into the tail vein. The animals infected with large (1 mg.) or small doses (0.1–0.01 mg.) of human tubercle bacilli died in 2½ or 3½ months. The animals killed earlier did not show gross lesions of organs. Microscopic investigation revealed small infiltrated foci containing tubercle bacilli. The injection of 1 mg. of bovine tubercle bacilli into mice produced within four weeks generalized tuberculosis with enormous quantities of bacilli in the organs, with particular localization of the tuberculous process in the lungs.

A. Griffith (1911, 1937) infected subcutaneously and intraperitoneally, rats, mice, and field-voles with human and bovine tubercle bacilli. The rats inoculated with large doses (10 mg.) of human bacilli died within 74 days and lesions were found only in the site of the inoculation. Two animals inoculated intraperitoneally died after 53 and 58 days, respectively, their tissues swarming with bacilli. White mice infected by the same route proved to be more susceptible to tubercle bacilli than rats. Field-voles were found to be highly susceptible to bovine infection but less so to human bacilli. The susceptibility of the field mouse to tubercle bacilli was found to be between that of the white mouse and that of the field-vole.

Peters (1912) examined and confirmed the findings of Trommsdorff on the possibility of using mice to differentiate between the bovine and human type of bacilli. According to him, 1 mg. of bacilli injected intravenously into a mouse enables the investigator to determine the type. In the case of the bovine type of bacilli the mice died within seven weeks with extensive tuberculosis of lungs, liver, and spleen. In the case of human bacilli the tuberculous process, eight or ninc weeks after the infection, was restricted to a few nodules in the lungs.

Weber (1912) opposed the opinion of Griffith who classified the mouse as an animal resistant to tuberculosis.

Boquet and Nègre (1921) investigated the different ways of infecting white mice and rats with tubercle bacilli. Intracutaneous infection with 0.0002 mg. of bacilli was less effective in a rat than in a mouse. Mice resisted subcutaneous infection with 0.01 mg. bacilli better than rats, but were more susceptible to an intraperitoneal infection. Infection through the digestive tract was less reliable. Apparently the rats and mice have equal susceptibility to this way of infection. The infected animals did not react to intradermal tuberculin injection; the Koch phenomenon was also negative in them. The conclusions made by the authors were that tuberculosis of rats and mice is of purely experimental interest and that these animals cannot replace the guinea pig and the rabbit in practical laboratory diagnosis of tuberculosis.

B. Lange (1922) confirmed Trommsdorff's view that the intravenous inoculation of tubercle bacilli is the surest way to produce the disease in mice. He was also unable to detect the sensitivity of infected mice to tuberculin; even a large dose of dead bacilli injected into these animals did not produce tuberculous allergy.

Ornstein and Steinbach (1925) found that the resistance of the albino rat to infection with a pathogenic human strain of bacilli (H37) is tremendous in comparison with that of the guinea pig.

Gunn, Nungester, and Hougen (1933–1934) compared the results of intraperitoneal and intravenous injection of bacilli into white mice (see Table 47). The intravenous route of inoculation produced a high rate of lung infections. The bacilli injected into the blood stream reach the heart directly and are projected into the lungs, avoiding the phagocytic reticuloendothelial cells of parenchimatous organs.

Table 47. Results of Intraperitoneal and Intravenous Infection of White Mice with Human Tubercle Bacilli, Strain H37

	Intraperitoneal		Intravenous	
	0.25 mg.*	0.025 mg.*	0.25 mg.*	0.025 mg.*
Number inoculated	13	8	6	8
Percentage with microscopic lesions	69	25	100	87
Percentage with macroscopic lesions in lungs	69	12	100	87
Average survival time (days)	79	120	24	59

Source: Gunn, Nungester, and Hougen (1933–1934).
* Moist weight of bacilli injected.

Gunn *et al.* did not observe in mice any differences in the gross and the microscopic lesions resulting from the inoculation of a bovine or a human strain of bacilli. A large dose of avian bacilli (1 mg.) invariably produced lesions of organs, but none of the twenty-eight mice inoculated died in the space of 46 weeks. Schwabacher and Wilson (1937) inoculated intravenously 200 million bacilli into white mice. Human and bovine strains were equally pathogenic; the survival time of the animals infected with human strains being from 25.5 to 32.3 days, and from 22.8 to 30.9 days for those infected with bovine strains. Later findings of Stamatin and Stamatin (1939) were not in agreement with these observations. They support the early findings of Trommsdorff that human and bovine strains show differences of pathogenicity in mice. The small amount of 0.001 mg. of bovine bacilli inoculated into mice produced progressive lesions.

Mouse in Experimental Tuberculosis

Glover (1944) found that mice are almost as susceptible as rabbits to infection with bovine tubercle bacilli through the respiratory route. Approximately 100 million bacilli produced infection; the chief lesions observed were in the lungs. Caseation was completely absent from the lesions. Ratcliffe (1952) kept mice for 30 minutes to 5 hours in a cloud of Ravenel or H37Rv tubercle bacilli; the animals developed lung tuberculosis in 4 to 8 weeks. Mice were found to be as susceptible to inhalation tuberculosis as guinea pigs and hamsters.

An infection may be easily performed intranasally, but it presents hazards for laboratory workers. Gray and Mattinson (1952) used the method of intranasal instillation of tubercle bacilli to produce pulmonary tuberculosis in mice and to compare the sensitivity of this way of animal infection with the sensitivity of cultivation methods. The intranasal way of inoculation created the danger of cross infection in animals (see p. 356). Pierce, Dubos, and Middlebrook (1947) tried the intracerebral route of infection. While under anesthesia, Swiss albino and dba mice were inoculated in the brain with graded amounts of bacilli in the final volume of 0.03 ml. of liquid. Even small doses of 10 to 100 bacilli multiplied in the brain within the first week but gross pulmonary lesions were detected only two or three weeks after the intracerebral inoculation. The pulmonary lesions of dba mice were more extensive than those of Swiss albino mice. Four different strains of tubercle bacilli, including H37Rv and Ravenel, were tested and no differences in their action were found. Stewart (1951) used the intracerebral way to infect mice in his study of virulence of tubercle bacilli.

Levaditi, Vaisman, and Barrat (1950) found cavities in the lungs of mice infected with tubercle bacilli.

The resistance of mice to tubercle bacilli is of a peculiar nature. Compared to the resistance of guinea pigs, it is higher to pathogenic bacilli but lower to attenuated (Branch, 1933), isoniazid-resistant (Karlson and Ikemi, 1954), and chromogenic bacilli (Lominski and Harper, 1953; Timpe and Runyon, 1954). Of the same nature is the increased sensitivity of hamsters to BCG strain.

The Tuberculin Reaction in Mice

The experimental data of recent years cast new light on the absence of tuberculin sensitivity of skin in tuberculous mice, a fact observed by earlier investigators (Römer; Fränkel and Baumann; Boquet and Nègre; B. Lange).

Hart, Long, and Rees (1952) found that intravenous injection of 1 to 2 mg. of purified tuberculin (PPD) into mice infected previously with tubercle bacilli (strain H37Rv) killed 50 per cent of the animals. In noninfected animals these doses of tuberculin were not harmful. Kirchheimer and Malkiel (1953) infected nine mice with a small amount of tubercle bacilli, of the pathogenic strain (H37Rv) and 60 days later injected into these mice 2 mg. of PPD tuberculin. All the mice died. Similar results were obtained in mice infected intraperitoneally with 10 mg. BCG. This sensitivity of tuberculous mice to tuberculin is apparently of specific nature. The cause of the insensitivity of the skin of tuberculous mice to tuberculin remains unknown. It may be connected with the lack of bactericidal activity and complement deficiencies of mouse serum (Muschel and Muto, 1956).

The Healing Process in Mouse Tuberculosis

The resistance to tuberculous infection and the process of recovery from tuberculosis of mice was investigated by E. Long (1934). According to him, the healing process can be best seen in the lungs.

Twenty-four hours after the intraperitoneal injection of 1 mg. of pathogenic tubercle bacilli, bacilli were detected in the liver and the spleen of the animals, but they were first seen in the lungs only 11 days after the infection. Large phagocytic cells filled the alveoli of the lungs. These cells were so packed with tubercle bacilli that their cytoplasm could not be seen. At a later period, 150–180 days after the infection, these cells containing bacilli had disappeared from the lungs. Pneumonic foci and necrosis of the lung tissue appeared, but caseation was seen in only one mouse. These observations on mouse tuberculosis are in agreement with the early findings of Yersin (1888) on tuberculosis of rabbits. The injected tubercle bacilli were stopped chiefly in the capillary vessels of liver and spleen. The cells, overfilled with bacilli, were floating free in the capillaries; toward the second week after the infection, almost all bacilli were found inside the cells.

Pagel (1940) investigated the tissue reaction in mice infected intracutaneously with tubercle bacilli. The destiny of tubercle bacilli injected into a rat was investigated by Wessels (1941). In the first week after the injection of 0.1 mg. of bovine bacilli, the bacilli were found in ever-increasing quantities in different organs of the rat, but as early as two weeks after the infection, the number of bacilli started to diminish in the liver of the infected animal. After two to four weeks striking differences developed between the bacilli content in the lungs and in other organs. At that time there was still an unrestrained increase of bacilli in the lungs but the decrease of bacilli took place in the liver and the spleen.

Gerstl and Thomas (1940–1941) inoculated 300 mice intraperitoneally with 1.0 to 1.5 mg. of bovine tubercle bacilli. Lesions developed in ten days and were characterized by the formation of epitheloid cell tubercles. In most animals the lesions regressed 80 days after the infection – even in the spleen, where, 20 to 30 days after the inoculation, tubercle formations had replaced most of the pulp, and the complete resolution of the lesions followed.

Pierce, Dubos, and Schaefer (1953) studied the multiplication and survival of tubercle bacilli in the organs of mice. The quantitative determination of the number of living bacilli in the tissue at different times after the infection led to the conclusion that only bacilli pathogenic to the guinea pig are capable of multiplying and of establishing infection in mice. At first, the population of tubercle bacilli in the lungs of infected mice was much lower than in the spleen, but their number began to increase continuously. The level of bacilli reached in the organs was found to be the expression of the pathogenicity of the strain.

These findings in mice infected with tubercle bacilli are in agreement with the observations we made about the fate of swine erysipelas bacilli in infected mice (1926). This atoxic septicemic microorganism, injected into mice, inundates its organs like the tubercle bacillus did in the experiments of Yersin, Long, and Wessels. The bacilli are early taken up by the endothelial and Kupfer's star cells of the liver. These cells separate from the mother substrate and float toward the lungs in the form of round, free bodies overfilled with bacilli, freeing the great parenchimatous organs from the bacilli and accumulating in the lungs. This phenomenon can be observed to best advantage when the resistance of the mice is increased through the injection of anti-infectious swine erysipelas serum. The mouse infected with pathogenic swine erysipelas bacilli dies when most bacilli seem to be eliminated from the organs. The work of Wessels (1941) demonstrates that a similar process takes place in rats infected with tubercle bacilli. Thus, because of its high phagocitary activity, the liver is the first organ where the number of bacilli rapidly declines, and the lungs are the place where they accumulate steadily, giving the impression of multiplication. The lungs are an important natural port of evacuation for undissolved intruders in the body. The bacilli are eliminated through the mouth with the secretions formed in the lungs or are swallowed and carried out with the feces.

The level of bacillary population attained in the organs of an infected animal is expressed by the difference between the bacilli originated in the organism and those eliminated from it. The breakdown of the mechanism of elimination in the lungs or the kidney may cause the increase of bacillary population in the organs and the death of the organism.

Influence of Hereditary Factors and Diet on Experimental Tuberculosis in Mice

Pierce, Dubos, and Middlebrook (1947) infected mice with 0.5 ml. of seven-day-old H37Rv culture grown in a Tween-albumin medium. Feeding and intravenous, intracerebral, and intraperitoneal inoculations were used. The extent of the pulmonary lesions and minimal lethal doses were studied in 18 different breeds of mice. These studies revealed considerable differences in the susceptibility of mice of different strains to infection with tubercle bacilli. Strains of mice were as follows in order of increasing susceptibility to tubercle bacilli: Swiss albino, Swiss albino CFW, the Rockefeller Institute strain, Chocolate, *Mus musculus domesticus* (Rockefeller Institute), C57 black, dba line 1, etc. In general, pigmented animals were found to be much more susceptible to tuberculosis than albino strains. In pigmented mice the lesions were more necrotic than in albino strains. The lesions of albino strains have a tendency to regress.

The influence of heredity on the susceptibility of mice to tuberculosis was demonstrated by Grumbach (1949b). Seven different strains of mice, five in each lot, were infected intravenously with 0.1 ml. of H37Rv strain grown in Tween-albumin medium. All but the mice of the strain Grunder died within 40 days. (See Figs. 38 and 39.) The lung volumes of the mice of strains Huber and Stark were considerably increased, the lung tissue showing total caseation. The lung volume of the mice of strain Grunder was not increased and the lung parenchyme showed few tuberculous lesions.

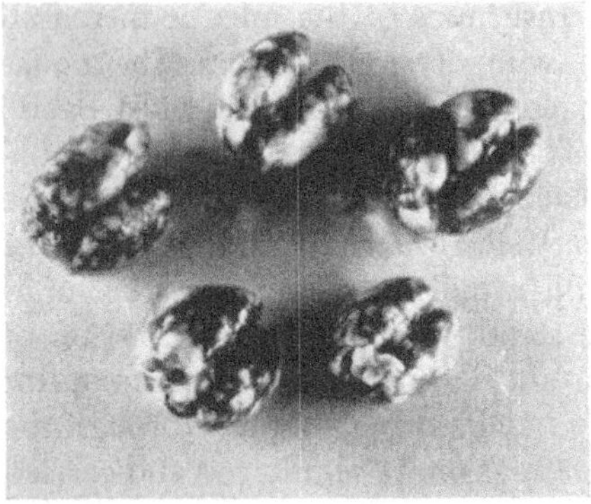

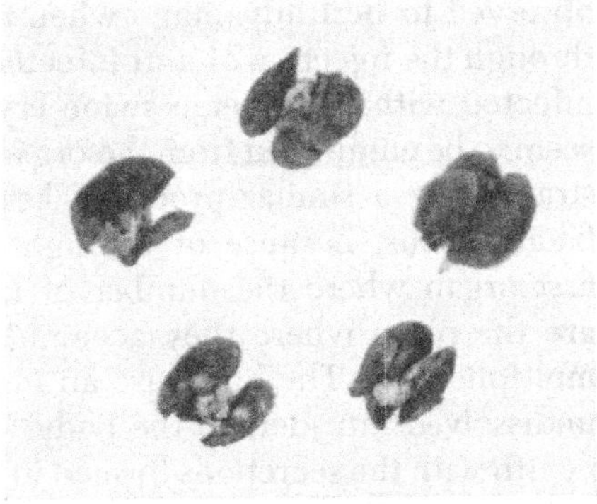

Figure 38. Spread of tuberculosis in the lungs of a mouse, strain Stark, infected intravenously with 0.1 ml. (approximately 100,000 bacilli) H37Rv bacilli (Grumbach, 1949a).

Figure 39. Spread of tuberculosis in the lungs of a mouse, strain Grunder, infected intravenously with 0.1 ml. (approximately 100,000 bacilli) H37Rv bacilli (Grumbach, 1949a).

The effect of diet on the experimental tuberculosis of mice was investigated by Dubos and Pierce (1948). The survival time of white mice infected with mammalian tubercle bacilli was markedly influenced by the food given to the animals during the experiment. A mixture of whole wheat and dried milk was most favorable to the increase of resistance to the infection; a mixture of corn flour and butter was most unfavorable. In the experiments of Hurni, Hirt, and Ragaz (1951), white mice were infected intravenously with 0.1 mg. of bacilli of human strain H37Rv and divided into two lots of 20 animals each (see Table 48). One lot was fed boiled corn and potatoes, the other lot received a complete diet consisting of a whole wheat, dried milk, yeast, and salt mixture.

Table 48. The Influence of Diet on the Experimental Tuberculosis of Mice Infected Intravenously with 0.1 mg. of Human Tubercle Bacilli, Strain H37Rv

	Corn and Potato Diet (20 Mice)	Complete Diet (20 Mice)
Necrotic lesions of organs	30%	0%
Alive after 28 days	13	17
Loss of weight	22.7%	5.9%

Source: Hurni, Hirt, and Ragaz (1951).

Hurni *et al.* also investigated the influence of the weight and age of mice on the results of experimental tuberculosis. The investigation of 308 infected and treated mice which weighed from 11 to 23 g. showed no statistically significant differences in the results obtained. (An 11 g. mouse is about 4 weeks old, a 20 g. one is 2–3 months old.) Because of this it is not necessary to divide 1–3 month old mice into strict weight groups when they are used in an experiment. Mice of either sex respond in a similar way to infection with tubercle bacilli (Donovick, McKee, Jambor, and Rake, 1949).

Grumbach (1953) found considerable differences in the survival time of mice infected intravenously with tubercle bacilli in summer and in winter. The mice infected in summer showed a considerably greater resistance to infection than those infected in winter. Milzer and Levine (1948) observed that pigmented mice inoculated intraperitoneally with 500,000 H37Rv bacilli and 5 per cent gastric mucin (type 1701-W, Wilson laboratories), developed tuberculous lesions of 2 to 3 mm. in ten days.

The Mouse in the Screening of Antituberculous Drugs

The use of mice instead of the classical guinea pig and rabbit in experiments with antituberculous agents (gold, silver compounds, dyes) was initiated by Kolle and Schlossberger (1923). Browning and Gulbransen (1926) confirmed the findings of Marmorek (1906), that one of the important advantages of mice over guinea pigs and rabbits is their low susceptibility to tuberculosis. Tubercle bacilli produce in mice protracted, chronic infection. Because of these peculiarities, the course and the appearance of mouse tuberculosis resemble human tuberculosis much more than does the galloping tuberculosis of the guinea pig. Gunn, Nungester, and Hougen (1933–1934) underlined the relative lack of susceptibility of the mouse to infection with tubercle bacilli and the value of this animal in experiments where the chronicity of the disease is desired. The rarity of spontaneous tuberculosis in the mouse and the uniform results obtained from intravenous administration of suitable doses of tubercle bacilli to them also impressed these investigators.

The mouse was used as a test animal by some early investigators of sulfonamides. Nitti and Jouin (1942) treated tuberculous mice with the compound 1162-F. The pulmonary lesions produced by the intravenous injection of tubercle bacilli were not influenced by this drug.

A further step ahead in the development of a screening procedure for therapeutic substances in the mouse was the work of Martin (1946). He found that small doses of tubercle bacilli (0.01 mg.) induce resistance to reinfection in mice, but that a dose of 1 mg. of pathogenic bacilli injected intravenously causes the death of 95 per cent of the infected animals in approximately 21 days. The rapid and uniformly fatal infection of animals may be used as the basis for the assessment of antituberculous drugs. The increase of the average survival time of sufficiently large numbers of treated animals by 1 or 2 days in comparison to that of untreated controls was found to indicate the activity of the drug.

Martin's method of evaluating the activity of antituberculous drugs by comparing the prolonged survival time of treated mice with the life span of untreated animals has been further developed in recent years.

In the series of works on the evaluation of the antituberculous activities of drugs published by various authors in the *Annals of the New York Academy of Science*, Donovick (1949) summarized the conditions under which mice can be successfully used as test animals in experiments of this sort. The results depend on the choice of (1) a suitable strain of tubercle bacilli, (2) a suitable strain of mice, (3) the right dose of infectant, and (4) the best way of infecting the animal. Donovick (1949) and Donovick, McKee, Jambor, and Rake (1949) found that only when the right strain of bacilli in an adequate dose and a suitable strain of mice are used does the death rate of mice follow a normal frequency distribution curve. Among the strains tested, the bovine Ravenel strain gave the most uniform death rate, but the size of inoculum played an important role. The strain was grown in Tween 80–albumin or Kirchner's medium with added Tween 80 and bovine serum. The cultures were diluted 1:10 and contained approximately 8×10^5 viable organisms per ml. One half ml. of the diluted culture was injected intravenously into the mice of CF1 strain. This strain of mice showed a uniform mortality rate. Under these conditions of experiment the percentage of dead animals plotted against the time gave a straight line, indicating a normal frequency distribution. The 50 per cent mortality time

(T_{50}) has been taken as endpoint in these studies. It was found that the 50 per cent mortality time of mice (T_{50}) and their average survival time coincided closely.

The use of the T_{50} value has an advantage over the use of the average survival time in that it permits the calculation of the endpoint before 100 per cent of the animals succumb, and also in that it indicates the death rate not of tuberculous origin. The infected animals were observed for 35 days but no tuberculous lesions in their organs were investigated, although the authors recognize that the data obtained from gross and microscopic examinations of animals are helpful in the evaluation of the activity of a drug.

Baker, Schlosser, and White (1949) also used the survival time of mice as the criterion to estimate the antituberculous activity of a drug. These authors started out by standardizing the components of the procedure. They recognized that the human strain H37Rv, cultivated in Tween 80–albumin medium, was unsatisfactory to produce a uniform death rate in intravenously infected mice. After nine months the bacilli cultivated in this medium have lost their pathogenicity for mice. These cultures did not reveal the "cord-formation" any more. The bovine strain D4 was chosen; 0.5 mg. of its wet weight produced acute tuberculous pneumonia in mice within two weeks and killed 100 per cent of the animals. The strain was maintained on agar–egg yolk medium. The results of the untreated control group and of the groups of mice that underwent the treatment were expressed in terms of the median survival time T_{50}.

The effect of Promizole, PAS, and streptomycin on the course of tuberculous infection in mice was studied. A significant prolongation of the life of animals treated with 300 to 3,100 mg. PAS per kg. per day was obtained. Streptomycin in doses ranging from 10 to 80 mg. was one hundred times more effective than PAS.

A considerable amount of information about the susceptibility of the mouse to tubercle bacilli has been accumulated since Koch, but ten years ago the histopathology of mouse tuberculosis was largely unknown. This lack of knowledge and the general assumption that mice are resistant to infection with tubercle bacilli prevented the wide use of mice in the screening of antituberculous substances.

The work of Youmans and McCarter (1945) and Raleigh and Youmans (1948) changed this view. Youmans and McCarter (1945) inoculated 30 white Swiss mice, weighing 25 g. intravenously with 0.1 mg. H37Rv strain. Half the animals were treated with streptomycin; the control animals remained untreated. After 28 days only 13.3 per cent of the control animals were alive, whereas 86.6 per cent of the treated mice had survived. All surviving animals were then sacrificed. It was possible to make a clear-cut differentiation of the antituberculous action of the antibiotic by examining the lungs of the animals. All control animals showed grossly recognizable tubercles in the lungs and a congestion of the organs. In the treated animals no gross lesions were observed. Microscopic examination of the lungs provided further important differentiation possibilities. In untreated animals the tubercles consisted of large areas of necrotic tissue surrounded by monocytic exudate and cells filled with large quantities of tubercle bacilli. (See Figs. 40 and 41.)

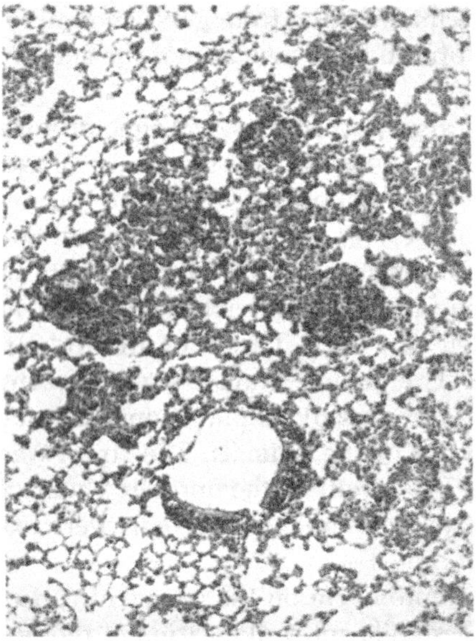

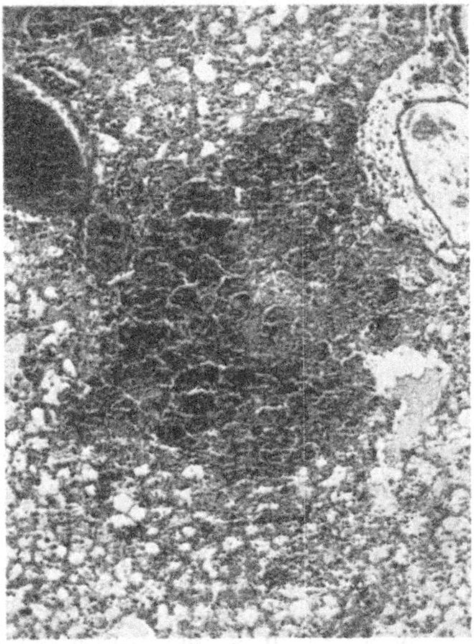

Figure 40. Proliferative pulmonary tuberculous lesions in mouse, × 75 (Youmans *et al.*, 1945).
Figure 41. Necrotic-exudative pulmonary tuberculous lesions in mouse, × 75 (Youmans *et al.*, 1945).

Raleigh and Youmans (1948) indicated that two features dominate the lung tuberculosis of mice: great enlargement of the organ with septal thickening, and extensive necrotic-exudative lesions with vascular congestion. These lesions, which develop between 14 and 21 days after the infection, swarm with tubercle bacilli. This type of lesion is found in 80 per cent of the animals that die in a short space of time. The other type of lesion, the proliferative one, is found in about 20 per cent of animals. Its main characteristic is that the lungs of the infected animals are not enlarged. Microscopically, the process is predominantly proliferative with little or no necrosis, and most alveoli are conserved intact. A few neutrophiles, a large number of foam cells, and a small number of acid-fast bacilli are found in the lesions. The other organs of mice – the liver, the spleen, and the kidneys—mostly reveal proliferative lesions. The animals with proliferative lesions survive the infection for a long time. The histopathology of mouse tuberculosis is characterized by negative findings, such as the absence of epitheloid cells, Langhans giant cells, and cavities, but by an increase in the amount of connective tissue.

Grün and Klinner (1952) described as follows the early phases of mouse tuberculosis. After tubercle bacilli have been injected into the blood stream, most of them reach the lungs and form emboli in the capillaries. As early as 30 minutes after the injection leucocytes start to surround the emboli. In the first hours after the injection, endothelium of the capillaries starts to proliferate, forming large mononuclear cells (macrophages). These cells take up most of the bacilli and separate from the walls of the blood vessels. In the form of round free cells, stuffed with tubercle bacilli, they fill up the alveolar spaces. According to Grün and Klinner, tubercle bacilli multiply in macrophages.

The observations of Grün and Klinner support our findings on the role of endothelial cells in the liberation of the organism from the septicemic intruders. The cells, overfilled with bacilli, are expelled from the lungs with sputum (see p. 345).

The whole cellular formation around the bacilli looks like a nodule in the lung parenchym. These nodules increase in size and infiltrate the adjacent alveolar spaces, forming lesions of considerable size. Contrary to Youmans and co-workers, Grün and Klinner do not admit the existence of exudative and proliferative forms of mouse tuberculosis. Both of these forms characterize human tuberculosis. The exudative processes are absent in the lungs of a tuberculous mouse.

Moeschlin, Jaccard, and Bosshard (1948) studied the results of the treatment of mouse tuberculosis with combined streptomycin, PAS, and sulfonamide. McKenzie, Malone, Kushner, Oleson, and Subbarow (1948) investigated the effect of nicotinic acid on mouse tuberculosis. Hurni, Hirt, and Ragaz (1951) used PAS and its derivatives in mouse tuberculosis. These investigations indicated that a series of 20 mice must be used for each dose of the substance studied. Each experiment should consist of 15 or 20 series, one of them involving an untreated control group.

The Russian workers Berezina and Petrova (1953) investigated the development of bronchogenic tuberculosis and the action of streptomycin on this disease in white mice. The mice were placed under ether anesthesia and infected by the intranasal route with six drops of a suspension of the bovine strain containing five million bacilli per ml. The histologic investigation of the organs revealed that the tuberculous process in the lungs started 24 hours after the infection in the form of lymphoid cell infiltration. Between the eleventh and twentieth day after the infection, caseous necrosis of the lung tissue developed. The liver and the spleen showed signs of tuberculous infection. Streptomycin (0.5 mg. during 30 days) in 40 per cent of animals infected intranasally prevented the development of lung tuberculosis.

The effect of drug action on the tuberculous process in mice can be detected by the decrease of the tuberculous involvement of the lungs and by the character of the histopathologic lesions. When only the survival time of animals is taken into account in an attempt to determine the activity of a drug, it may take four to six months till a sufficiently large number of animals die. By killing the animals earlier and by comparing their histologic lesions at different intervals, the goal may be reached within four weeks. The survival time, the weight changes, and the histopathologic lesions of the animals provide information about the activity of the substance studied, but the histopathology is of the greatest importance in the assessment. An effective drug, such as streptomycin, will prolong the survival time of the mice or prevent their death; very few or no gross lesions will be seen, although microscopic examination may reveal small proliferative foci in the lungs. A less effective substance will produce gross pulmonary lesions of the proliferative type. An ineffective compound will produce exudative-necrotic lesions similar to those of the controls. The animals will lose weight, the survival time will be short.

Stewart (1950) found that mice inoculated with 0.02 mg. human tubercle bacilli, strain 905, died in 25 to 100 days. The survival time varies considerably. Mice dying within 21 days showed necrotic lesions, whereas in those that survived for 35 days the severity of the disease was arrested. When mice were inoculated with 0.0004–0.01 mg. of the same bacilli, the survival time lengthened, the severity of the lesions decreased. In the infected mice no true tubercles were found. Thickening of the alveolar septa by congestion was observed and mononuclear infiltration formed gray nodules in the lung. No giant cells and fibroblasts were found. The number of tubercle bacilli present in the lesions was in direct relation to the progress of the infection. These findings of Stewart's were corroborated by Youmans and Youmans (1951). The survival time of mice infected with tubercle bacilli is inversely proportional to the number of bacilli inoculated.

The two methods of assessment – one, favored by Martin, Donovick, and Baker, taking into account the prolongation of the survival time of treated animals over untreated controls, and the other, favored by Marmorek and Youmans, taking into account the extension and character of the lesions of the organs (lungs) of treated and untreated animals – are different not only in procedure but also in character. The first method, by which the death of mice is caused within two weeks from large (0.5 mg.) doses of pathogenic tubercle bacilli, approaches in its idea Ehrlich's classical method of assessing diphtheria antitoxin. The other method employs small (0.1 mg.) doses of pathogenic but less virulent strains of tubercle bacilli (chiefly

H37Rv), so as to produce chronic infection and to permit the pathologic lesions in the organs to reach different degrees of development in the treated and untreated animals. The results of the assessment of a drug may differ depending upon whether the first or the second method is used.

The efficacy of the two methods of estimating the therapeutic value of antituberculous drugs was compared by the author of the first procedure, A. Martin, together with Stewart (1950). Mice were infected with 0.02 mg. of the human strain of tubercle bacilli and the activity of three antituberculous drugs—PAS, streptomycin, and thiosemicarbazone 8388—was evaluated according to the procedures of these two methods. PAS (40 mg.) was added to the food, streptomycin (1,000 units) and thiosemicarbazone (1,000 units) were injected subcutaneously. The efficacy was assessed by recording all deaths and noting the presence or absence of pathologic lesions and their character. The survival time reflected the progress of the disease, but the correlation in prolonged experiments between pathologic findings and the mortality rate was not exact. Thus, on the sixtieth day of observation, mice treated with PAS showed 67 per cent mortality, whereas mice treated with streptomycin had 5 per cent mortality, although in both cases the pathologic lesions were equally advanced. The last mouse of the PAS group died on the eighty-fourth day, while 80 per cent of the mice treated with streptomycin lived over 182 days.

The conclusion of Martin and Stewart is that these findings support the view of Youmans and co-workers that exact information on the action of an antituberculous drug in murine tuberculosis can be obtained by the histopathologic examination of the organs. The prolonged survival time of mice in comparison with that of control animals indicates that a substance is an active antituberculous agent, but it does not reveal the degree of the activity of the drug. This activity is indicated by the nature and extension of pathologic lesions in the organs, mainly the lungs.

Grumbach (1952) investigated the location and extension of lesions in a genetically pure C3H carcinoma strain of mice infected intravenously with five million bacilli of the H37Rv strain. The deaths of 26 mice reared under identical conditions were not uniform, occurring between the second and the eleventh week, but the extension of the lesions was quite uniform and independent of the survival time of the animals. When the dose of the H37Rv strain reached 7.8 mg. (wet weight) the mice died immediately. These findings permitted Youmans and Youmans (1951) to calculate the generation time of tubercle bacilli (see p. 93) in mice as being 4.6 days, compared to 14 hours in a liquid medium.

Siebenmann (1951) expressed the opinion that there exists a close correlation between the numbers of tubercle bacilli in the lesions of the organs of mice and the advance of the disease. Because of this the results of a simple counting of tubercle bacilli in the organs may be used to determine the antituberculous activity of a substance. The quantity of bacilli found in the tissue of mice was taken into consideration to evaluate the antituberculous activity of drugs by Stewart (1950), but he recognized that the quantity of bacilli in the lesion may be taken into account only together with the extension and character of the lesions themselves. He recognized, like Browning and Gulbransen (1926), that the death of animals and the amount of bacilli found in their tissue are not always parallel phenomena.

Mass feeding of a drug may be of some use in estimating the drug's toxicity and in obtaining a general impression of its action. The weight differences of the uneaten food between the beginning and the end of the experiment permit the approximate estimation of the drug intake by the whole population of mice, but do not allow one to draw any conclusions about the action of the drug on each animal. To make possible such conclusions, the mice must be housed in individual cages, or the drug must be dissolved in a liquid and introduced into the esophagus by means of a blunt syringe.

As was pointed out by Donovick (1949), consideration must be given to the problem of whether or not a substance to be tested will pass through the blood-brain barrier following its administration to the animal. In most cases such information would not be available and the intracerebral route of infection of mice may lead to errors in the assessment of the chemotherapeutic value of a drug.

The findings about the role of mice in the screening of antituberculous drugs can be summarized as follows. The mice react uniformly to tubercle bacilli administered through the intravenous route and through this pathway of infection a great number of bacilli reach the lungs. Specific lesions develop in the lungs of mice in four weeks. To test a drug in mice, only a small quantity is needed. A statistically significant number of infected mice can easily be provided for every test. Natural tuberculous infection is exceptionally rare in mice. These qualities make the mouse the ideal animal for testing the antituberculous value of a drug. A drug which has an antituberculous action in mice promises to be effective in human tuberculosis.

Cornea of Mouse in the Study of Experimental Tuberculosis

The procedure for screening antituberculous substances in the cornea of the rabbit developed by Robson (1944) and Gardiner, Rees, and Robson (1949) (see p. 336) was tried out on mice by Rees and Robson (1950).

Albino mice, 18–25 g. in weight, were used in the experiments. The bovine strain of tubercle bacilli, the same as was used for the inoculation of the rabbit's eye, was employed to infect the corneas of mice. A dose of 1,000 tubercle bacilli was found to be the minimum necessary to produce consistent tuberculous lesions in the corneas of mice. To produce tuberculous infection in all the mice inoculated a considerably larger dose of bacilli was required than in experiments with the cornea of rabbits.

The injection, as in experiments with the corneas of rabbits, was made with a fine needle and a tuberculin syringe. Deep anesthesia of the animal is needed; however, it was found that ether anesthesia alone produces high mortality rate. Because of this, the mice were given, by means of a stomach tube, ¼ hour before the infection, 0.4 g. per kg. body weight, a 6 per cent suspension of α-bromoisovalerylurea in gum acacia with an ensuing short exposure to ether. By means of fine eye forceps, the eye was fixed, and the needle of the syringe was introduced with a rotating movement into the periphery of the cornea. Using a point source of light and a lens placed between the mouse and the operator, it was possible to inoculate some forty animals in about two hours. The amount of liquid injected was estimated to be approximately 0.01 ml.

In twelve days, the primary lesions appeared as minute gray nodules. Their size increased rapidly, and by the thirtieth day the lesions were caseous in appearance and pannus had developed. Hypopyon was seen sometimes, but, in contrast to corneal infections in the rabbit, ulcerations of the lesions were rare. After the thirtieth day of infection, the regression and healing of the lesions started.

The incubation period, the time needed for the lesions to appear, and the progression of the lesions in the cornea of a mouse, is a uniform process when a reliable technique of inoculation is used. These phenomena – the duration of the incubation period and the subsequent development of lesions – can be used for the assessment of antituberculous substances in the corneas of mice.

Rees and Robson studied the action of streptomycin and of sodium *para*-aminosalicylate on the tuberculous corneal lesions of mice.

In another series of experiments, the feeding of 5 g/kg of *para*-aminosalicylate to the mice was started 24 hours before the infection. All 10 control animals developed corneal infection between the eleventh and seventeenth day, while 10 out of the 12 treated animals developed lesions between the twenty-fifth and the thirty-second day. The remaining 2 animals were free from lesions after 105 days of observation.

The regression of the lesions in the untreated mouse cornea is a natural phenomenon of healing and must be taken into consideration when the test of the drug is made in a cornea infected 30 days earlier.

Keeping Infected Mice

Kirchheimer, Hess, Williston, and Youmans (1950) found pathogenic tubercle bacilli in feces collected in the course of one day from mice infected intravenously 14, 21, and 26 days previously with 0.2–0.05 mg. of H37Rv and Ravenel strains of tubercle bacilli. Bacilli were also detected in the gastric washings of these mice (see p. 177). Direct microscopic examination revealed the presence of tubercle bacilli in the blood and urine of infected mice (Grün and Klinner, 1952). Thus, tuberculous mice may be the source of tuberculosis infection in laboratory workers.

Mice can be infected with tuberculosis when exposed to tuberculous animals, as shown in Table 49.

Table 49. Tuberculous Infection in Healthy C57 and Albino Strains of Mice Exposed to Tuberculous Guinea Pigs and Mice

Animal and Nature of Exposure	Duration of Contact	No. Exposed	No. Infected	Degree of Lesions
Guinea pig				
Ulcerated lesions following subcutaneous inoculation with sputum from tuberculous patient........	4 weeks	5	3	+++
Guinea pig				
Closed lesions following intramuscular inoculation with tubercle bacilli	4 weeks	5	1	+
Mouse C57				
1,400 H37Rv bacilli intranasally..	2 weeks	5	1	+++
Albino mouse				
1,400 H37Rv bacilli intranasally..	2 weeks	5	1	++

Source: Gray and Mattinson (1952), abbreviated.

Grün and Klinner (1952) arrived at results different from those cited above. A large number of tubercle bacilli were seen in the urine of tuberculous mice by direct microscopy. Ten pairs of mice, one of each pair healthy, the other tuberculous, were kept together until the death of the infected animal. Some months later the noninfected animals were killed and none of them showed tuberculous lesions.

Römer (1903) injected tubercle bacilli into jugular veins of mice. At present, a more simple tail injection technique is in use. Kassel and Levitan (1953) devised a technique for repeated drawing of blood samples from the external jugular veins of mice. The mouse is firmly held by the loose skin of the neck between the thumb and index finger of the left hand, so that the neck and the thorax of the animal are well exposed. To fix the animal's head in its hyperextension, a gauze ribbon is put into its mouth and held across the back of the hand. After depilation, both jugulars can be easily located. The syringe and the needle (26 gauge) are wetted with an anticoagulant. The needle is introduced into the vein 1–2 mm. lateral to the sternoclavicular junction, and blood is withdrawn slowly in order to prevent the collapse of the vein.*

* For additional information on the mouse in experimental biology see the staff of the Roscoe B. Jackson Memorial Laboratory, *Biology of the laboratory mouse* (Dover, N.Y., 1956). U.S.A.

XXVIII

The Hamster in Experimental Tuberculosis

ONE of the many different animals infected with tubercle bacilli by Koch (1882) was the hamster. It was probably the European *Cricetus cricetus.*

The striped hamster, *Cricetus griseus* Thomas and Milne Edwards, is a small rodent, weighing about 30 g. It is abundant in China and was first used in experiments with tubercle bacilli by Korns and Lu (1927) of the Peking Union Medical College. These investigators inoculated the striped hamster, as well as white mice and guinea pigs, with tubercle bacilli of human, bovine, and avian types. The hamsters and mice were injected subcutaneously with 0.1 mg., the guinea pigs with 1.0 mg. of tubercle bacilli. (The guinea pigs weighed ten times more than the hamsters and the dose of bacilli inoculated into the guinea pigs was ten times stronger.) It was possible to make the diagnosis of tuberculosis in the hamsters six weeks after the inoculation; the majority of mice showed at that time only slight signs of infection. The lesions in hamsters were not so extensive as in guinea pigs; they were localized chiefly in the lungs, their tendencies to caseate being less pronounced than in guinea pigs. Tubercle bacilli were more abundant in the lungs, tracheo-bronchial lymph nodes, and spleens of hamsters than in the same organs of guinea pigs.

In their later work Korns and Lu (1928) inoculated striped hamsters with pathologic material (sputum, exudates, pus) from patients for the purpose of diagnosing tuberculosis. Microscopic examination revealed that the lesions in hamsters were almost wholly proliferative. Little caseation and only slight tendencies to giant cell formation were seen in the lesions which, however, contained an abundance of tubercle bacilli. This feature of the lesions made the diagnosis of tuberculosis in hamsters easier than in guinea pigs.

Rapid multiplication of tubercle bacilli in the Chinese hamster, especially when kaolin was added to the inoculum, was observed by T' ung and Wong (1940).

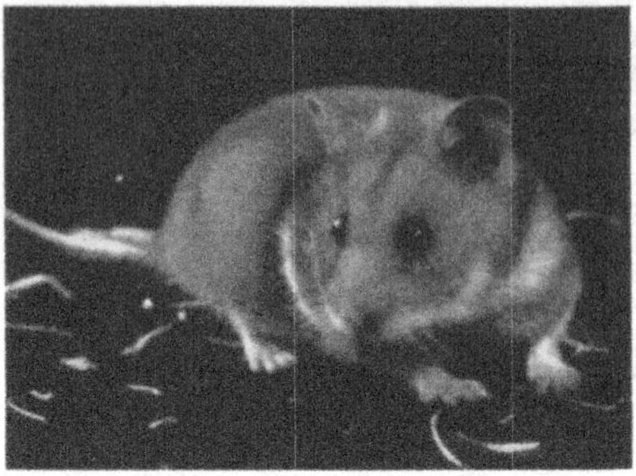

Figure 42. The golden hamster (Rolle, 1954).

The Syrian or golden hamster, *Cricetus* or *Mesocricetus auratus* Waterhouse, is probably a variant of the Chinese hamster. Balfour-Jones (1937) found the golden hamster susceptible to infection with acid-fast bacilli cultivated from the leprosy lesions of a wild rat. Griffith (1939, 1941) produced additional information about the susceptibility of the golden hamster to acid-fast bacilli. In his experiments six hamsters were inoculated subcutaneously with 1.0 mg. of bovine, 1–2 mg. of human, and 5 mg. of avian variants of tubercle bacill. All types gave rise to generalized progressive tuberculosis. The bovine type of bacilli caused the most extensive lesions. In his work of 1941, published posthumously, Griffith says that it is possible to infect the hamster with tubercle bacilli by feeding. Ungar (1942) described the tuberculous lesions of the hamster as similar to those of the guinea pig. Tubercle bacilli of human type (0.001 mg.) produced in 16–20 days post-mortem findings visible to the naked eye, consisting of enlarged lymph nodes and miliary eruptions in liver, kidney, and lungs.

Corper and Cohn (1944) compared the degree of susceptibility to tubercle bacilli of the golden hamster and the guinea pig. The animals were inoculated with graded amounts of tubercle bacilli.

The susceptibility to tubercle bacilli was found by gross examination to be much greater in the guinea pig than in the golden hamster, as shown in Table 50.

Glover (1946) inoculated guinea pigs and hamsters subcutaneously with serial dilutions from 10^{-4} to 10^{-8} mg. of bovine bacilli, 0.001 mg. of which had made rabbits tuberculous in the space of 45 days. The inoculated animals were all dead 180 days after the infection. The histopathologic examination showed that the golden hamster is as susceptible to tubercle bacilli of bovine type as the guinea pig. For the hamster the minimal infective dose of the bovine strain was 10^{-7} mg.; of the human strain, 10^{-6} mg. The caseous lesions were not common in them, however. Proliferative adenitis with lesions containing a large amount of bacilli was seen constantly. Giroux (1947) inoculated hamsters weighing 110–120 g. with 0.1–

0.5 mg. of tubercle bacilli of human and bovine types, and found that the hamster is less susceptible to tubercle bacilli than the guinea pig. The infected hamsters remained alive for four months.

Hussel (1950) inoculated subcutaneously 16 hamsters and 16 guinea pigs with a feebly virulent bovine strain of tubercle bacilli. The inoculated guinea pigs gave good positive tuberculin reaction on the eleventh day; in hamsters the reaction was positive on the twenty-fourth day. In 12 of the hamsters the tuberculosis diagnosis was positive thirty days after the infection, all guinea pigs showing at that time gross tuberculous lesions. Hussel concludes that the guinea pig is superior to the hamster for diagnosis of tuberculosis.

Table 50. Results of Subcutaneous Inoculation with Graded Amounts of Virulent Human Tubercle Bacilli (H37Rv) into Guinea Pigs and Golden Hamsters (Gross Examination)

Tubercle Bacilli Inoculated	Days after Infection	Tuberculosis Involvement *	
		Guinea Pigs	Hamsters
1.0 mg.	39	4	0
	57	4	1
	57	4	1
0.001	39	2	0
	57	3	0
	57	2	0
0.000001	57	1	0
	57	2	0
	57	2	0

Source: Corper and Cohn (1944).
* 0 = none, 4 = massive.

Reuss (1951), in the Institute of Professor K. Wagener at Hanover, carried out a comparative study of the adequacy of the hamster and of the guinea pig for the routine laboratory diagnosis of tuberculosis. Specimens of milk, tracheal contents of cows, and gastric washings of children were divided and inoculated subcutaneously into hamsters and guinea pigs. The palpation of the lymph glands, enlargement of which is an early sign of infection, was impossible in the hamster, because the glands are embedded in fatty tissue. The surviving animals were killed six weeks after the inoculation of the material. It was possible to compare the inoculation results of 253 specimens, as shown in Table 51.

The susceptibility of the golden hamster to tubercle bacilli in pathologic material was much less than that of the guinea pig. The mortality rate of hamsters from diseases other than tuberculosis was 31.7 per cent, that of guinea pigs 34.4 per cent. Moreover, the hamster can sometimes be aggres-

Table 51. The Results of Routine Tuberculosis Diagnosis in Guinea Pigs and Hamsters

Specimens	Number	Tubercle Bacilli Positive in Guinea Pigs No.	%	Tubercle Bacilli Positive in Hamsters No.	%
Market milk....................	104	6	5.7	3	2.8
Milk from individual cows......	92	13	13.9	10	10.9
Tracheal contents (cows)........	36	22	61.1	6	18.2
Gastric washings (children)......	21	8	38.0	3	14.3
Total	253	49		22	

Source: Reuss (1951).

sive. These reasons forced the Institute to give up the use of the hamster for routine diagnosis of tuberculosis. These findings were confirmed by Starck and Viehmann (1955).

Eicke (1952) injected tubercle bacilli into hamsters and guinea pigs and found that the Mantoux reaction was always negative in hamsters and that the palpation of their lymph nodes was not possible. The animals showed very few gross lesions of organs or none at all. Only a microscopic examination of the organs revealed tuberculous infection. It was concluded that the hamster has no advantage over the guinea pig in tuberculosis diagnosis. Rudat (1953) arrived at identical conclusions.

Through the addition of mucin to the injected tubercle bacilli the rapidity of development and the size of the lesions in the hamster were increased (Keil, Botta, and Stephan, 1953).

Rolle (1949) observed that tuberculin injected into tuberculous cattle produced in 14–24 hours an increase in polymorphonuclear leucocytes. This reaction was negative in animals not infected.

To investigate the practical value of polymorphonuclear reaction, Rolle and Wochinger (1951) inoculated hamsters with material of possible tuberculous origin but microscopically negative for tubercle bacilli. Tuberculin was injected into the hamsters four weeks after the inoculation of the material. When the reaction was negative, the injection of tuberculin was repeated in eight weeks. At that time the animals were sacrificed and a post-mortem examination was performed (see Table 52). The authors conclude that in the golden hamster the polymorphonuclear reaction is in agreement with the results of the post-mortem examination and that this reaction can be applied to secure the early diagnosis of tuberculosis.

Hauduroy and Rosset (1951) infected hamsters subcutaneously with BCG bacilli (the dosage was not specified) and found that the animals died one year after the infection. The lesions of the livers, spleens, and lungs of these animals contained epitheloid and giant cells but the nodules were not of classical structure. These investigators state that the golden hamster has a specific susceptibility to BCG, which is capable of provoking tuberculous lesions in these animals.

The findings of Hauduroy and Rosset were tested by van Deinse and Sénéchal (1954). When 50 mg. of living or dead BCG bacilli were inoculated intraperitoneally into hamsters, the animals died at the same time and with the same symptoms according to van Deinse and Sénéchal. The death was not caused by the pathogenicity of the BCG strain but by the high sensitivity of the hamster to tuberculin.

Giroux (1947) indicated that the golden hamsters attain sexual maturity in 36 days and that the gestation period of the guinea pig lasts for 75 days, that of the hamster for 16 days. Two-month-old animals are about 15 cm. long and weigh about 125 g. and may be used for the purpose of breeding. An experiment revealed that hamsters in Canada are in partial hibernation from October until April, although kept in a room at 17°–18°C. During the hibernation period there was no reproduction. This influenced unfavorably the final count in their fertility.

Table 52. Polymorphonuclear Reaction to Injection of 0.1 ml. of Tuberculin into Golden Hamsters Previously Inoculated with Material of Possible Tubercular Origin

Material and Length of Infection	Number of Polymorphonuclears Present		Results of Post-Mortem Examination
	Before Injection	After Injection	
Milk sediment			Positive
4 weeks	20	24	
8 weeks	24	76	
Milk sediment			Positive
4 weeks	30	32	
8 weeks	22	63	
Pus			Positive
4 weeks	26	72	
Milk sediment			Negative
4 weeks	21	33	
8 weeks	36	40	

Source: Rolle and Wochinger (1951).

Bürki (1951) found that the hamster can be infected with the anthrax, *Salmonella*, and *Brucella* bacilli, but that it does not have veins easily accessible to intravenous inoculation. According to Bürki, the heart puncture is hazardous in the hamster.

Tuberculosis infection spreads as easily in a hamster colony as in a mouse colony. Chute, Kenton, and Sommers (1954), reported a case which took place in a cancer research laboratory where 200 golden hamsters were kept in 48 open-wire-type cages. Four of these animals were inoculated in the cheek pouch with prostate tissue taken from a suspected cancer patient. The food holders and water bottles of the healthy and the inoculated animals were not kept apart. Within four months the inoculated animals died and a tuberculosis epidemic swept through the animal colony. The colony was destroyed; 70 animals were autopsied and in 35 of them culture and animal inoculation revealed tuberculosis caused by the human type of bacilli. The infected animals developed heavy amyloidosis of the kidneys.

XXIX

Chorioallantoic Membrane and Chick Embryo in Experimental Tuberculosis

SINCE it has been demonstrated that membranes of chick embryo are susceptible to infection with microorganisms, the developing egg has been much used in the studies of bacteriologic, chemotherapeutic, and histologic problems. (See Fig. 43.)

The most outstanding feature of this method is the use of living developing embryonic tissue as the medium of culture. A large number of organisms which can be brought to development only in a living organism or in tissue culture, multiply readily in a developing chick embryo.

Like every great discovery, the chick embryo method opened wide possibilities for research. It rendered unrivaled service to the cultivation of viruses, which for their growth require the presence of living tissue, and provided a means of realizing the preparation of typhus, influenza, rabies, and other vaccines. The chick embryo method also made possible the study of pathologic lesions which were known only in living beings.

Only fresh and fertilized eggs, not more than ten days old, should be used for the chorioallantoic membrane experiments. The temperature of incubation of the eggs should be kept between 37.5° and 38°C., the humidity must be at 50 to 70 per cent. The eggs should be turned twice daily.

As the incubation proceeds, it is necessary to know whether the embryo has developed, to know if it is alive, and to determine its position inside the shell, as well as to know the extent of the development of the chorioallantoic membrane, the origin of the allantoic vein, and the location of the air space. This information can be obtained by transillumination of the egg.

The Embryo and Its Membrane

The chorioallantoic membrane is the respiratory organ of the embryo; it is richly supplied with blood vessels and capillaries. The air penetrates

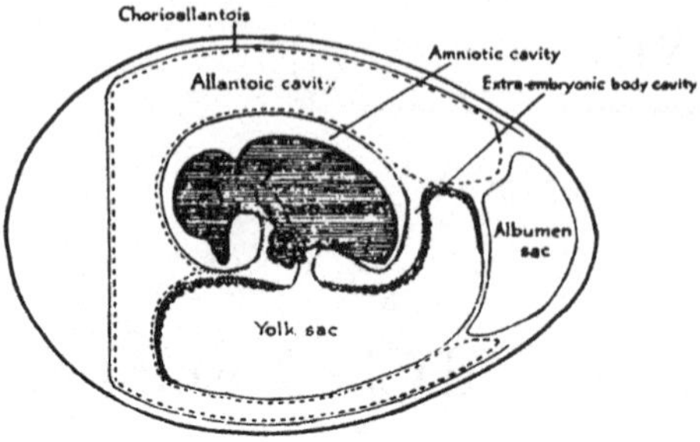

Figure 43. Membranes and cavities in 12-to-15-day-old chick embryo (Beveridge and Burnet, 1946).

through the shell. The main arteries come from the yolk stalk to the membrane. The large allantoic vein (Fig. 44) is easily recognizable when the egg is transilluminated by its source at the junction of the two chorioallantoic veins. (The junction of these veins may be used as a fixed point to recognize the position of the embryo inside the shell.) Chorioallantoic membranes show a wide range of variations in the arrangement of their blood vessels.

The chorioallantoic membrane on the side adjacent to the shell is covered with a layer of epithelial cells. This is the ectodermal layer of the embryo.

Beneath the ectoderm there is a relatively wide mesodermal layer which is a network or loose syncytium of polygonal or spindle-shaped cells embedded in a homogeneous intercellular substance. The mesoderm is interwoven with blood vessels and capillaries connected with those of the ectoderm. The subsurface of the mesoderm is covered with a flattened layer of cells resembling those of the ectoderm. This is the third cell layer of the chorioallantoic membrane, the entoderm. (See Fig. 45.)

The allantois originates from the body of the embryo; it is a reservoir of body excretions. The yolk sac contains the yolk. Starting with the twelfth day of incubation the egg yolk progressively becomes thicker. On the sixteenth to eighteenth day of embryonic life the lungs of the embryo take over respiration. At that time the chorioallantoic membrane dries out and loses its respiratory function.

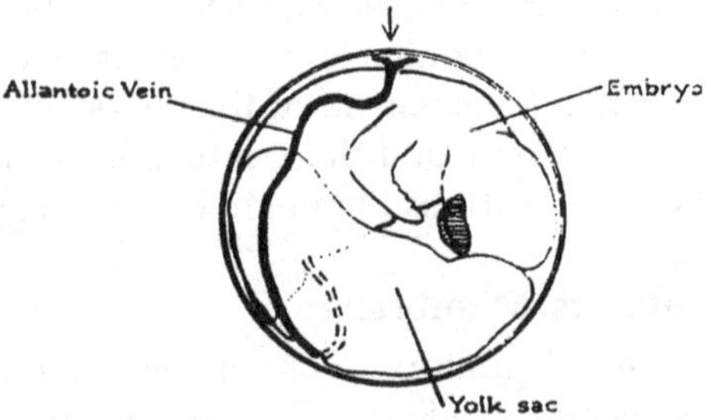

Figure 44. The origin of the allantoic vein as seen from the air sac end of the egg (Beveridge and Burnet, 1946).

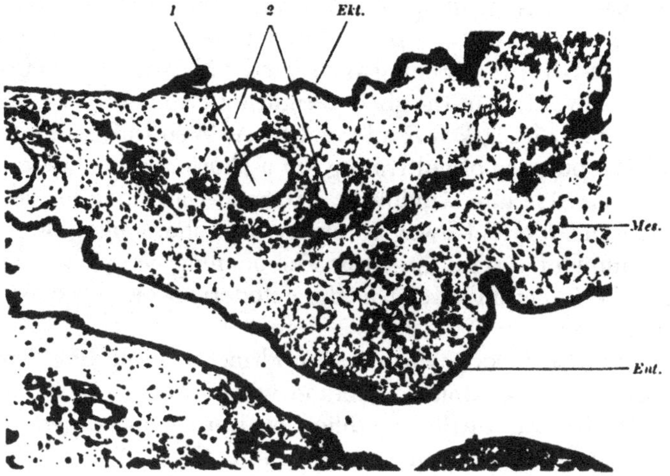

Figure 45. Section of 15-day-old chorioallantoic membrane. Ekt.: ectoderm. Mes.: mesoderm. Ent.: entoderm. 1. Artery. 2. Vein. (Schürmann, 1952.)

Inoculation

Levaditi (1906) says that Borrel in 1905 successfully infected chick embryos with chick spirilles discovered in Brazil by Marchoux and Salimbeni. Injecting into a developing egg the blood of a chick infected with the spirilles, Borrel obtained a highly infected chicken.

Levaditi (1906) confirmed the findings of Borrel with the statement that the spirilles remained alive and multiplied only in the developing egg when the embryo was formed. All attempts to bring the spirilles to development in the nondeveloping egg were unsuccessful. The presence of living cellular elements was essential to the cultivation of the spirilles in the egg.

Rous and Murphy (1911) pointed out the similarity between the neoplastic cells and the cells of embryonic tissue and observed that the study of these cells might shed new light on the problems of malignant growth. These authors studied the development of sarcoma in the chick embryo infected with a transmissible agent of avian sarcoma.

Levaditi and Rous introduced the inoculum into the embryo by piercing the membrane with a needle or a capillary pipette. By this procedure the inoculum was frequently accidentally introduced into parts of the embryo unsuitable for the growth of the inoculated organism. Consequently the pathologic changes could not develop, and the procedure damaged the embryo severely, often causing its premature death.

A method of operating on the desired parts of the chick embryo, so as to make possible the study of problems of experimental embryology, was developed by E. Clark (1920) at the department of anatomy at the University of Missouri. A small opening was made in the shell of an incubated egg by means of a needle or a knife. After the operation, a piece of flamed mica was placed over the opening and sealed with wax. The incubation was continued, the window in the shell permitting observation of the embryo.

The technique of Clark was adopted by A. Woodruff and Goodpasture (1931), for the purpose of cultivating, on a chorioallantoic membrane, the fowl-pox virus. A square window 7 $\times$ 10 mm. was made in the shell; the shell membrane was cut away to expose the chorioallantoic membrane, which was implanted with the virus. The opening was closed with a glass coverslip. The infection spread in the ectodermal and entodermal layers of the membrane.

In the same year Goodpasture, A. Woodruff, and Buddingh successfully infected the chorioallantoic membrane with vaccine virus. The original method of Clark was further modified by Burnet and others. A dentist's drill was generally used as a means of opening the shell.

Goodpasture (1933) indicated that chick embryo tissue might be of use in the study of human bacterial infections. Gallavan (1937) reproduced encephalitis and meningitis in chick embryos following the inoculation of chorioallantoic membranes with *Haemophilus influenzae*; Goodpasture and Anderson (1937) infected the chick embryo with cultures of streptococci, *Salmonella*, and *Brucella*. Morrow, Syverton, Stiles, and Berry (1938) successfully cultivated *Leptospira icterohaemorrhagiae* in the chorioallantoic membrane. The organism regularly invaded the embryo, killing the embryos in six or seven days. Human fungus infections were studied in chorioallantoic membrane (Moore, 1941); Cromartie (1941) used the chorioallantois to investigate the problems of active and passive immunity to diphtheria. The method was successfully applied to investigations of tuberculosis bacteriology, in studies of the action of antituberculous drugs, and in the histology of tuberculous lesions.

The actual technique of inoculation of the membrane permits the infection of separate germinal layers or tissue of the embryo to accommodate the growth of dermotropic viruses (vaccine) on the ectoderm, the neurotropic ones (rabies) in the nerve tissue, and rickettsiae in the yolk sac.

Intravenous Infection

The intravenous infection of the embryo was first practiced by Polk, Buddingh, and Goodpasture (1938), who demonstrated the presence of a hemolytic amboceptor in the extraembryonic fluids of a chick embryo over a period of six days following intravenous injection. To carry out the intravenous infection, the course of a large allantoic vein must be located by transilluminating of the egg. An area of about one square centimeter is marked on the shell over the vein and the shell is opened at that spot. The injection into the vein may be made with a 27-gauge needle mounted on a tuberculin syringe. The direction of the injected liquid must coincide with that of the blood flow in the vessel.

Eichhorn (1940) indicated that 10-to-11-day old embryos are the youngest in which one can carry out satisfactory intravenous injections. If a faulty technique is employed, the death rate of embryos from hemorrhage of a punctured vein may reach 30 per cent.

H. Lee, Stavitsky, and Lee (1946) introduced a technique of inoculation by exposing large areas of the incubated egg to full visibility. The shell over the margin of the air space was cut away and the chorioallantoic membrane under the air space was exposed, making possible injections into the vein, the amniotic fluid, the allantoic fluid, the yolk sac, or into the chorioallantoic membrane. Blood samples or extra-embryonic liquids may be collected.

The possibility of intracerebral infection of embryos was indicated by Buddingh and Polk (1939). These investigators performed intracranial infection on 14–16-day-old embryos with 0.025 ml. of meningococci culture. The infection was mostly localized within the meninges, cranial sinuses, and cerebrospinal fluid of the embryos. J. Dawson (1941) used the intracerebral inoculation method to develop the chick-embryo-adapted rabies virus.

H. Lee *et al.* found that chick embryos have considerable resistance to outside contamination, and work with them is possible in an open room without special measures of protection against contamination.

Advantages and Limitations of the Chorioallantoic Method

Advantages. According to Burnet (1936), Beveridge and Burnet (1946), Schürmann (1952) and others, the advantages of the chick embryo method may be summarized as follows: (1) the tissues of the developing embryo are a sterile living culture medium; (2) the developing embryo in the egg is protected from outside influences and is an organism largely independent of the outer world; (3) the developing embryo has not been in touch with the infectious agents, and its reaction to the infection is virginal; (4) the embryo is incapable of producing antibodies – the complement is absent from the serum of an embryo (this fact may be of value to serological studies); (5) the mesoderm of a developing chorioallantoic membrane is an undifferentiated tissue of high reactivity; (6) physiologic and pathologic processes in the membrane, as in the embryo itself, proceed at a high speed and their course and final stage may be easily and repeatedly observed in a considerably shorter time than in an inoculated animal; (7) the pathogenic organisms introduced into an embryo cannot be excreted; it is possible to study the quantitative side of the problem; (8) the eggs are inexpensive; the methods of infection and incubation are not difficult.

M. Moore (1942), pointed out the scientific value of inoculating the chorioallantoic membrane of a developing chick with mycobacteria. The procedure, said Moore, permits a day-by-day or even hour-by-hour examination of the evolution of the lesions and tracing of the origin of various types of cells or tissues involved in the formation of the lesions, as well as following the fate and the morphologic changes of the inoculated organism.

Limitations. The authors cite the following limitations: (1) the necessity of using bacteriologically pure material for inoculation purposes; (2) the early death of the embryos; (3) the necessity of determining in some cases the optimal age of the embryos to be inoculated, the optimal temperature of the incubation, etc.; (4) the difficulty of separating the specific lesions from the nonspecific irritative ones; (5) although the embryonated egg method is an *in vivo* procedure, the course of infection and the formation of lesions in it are rapid, the time of observation is short – approximately ten days – and the environment so specific (avian embryo) that the interpretation of the observed phenomena is often difficult, if at all possible. This must be especially emphasized in the cases of infection of embryonated egg with mammalian tubercle bacilli.

Tuberculosis of the Chorioallantoic Membrane

Cadiot, Gilbert, and Roger (1891) succeeded in infecting chickens with human tubercle bacilli only occasionally. Chickens are extremely resistant to the organisms of human and bovine tuberculosis. The intracerebral inoculation of tubercle bacilli produced localized tuberculous lesions in the chick (Feldman, 1934).

The response of the chorioallantoic membrane of the chick embryo to the inoculated tubercle bacilli is different from that of the chick. It is possible to infect the chorioallantoic membrane of the chick embryo with tubercle bacilli of avian type, but even more easily and profoundly with tubercle bacilli of human and bovine types. There is no explanation for the different susceptibility of a fowl and its embryo to tubercle bacilli.

The credit for first having used the developing chick embryo to study tuberculosis is due to Maffucci (1889). In his experiments, from a total of 18 eggs inoculated with the culture of an avian strain of tubercle bacilli, 8 chickens were hatched. One of them lived for 78 days, another for 4½ months. All of them died from heavy tuberculous infection of the lung, the liver, and the spleen. These organs showed widely spread caseation necrosis and contained an abundance of tubercle bacilli.

As was first shown by Goodpasture and Anderson (1937), the six-to-eight-day-old chorioallantoic membrane of a chick can be infected with tubercle bacilli of avian type, but six-day-old embryos, when infected, do not survive for more than four days. The infected membranes did not show gross lesions at 24 hours, but 48 hours after the infection they appeared thickened and gelatinous. At that time an increase in polymorphonuclear leucocytes and mononuclear cells was noted, probably followed by the formation of giant cells. The lesions were localized more within than on the membranes. The bacilli easily invaded the mesoderm of the membrane, and multiple foci, composed of mononuclear cells and fibroblasts, were found there.

In the experiments of Goodpasture and Anderson three chicks hatched from the infected eggs. Contrary to the early findings of Maffucci, tubercle bacilli were not found in the peritoneal fluids, the liver, nor in the spleen of the chicks.

Since the publications of Goodpasture and his co-workers, the membranes of developing chick embryo have been widely used in tuberculosis research.

Costil and Bloch (1938) studied the behavior of ten-day-old chorioallantoic membranes implanted with $^{1}/_{10}$ mg. of tubercle bacilli of human type (two strains) and of avian type (three strains). The infected eggs were incubated at 39.5°C. and opened between the third and tenth day after infection. In the case of the human strains edema appeared in the infected membranes but regressed on the fifth day and the membranes desiccated progressively. Starting with the seventh day, some white nodules appeared on the membranes and on the tenth day of infection the dry membranes were covered with nodules of different sizes, some of them the size of a pinhead. The avian strains in the first seven days of infection produced the same changes in the membranes as bacilli of human type. At the end of the incubation no gross tuberculous lesions were seen in the membranes infected with the bacilli of avian type.

Emmart and Smith (1941) investigated the changes which occur in the chorioallantoic membranes of the chick embryo after they have been implanted with tubercle bacilli. Three human and one bovine strains were used in their work. The incidence of tubercle formation on the membranes differed greatly with each individual strain. With the feebly virulent Saranac strain H37 only 13 per cent of the membranes gave signs of tubercles; with the Phipp's Institute H37 strain 75 per cent were infected; and with the most virulent strain of all, A27, 100 per cent of the membranes were infected. In the case of the virulent A27 strain, out of 32 embryos inoculated with 1 mg. of tubercle bacilli each, only 8 embryos survived for six days. In this case all membranes contained a great number of tubercles one to four mm. in diameter. The epithelial proliferation was extensive; the cell aggregates in the mesoderm were numerous. The tubercles showed caseation necrosis.

The bovine Ravenel strain of tubercle bacilli, which, in a dose of 0.015 mg., kills a rabbit in 30 to 50 days if injected intravenously, showed a lower incidence of tubercle formation than was expected when implanted on a choriallantoic membrane. Mesodermal proliferation and epitheloid cells were present but caseation necrosis was absent.

The implantation of dead tubercle bacilli on the membranes produced neither gross nor microscopic tubercle formation, although some cellular proliferation in the mesoderm and epitheloid cell aggregates was observed.

The membranes implanted with 2.0 mg. of purified tuberculin (PPD) were characterized by thickening and distinct proliferation of the epithelial layer, moderate proliferation of the mesoderm, and the appearance of epitheloid cells. The reaction of the membranes to tuberculin was slightly more extensive than their reaction to the implantation of heat-killed tubercle bacilli.

In their next work, Emmart and Smith (1943) compared the action of the pathogenic H37Rv strain (Fig. 46) and the H37Ra strain of reduced pathogenicity on the chorioallantoic membrane. In 96 per cent of the membranes inoculated with the H37Rv strain, tubercles were found at all stages of development, whereas the membranes inoculated with the apathogenic strain showed initial tubercle formations in only 18 per cent of the cases.

M. Moore (1942) worked with six strains of bacilli of human type, three bovine, four avian, two strains from the cold-blooded animals, and with bacilli of rat leprosy pressed from the eight-to-ten-month-old lepromatous

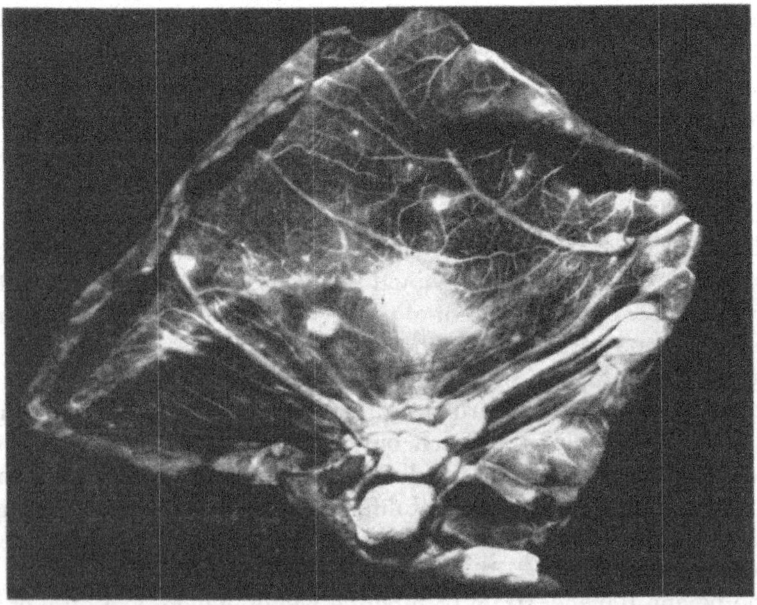

Figure 46. Gross lesions of 15-day-old chorioallantoic membrane 6 days after inoculation with H37Rv, × 1.3 (Emmart and Smith, 1943).

nodules of rat leprosy. Pathogenic tubercle bacilli rapidly invaded the mesoderm, formed tubercles, and caused caseation necrosis. Pathogenic bacilli planted on the ectoderm were taken up by the wandering cells and carried into the mesoderm. The fusion of the mononuclear cells produced giant cells seen chiefly at the margin of the lesion. Less virulent bacilli invaded the mesoderm slowly. *Mycobacterium leprae murium* caused nodular lesions which contained a large number of macrophages with vacuoles and a great number of leprosy bacilli in their cytoplasm, resembling the "foam" cells of leprosy.

The response of the chick embryo and its membranes to infection with tubercle bacilli of avian type was investigated by Canat and Opie (1943). The bacilli introduced into the membrane or into the tissue of the embryo invaded the ectodermal and mesodermal layers and the embryo itself, causing accelerated proliferation of the cells. In embryos up to six days of age, mononuclear wandering cells appeared and circumscribed nodules were formed. The lesions did not have the structure of tubercles because the epitheloid cells were not formed.

Fite and Olson (1944) compared the action of 41 strains of human, bovine, avian, and saprophytic strains of mycobacteria on the chorioallantoic membrane of chick embryos. Doses of 1.0 and 0.01 mg. produced nodules. The pathogenic bacilli migrated through the ectoderm but no growth of bacilli on the ectoderm was observed. Dead and saprophytic strains frequently caused lesions indistinguishable from those produced by pathogenic strains.

Dubos, Davis, Middlebrook, and Pierce (1946) inoculated developing chick embryos with cultures of human, bovine, and avian strains of tubercle bacilli, diffusely grown in liquid Tween-albumin medium. The injections were either made into the yolk sac of seven-day-old embryos or on the chorioallantoic membranes of ten-day-old embryos. All human and bovine strains produced lesions of the chorioallantoic membrane but only one of the four avian strains tested produced infection. The avian tubercle bacilli inoculated into the yolk sac never multiplied. The yolk sacs inoculated with the mammalian tubercle bacilli produced abundant cultures; the number of bacilli reached 10^8 per ml. The membranes inoculated with 0.001 or 0.002 mg. of bacilli produced a considerable number of gross lesions, whereas the membranes inoculated with 0.0001 mg. remained apparently normal.

Eggerth, Dresher, and McOsker (1948) confirmed the great variations in the minimal infective dose of tubercle bacilli for chorioallantoic membrane. Emmart and Smith (1941) needed doses of pathogenic tubercle bacilli as large as 1 mg. to infect chorioallantoic membranes; Dubos (1946) found 0.001 mg. of tubercle bacilli to be the minimal effective dose for the membranes.

The resistance of the chorioallantoic membrane to infection with tubercle bacilli increases with age. The membranes are most susceptible to infection on the sixth or seventh day of incubation, when 10^{-7} mg. bacilli are able to produce infection in them; 10–12-day-old membranes needed 10^{-4} mg. of bacilli to cause infection.

Tubercle bacilli inoculated into the yolk sac according to the technique of Cox (1938) grew well. In confirmation of an early work of Sclavo (1894) (see p. 197), Eggerth *et al.* obtained in 16 days excellent growth of tubercle bacilli in the yolk of nonfertile eggs inoculated with 10^{-8} mg. of bacilli when the inoculated eggs were shaken daily.

The bacilli inoculated into the allantoic cavity or the amniotic sac produced infections which also spread over the chorioallantoic membrane.

Histogenesis of a Tubercle in the Chorioallantoic Membrane and Its Transformations

The response of a developing tissue to the invading tubercle bacilli was first studied in tissue cultures. Maximow (1924) reported the results of his investigation of mammalian tissue cultures infected with tubercle bacilli. The tissue cultures infected with saprophytic organism died in a short time; in tissue cultures infected with tubercle bacilli no degeneration or death of cells occurred during three weeks of observation, both the tissues and the tubercle bacilli prospered simultaneously. The most active elements in the cultures were the reticular cells and the lymphocytes. These wandering cells engulfed large quantities of tubercle bacilli and transformed themselves into large polyblasts and epitheloid cells which, by assembling together, formed primary tubercles. Through the fusion of wandering cells, giant cells of the Langhans type were formed. The tubercle bacilli produced specific formative stimuli on the tissue cells, leading to the formation of tubercles. The end result of the tuberculous process – caseation – was also seen in the tissue cultures.

Gross lesions of chorioallantois. When a seven-day-old membrane is implanted with pathogenic tubercle bacilli and incubated for eight more days and then observed, the membranes are strewn over with grayish nodules of pinhead dimensions. The first nodules could be seen as early as the third day of infection. On the first day the membrane at the site of infection shows clear edema which may be of nonspecific, irritative origin. On the second and third days of infection the edema becomes muddy. The invasion by tubercle bacilli of the noninoculated regions of the membrane is seen on the fifth day of infection and it proceeds along the blood and lymph vessels.

Microscopic lesions of chorioallantois. The histologic investigation of the membranes by Costil and Bloch (1938) revealed that the start of the reaction to the infection was exudation. In the case of bacilli of human type, on the third day of infection, formations of small nodules composed of leucocytes and containing large quantities of bacilli were observed. Between the seventh and tenth day, these nodules, which could be seen on the surface of the membrane, showed a Langhans-type structure. The bacilli of avian type did not produce nodules but rather caused the infiltration of membranes by monocytes.

The microscopic examination of the membranes by Emmart and Smith (1941) revealed that there were no morphologic changes in the membranes that could be associated with the action of only one or another specific strain of bacilli. Generally, the proliferation or thickening of the epithelial layer with a following desquamation was observed. Invagination of the epithelium occurred; then the "pearls" detached from it, and were seen embedded in the mesoderm of the membrane.

In the mesoderm, where the chief activity of the infection occurred, the cellular proliferation produced dense foci composed of monocytes, leucocytes, and eosinophile cells. As the tubercle formation developed, the monocytes increased in number and large phagocytes appeared.

The histogenesis of tubercle bacilli in chorioallantoic membranes was recently investigated by Schürmann (1952). Seven-day-old membranes were infected with human and bovine strains of tubercle bacilli. The infected eggs were incubated and samples of the eggs investigated every 24 hours until the remaining eggs hatched.

The tubercle bacilli planted on the chorioallantoic membrane needed two or three days to invade the mesoderm. Part of the epithelial cells of the membrane at the site of inoculation died, others were stimulated to a papillary growth. The first response of the mesoderm to the invading tu-

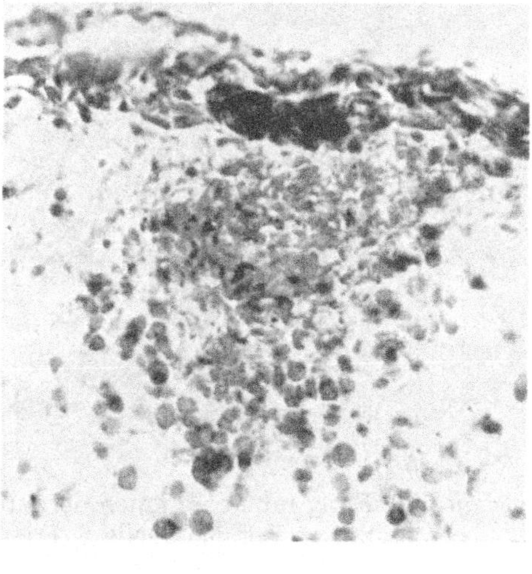

Figure 47. Beginning tubercle formation in chorioallantoic membrane, × 570 (Emmart and Smith, 1943).

bercle bacilli was exudation. The exudate from the terminal vessels accumulated in the reticulum of the mesoderm. The accumulating monocytes and eosinophiles increased in number and made the clear exudate turbid. The size of the lesions was in direct relation to the amount of bacilli inoculated.

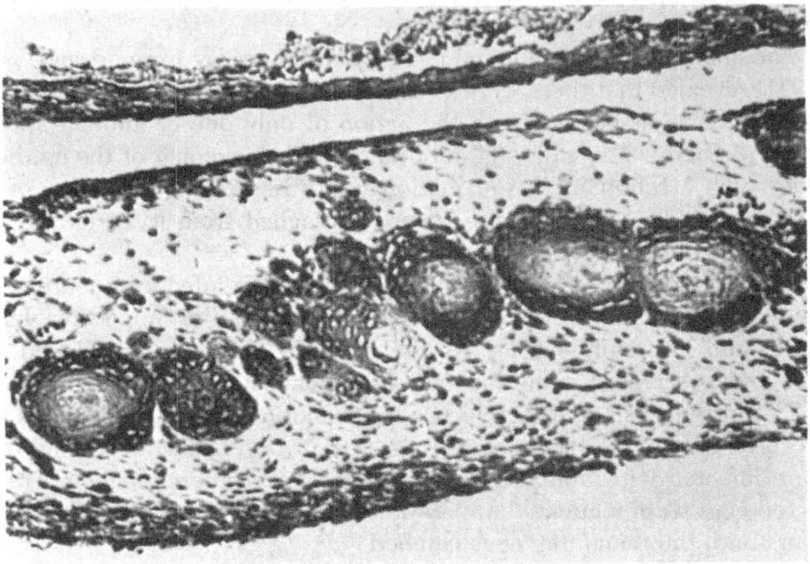

Figure 48. "Pearl" formation in chorioallantoic membrane inoculated with tubercle bacilli of bovine type, × 190 (Moore, 1942).

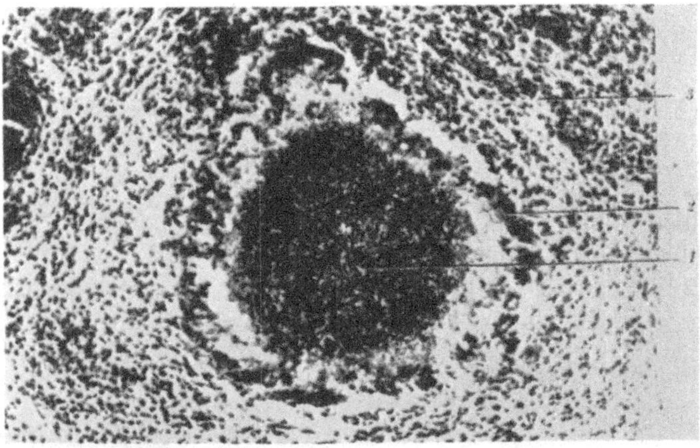

Figure 49. Early tubercle in mesoderm of chorioallantoic membrane. 1. Exudate center. 2. Layer of giant cells. 3. Pre-epitheloid cells. (Schürmann, 1952).

Chorioallantoic Membrane and Chick Embryo

In the early exudative phase of infection the cells of the mesoderm were active; they started to proliferate and enclosed the lesions with the syncytium of cells. Thus, the exudative response of the mesoderm to the infection was replaced by a productive one. The necrotic lesions in the infected mesoderm developed early, during the exudative phase. In the centers of the cell clusters, amorphous masses of degenerated leucocytes and a debris of nuclei appeared. In the necrotic lesions the Ziehl-Neelsen staining method revealed only a few acid-fast bacilli.

The tubercles of the chorioallantoic membrane eight days after the infection consisted of large exudate centers with an abundance of leucocytes; these centers being surrounded by the wall of giant cells. Many tubercle bacilli were engulfed by the cells but the center of the tubercle contained only a few of them, although the caseation necrosis developed there.

Chorioallantoic Membrane in the Screening of Antituberculous Drugs

Following the comparative studies of the action of pathogenic H37Rv strain and H37Ra strain of tubercle bacilli of reduced virulence on chorioallantoic membranes, Emmart and Smith (1942) used the chorioallantoic membrane and guinea pig inoculations to compare the changes in virulence of tubercle bacilli subjected to the action of Promin (p,p′-diaminodiphenilsulfone-N-N′-dextrose sulfonate).

The differences in virulence were well revealed in the experiments with bacilli treated for 104 days with Promin. Membranes inoculated with these bacilli showed in 58 per cent of the cases only slight development of tubercles. In the control experiments all membranes were infected, 75 per cent of them showing extensive tubercle development. The results obtained in guinea pigs were comparable to those obtained in chorioallantoic membranes.

Emmart (1945) investigated the action of streptothricin and streptomycin on the tuberculosis of the chorioallantoic membrane by dropping ⅕ ml. of the dissolved drug on the surface of the infected chorioallantoic membranes. After 6 days of incubation the number of surviving embryos was estimated. When 278 units of streptothricin were used, the survival rate was 46 per cent, while 1,000 units of streptomycin gave 68 per cent survival. Streptothricin was approximately four times more toxic to membranes than streptomycin.

Emmart and Seibert (1945) studied the action of the sera of tuberculous rabbits and the sera of rabbits sensitized with tuberculin on the development of tubercles in the chorioallantoic membranes.

Lee and Stavitsky (1947), and Lee (1949) studied the possibility of using chick embryo for preliminary screening of tuberculostatic substances. In the hope of avoiding irregularities, the intravenous route of infection was used in the experiments. This method gave a uniform degree of infection when $\frac{1}{20}$ mg. of tubercle bacilli suspended in 0.05 ml. of saline solution was injected into 11- or 12-day-old embryos. The mortality rate of the infected embryos was one fifth to one third of the embryos inoculated. The infection consistently resulted in the involvement of liver and spleen of the embryos. The surviving eggs were opened on the twentieth day of incubation, the embryos removed, and their livers taken out for microscopic investigation. The weight of the spleen was determined; the infected spleens had increased four to five times in size and weight. The lesions of the liver consisted in nodules composed of mononuclear cells containing large quantities of bacilli. The degree of the involvement of these organs was found to be a reliable criterion for estimating the effectiveness of the tuberculostatic action of the drug. Streptomycin, administered three times, in doses of 2,000 μg, at intervals of 48 hours, prevented the development of splenomegaly and lesions of the liver when the administration was started at the time of the infection.

In a chick embryo the degree of the splenic enlargement and the liver involvement permitted the investigators to interpret the tuberculostatic action of a drug in ten days.

When an unknown drug is screened, first of all the toxicity – the largest dose permitting the survival of the embryo for a ten-day period – must be established. The chick embryo method cannot replace the screening of drugs in animals, but it may be useful for the preliminary screening of an antituberculous substance promising *in vitro*.

Embryonated Egg in the Diagnostic Cultivation of Tubercle Bacilli

McNelly and Riddell (1949) investigated the possibility of using the embryonated egg as a medium for the primary isolation of tubercle bacilli from 100 sputum samples and compared the results obtained from the cultivation of aliquots of the sputa on the medium of Petragnani and in Dubos' liquid medium. Trisodium phosphate or acid was used to decontaminate the sputa. The embryonated eggs were inoculated with the material on the chorioallantoic membranes and into the yolk sacs. After the incubation the yolk was withdrawn, and smears were stained and investigated for tubercle bacilli. The liquid Dubos' medium was inspected daily for turbidity, and smears from the medium were made as soon as cloudiness appeared. Guinea pigs were inoculated with 0.5 ml. of suspensions of yolk and membranes to test the pathogenicity of the cultures.

The authors recognized the primary cultivation of tubercle bacilli in embryonated eggs as a promising procedure, since the results, as shown in the accompanying tabulation, were obtained in four to seven days. The question whether embryonated eggs can be successfully used for the diagnostic cultivation of material containing few tubercle bacilli still remains to be answered.

Membranes and cultures positive	71
Membranes and cultures negative	14
Membranes positive, cultures negative	12
Membranes negative, cultures positive	3

Klose, Knothe, and Schürmann (1951) found that primary cultivation on the usual media and animal inoculation are more reliable procedures for detecting mycobacteria than the inoculation of embryonated eggs.

Brueck and Buddingh (1952) inoculated pathologic material into the yolk sac of 5–8-day-old embryos. Spinal fluids obtained with aseptic precautions were injected in amounts from 0.2 to 0.5 ml. per yolk sac; gastric washings and sputa were decontaminated with a 4 per cent sodium hydroxide solution, and 100 units of penicillin were added to each ml. of material. Gram-negative contaminants were controlled by the addition of chloromycetin. Six eggs were injected with each sample of material and the eggs were candled daily. Starting with the fourth day after the inoculation, one embryo from each sample of material was examined daily. The presence of acid-fast bacilli was demonstrated in a fatty layer which appeared when 1 ml. of yolk was shaken with a 15 per cent phenol solution. Fifty specimens were cultivated and acid-fast bacilli were demonstrated in them after four to six days of incubation. This method could be of some value in the early diagnosis of tuberculosis.

Action of Embryo Extract on the Tubercle Bacilli

Friedmann (1945) reported that the growth of tubercle bacilli in a chick embryo medium prepared from 11–12-day-old chick embryos, which had been subjected to mincing and extracted with Tyrode solution, was greatly enhanced, and that the cultures developed in three to eight days.

Brieger and Fell (1946), in order to investigate the behavior and reproduction of tubercle bacilli in the tissue fluids, cultivated two pathogenic avian strains of tubercle bacilli in an 11-day-old chick embryo extract. The behavior of bacilli in hanging drops was observed on a warm stage for several days. The bacilli grew very actively, elongated during the first 24 hours, and formed filamentous cultures which broke down into short rods. No mode of reproduction of bacilli other than ordinary fission was discovered.

Bloch (1948) investigated the effect of chick embryo extract on tubercle bacilli cultivated in Dubos' liquid medium. The addition of 0.5 to 1.0 per cent of extract rendered growth more abundant, increased the serpentine pattern of the cultures, and even induced this property in the nonlethal variant H37Ra. The lungs of mice infected with these cultures grown on chick embryo extract showed tuberculous lesions. Heating at 100°C. destroyed in 6 minutes the active principle of the embryo extract. The active substance did not pass through cellophane membranes and was not soluble in ether, alcohol, or acetone. The extracts from the old (17-day) embryos were almost completely inactive.

The findings of Friedmann and Bloch concerning the growth activation of chick embryo extract of tubercle bacilli were not corroborated by Abramson (1952). He added chick embryo extract prepared according to the method of Friedmann and Bloch in the amount of 1 per cent to Tween-albumin medium. The medium was inoculated with H37Rv and H37Ra strains of tubercle bacilli, and the mean generation time of the cultures was determined. The chick embryo extract did not shorten the generation time of H37Rv and H37Ra strains in Tween-albumin medium. These observations confirmed the findings of Youmans and Youmans (1949), that the 14.4-hour period is the mean generation time of tubercle bacilli in a liquid medium containing serum.

Differentiation of Types and Pathogenicity of Tubercle Bacilli and Interpretation of the Lesions Produced by Tubercle Bacilli in Chorioallantoic Membranes

The early investigators of tuberculosis of the chorioallantoic membrane, such as Costil and Bloch (1938), put great emphasis on the peculiarities of the lesions produced by different types of mycobacteria in the ectoderm and mesoderm of the chorioallantoic membrane. According to Costil and Bloch, tubercle bacilli of avian type multiply on the surface of the membrane, sometimes producing necrosis but never invading the deeper parts of the membrane. The invasion of the mesoderm was regarded as a specific property of the mammalian mycobacteria (Emmart and Smith; M. Moore). These views on the different action of avian and mammalian strains on membranes were supported by some later investigators: "There is thus marked difference between the avian and human infection as far as the ectoderm is concerned and no explanation has been given for the fact that avian bacilli multiply so actively on the ectoderm and destroy it in places, while human and bovine bacilli produce keratinization and often desquamation of the epithelium and do not grow so profusely on the surface of the membranes" (Brieger, 1951).

To other investigators the differences in action of various types of mycobacteria on chorioallantoic membrane are quantitative and cannot serve as a criterion for differentiating types of mycobacteria. Canat and Opie (1943) state that "avian tubercle bacilli, introduced into the membranes or into the tissue of early chick embryos, invade both ectodermal and mesodermal cells." Fite and Olson (1944) were not able to observe any signs of growth of bacilli on the ectoderm. The attempts of some investigators (Emmart and Smith; M. Moore) to use the chorioallantoic membrane to determine the differences between the pathogenicity of tubercle bacilli on the grounds of the abundance or size of the lesions must be recognized as unsuccessful. According to Fite and Olson (1944), the chorioallantoic membrane failed to differentiate the mycobacteria of intermediate pathogenicity. The lack of invasiveness of the chorioallantoic membrane permits only the differentiation of the saprophytic or nonpathogenic mycobacteria from pathogenic ones. Tubercle bacilli of avian type on chorioallantoic membranes show the properties of nonpathogenic organisms.

M. Moore (1942) observed that the fish strain *Mycobacterium marinum* rapidly invades the mesoderm and stimulates the appearance of a great number of polymorphonuclear leucocytes and epithelial cells but does not produce giant cells, unlike the snake strain *M. thamnopheos*, which produces a great number of giant cells in the mesoderm (Fig. 50). If these observations are correct, they confirm the view that there is no relation between the pathogenicity of the bacilli as observed in susceptible animals and their action on the chorioallantoic membrane. Neither of the above mycobacteria has ever been proved pathogenic either to chick or to mammals.

Doubts have been raised about the interpretation of the histologic structures appearing in membranes and embryos infected with mycobacteria.

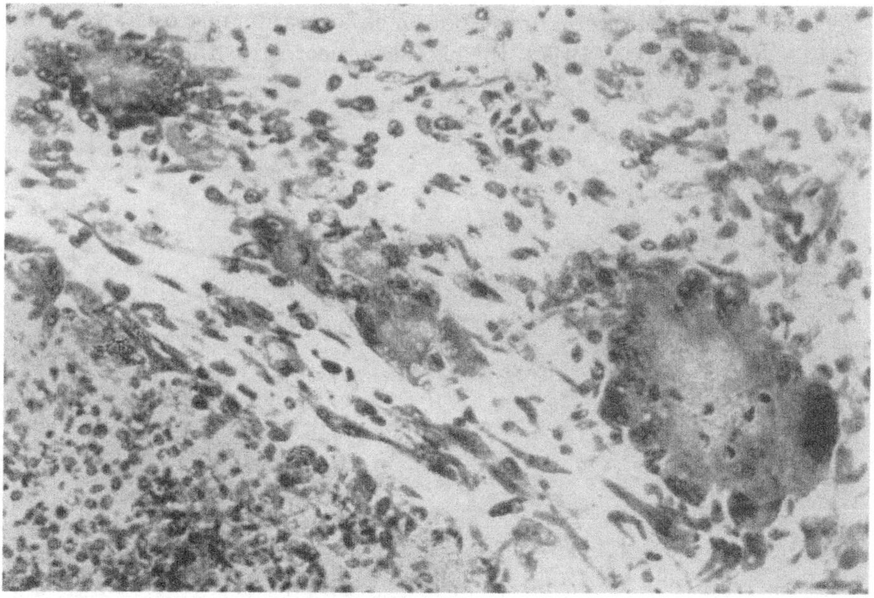

Figure 50. Giant cell formation in chorioallantoic membrane infected with *Mycobacterium thamnopheos*, × 630 (Moore, 1942).

Canat and Opie (1943) made the following statement: "The lesion that is formed by proliferation of fibroblasts and the accumulation of mononuclear phagocytes does not resemble a tubercle because it lacks the epitheloid cells that give the tubercle its characteristic form." Fite and Olson (1944) state that the difference between the action on the membrane by dead and by living bacilli was in most cases merely quantitative. The response of the tissue to dead bacilli was in many ways like that to living bacilli. Mechanical factors may be involved in the distribution of lesions. Lee and Stavitsky (1947) abstain in their work from using the word "tubercle" to indicate the formations found in the liver and spleen of embryos infected intravenously with tubercle bacilli. A membrane inoculated with a mold produced a histologic picture nearly identical with that seen in membranes inoculated with human tubercle bacilli. The nonspecificity of response on the part of the embryonic tissue inoculated with tubercle bacilli should be kept in mind.

Some investigators doubt that tuberculous caseation necrosis (Fig. 51) occurs in embryonic tissue. The phenomenon described as caseation necrosis by Emmart, Smith, Moore, and others in the membranes was interpreted differently by some other workers. Fite and Olson emphasize that the "necrosis" in the mesoderm depends entirely upon the invaginated areas of the ectoderm and consists of the ectodermal cells infiltrated with leucocytes. According to Fite and Olson, it is misleading to designate the necrotic areas in ectoderm or mesoderm as "caseation necrosis." According to Lee and Stavitsky (1947), the caseation necrosis is the response of the

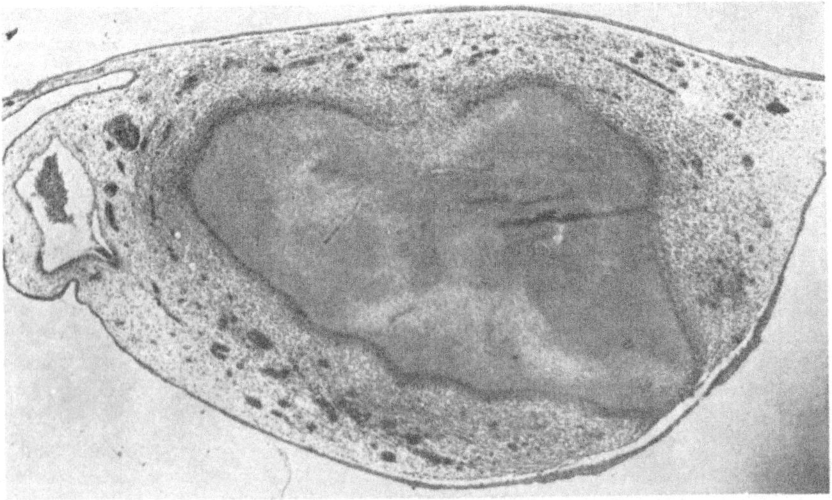

Figure 51. Caseous degeneration of a tubercle of the chorioallantoic membrane, × 18 (Emmart and Smith, 1943).

tissue to the preceding tuberculin sensitization but there is no evidence for its occurrence in the chick embryo.

The foregoing shows that the chorioallantoic membrane of a chick embryo is an extremely interesting and rewarding site for studying diverse problems of tuberculosis bacteriology, histology, and pathology. The existing data are not sufficient to enable one to differentiate in a chorioallantoic membrane the types and the pathogenicity of mycobacteria by the character of the lesions produced. More objective knowledge about the response of embryonic tissue to invading mycobacteria, with less emphasis on the similarity of this response to human or bovine tuberculous lesions, is necessary.

XXX

Hazards and Precautions in the Laboratory

THE greatest of all dangers is perhaps becoming acclimatized to a danger. Human nature is endowed with the power of adaptation, and daily work with tubercle bacilli may lead to laxness in the routine. Remaining aware of a persisting danger during long years of work, often in the same place and with the same microorganism, is one of the peculiarities of the true scientific mind.

Laboratory accidents and the infection of bacteriologists and pathologists have considerably increased with the growing number of persons working in diagnostic and research laboratories. The hazards of laboratory infection are far beyond those met in ordinary life, as was shown by viral laboratory infections (Sulkin and Pike, 1951).

The gateways permitting tubercle bacilli to enter the human organs are (1) the skin, (2) the subcutaneous tissue, (3) the respiratory tract, (4) the alimentary tract, (5) the urinary and genital system, (6) the eyes.

In experimental inoculations, as well as in naturally acquired infection, the lymphatic vessels are the chief channels of dissemination of tubercle bacilli. Sometimes the bacilli can reach the blood stream and lead to miliary dissemination into the distant organs.

To illustrate the accidents possible in tuberculosis laboratories we will select from the bulk of all that has been published on this subject a few cases on which there is precise information.

The questionnaire of Sulkin and Pike (1951), mailed to 5,000 laboratories in the United States, revealed 1,342 infections presumably acquired during laboratory work. The authors made an attempt to classify the infections as definitely, probably, and possibly acquired in a laboratory. The large majority of infections occurred among the trained scientific personnel. The greatest number of infections originated from the clinical specimens and the largest number of accidents was due to the use of syringes. Tuberculosis work produced 153 accidents, with 24 definite cases of infection acquired in a laboratory. Out of these 153 accidents, 139 cases ended with complete recovery, 10 cases caused complications and poor health, and 4 cases brought about the death of the worker. The most frequent localization of tuberculosis was in the lung.

The analysis of these laboratory infections by E. Long (1951) indicates that the surprising fact revealed by Sulkin and Pike – that the largest proportion of infections occurs among the trained workers – is probably due to these workers' frequent exposure to the source of infection.

Accidental Self-Inoculation

Bablet, Ducourtioux, and Bloch (1936) described an accidental intradermal laboratory self-inoculation of tubercle bacilli of bovine strain Vallée into the fleshy part of the thumb. The virulence of this strain, cultivated during many years in the laboratory of the Pasteur Institute in Paris, was regarded as weak, a dose of 0.01 mg. injected intravenously being almost inoffensive to a rabbit.

In the first week after the accident, which occurred on April 11, a nodule developed under the skin, increased slowly, was painful to pressure, and reached the dimensions of a big pea. In the third week, the ganglions in the armpit were palpable, one of them reaching the size of a nut. On June 12, two months after the infection, the ganglions were removed with an electric knife and electrocoagulation and curettage were carried out. In the removed tissue, acid-fast bacilli were discovered by direct examination. Four guinea pigs and Löwenstein's medium were inoculated with the material. After 24 days of incubation, 17 round, white, smooth colonies of acid-fast bacilli resembling those of the strain Vallée developed on the medium. Guinea pigs developed tuberculosis in five months and the rabbits inoculated with 0.01 mg. of the culture died in two to three months of generalized tuberculosis.

Tegström published the story of his case in 1942. He had always been in good health; there had been no indication of tuberculosis in his family. In 1938, Pirquet reaction was negative on him. In that year, he was intracutaneously vaccinated with 0.05 mg. of BCG. The tuberculin reaction changed from negative to slightly positive. An X-ray picture of his lungs taken shortly before the accident did not show pathologic changes. In the summer of 1940 he worked at the Bacteriologic Institute of Uppsala, Sweden, and on August 29, when cutting an enlarged lymph gland of a tuberculous guinea pig, a small speck of pus happened to squirt into his right eye. The eye was thoroughly washed with soap and water and a tepid solution of boric acid. On September 22, 24 days after the accident, Tegström felt some pain in the area of the right ear. On the morning of September 25, the edges of the eyelids of the right eye stuck together and a secretion appeared. The preaurical lymph gland was swollen, but the glands of the neck were not enlarged. On the tarsus of the upper eyelid a circular ulcer 3 mm. in diameter appeared. A smear from the ulcer revealed acid-fast bacilli. The material, inoculated on Hohn's medium, produced a culture of acid-fast bacilli. Two guinea pigs inoculated with it were tuberculous in two months. Rabbits inoculated with 0.01 mg. of bacilli revealed the human type of bacilli. The diagnosis was conjunctival tuberculosis.

From September 28, 1940 to March 29, 1941, the eye was treated once a week with Finsen rays. Two weeks after the treatment, the swelling of the preauricular gland disappeared almost completely and the conjunctival ulcer cleared. Six weeks after the beginning of the treatment, the lymph gland was almost impalpable, insensitive; the conjunctival ulcer had healed. In February 1941, the conjunctival infection and the remainders of lymphadenitis had disappeared. However, Tegström admits that after long work periods, his right eye is more tired than the left.

Six of Grady's Cases

Grady (1951) reviewed the literature available on inoculation tuberculosis and added his own 8 cases to the 70 reported by Stokes in 1925. Out of Stokes' 70 cases, 41 were cases of wound tuberculosis developed after ritual circumcisions.

Six of the eight cases of inoculation tuberculosis reported by Grady occurred in physicians who were residents in pathology. The accidents took place during the autopsies of tuberculous patients. The site of inoculation was the arm or the fingers; the left arm in three cases, the right one in the other three. In three cases the physicians were not aware of the accident. The first indication of infection appeared in 10 to 30 days in the form of induration or ulceration of the skin. The diagnosis was secured by the discovery of the tubercle bacilli or by a histologic investigation of the biopsy material. The victims of all eight accidents were hospitalized.

First case. The first signs of infection were observed approximately 20 days after the physician had performed the autopsy. The site of the infection was the dorsum of the left hand. The physician had not been aware of the accident. Caseation developed, the abscess was aspirated, and excision by cautery was performed. Streptomycin and PAS were administered. Recovery was achieved after five months of treatment.

Second case. One month after an autopsy the infection developed as a local ulceration in the left forefinger. The physician had not been aware of the accident. Streptomycin was given for four months, and excision of the ulcer performed. After five months of treatment, the ulcer had healed, but the movement of the finger remained limited.

Third case. The site of infection was a superficial scratch on the right wrist, which was washed with alcohol. One month later the physician developed fever. One year later lymph nodes and lymph chains were removed, and the wound was cauterized with phenol. After three years of treatment, the physician returned to regular work. His hand was still sore, and febrile reactions remained.

Fourth case. Infection occurred in a slight scratch made when a needle pierced the glove on the right thumb. After three weeks induration, ulceration had developed at the site of infection. Streptomycin was given for thirty days, the finger was immobilized. Adenitis did not develop; recovery took place in two months, with limitation of the movement of the finger.

Fifth case. The physician was not aware of the accident. There was swelling of the right index finger and pain in the axilla. The ulcer and surrounding skin were removed. After five weeks, the patient developed bilateral minimal pulmonary tuberculosis.

Sixth case. The site of infection was the left thumb, where ulceration developed. The thumb was immobilized. The ulceration was cured after three months, but three months after that the patient was hospitalized; infiltration of the left lung appeared. The gastric contents were positive for tubercle bacilli.

To these cases reported by Grady we add the history of an accident that occurred in our laboratory. A laboratory technician, a girl of eighteen, who had received 0.2 g. of BCG per os one year earlier, broke a glass tube containing about 1 ml. of sputum strongly positive for tubercle bacilli. The site of the wound was the left forefinger; it was open, 1.5 cm. long and 0.3 cm. deep. The content of the tube had been spilled over the wound.

The wound was allowed to bleed profusely for some minutes, then it was washed in a strong stream of water and partly excised. A large quantity of thiosemicarbazone was put into it and the wound closed. The girl was given 0.5 g. streptomycin daily during four days. The wound healed without complications. The spilled sputum was cultivated and produced an abundant culture of tubercle bacilli. After one year of observation the girl did not show any indication of tuberculous infection.

The Japanese investigators Tamura, Ogawa, Sagawa, and Amano (1955) have given an account of an epidemic of cutaneous and lymphatic tuberculosis which followed the antityphoid vaccination of schoolchildren. Out of 631 vaccinated children, 102 were infected. The presumable source of the infection was the tuberculous physician who performed the vaccination.

The review of the literature and cases reported above show the grave consequences of the inoculation of tubercle bacilli into human beings. The results of treatment of the cases reported suggest that washing the wound with a stream of water and a wide excision of the site of inoculation or of the developed ulcer along with secondarily infected lymph nodes is the best treatment. Antibiotic and chemotherapeutic treatment must be added to the surgery.

Premeditated Self-Inoculation

A few carefully described cases of self-inoculations with laboratory strains of tubercle bacilli—inoculations known to be premeditated—have given rare opportunities for following the course of tuberculous infection in man under determined experimental conditions.

The case most adequately investigated, bacteriologically and clinically, is described by Jones, Platt, and Amill (1949). A thirty-year-old unmarried woman, an experienced bacteriologist, entered the hospital on January 15, 1948, in a feverish state, but for the succeeding eight days remained asymptomatic and afebrile. Cultures and the inoculation of urine into guinea pigs did not reveal any infection. On the ninth day, the woman began to have severe chills, and then admitted that on January 14, 1948, she had intravenously injected into her left cubital vein 1 ml. of a heavy suspension of pathogenic tubercle bacilli, with the intention of committing suicide.

The skepticism that met this confession delayed the therapy for six days. The physical examination was negative, except for a tender area in the left antecubital fossa. Between the sixteenth and the twenty-first day after the self-inoculation, miliary infiltration appeared in both lungs. At this time, a large number of acid-fast bacilli were seen on examination of the material extracted from the lesion of the left antecubital fossa. Cultures of this material were positive for tubercle bacilli. The tuberculin skin test with 1:100,000 O.T. was negative; cultures and inoculation of the patient's sputum, blood, urine, and cerebrospinal fluid into guinea pigs remained negative for tubercle bacilli. No splenic enlargement was observed. The patient started complaining about severe pain at the site of the inoculation. The wound opened of itself and thick, yellowish pus was discharged. Following this, the pain subsided and the patient's temperature dropped to 37.8°C.

The tubercle bacilli isolated from the patient showed sensitivity to less than 1 microgram of streptomycin. The patient received a total of 241 g. of streptomycin during a period of 105 days, in maximum doses of 3 g. She was discharged 125 days after hospitalization. In October 1948, her health was good enough to permit her to get married.

At the start of the treatment of this patient the total excision of the site of inoculation was suggested, but this measure was not adopted. It appears that this intervention might have been beneficial to the patient, because streptomycin therapy has shown no effect as long as the local abscess has not been evacuated.

Recently another well-defined case of self-inoculation with tubercle bacilli was published by Chien and Wiggins (1954). A single diabetic woman, 21 years old, a bacteriology technician, was admitted to the hospital with painful swellings of a week's duration in her left thigh (Fig. 52). She admitted that she had, with suicidal intention, inoculated herself with 1 ml. of a heavy suspension of tubercle bacilli prepared from a four-week-old culture. The patient had made the injection of tubercle bacilli three times and the fourth time injected a suspension of *Pseudomonas aeruginosa.*

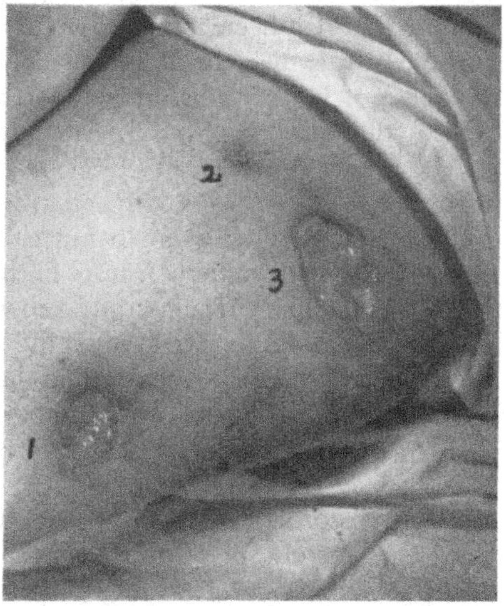

Figure 52. Wounds inflicted in girl's thigh by self-inoculation. 1, 2. Tubercle bacilli. 3. *Pseudomonas aeruginosa.* (Chien and Wiggins, 1954.)

The swellings gradually increased and were opened. Biopsy ten days after the inoculation revealed multiple tubercle formations. Cultures of tubercle bacilli were obtained from the inoculation site.

The patient was treated with 1 g. dihydrostreptomycin and 12 g. PAS for 43 days with added injections of chloramphenicol to combat the *Pseudomonas* infection.

No tuberculosis developed in the lungs or other organs, with the exception of an enlargement of a single lymph node in the inguinal area. After seven months of hospitalization the woman was released and was well one year later. She was again employed as a laboratory technician.

Mikhail and Tattersall (1954) related the case of an 18-year-old laboratory technician who, after receiving a BCG vaccination, inoculated three times, at intervals of three days, a suspension of pathogenic tubercle bacilli of human type into his abdominal wall. Streptomycin-sensitive tubercle bacilli were cultured from pus taken from the inoculation site. Streptomycin in a dose of 1 g. and 20 g. of PAS were administered daily for 54 days. One of the lesions was removed by surgery. Five months after the self-inoculation the abdominal lesions were healed.

Droplets and Dust as Agents Transmitting Tubercle Bacilli

The transmission of tubercle bacilli through the air was recognized by Koch (1882) as one of the common ways of spreading tuberculosis ("*Es ist also hiernach sehr wahrscheinlich, dass die Tuberkelbacillen, gewöhnlich mit der Athemluft an Staubpartilkelchen haftend, eingeathmet werden*"). In one of Koch's experiments, four guinea pigs, inoculated with sputum that had been conserved in dry conditions for eight weeks, were as tuberculous as the control animals inoculated with fresh sputum.

A case of human inhalation tuberculosis acquired in laboratory conditions in the course of early experiments with inhalation tuberculosis in animals is reported by Cornet (1889). A strong, healthy caretaker in his early forties was admonished not to enter the room where tuberculosis inhalation experiments on dogs were being carried out. Notwithstanding this, he entered the room to demonstrate on his own person the innocuousness of these experiments. He acquired tuberculosis and died in 14 weeks. The examination of the body revealed the same type of inhalation tuberculosis as was observed in the dogs used in the experiments.

After the work of Koch, all the importance in the transmission of tuberculosis was put on the dry, infectious dust particles until Flügge (1897) emphasized as transmission agents the liquid droplets eliminated by sick persons. According to the early investigations of Cornet (1889) tubercle bacilli are widely spread in the surroundings of their source, the tuberculous patient. In the dust of seven tuberculosis hospitals pathogenic tubercle bacilli were found in 20 samples out of a total of 94 investigated (21.3 per cent). The dust collected in the rooms of patients living in private houses produced tuberculosis in 34 guinea pigs out of 170 inoculated (20 per cent). Tubercle bacilli were not found in the dust of streets.

The conditions of interhuman transmission of tuberculosis were clarified by Chaussé (1912, 1914, 1916). He indicated that a dry sputum rich in tubercle bacilli, in the conditions of a private apartment, is virulent for guinea pigs until the tenth day through inhalation, and for 30 to 40 days by subcutaneous inoculation. The experiments with guinea pigs who lived in the same rooms with tuberculous patients showed the extraordinary infectiousness of the disease: out of 19 guinea pigs placed at a distance of 3 m. from the mouths of the patients 15 were tuberculous after one month of exposure. All animals gave signs of pulmonary tuberculosis of the inhalation type.

Droplets are not easily formed from mucous sputum. To separate respirable droplets less than 50 microns in diameter from such material, the velocity of the air stream must be from 30 to 35 m. per second. These conditions are fulfilled on the vocal cords during the moment of coughing. By exposing 152 guinea pigs to the cough of tuberculous patients, Chaussé obtained 31 per cent infected animals. It is not possible in practice to separate the infection acquired from droplets from that conveyed through infectious dust. The heaviest droplets – the most powerful carriers of infection – rapidly settle down and are transformed into infectious dust. The brushing of clothes and handling of infected linen easily produce infectious dust. B. Lange and Keschischian (1925) and B. Lange and Nowosselsky (1925), reviewing the abundant material published on these problems, and on the basis of their own experiments, reached the conclusion that projected infectious droplets are rarely under 20 microns in diameter and are not inhaled into the lungs. The bulk of tuberculous lung infection must be attributed to the inhalation of infectious dust.

The expression "droplet nuclei," coined by Wells in 1936 to indicate some new properties of the droplets, in reality designates nothing other than the droplets or the infectious dust alluded to by Koch, Chaussé, Lange, and other early workers.

The experiments of Lurie (1930), on the dissemination of infection by tuberculous guinea pigs confirmed the results obtained by Chaussé on the spreading of the infection by tuberculous human beings: out of 103 guinea pigs which lived for 32 months in separate cages in the same room with tuberculous guinea pigs, 15 developed inhalation tuberculosis. The infection was equally distributed in the room, independent of the proximity of the animals to the source of contagion. Apparently the tubercle bacilli were uniformly spread in the air of the room. The chief source of tubercle bacilli in the air were the infectious ejections of the animals.

Bogen and Dunn (1941) exposed Petri dishes containing a 5 per cent glycerol solution to the air in different places in a tuberculosis sanatorium. The culturing and the inoculation into guinea pigs of specimens collected in admitting wards revealed 2 positive specimens out of 18; in laboratories where infectious sputum was handled, 3 dishes were positive out of 35 exposed. Although 10 per cent of Petri dishes of 65 $cm.^2$ surface were infected after some hours of exposure, the authors consider that the danger of airborne tuberculosis infection in these places is negligible.

Droplets containing tubercle bacilli were expelled by 10 out of 20 patients with open tuberculosis; out of 410 droplets collected during 120 coughs, 36 were found to contain from 1 to 40,000 tubercle bacilli. Tubercle bacilli were found in the mouth, on the teeth, and on the tonsils of patients with open tuberculosis (Duguid, 1946).

The swabbing procedure demonstrated the presence of tubercle bacilli in the mouth, and on the teeth, tongue, and tonsils of patients with open tuberculosis, although they are not so abundant there as in the larynx (Duguid, 1946; Adler, Toman, Tomanova, 1950). Tubercle bacilli, expelled from their breeding place in the lungs, infect respiratory passages and the mouth, pass into the stomach and the intestines, and are eliminated with the sputum and the feces. Mühlenbach and Tomek (1952) found tubercle bacilli in the surroundings of tuberculous patients, chiefly on bed linen and utensils. Griffith and Denaro (1956) investigated the degree of contamination by tubercle bacilli of eating utensils used by patients whose sputa contained tubercle bacilli. Out of a total of 304 forks used by these patients, 41, or 13 per cent, yielded cultures of tubercle bacilli.

Meyer-Lie (1953) investigated the content of tubercle bacilli in the air and the dust of sanatorium wards (see Table 53). Air was collected with Bourdillon's sampler between the beds, at the level of the patients' heads. Löwenstein's medium was exposed in Petri dishes for three minutes, at the same sites. Dust was collected with sterile linen pieces, inoculated into guinea pigs, and planted on Löwenstein's medium. Tubercle bacilli were found in the air and the dust of many rooms, especially in the examination room where dressings were changed.

Table 53. Results of Investigation for Tubercle Bacilli of Dust and Air from Sanatorium Wards

Transmitting Agent	No. of Samples	Positive for Tubercle Bacilli	
		No.	%
Dust (guinea pigs)	128	20	15.63
Dust (culture)	256	26	10.15
Air (culture)	256	9	3.52

Source: Meyer-Lie (1953).

The interest in the problems of droplet infection of tuberculosis has been revived through the application of high-speed photography and through the recent works of Wells, Lurie, and co-workers. Weyrauch and Rzymkowski (1938) obtained, with a Contax camera and powerful lens, photographs showing abundant projections of droplets from the mouth and the nose during the acts of speaking (pronouncing *t* and *p*), coughing, and sneezing.

High-speed photography (exposure time of $\frac{1}{30,000}$ second) with electric illumination in intermittent flashes, developed by Turner, Jennison, and Edgerton (1941), was capable of catching the movement of very fine droplets expelled by sneezing or coughing (Fig. 53). The number of droplets expelled by a violent sneeze or a cough may reach tens of thousands; their diameter is usually less than 2 mm., many of them being less than 0.1 mm. The involuntary closing of the mouth near the end of the sneeze produces the smallest droplets, but most of the droplets are propelled not farther than 1 m. from the mouth. Johansson and Ferris (1946) showed the production of infectious droplets by such ordinary bacteriological manipulations as the pipetting of liquids.

Wells and Lurie found that the number of tubercle bacilli in aerosol,

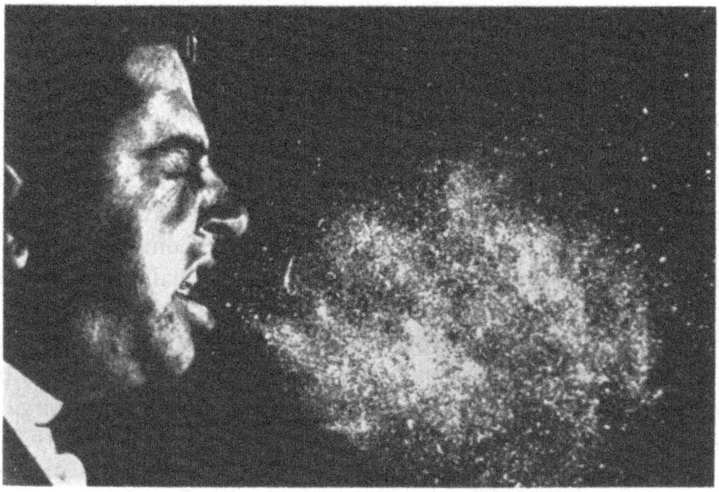

Figure 53. Photograph of particles expelled by sneezing (Turner, Jennison, and Edgerton, 1941).

calculated as aspired by rabbits, was in agreement with the quantity of bacilli cultivated from the lungs of the animals. Their conclusion was that the particles larger than 5 microns were removed from the aerosol in the upper respiratory passages of the animals. The settling velocity of water particles was about 15 cm. per minute when the diameter of the particles was 9 microns. All droplets that had a settling velocity of less than 3 cm. per minute in still air penetrated into the lung alveoles. Of the droplets settling at the rate of 30 cm. per minute, fewer than 10 per cent reached the lung alveoles.

Ratcliffe (1952) under experimental conditions similar to those of Wells and Lurie, investigated the airborne tuberculous infection of mice, hamsters, rats, guinea pigs, and rabbits. Infectious liquids containing from 30,000 to over 4,000,000 virulent tubercle bacilli per ml. were used in his experiments, but 99 per cent of the bacilli died during their transfer from water into the aerosol phase. The inhalation of aerosols by animals lasted from 30 minutes to 5 hours. Mice inhaled 1.25, hamsters 3.5, rats 6.0, guinea pigs 15.0, and rabbits 40.0 liters of aerosol per hour per animal. (Wells and Lurie calculate that 5.6 liters of air per minute participate in the respiration of an adult man of 60 kg., breathing at the rate of 16 times a minute.) Ratcliffe concludes from his experiments that infectious aerosol penetrates into the alveolar tissue of all these animals and that they are equally susceptible to inhaled infection.

These experiments on droplet infection, conducted with modern laboratory methods, could hardly be applied to human conditions. Results obtained with heavy aerosols charged with pathogenic bacilli, produced by high-speed machines, and inhaled by animals squeezed together in narrow boxes, are not sufficient to refute or change the observations and experiments of Koch, Chaussé, Lange, and many others, conducted under natural conditions, on the role of dust in the transmission of tuberculosis. Pulmonary tuberculosis develops as the result of inhalation of a few bacilli, as was particularly stressed by Jensen, Bindslev, and Holm (1935). In allergic guinea pigs, the inhaled tubercle bacilli produced local active cell reaction and remained isolated in the cells for a long time. Contrary to this, in nonallergic organisms, the bacilli did not produce local tissue reaction but multiplied actively within the cells.

Without pretending to explain the spread of tuberculosis among humans, the inhalation experiments, by providing the possibility of infallibly producing quantitative airborne tuberculosis in experimental animals, offer good service to the study of methods for preventing airborne contagion. A survey of the problems of airborne contagion can be found in a recent book by W. F. Wells (1955).

Germicidal Action of Ultraviolet Light

The germicidal action of light on bacteria was demonstrated by Roux in 1887. Barnard and Morgan (1903) established that the germicidal action of light is limited to the ultraviolet part of the spectrum, to the 300 mμ and shorter waves. Gates (1930) gave a quantitative estimation of factors involved in the germicidal action of ultraviolet light. The influence of wave length of radiation, intensity, and time of exposure on lethality of microorganisms was measured. To estimate these factors, monochromatic radiation was used. The test objects were laboratory strains of *Escherichia coli* and *Staphylococcus aureus*. The death rate of bacteria from radiation or a chemical disinfectant is similar in its course to the monomolecular chemical reaction. In the initial period of exposure to radiation, the bacteria do not die. A summation of energy up to a given level is necessary to cause their death. The resistant organisms that survive need an increased amount of radiation energy to be destroyed.

The light waves ranging from 302 mμ to 313 mμ in length have bacteriostatic action. Bactericidal action was observed in the wave lengths down to 225 mμ. The waves of 3.5 m. had no appreciable effect on *Escherichia coli* and *Staphylococcus aureus* (Hasché and Loch, 1938). Besides the wave length, the intensity of radiation, which depends upon the energy used in the burner, is another important factor of ultraviolet radiation action on living organisms.

Humidity strongly influences the bactericidal action of ultraviolet light on the bacteria suspended in the air. At low humidity, the killing power of the ultraviolet light is many times higher than at high humidity (Wells and Wells, 1936).

The resistance of bacteria to ultraviolet light is different at different stages in the life cycle of the bacteria, being higher in resting forms than in forms that are multiplying.

E. Mayer and Dworski (1932) studied the action of ultraviolet radiation on tubercle bacilli. In their experiments, a suspension of tubercle bacilli in a concentration of approximately 2,750,000 per ml., placed in a quartz cell at a distance of 2.5 cm. from the burner, was submitted to radiation and, after 2, 4, 5, 7, and 10 minutes, samples of 0.1 ml. were inoculated into two guinea pigs. When the intensity of radiation reached 5.93×10^6 ergs per second per $cm.^2$, tubercle bacilli were destroyed in 4 minutes. Dried bacilli on glass slides were destroyed in the same length of time and by the same intensity of radiation as bacilli in water suspension. Smithburn and Lavin (1939) used a burner, 90 per cent of whose radiation was 245 mμ. Tubercle bacilli (pathogenic H37Rv strain, 0.05 mg. per ml.) were killed after one minute of exposure to the lamp. One mg. of bacilli per ml. was destroyed after 10 minutes of exposure. The bacilli treated retained their acid-fastness.

According to the investigations of other authors, mycobacteria subjected to ultraviolet light lose their acid-fastness, which is followed by the loss of Gram-positiveness. *M. lacticola* loses its acid-fastness in the space of two hours, and its Gram-positiveness in six hours of exposure to ultraviolet irradiation (Bartholomew and Mittwer, 1952). This confirms the early observation of Cernovadeanu and Henri (1910) and E. Mayer and Dworski (1932).

Wells and Lurie (1941), who experimented with a virulent bovine Ravenel strain of tubercle bacilli, stated that up to 95 per cent of the bacilli in a heavily infected aerosol were killed when exposed for three seconds at a distance of 5 cm. to an almost monochromatic ultraviolet light of 253.7 mμ wave length. Rabbits exposed to the inhalation of irradiated bacilli survived from 2 to 3 times longer than the control animals exposed to nonirradiated bacilli under the same conditions. Lurie (1944) investigated the protective action of ultraviolet light on rabbits of high and low natural resistance to tuberculosis. The rabbits were exposed to natural airborne contagion spread by a group of tuberculous rabbits infected with the bovine Ravenel strain of tubercle bacilli. The cages of the noninfected animals were placed at a distance of 15 cm. from the cages of the infected ones. The space between the cages of the infected and the noninfected animals was irradiated by a lamp emitting, from a distance of 2 m., monochromatic ultraviolet light of 253.7 mμ wave length. When the intensity of the irradiation was high, it protected all the rabbits from the infection which caused tuberculosis in 73 per cent of control rabbits in nonirradiated cages. The source of infection was the urine and the feces of the infected animals. The tubercle bacilli–laden particles transmitting the infection were very small in size.

Precipitation by Aerosols

Our investigation of pine oil (1938) showed the bactericidal action of this oil on the tubercle bacilli. The fractional distillation of this oil produced liquids with high germicidal properties and of an agreeable odor and insignificant toxicity to human beings and experimental animals. The aerosol of pine oil settles down in a few hours in the form of a fine film and precipitates the microorganisms from the air. (Our experiments were made on heavily infected air in a guinea pig stable.) These observations were corroborated by Allweiss (1940). Recent investigations by Rolle and Mayr (1952) showed that 1 ml. of pine oil dispersed in 1 cubic meter of space produces in 40 minutes a considerably reduced growth of tubercle bacilli exposed on slides to the aerosol. Three ml. of oil, atomized in the same space, destroyed the tubercle bacilli after 1 hour of exposure. The domestic animals in the stables where these disinfection experiments were performed did not show any reaction to the aerosol when the concentration was not too heavy. Introduced into the mouth or eaten along with food, the oil caused inflammation of the intestines. The authors' experiments on themselves showed that a 30-minute stay in a room filled with not very heavy aerosol of pine oil did not have any harmful effect.

Aerosols of glycols were tested for the same purpose. Potter (1944) observed that tubercle bacilli were killed in 5 minutes when exposed to an 80 per cent concentration of propyleneglycol in the air, and in 15 minutes when the bacilli were exposed to triethyleneglycol. Lester, Robertson, and Puck (1949) reported that the aerosol of glycol at a 50 to 100 per cent saturation in air of relative humidity between 15 and 40 per cent, killed, in the first few minutes of exposure, between 30 and 90 per cent of suspended streptococci, staphylococci, and pneumococci; as the humidity rose above 50 per cent, the bactericidal effect diminished. Rolle and Mayr (1952) found the bactericidal action of triethyleneglycol on tubercle bacilli to be inferior to that of pine oil.

Protective Value of Gauze Masks

The protective value of gauze masks in the preservation of rabbits from airborne contagion of tuberculosis was studied by Lurie (1949a) and Abramson (1956). The gauze mask of 3 to 5 layers of material blocked practically all the interthread spaces. Twelve out of twenty rabbits provided with such masks were protected during quiet breathing from 29 to 1,027 tubercle bacilli units which were found deposited in the lungs of control animals breathing without masks. The animals in these experiments were exposed to heavily infected air but, notwithstanding this, more than half of them were protected from the infection. The exposure of human beings to such heavy infection is improbable.

The depth of breathing is a determining factor in the mask's effective ness in preventing infection. The mask does not stop the passage of tubercle bacilli projected by the coughs of tuberculous patients. The retention of tubercle bacilli by a gauze mask is a result of the adherence of the bacilli to the threads (Shapiro, 1950).

Safety Measures in a Tuberculosis Laboratory

The safeguarding of workers in a tuberculosis laboratory is a grave problem. The greatness of the risk of being exposed to tubercle bacilli in a laboratory depends largely upon the bulk of material manipulated. Efforts must be made to introduce a safe technique. Such a technique is often expensive but protection of the individual against infection with tubercle bacilli overrides all other considerations (Anderson, 1950).

An orderly, disciplined, and trained staff will reduce the laboratory hazards and minimize accidents, but the condition of a laboratory and the quality of its workers depend largely upon the experience and devotion to the cause of the head of the institution.

A general review of safety measures to be taken in a tuberculosis laboratory was made by Fish and Spendlove (1950). The following is a synthesis of these measures, based on the statements of many authors and on our own experience.

1. *Medical examination*

a. A medical examination and a chest X-ray is to be required before employment, with successive X-ray screening every three months.

b. Workers should be tested with tuberculin. Tuberculin-negative persons could be vaccinated with BCG or excluded from direct work with tubercle bacilli.

c. Illness and accidents must be reported immediately.

2. *Rest facilities*

a. Workers in a tuberculosis laboratory are not to be subjected to excessive strain.

b. Rest periods should be allotted during the work.

c. Washing, shower, and clothes- and shoe-changing facilities must be available to the workers. This is of particular importance to employees with small children at home.

3. *Laboratory equipment and procedures.* It is of extreme importance to avoid by all means the contamination of the laboratory and of one's own working place. There is no equipment or procedure that will eliminate infection if the worker is careless. It is preferable to avoid dangerous procedures after sleepless nights, and during headaches or other indispositions.

a. In a tuberculosis laboratory, there must be a room where all heavy transfers and manipulations of viable tubercle bacilli are performed. This room is regarded as contaminated and no other work is done there. It should have good ventilation, rubber or linoleum floor covering, and a germicidal ultraviolet ceiling lamp. Closed containers for the infected material are to be kept in the room, as well as a disinfectant solution. (The composition of our solution is alcohol (95 per cent), 700 ml.; water, 300 ml.; mercury bichloride, 1 g.; methylene blue solution, a few drops.) In the contaminated room there is a cabinet for sterile glass and all other necessary material, so that the worker can avoid leaving the room during the work.

b. A worker entering the contaminated room steps into a pair of easy slippers at the door, puts a coat over his clothes, dons goggles or glasses, a gauze mask, and a surgical hat. After work, these articles are exposed to ultraviolet light and are taken out of the room only for sterilization.

c. Rubber gloves, though recommended by some workers, are rarely used. The protection they give in tuberculosis work is more apparent than real. They impede the work and tire the worker. The intact skin is impenetrable to tubercle bacilli. Abundant running water and soap safeguard soiled skin against infection. No infectious material is to be handled with wounded hands.

d. Smoking or eating is not permitted in a contaminated area.

e. The grinding of infectious material in ordinary mortars, strong shaking, and the blowing of infectious liquids from pipettes are avoided even in the contaminated room.

f. The bacteriologic needles and syringes are dangerous sources of infection. A heap of a fresh culture of tubercle bacilli on a needle rapidly brought in contact with a flame explodes ("shoots") and scatters infectious fragments. To avoid this, we use a combustion chamber on an ordinary Bunsen burner to sterilize needles (Fig. 54). All manipulation of live tubercle bacilli is carried out over a pan covered with absorbent paper which has been soaked in a disinfectant solution.

g. The needle on the syringe is tightly wrapped with cotton to prevent the stream of infectious liquid from shooting out during the injection.

h. Fermented, heated, or shaken liquids may be projected when the container is opened suddenly. To avoid this, the containers must be wrapped in a towel soaked in a disinfectant solution before opening.

i. Safety hoods provided with ventilation and ultraviolet light are recommended by some investigators for handling infectious material. They may be useful for short operations in diagnostic laboratories with a large staff, or for workers with little experience. Work within a hood is tiresome and inaccurate; therefore the use of the hood has been rejected in most tuberculosis research laboratories.

4. Decontamination and cleaning

a. Disinfection is not a safe procedure of decontaminating laboratory glass or material, but there is often no other way of eliminating the hazard from spilled infectious material. The spilled material is covered with an absorbing paper or cotton which is left there overnight and is from time to time soaked with disinfectant liquid.

b. All contaminated laboratory glass, instruments, linen, etc., should be first autoclaved or boiled, and then washed.

c. The laboratory floor must be mopped with soapy water every evening after work, and rubbed with dust-preventing floor polish. There are many disinfecting floor polishes (Grün, 1932). Their real value is uncertain. Dry sweeping of the floor or dusting of a laboratory should be avoided.

d. Every morning before work, the worker should clean his working place with absorbent cotton soaked in a disinfectant liquid. Once a week a general cleaning of the laboratory is performed.

e. The animal autopsy room is considered a contaminated area.

The protection of the workers against airborne tuberculosis is based on (a) the destruction by ultraviolet light of the tubercle bacilli dispersed in the air; (b) the precipitation to the ground with aerosols of floating bacilli; and (c) the use of protective masks in the infected area. Sunlight and ventilation were early recognized as factors preventing tuberculosis infection.

Solotorovsky, Robinson, and Kniazuk (1953) gave some suggestions how to build and operate a tuberculosis laboratory. Unfortunately their advice is of a more theoretical than practical value. The use of hoods, heavy gowns, rubber gloves, and goggles, recommended by these authors, may be useful in certain dangerous steps of the work. According to Hughes (1952), one such dangerous operation is the pouring of tuberculous material from the

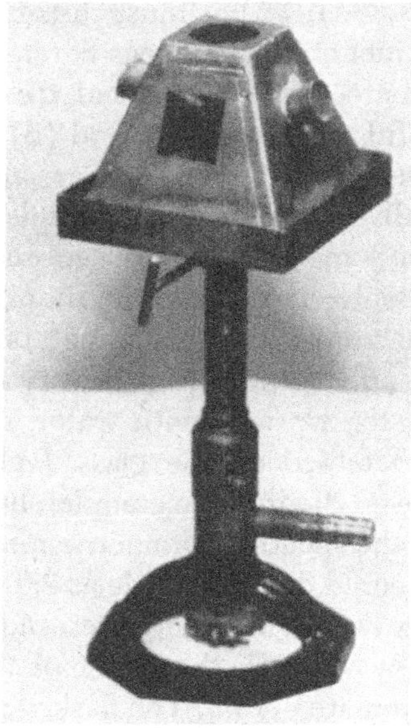

Figure 54. Combustion chamber for sterilizing bacteriological needles (Darzins, 1952).

original container into small centrifuge tubes. This transfer of material frequently contaminates the surroundings.

Work in a tuberculosis laboratory is not different from work in any other bacteriologic laboratory handling pathogenic microorganisms. The builder of a tuberculosis laboratory must realize that there is a restricted number of protective measures one can impose on or require from the workers. When this is not taken into consideration, these measures will become a real burden to the workers, and they will be avoided, carried out carelessly, or work will slow down.

The human element, not the machines, determines the successes and the disasters in the laboratory. Therefore all emphasis must be put on the selection and training of this element. Recommendations to house not in separate rooms, but together in one room, the tuberculous and the healthy guinea pigs, and to protect the healthy ones from infection by means of a screen of ultraviolet light, show an excessive belief in the protective power of devices.

Fremming, Benson, Young, Nye, and Smith (1955) indicated what measures they had to take to prevent the spread of infection from a tuberculous monkey colony used in experiments with antituberculous drugs.

Cleaning and Sterilization of Glassware

Clean glassware is of great importance for the growing of small inocula of tubercle bacilli. The ideal cleaning solution for use in a tuberculosis laboratory must possess the following properties: (1) it must kill tubercle bacilli in the contaminated container within a reasonable length of time (overnight); (2) it must dissolve the infectious material adhering to the container and make it easily removable by running water; (3) its use must eliminate further chemical treatment of glassware; (4) it must not be harmful to the workers; and (5) it must not attack the glass.

These ideal conditions are not met by any of the cleaning solutions actually in use in tuberculosis laboratories.

For some cleaning procedures, especially where organic material must be dissolved, oxidizing solutions are used. A particularly well-known solution is the one containing potassium dichromate and sulfuric acid. Dichromate adheres to the glass very tightly, and is difficult to remove entirely. After ten rinsings with water, considerable amounts of dichromate were still detected on the glass. Only boiling with several changes of water removed dichromate completely (Laug, 1934). R. Henry and Smith (1946) used the spectrophotometric method to detect dichromate. By this method they could detect as little as 0.01 μg. of dichromate per ml. When a 250 ml. Pyrex flask which had been in contact for 48 hours with dichromate was rapidly washed, the water of the eleventh washing contained 0.1 μg. of dichromate per ml. The flask was then filled with water and, after 22 hours at room temperature, the water, when concentrated to 10 ml., still contained 0.2 μg. of dichromate.

Butler and Johnston (1954) used radioactive Cr^{51} to measure the amount of chromium retained on quartz, Pyrex glass, and commercial plate glass. The Cr^{51} was converted to dichromate cleaning solution and the scintillation spectrometer and Geiger counter were used to determine the amount of radioactive chromium retained on the glass surfaces. The limit of detection of $K_2Cr_2O_7$ in these procedures was 10^{-4} μg. Each piece of glass was soaked in the radioactive cleaning solution for 24 hours, rinsed for about a minute in running water, dried, and thereupon the radioactivity was determined. Under these conditions Pyrex glass was found to retain more chromium than other brands of glass. Continued washing or strenuous rubbing with Kleenex did not alter the retention. The retention was considerably increased when the glass surface was soiled with grease from hands. The retention was due to the adsorption of the chromium ion rather than adsorption of the dichromate ion. The quantities of chromium retained on glass surfaces were negligible. All glass retained a 0.03 monolayer of chromium; when soiled with grease, the retention increased to 0.5 monolayer of chromium.

Instead of dichromate solution, a mixture of nitric and sulfuric acids may be used (Tobie, 1941). Unfortunately, this mixture produces harmful fumes.

Earle (1943) devised a method and a solution for cleaning glassware of methylcholantrene and other carcinogenes active in high dilutions. He ruled out the dichromate–sulfuric acid mixture because of the unsatisfactory growth of cell cultures in containers cleaned with this solution. The cleaning solution of Earle consists of 80 per cent sulfuric acid mixed with small quantities of nitric acid (100 ml. of concentrated nitric acid to 13 gallons of sulfuric acid). The mixture is to be heated by means of steam. Heavy fuming was avoided by using 80 per cent sulfuric acid. Earle further advised that glassware, before being placed in the acid solution, must be free from the salts of heavy metals.

Because of the difficulty of removing dichromate from glass, an acid permanganate mixture was recommended by Goldie (1947a) for cleaning glassware contaminated with tubercle bacilli. It was to have the following composition: 50 g. of potassium permanganate dissolved in 5 liters of water and 50 ml. of commercial sulfuric acid slowly added to the solution. The cleaning action of permanganate was attributed to the developing permanganic anhydride Mn_2O_7. Contaminated glass must be exposed overnight to this mixture, then transferred to a solution prepared by dissolving 120 g. oxalic acid in 5 liters of hot water, where it remains one more night. After the exposure, the glass is rinsed in running water for half an hour. The acid permanganate solution destroys tubercle bacilli; old glass, however, requires mechanical cleaning. The alkaline permanganate solution, like the dichromate solution, attacks skin and is poisonous.

Soap, ordinarily used in cleaning solutions, is noxious to the growth of tubercle bacilli. Soap is particularly dangerous in liquid media. If possible, cleaning solutions not containing soap must be used. (The cleaning solution or detergent not containing soap may be of the following composition: sodium metasilicate 0.7 part, tetrasodium pyrophosphate 0.07 part, and trisodium phosphate 0.07 part, dissolved in 100 parts of hot water.)

After the cleaning solution has been applied, the glassware must be repeatedly washed in running tap water and then thoroughly rinsed in distilled water. If hot running water is used, it may contain detergent from the boiler. In our laboratory, all infected glassware is first autoclaved, then left soaking in warm detergent solution and cleaned mechanically. The clean glass is thoroughly rinsed with hot, cold, and distilled water. Only pipettes, when heavily covered with blood or other organic matter, are soaked in acid dichromate solution.

As was particularly emphasized by Drea (1946) some ordinary laboratory cleaning procedures and sterilization methods leave behind products highly noxious to the growth of tubercle bacilli. The glassware cleaned with a dichromate solution (500 ml. saturated solution of $K_2Cr_2O_7$ and 800 ml. of crude, concentrated H_2SO_4), when thoroughly rinsed, did not prevent the growth of small inocula of tubercle bacilli, but cotton, used to plug the containers, if heated in a dry oven at the temperature from 160° to 170°C., produces noxious dry distillation products. These tar compounds cover the inner surface of the glass and then spread as a fine film over the surface of liquids, or are dissolved in the media prepared in containers. Paraffins and other products of dry distillation escaping from the heated cotton are responsible for the delay in the growth of tubercle bacilli.

Drea (1946) gives the following tests for glass cleanness: (1) in a clean glass no gas bubbles will adhere to the glass walls if it is filled with hot tap water; (2) the vapors of hot water poured into a cool dry flask will not condense in the form of minute drops on the wall above the water level.

Bibliography and Indexes

Bibliography

The number in parentheses indicates the title of the journal in the list of periodicals (p. 457). The numbers after the parentheses give the year, the volume, and the page of the periodical respectively, unless otherwise stated.

Abbott, J. N.: Technics and circumstances in the bacteriologic diagnosis of tuberculosis. (19), 1950, 40, 833.

———: Effective use of penicillin to reduce contamination in sputum concentrates to be examined for tubercle bacilli. (19), 1951, 41, 287.

Abel, G.: Vergleichende Untersuchungen über die Widerstandsfähigkeit von Tuberkelbazillen und säurefesten Saprophyten bestimmten Chemikalien (Antiformin, organischen und anorganischen Säuren) gegenüber. (245), 1939, 143, 225.

Abelson, P. H., and E. Aldous: Ion antagonisms in microorganisms: Interference of normal magnesium metabolism by nickel, cobalt, cadmium, zinc, and manganese. (135), 1950, 60, 401.

Abolins, L.: Alkaline phosphatase in various cell types of the anterior pituitary of the guinea pig. (175), 1948, 161, 556.

Abraham, E., E. Chain, C. Fletcher, A. Gardner, N. Heatley, M. Jennings, and H. Florey: Further observations on penicillin. (161), 1941, 241, 177.

Abramson, S.: The failure of chick embryo extract to accelerate the growth of tubercle bacilli. (22), 1952, 65, 783.

———: Experimental air-borne infection. (22), 1956, 73, 315.

Abreu, M. de: O lavado pulmonar no diagnóstico étiopatogênico ou evolutivo da tuberculose. (202), 1945, 27, 457.

———: Pulmonary lavage. A method for demonstrating tubercle bacilli. (22), 1946, 53, 570.

———: 1100 lavados pulmonares no diagnóstico bacteriológico da tuberculose. (201), 1947, 55, 59.

Académie nationale de médecine (France): Conclusions de l'académie à propos de l'expérimentation sur l'homme. (82), 1952, 136, 562.

Ackart, W. B., and T. J. Murray: A medium for the rapid cultivation of *Mycobacterium avium*. (135), 1951, 62, 75.

Adair, C. V., B. Drobeck, and P. A. Bunn: Use of rabbit eye as tissue to study tuberculosis. 2. Effect of certain antituberculous agents upon ocular tuberculosis. (22), 1951, 64, 207.

Adams, W. E., and A. J. Vorwald: The treatment of pulmonary tuberculosis by bronchial occlusion. An experimental study. (155), 1934, 3, 633.

Adler, H., K. Toman, and G. Tomanova: Tonsillar swab culture in lung tuberculosis. (6), 1950, 25, 78.

Agnello, V.: Influenza degli essudati pleurici sulla vitalità del bacillo di Koch. Ricerche sperimentali. (163), 1935, 6, 817.

Bibliography

Ahrens, W., and H. Wanke: Lässt sich die mikroskopische Tb-Sputumdiagnose durch Anwendung schnellaufender Zentrifugen verbessern? (102), 1954, 9, 1153.

Aitoff, M.: Quelques remarques sur le cord factor des souches avirulentes du bacille tuberculeux. (29), 1956, 91, 383.

Ajl, S. J., and C. H. Werkman: Replacement of carbon dioxide in heterotrophic metabolism. (45), 1948, 19, 483.

———: Anaerobic replacement of carbon dioxide. (191), 1949, 70, 522.

Akademia Nauk (Academy of Sciences), Moscow, U.S.S.R.: Rezoliutsia Konferentsii Akademii meditsinskikh nauk SSSR i Otdelenia biologicheskikh nauk Akademii Nauk SSSR. (225), 1952, 34, 318.

———: Postanovlenie prezidiuma Akademii Nauk SSSR ot 12 iunia 1953, No. 301. (225), 1953, 36, 28.

Aksjanzew, M. I.: Über das Oxydoreduktionspotential einiger Tuberkelbazillenstämme im Zusammenhang mit ihrer Virulenz. (242), 1933, 68, 249.

Allgöwer, M., and H. Bloch: The effect of tubercle bacilli on the migration of phagocytes *in vitro*. (22), 1949, 59, 562.

Allilaire, E., and E. Fernbach: Quelques observations sur la culture du b. tuberculeux en milieu non glycériné. (99), 1920, 171, 375.

Allweiss, P.: Über die Wirkung ätherischer Öle auf Tuberkelbazillen. (235), 1940, 122, 383.

Almquist, E.: Über eine Methode, das spezifische Gewicht von Bakterien und anderen Körperchen zu bestimmen. (235), 1898, 28, 321.

Altevogt, R., and B. Kuckhern: Ein neuer Versuch zur Typendifferenzierung von Tuberkelbazillen. (245), 1955, 162, 90.

American Trudeau Society and the American National Tuberculosis Association: Report of the committee on evaluation of laboratory procedures. (22), 1946, 54, 428.

———: The effect of cortisone and/or corticotropin on tuberculous infection in man and on experimental tuberculous infections in animals. (22), 1952, 66, 254, 257.

———: Report of panel discussion on survival and revival of tubercle bacilli in healed tuberculous lesions. (22), 1953, 68, 477.

Anderson, R. J.: Protection for the laboratory worker. (194), 1950, 65, 463.

Andrade, L. de: Contribução ao estudo das Micobactérias. Fluoromicroscopia e reação citoquímica de Dubos. (167), 1951, 49, 7.

Andreasen, A. A., and T. J. B. Stier: Anaerobic nutrition of *Saccharomyces cerevisiae*. 2. Unsaturated fatty acid requirement for growth in a defined medium. (137), 1954, 43, 271.

Andrejew, A.: Contribution à l'étude du métabolisme respiratoire des bacilles paratuberculeux. 1. Métabolisme respiratoire du bacille de la fléole. (29), 1946a, 72, 365.

———: Sur la végétation du bacille de Koch en profondeur. (29), 1946b, 72, 891.

———: Les échanges respiratoires de bacilles tuberculeux de souches différentes. (29), 1947, 73, 235.

———: L'utilisation par oxydation de quelques substances azotées par le bacille de Koch. (29), 1948, 74, 464.

———: Effet du benzoate et du salicylate sur la respiration des bacilles tuberculeux virulents et avirulents. (29), 1951, 81, 550.

———, and A. J. Rosenberg: Métabolisme intermédiaire des Mycobactéries. 1. Les cytochromes des bacilles tuberculeux humains (H37Ra), bovins (BCG), aviaires (A_{17}) et de *M. phlei*. (85), 1952, 34, 279.

Andrewes, F. W., and K. J. P. Orton: A study of the disinfectant action of hypochlorous acid, with remarks on its practical application. (245), 1904, 35, 645.

Angevine, D. M., and R. W. Huntington: Experimental ocular tuberculosis in normal and immunized rabbits. (17), 1941, 17, 155.

Angulo, J. J., J. H. L. Watson, and J. Olarte: Artifacts, with other nonspecific appearances resembling virus particles, and the so-called filamentous forms of influenza and fowl pest viruses in human skin tissue fluid examined with the electron microscope. (135), 1950, 60, 129.

Ardenne, M. von: Ergebnisse einer neuen Elektronen-Übermikroskop-Anlage. (176), 1940, 28, 113.

———: Elektronen-Übermikroskopie lebender Substanz. (176), 1941, 29, 521, 523.
Arena, A., and A. Cetrángolo: La tuberculosis humana de origen bovino en la Argentina. (24), 1946, 8, 36.
Arloing, F.: Évolution de l'infection tuberculeuse expérimentale par le bacille de Koch en culture homogène chez les mammifères, les oiseaux, et les vertébrés à sang froid. (98), 1910, 68, 701.
Arloing, S.: Sur l'obtention de cultures et d'émulsions homogènes du bacille de la tuberculose humaine en milieu liquide et sur une variété mobile de ce bacille. (99), 1898, 126, 1319.
Armand-Delille, P. F., A. Mayer, G. Schaeffer, and E. Terroine: Culture du bacille de Koch en milieu chimiquement défini. (98), 1913, 74, 272.
Armand-Delille, P. F., and J. Vibert: Le diagnostic bactériologique de la tuberculose pulmonaire des jeunes enfants par l'examen du contenu gastrique. (82), 1927, 97, 373.
Armstrong, A. R.: Trisodium phosphate in culturing for tubercle bacilli. (96), 1948, 59, 73.
———: The place of Dubos' oleic-acid albumin medium in routine laboratory practice. (93), 1950, 12, 60.
———: The laryngeal swab specimens in the cultural diagnosis of pulmonary tuberculosis. (96), 1951, 65, 575.
Aronson, J. D., and C. E. Whitney: The types of tubercle bacilli found in tuberculous lesions and in nontuberculous tissue in man. (145), 1930, 47, 30.
Asnis, R. E., and A. F. Brodie: A glycerol dehydrogenase from *Escherichia coli.* (136), 1953, 203, 153.
Asselineau, J.: Lipides du bacille tuberculeux. Constitution chimique et activité biologique. (9), 1952, 5, 1.
———, and E. Lederer: Sur des différences chimiques entre des souches virulentes et non virulentes de *Mycobacterium tuberculosis.* (99), 1950, 230, 142.
———: Sur la constitution du "cord-factor" isolé d'une souche humaine de bacille tuberculeux. (69), 1955, 17, 161.
Aubert, E.: "Cold" stain for acid-fast bacteria. (94), 1950, 41, 31.
Augier, J., and R.-O. Prudhomme: Écrans liquides adaptés à la microscopie en fluorescence utilisant l'auramine comme fluorochrome. (29), 1948, 75, 223.
Averbakh, M. M.: K gistokhimitsheskoi kharakteristike morphologitsheskikh reaktsii pri letshenii eksperimentalnogo tuberkuleza antibiotikami i khimiopreparatami. (186), 1956, No. 1, 43.
Avery, O. T., C. M. MacLeod, and M. McCarty: Studies on the chemical nature of the substance inducing transformation of pneumococcal types. Induction of transformation by a desoxyribonucleic acid fraction isolated from pneumococcus Type III. (139), 1944, 79, 137.
Axen, A.: Beitrag zum kulturellen Nachweis von Tuberkelbazillen in serösen Körperflüssigkeiten vermittels flüssiger Nährböden. (158), 1933, 1, 273.
Azzi, A.: Sulla resistenza del bacillo del tubercolo nello sputo all'azione dell'acido solforico. (57), 1924–1925, 47, 139.
Baas-Becking, L. G. M., and G. S. Parks: Energy relations in the metabolism of autotrophic bacteria. (183), 1927, 7, 85.
Babes, V.: Über isoliert färbbare Antheile von Bacterien. (235), 1889, 5, 173.
———: Les corpuscules métachromatiques des bacilles acidorésistants. (98), 1910, 68, 315.
Bablet, J., M. Ducourtioux, and F. Bloch: Auto-inoculation intradermique d'une souche de laboratoire de tuberculose bovine; modification consécutive de la virulence. (98), 1936, 123, 1086.
Badoux, V.: La microculture rapide du BK sur les lames, son intérêt pour la démonstration de la sensibilité aux antibiotiques. (133), 1951, 29, 1164.
Bainbridge, F.: The action of certain bacteria on proteins. (143), 1911, 11, 341.
Baker, M. J., M. E. Schlosser, and H. I. White: A method for evaluating antitubercular activity in mice. (36), 1949, 52, 678.

Bibliography

Balander, A. J.: De la contagiosité des formes dites "fermées" de tuberculose. (185), 1936, 44, 1274.

Baldwin, E. R.: Nonpathogenic acid-fast bacilli. (22), 1942, 45, 756.

———, S. A. Petroff, and L. S. Gardner: Tuberculosis. Bacteriology, Pathology and Laboratory Diagnosis. Lea, Philadelphia, 1927. U.S.A.

Balfour-Jones, S.: The experimental transmission of rat leprosy to the golden hamster (*Cricetus auratus*). (148), 1937, 45, 739.

Ball, E. G.: Studies on oxidation-reduction. Phthiocol, pigment of human tubercle bacillus. (136), 1934, 106, 515.

Bance, J.: Contribution à l'étude comparée du métabolisme des bacilles tuberculeux BCG, humain, bovin et aviaire cultivés sur milieu de Sauton. (41), 1942, 31, 71.

Barnard, J. E.: The limitations of microscopy. (154), 1919, p. 1.

———: The microscopical examination of filterable viruses, associated with malignant new growth. (161), 1925, 209, 117.

———: Morphology of bacteria in the living state. A system of bacteriology in relation to medicine. Medical Research Council, London, 1930, 1, 115.

———, and H. R. de Morgan: The physical factors in phototherapy. (81), 1903, 2, 1269.

Barnett, M., S. R. M. Bushby, and D. A. Mitchison: Isoniazid-resistant strains of tubercle bacilli. Their development and stability. (161), 1953, 264, 314.

Báron, J., and M. Pólányi: Über die Anwendung des zweiten Hauptsatzes der Thermodynamik auf Vorgänge im tierischen Organismus. (68), 1913, 53, 1.

Bartholomew, J. W., and T. Mittwer: Cell structure in relation to the Gram reaction as shown during lysis of *Bacillus subtilis*. (140), 1951, 5, 39.

———: Effect of ultraviolet irradiation on Gram positiveness. (135), 1952, 63, 779.

Bartholomew, J. W., and W. Umbreit: Ribonucleic acid and the Gram stain. (135), 1944, 48, 567.

Bartsch, E.: Die Tuberkelbakterienfärbung nach Osol. Ein Vergleich mit der Färbung nach Ziehl-Neelsen. (237), 1935, 47, 221.

Basch, F. P., P. Holinger, and H. G. Poncher: Physical and chemical properties of sputum. 1. Factors determining variations in portions from different parts of the tracheobronchial tree. (13), 1941, 62, 981, 1149.

Bassermann, F. J.: Beitrag zum Nachweis von Kernäquivalenten in Tuberkelbazillen. (245), 1952, 158, 104.

———: Elektronenoptische Untersuchungen zur experimentellen Tuberkelbacillenphagocytose. (63), 1954, 112, 162.

Bastin, R.: Action du sérum sanguin et du sang total sur le départ des cultures du bacille tuberculeux. (98), 1948, 142, 11.

Baudran, G.: Bacilles de Koch. Milieux aux glycérophosphates. Doses maxima de fer et de manganèse. (99), 1910, 150, 1200.

Bazzicalupo, C., A. Portella, and M. Contieri: Action of propylene glycol upon experimental tuberculosis in guinea pigs. (191), 1951, 78, 671.

Beattie, M.: Cultivation of *Mycobacterium tuberculosis*. A comparison of hydrochloric acid and trisodium phosphate in the preparation of sputum and of the use of fluid Dubos-Davis medium and Petragnani medium. (146), 1949, 34, 733.

Beaven, G. H., and E. R. Holiday: Ultraviolet absorption spectra of proteins and amino acids. (8), 1952, 7, 319.

Beck, F., and D. Yegian: A study of the tubercle bacillus in resected pulmonary lesions. (22), 1952, 66, 44.

Beckh, A., and Penzoldt: Über die antibakteriellen Wirkungen einiger Anilinfarbstoffe. (49), 1890, 26, 310.

Becquerel, P.: Influence des sels d'uranium et de thorium sur le développement du bacille de la tuberculose. (99), 1913, 156, 164.

Beerstecher, E., Jr.: Petroleum microbiology. Elsevier Press, Houston, Texas, 1954. U.S.A.

Beggi, D., and V. Picasso: Ricerche comparative su alcuni metodi d'arricchimento per il bacillo di Koch. (206), 1933, 49, 1925.

Bibliography

Behmann, H.: Tuberkelbazillennachweis im Kehlkopfabstrich. (172), 1930, 77, 62.
Behrens, M.: Über die Lokalisation der Hefenucleinsäure in pflanzlichen Zellen. (241), 1938, 253, 185.
Behring, E. von: Über die Bestimmung des antiseptischen Wertes chemischer Präparate mit bes. Berücksichtung einiger Quecksilbersalze. (103), 1890, 15, 837.
Bekker, J. H.: Über den fluoreszenzmikroskopischen Nachweis von Tuberkelbazillen in Sputum. (245), 1941, 148, 125.
Beller, K.: Der Nachweis des *Typus bovinus* bei Lupuserkrankungen und anderen tuberkulösen Prozessen des Menschen. (245), 1942, 148, 118.
Benassi, C. A., and B. Perisinotto: Ricerche cromatografiche sui metaboliti del triptofano in colture di *Mycobacterium tuberculosis.* (74), 1952, 31, 90.
Berezina, E., and M. Petrova: Deistvie streptomicina na bronkhogennyi tuberkulez belykh myshei. (186), 1953, No. 6, 45.
Berg, W. N.: The law of small numbers as applied to virulence measurement. (22), 1941, 43, 685.
Bergey, D. N.: Manual of determinative bacteriology, 6th ed. Williams & Wilkins, Baltimore, 1948. U.S.A.
Bernard, Claude: Introduction à l'étude de la médecine expérimentale. Delagrave, Paris, 1912. France.
Bernard, E., and B. Kreis: La méthode de culture sur lames du bacille de Koch. Son intérêt pour la recherche de la streptomycino-résistance. (205), 1949, 13, 124.
Bernheim, F.: The effect of salicylate on the oxygen uptake of the tubercle bacillus. (212), 1940, 92, 204.
———: The effect of various substances on the oxygen uptake of the tubercle bacillus. (135), 1941, 41, 387.
———: The oxidation of benzoic acid and related substances by certain *Mycobacteria.* (136), 1942, 143, 383.
———: The effect of salicylic acid on the growth, morphology and virulence of *M. tuberculosis.* (22), 1948, 58, 210.
———: Metabolism of *Mycobacteria.* (9), 1951, 4, 5.
———: The effect of substituted benzoic acids on adaptive enzyme formation in a *Mycobacterium.* (136), 1953, 203, 775.
———, W. E. DeTurk, and H. Pope: The nitrogen metabolism of certain strains of *Mycobacterium tuberculosis.* (135), 1953, 65, 544.
Berry, J., and H. Lowry: A slide culture method for the early detection and observation of growth of the tubercle bacillus. (22), 1949, 60, 51.
———: Efficiency of slide culture of tubercle bacilli. (12), 1950, 20, 1037.
Bergström, S., H. Theorell, and H. Davide: Effect of some fatty acids on the oxygen uptake of *Mycobact. tubercul. hum.* in relation to their bactericidal action. (175), 1946, 157, 306.
Bertalanffy, L. von, and I. Bickis: Identification of cytoplasmic basophilia (ribonucleic acid) by fluorescence microscopy. (142), 1956, 4, 481.
Bertalanffy, L. von, F. Masin, and M. Masin: Use of acridine orange fluorescence technique in exfoliative cytology. (212), 1956, 124, 1024.
Bertrand, G.: Importance de traces d'élements dans les processus biologiques. (31), 1938, 4, 65.
Besredka, A.: Étude sur le bacille tuberculeux. (99), 1913, 156, 1633.
———:Culture des bacilles tuberculeux dans du jaune d'oeuf. (29), 1921, 35, 291.
———, and F. Jupille: Le bouillon à l'oeuf. (29), 1913, 27, 1009.
Bessis, M.: Ultra-structure du protoplasma des thrombocytes au microscope électronique. (98), 1948, 142, 647.
Bettag, O. L.: Personal communication, 1952.
Beveridge, W., and F. Burnet: The cultivation of viruses and rickettsiae in the chick embryo. (165), 1946, No. 256.
Bezançon, F.: Sur le caractère relativement aérobie du bacille tuberculeux. (205), 1924, 5, 215.
———, P. Braun, and A. Meyer: La recherche systématique du bacille de Koch par la

culture des exudats pharyngo-laryngés prélevés par écouvillonnage. (82), 1937, 117, 506.
Bezançon, F., and V. Griffon: Culture du bacille tuberculeux sur le jaune d'oeuf gélosé. (98), 1903, 55, 603.
Biedert: Ein Verfahren, den Nachweis vereinzelter Tuberkelbacillen zu sichern, nebst Bemerkungen über die Färbbarkeit der Bacillen und Aetiologie der Tuberkulose. (66), 1886, 23, 713.
Bienstock, B.: Zur Frage der sogenannten Syphilisbacillen- und der Tuberkelbacillenfärbung. (116), 1886, 4, 193.
Bier, O., and N. Planet: Influencia da agitação sobre o desenvolvimento das culturas bacterianas. (58), 1937, 8, 107.
Bishop, F. W., L. G. Suhrland, and C. M. Carpenter: A comparative study by electron microscopy of the morphology of *Mycobacterium leprae* and cultivable species of *Mycobacteria.* (126), 1948, 16, 361.
Bisset, K. A.: Observations upon the bacterial nucleus. (143), 1948, 46, 264.
———: The nuclear cycle in bacteria. (143), 1949, 47, 182.
———: The cytology and life-history of bacteria. Williams & Wilkins, Baltimore, 1955. U.S.A.
Bloch, H.: Über den Stoffwechsel von Tuberkelbazillen. 2. Mitteilung: Die Ersetzbarkeit von Glyzerin. (210), 1944, 7, 489.
———: The effect of chick embryo extract on the growth and morphology of tubercle bacilli. (139), 1948, 88, 355.
———: Studies on the virulence of tubercle bacilli. (139), 1950, 91, 197.
———: Acid-fast bacteria. (38), 1953, 7, 19.
———, E. Matter, and E. Suter: The effect of glycerol and related substances on the growth and the oxygen uptake of the tubercle bacillus. (22), 1947, 55, 540.
Bloch, H., and H. Noll: Studies on the virulence of tubercle bacilli. Variations in virulence effected by Tween 80 and thiosemicarbazone. (139), 1953, 97, 1.
Bloch, R. G., G. Gomori, and M. Sperry-Braude: The effect of iron on experimental tuberculosis. (22), 1948, 58, 671.
Bloch, R. G., K. Vennesland, and C. Gurney: The effect of cortisone on tuberculosis in the guinea pig. (146), 1951, 38, 133.
Bluhm, L.: Is there any risk of infection from gastric lavage positives? (6), 1947, 21, 70.
Blume, C. A.: Zur bakteriologischen Frühdiagnose der Lungentuberkulose. (66), 1905, 42, 1072; (66), 1906, 43, 981.
Böcker, E.: Über das Wachstum von Tuberkelbazillen in eidotterhaltigen flüssigen Nährböden. (235), 1922, 95, 344.
———: Über die submerse Vermehrung der Tuberkelbacillen in flüssigen Nährböden. (235), 1923, 99, 121.
Boer, O.: Über die Leistungsfähigkeit mehrerer chemischer Desinfectionsmittel bei einiger für den Menschen pathogenen Bakterien. (235), 1890, 9, 477.
Bogen, E., and E. Bennett: Tubercle bacilli in sputum; criteria for negativity and significance of number of bacilli found. (22), 1939, 39, 89.
Bogen, E., and W. Dunn: Tubercle bacilli in air and dust. (22), 1941, 43, 435.
Boissevain, C. H.: The action of unsaturated fatty acids on tubercle bacilli. (22), 1926, 13, 84.
———: Growth promotion of the tubercle bacillus by serum albumen. (191), 1940, 44, 110.
———: Survival of tubercle bacilli in solutions containing glycerol or its oxidation products. (191), 1943, 54, 342.
———, and H. W. Schultz: A lipoid growth factor for the tubercle bacillus. (22), 1938, 38, 624.
Boivin, A.: Directed mutation in colon bacilli, by an inducing principle of desoxyribonucleic nature: its meaning for the general biochemistry of heredity. Cold Spring Harbor symposia on quantitative biology, New York, 1947, 12, 7. U.S.A.
———: Les acides nucléiques dans la constitution cytologique et dans la vie de la cellule bactérienne. (98), 1948, 142, 1258.

———, R. Tulasne, R. Vendrely, and R. Minck: Le noyau des bactéries. (185), 1948, No. 37, 440.

Boivin, A., and R. Vendrely: Les nucléoprotéides, constituants des cellules bactériennes. (98), 1943, 137, 432.

Bonfiglioli, H., A. Cetrángolo, and C. Acuña: Determinación de la estreptomicino-resistencia del Mycobacterium tuberculoso con la técnica de Pryce. (184), 1950, No. 41, 2458.

Boquet, A.: Sur la culture du bacille tuberculeux en milieux synthétiques à base de sels d'ammonium. (98), 1944, 138, 340.

———, and J. Bretey: Sur le développement de l'allergie chez le cobaye tuberculeux. (98), 1933, 113, 807.

———: Développement et évolution de la sensibilité à la tuberculine chez le cobaye. (29), 1934, 52, 252.

———: Influence du nombre de bacilles inoculés sur le développement de la tuberculose expérimentale. (205), 1950, 14, 440.

Boquet, A., and L. Nègre: Contribution à l'étude de l'infection tuberculeuse chez les petits rongeurs. (29), 1921, 35, 142.

Boquet, P., and Y. Lehoult: Action du venin de *Naja tripudians*, de *Vipera aspis* et de *Vipera ruselli* (*Daboia*) sur le cytoplasme des bactéries. (29), 1948, 74, 339.

Borch Jørgensen, B., and O. Horwitz: Dermatological complications of BCG vaccination. (6), 1956, 32, 179.

Borrel, A., L. Boez, and A. de Coulon: Exaltation de virulence de bacilles tuberculeux atténués. (98), 1923a, 89, 1109.

———: Facteurs accessoires de la croissance du bacille tuberculeux. (98), 1923b, 89, 191.

Borries, B. von: Personal communication, 1952.

———, and V. Glaser: Über die Temperaturerhöhung der Objekte im Übermikroskop. (159), 1944, 106, 123.

Borries, B. von, and E. Ruska: Vorläufige Mitteilung über Fortschritte im Bau und in der Leistung des Übermikroskopes. (228), 1938, 17, 99.

———: Ein Übermikroskop für Forschungsinstitute. (176), 1939, 27, 577.

———: Neue Beiträge zur Entwicklungsgeschichte der Elektronenmikroskopie und der Übermikroskopie. (117), 1948, 2, 267.

———, and H. Ruska: Bakterien und Virus in übermikroskopischer Aufnahme. (158), 1938, 17, 921.

Bossan, E., and M. Baudy: Nouveau procédé d'isolement du bacille tuberculeux dans les crachats. (98), 1922, 87, 954.

Bossan, E., and H. Roset: Culture du bacille tuberculeux en milieux liquide aéré. (98), 1923, 88, 1086.

Boughton, B. W., and M. R. Pollock: Long-chain unsaturated fatty acids as essential bacterial growth factors. Further studies with *Corynebacterium Q*. (67), 1952, 50, XXXI.

Brachet, J.: La détection histochimique des acides pentosenucléiques. (98), 1940, 133, 88.

———: The use of basic dyes and ribonuclease for the cytochemical detection of ribonucleic acid. (196), 1953, 94, 1.

Branch, A.: Study of acid-fast organisms other than mammalian tubercle bacilli isolated from disease in man. (221), 1933, 14, 337.

Brandt, K. M.: Physikalische Chemie und Cytologie der Presshefe. (Ein Sammelbericht und neue Untersuchungen im ultravioletten Licht und an gefärbtem Material). (193), 1942, 36, 77.

Braun, A. C.: Thermal studies on the factors responsible for tumor initiation in crown-gall. (11), 1947, 34, 234.

Braun, H.: Zur Frage des Verwendungsstoffwechsels des *Typus humanus* und des *Typus bovinus* des *Mycobacterium tuberculosis*. (210), 1955, 18, 989.

———, A. Stamatelakis, and S. Kondo: Der Verwendungsstoffwechsel säurefester Bakterien. 1. (68), 1924, 145, 381.

———, and R. Goldschmidt: Der Verwendungsstoffwechsel säurefester Bakterien. 2. Mitteilung: Der Verwendungsstoffwechsel der Kaltblütertuberkelbazillen (Blindschleichentuberkelbazillus und Schildkrötentuberkelbazillus Friedmann). (68), 1924, 146, 573.
Braunsteiner, H., F. Mlczoch, and W. Zischka: Elektronenmikroskopische Untersuchungen über die Wirkung von INH (Rimifon) auf die Tuberkelbazillen. (211), 1953, 10, 91.
Bretey, J.: Expérience d'infection par un seul bacille tuberculeux isolé au micromanipulateur. (29), 1944, 70, 357.
———, and A. Andrejew: Respiration des bacilles tuberculeux dans le milieu de Dubos. Tween 80. (98), 1949a, 143, 171.
———: Fraction V. (98), 1949b, 143, 173.
Breusch, F. L.:The biochemistry of fatty acid catabolism. (7), 1948, 8, 343.
Brieger, E. M.: New approaches to the study of experimental infection. (9), 1951, 4, 236.
———, V. Cosslett, and A. Glauert: Action of antibiotics on avian tubercle bacilli studied with the electron microscope. (175), 1953, 171, 211.
Brieger, E. M., and H. B. Fell: Warm-stage observations on the initial development of the avian tubercle bacillus cultivated in embryo extract. (143), 1946, 44, 158.
Brieger, E. M., and A. Glauert: A phase-contrast study of reproduction in mycelial strains of avian tubercle bacilli. (140), 1952, 7, 287.
Brieger, E. M., and C. F. Robinow: Demonstration of chromatinic structures in avian tubercle bacilli in the early stages of development. (143), 1947, 45, 413.
Briggs, G. O. A., and M. H. Jennison: Detection of *Mycobacterium tuberculosis* by means of fluorescence microscopy. (221), 1947, 28, 189.
Bringmann, G.: Elektronenmikroskopische Studien über die Kernäquivalente und die Zellorganisation von *Bacillus polymyxa Prazmowski* und anderen Bazillen. (245), 1951, 156, 547.
———: Elektronenmikroskopische Analyse der Wirkung von Neoteben auf *Mycobacterium avium Chester*. (245), 1953, 159, 521.
———: Zur Interpretation elektronenemikroskopischer Bakterienbilder insbesondere der Coli-Gruppe. (235), 1954, 139, 155.
Brodhage, H.: Versuche und Erfahrungen über das Wachstum von Tb-Bazillen in dem Dubosschen Nährmedium. (235), 1950, 130, 657.
Browaeys, J.: Sur l'assimilation par le bacille Grassberger d'impuretés étalées en couches minces à la surface de l'eau. (98), 1946, 140, 729.
Brown, L., and D. Smith: The cultivation of tubercle bacilli directly from sputum by the use of antiformin. (147), 1910, 22, 517.
Browning, C. H., and R. Gulbransen: Studies on experimental tuberculosis in mice. The susceptibility of mice to inoculation with tubercle bacilli. (143), 1926, 25, 323.
Bruce, H. M.: Feeding and breeding of laboratory animals. 14. Size and breeding group and production in mice. (143), 1954, 52, 60.
Brucke, K.: Erkennung von Dissimulation offener Lungentuberkulose mittels Tuberkelbazillennachweis im Larynxabstrich. (172), 1931, 78, 1173.
Brueck, J. W., and G. Buddingh: Isolation of *M. tuberculosis* by inoculation of the yolk sac of embryonated eggs. (191), 1952, 80, 589.
Brügger, H.: Über die aktive Behandlung der offenen Lungentuberkulose bei Kindern und Jugenlichen. (172), 1941, 88, 466.
Brun, J., and J. Viallier: Isolement direct en milieu de Dubos, de souches de *Mycobacterium tuberculosis,* à partir de produits pathologiques. (98), 1949, 143, 263.
Buc, E.: Sur la croissance du bacille tuberculeux dans les milieux liquides. (205), 1924, 5, 520.
———: Procédé de culture du bacille de Koch dans les épanchements pleuraux. (98), 1928, 98, 1495.
Buchner, H., K. Longard, and G. Riedlin: Über die Vermehrungsgeschwindigkeit der Bakterien. (245), 1887, 2, 1.
Buddingh, G. J., and A. D. Polk: Experimental meningococcus infection of the chick embryo. (139), 1939, 70, 485.

Bürki, F.: Der Goldhamster als Versuchstier in der mikrobiologischen Laboratoriumspraxis. (235), 1951, 133, 160.
Büttner, H.: Zur Kenntnis der Mykobakterien, insbesondere ihres quantitativen Stoffwechsels auf Paraffinnährböden. (51), 1926, 97, 12.
Buhler, V. B., and A. Pollak: Human infection with atypical acid-fast organisms. (12), 1953, 23, 363.
Bukatsch, F., and M. Haitinger: Beiträge zur fluoreszenzmikroskopischen Darstellung des Zellinhaltes, insbesondere des Cytoplasmas und des Zellkernes. (193), 1940, 34, 515.
Bunn, P., and B. Drobeck: Use of rabbit eye as tissue to study tuberculosis. Development of localized ocular lesion. (22), 1951, 64, 197.
Burckhardt, J. L.: Über fakultativ offene Lungentuberkulose. (209), 1941, 22, 604.
Burgos, R.: Valor comparado del lavado traqueobrónquico y del contenido gástrico en la investigación del bacilo de Koch. (122), 1948, 8, 33.
Burkl, W.: Fluoreszenzmikroskopischer Nachweis der Sexualhormone im Rattenhoden. (244), 1954, 40, 379.
Burnet, F. M.: The use of the developing egg in virus research. (165), 1936, No. 220.
Burns, H. A.: Tuberculosis in institutions for the mentally ill. (106), 1945, 11, 304.
Bush, G. P., and L. H. Hattery: Teamwork in research. American University Press, Washington, D.C., 1953. U.S.A.
Butler, E. B., and W. H. Johnston: Retention of chromium by glass following treatment with cleaning solution. (212), 1954, 120, 543.
Byham, B. B.: An evaluation of certain culture media for tubercle bacilli. (12), 1950, 20, 678.
Cadéac and Bournay: Rôle microbicide des sucs digestifs sur le bacille de Koch. Transmission de la tuberculose par les matières fécales. (98), 1893, 45, 599.
Cadiot, Gilbert, and Roger: Tumeurs blanches produites chez le lapin par inoculation intra-péritionéale de tuberculose aviaire. (98), 1891, 43, 66.
Calcinai, M.: Attività ossido-riducente di BB. di Koch provenienti da culture in varie fasi di sviluppo. (74), 1938, 17, 845.
Caldwell, P. C., and C. Hinshelwood: The nucleic acid content of *Bact. lactis aerogenes.* (152), 1950, p. 1415.
Calmette, A.: Existe-t-il dans la nature ou peut-on créer artificiellement des formes saprophytiques du bacille de Koch qui soient capables de se transformer en bacilles tuberculeux virulents? (205), 1924, 5, 716.
———: L'infection bacillaire et la tuberculose chez l'homme et chez les animaux. Masson, Paris, 1936. France.
———, A. Boquet, and L. Nègre: Rôle du facteur terrain dans l'évolution de la tuberculose expérimentale chez le lapin et chez le cobaye. (99), 1923, 176, 1197.
Calmette, A., and C. Guérin: Sur l'évacuation de bacilles tuberculeux par la bile dans l'intestin chez les animaux porteurs de lésions latentes ou "occultes." (99), 1909, 148, 601.
Calmette, A., L. Massol, and M. Breton: Milieux de culture pour le bacille tuberculeux. (98), 1909, 67, 580.
Campbell, J. I. R., and F. N. Stokes: Tricarboxylic acid cycle in *Pseudomonas aeruginosa.* (136), 1951, 190, 853.
Campbell, L. Kempf: The alanine and histidine metabolism of the tubercle bacillus. (22), 1925, 11, 458.
Camroe, J., and R. Dripps: The oxygen tension of arterial blood and alveolar air in normal human subjects. (18), 1944, 142, 700.
Canat, E. H., and E. L. Opie: Inflammation in embryonic life. 2. Infection of chick embryos with avian tubercle bacilli. (17), 1943, 19, 385.
Cancela Freijo, J.: El concepto bacteriológico de curación de la tuberculosis. (122), 1946, 6, 360.
Canetti, G.: Les bacilles de Koch existant dans les lésions des phtisiques sont-ils vivants ou morts? (205), 1946, 10, 26.
———: The tubercle bacillus. Springer, New York, 1955. U.S.A.

Cantonnet, B. P., L. T. Murguía, H. Cantonnet, and H. Lieutier: El valor del lavado gástrico y de los medios de cultivo en la infección tuberculosa. (198), 1938, 7, 563.
Capaldi, A.: Zur Verwendung des Eidotters als Nährbodenzusatz. (245), 1896, 20, 800.
Carrel, A., and L. E. Baker: The chemical nature of substances required for cell multiplication. (139), 1926, 44, 503.
Carson, S. F., and S. Ruben: Carbon dioxide assimilation by propionic acid bacteria studied by the use of radioactive carbon. (188), 1940, 26, 422.
Carvalho, A. de: Was leistet die mikroskopische Untersuchung, das Kulturverfahren und der Tierversuch bei der Ermittlung kleinster Tuberkelbazillenmengen im Untersuchungsmaterial? (242), 1932, 63, 305.
———, and C. Vidal: L'influence du sang humain sur le développement du bacille de Koch dans les milieux de culture liquides. (98), 1936, 121, 264.
Carvalho, L. de, and A. de Carvalho: Mode d'action du pneumothorax. (205), 1935, 1, 578.
Caspersson, T.: Über den chemischen Aufbau der Strukturen des Zellkerns. (213), 1936, 73, Supplement 8.
———: Cell growth and cell function. A cytochemical study. Norton, New York, 1950. U.S.A.
———, and K. Brandt: Nucleotidumsatz und Wachstum bei Presshefe. (193), 1941, 35, 507.
Caspersson, T., and J. Schultz: Pentose nucleotides in the cytoplasm of growing tissues. (175), 1939, 143, 602.
Cassel, W. A.: The use of perchloric acid in bacterial cytology. (135), 1950, 59, 185.
Cattaneo, C., M. Morellini, V. Ortali, and G. Penso: Studi e ricerche sui micobatteri. L'azione dell'acido p-aminosalicilico sui micobatteri. Differenziazione dei bacilli tubercolari dai paratubercolari. (163), 1950, 20, 291.
Cernovadeanu, P., and V. Henri: Étude de l'action des rayons ultraviolets sur les microbes. (99), 1910, 150, 52.
Chapman, G. B., and J. Hillier: Electron microscopy of ultra-thin sections of bacteria. 1. Cellular division in *Bacillus cereus*. (135), 1953, 66, 362.
Chargaff, E.: Structure and function of nucleic acids as cell constituents. (114), 1951, 10, 654.
———, and D. H. Moore: A bacterial glycogen: the isolation from avian tubercle bacilli of a polyglucosan of very high particle weight. (136), 1944, 155, 493.
Chargaff, E., and H. F. Saidel: On the nucleoproteins of avian tubercle bacilli. (136), 1949, 177, 417.
Chaussé, P.: La vitalité du bacille tuberculeux éprouvée par inoculation et par inhalation. (99), 1912, 155, 486.
———: Teneur bacillaire et conditions de pulverisabilité de la salive et des crachats tuberculeux par les courants aériens. (29), 1914, 28, 608.
———: Nouvelles recherches sur la contagion de la tuberculose par l'air expiré pendant la toux. (29), 1916, 30, 613.
Chauveau, A.: Tuberculose expérimentalement produite par l'ingestion de viande tuberculeuse. (118), 1868, 20, 550.
Chaves, A. D., L. R. Peizer, and D. Widelock: A comparative study of the effectiveness of laryngeal swabs and gastric aspiration for the detection of *M. tuberculosis* in chest clinic patients. (22), 1953, 67, 598.
Chaves, C. B., and M. P. Magarão: O método agitação-precipitação no diagnóstico bacteriológico da tuberculose. (59), 1954, 13, 147.
Chien, J. T. T., and M. L. Wiggins: Self-inoculation with *M. tuberculosis* and *Ps. aeruginosa* by a diabetic woman. (22), 1954, 69, 818.
Choucroun, N.: Biological effects of a toxic and sensitizing substance isolated from paraffin oil extract of dead tubercle bacilli. (212), 1943, 98, 327.
Churchman, J. W.: The selective bactericidal action of gentian violet. (139), 1912, 16, 221.
———: The mechanism of selective bacteriostasis. (188), 1923, 9, 78.
———: Inhibiting properties of anilin dyes. (216), 1926, 1, 27.

———: The structure of *B. anthracis* and reversal of the Gram reaction. (139), 1927, 46, 1007.
———, and L. Siegel: Cultural separation of bacteria on the basis of triphenyl methane coefficients. (216), 1928, 3, 73.
Chute, R. N., H. B. Kenton, and S. C. Sommers: A laboratory epidemic of human-type tuberculosis in hamsters. (12), 1954, 24, 223.
Clark, E.: Technique of operating on chick embryos. (212), 1920, 51, 371.
Clark, M. E.: Examination for evidence of tuberculosis. Annual report of the division of laboratories and research. State Department of Health, New York, 1952, p. 67. U.S.A.
Claude, A.: Particulate components of cytoplasm. Cold Spring Harbor symposia on quantitative biology, New York, 1941, 9, 263. U.S.A.
———: The constitution of mitochondria and microsomes, and the distribution of nucleic acid in the cytoplasm of a leukemic cell. (139), 1944, 80, 19.
———, and E. F. Fullam: An electron microscope study of isolated mitochondria. (139), 1945, 81, 51.
Čmelik, S.: Über die Lipoide der tuberkulösen Foci beim Menschen. (68), 1952, 322, 288.
Cohen, M. B., and J. S. Fleming: The diagnosis of epidemic meningitis and the control of its treatment by rapid bacteriological and serological methods. (145), 1918, 23, 337.
Cohen, S., J. C. Snyder, and J. H. Mueller: Factors concerned in the growth of *Corynebacterium diphtheriae* from minute inocula. (135), 1941, 41, 581.
Cohn, M. L.: Growth of human tubercle bacilli under restricted air conditions. (22), 1944, 49, 463.
———, C. Kovitz, U. Oda, and G. Middlebrook: Studies on isoniazid and tubercle bacilli. 2. The growth requirements, catalase activity, and pathogenic properties of isoniazid-resistant mutants. (22), 1954, 70, 641.
Coletsos, P. J.: De certains difficultés dans le diagnostique bactériologique des tuberculoses paucibacillaires. (29), 1947, 73, 188.
Cornet, G.: Die Verbreitung der Tuberkelbacillen ausserhalb des Körpers. (235), 1889, 5, 191.
Corper, H. J., and M. L. Cohn: The nutrient quality of eggs for growing tubercle bacilli. (14), 1933, 18, 1.
———: Media for tubercle bacilli. An evaluation of different media for diagnostic cultures of tubercle bacilli. (22), 1942, 46, 560.
———: The biological diagnosis of tuberculosis: quantitative animal evaluation tests on the Syrian hamster and guinea pig. (12), 1944, 14, 571.
Corper, H. J., L. Fiala, L. Kallon: The routine cultivation of tubercle bacilli from the sputum by Petroff's method. (145), 1919, 3, 185.
Corper, H. J., H. Gauss, and O. B. Rensch: Studies on the influence of carbon dioxide on the resistance to tuberculosis. (22), 1921, 5, 562.
Corper, H. J., and R. E. Stoner: An improved procedure for the diagnostic culture of mammalian tubercle bacilli. (146), 1946, 31, 1364.
Coryllos, P. N., and G. L. Birnbaum: Alveolar gas exchanges and atelectasis. Mechanism of gas absorption in bronchial occlusion. (47), 1930, 21, 1214.
Costil, L., and F. Bloch: Réaction de la membrane chorio-allantoïde de l'embryon de poulet aux bacilles tuberculeux humains et aviaires. (98), 1938, 128, 40.
Coulaud, E.: État allergique durable, obtenu chez les animaux de laboratoire, par injection sous-cutanée de bacilles tuberculeux morts, enrobés dans la paraffine solide. (205), 1934, 2, 850.
Cox, H. R.: Use of the yolk sac of developing chick embryo as medium for growing *Rickettsiae* of the Rocky Mountain spotted fever and typhus groups. (194), 1938, 53, 2241.
Cromartie, W. J.: Infection of normal and passively immunized chick embryos with *Corynebacterium diphtheriae*. (17), 1941, 17, 411.
Cruickshank, D. B.: Towards fluorescence microscopy. (221), 1947, 28, 97.

———: Bacteriology of tuberculosis, in Modern Practice of Tuberculosis, T. H. Sellors and J. L. Livingstone, eds. Butterworth, London, 1952, 1, 53. England.
Cummings, M. M.: Detection of the tubercle bacillus. Survey of current laboratory procedure. (91), 1949–1950, 2, 705.
———, M. C. Drummond, and H. B. Schwartz: A slide culture method for streptomycin sensitivity testing. (106), 1950, 17, 202.
Cunha, A. da, and J. Muniz: Réaction nucléaire de Feulgen chez les spirochètes et les bactéries. (98), 1929, 100, 951.
Curran, H. R., and F. R. Evans: The killing of bacterial spores in fluids by agitation with small inert particles. (135), 1942, 43, 125.
Cutinelli, C.: Ricerche sul metabolismo glucidico del bacillo di Koch. (74), 1940, 19, 146.
———: Gli acidi grassi nello sviluppo del bacillo di Koch. (56), 1941, 8, 487.
Dabelstein, H.: Das Fluoreszenzmikroskop in der laufenden Tuberkulosediagnostik. (245), 1939, 143, 242.
Daddi, G., and B. Nuti: Valore della prova colturale ripetuta nei malati negativi all'esame microscopico diretto. (33), 1949, 12/1, 77.
Dade, I.: Zur Frage der Typendifferenzierung von Tuberkelbakterien. (63), 1954, 112, 149.
Daels, F.: Beitrag zum experimentellen und anatomo-pathologischen Studium der Augentuberkulose. (224), 1907, 190, 90, Beiheft.
Daniels, M.: Scientific appraisement of new drugs in tuberculosis. (22), 1950, 61, 751.
Darzins, E.: Sur la fonction du tissue-réticuloendothélial dans l'organisme malade. (98), 1926a, 94, 623.
———: L'imprégnation à l'argent des Bacilles tuberculeux et du Bacille bilié de Calmette et Guérin (BCG). (98), 1926b, 95, 194.
———: Recherches sur les bacilles paratuberculeux de Moeller et de Grassberger. (29), 1932, 49, 743.
———: Recherches sur l'action de l'huile de pin et de l'huile de chaulmoogra sur les bacilles acido-résistants et sur la tuberculose éxperimentale du cobaye. (29), 1938, 61, 172.
———: Influence des carotenoïdes sur la croissance et l'acido-resistance des bacilles paratuberculeux de la fléole. (29), 1939, 63, 455.
———: Der animale Bakterienwuchstoff. (235), 1948, 128, 662.
———: The early diagnosis of tuberculosis and the direct determination of streptomycin resistance of tubercle bacilli. (6), 1951, 25, 474.
———: The epizootic of tuberculosis among the gias in Bahia. (6), 1952, 26, 170.
———, and G. Fahr: Cord-forming property, lethality and pathogenicity of *Mycobacteria*. (106), 1956, 30, 642.
Darzins, E., and T. Vitols: Bacteriologic diagnosis of tuberculosis in mentally ill patients. (106), 1956, 29, 324.
Davies, R.: The influence of normal blood and certain of its constituents on the growth and viability of the tubercle bacilli. (221), 1939, Supplement 5.
———: The effect of carbon dioxide on the growth of the tubercle bacilli. (77), 1940, 21, 243.
Davies, T. W., and C. J. Doherty: Gastric lavage in the diagnosis of tuberculosis in children. A survey of 75 cases. (81), 1942, 1, 212.
Davis, B. D.: Absorption of bacteriostatic quantities of fatty acids from media by large inocula of tubercle bacilli. (194), 1948, 63, 455.
———, and R. J. Dubos: Serum albumin as a protective rather than nutritive growth factor in bacteriological media. (114), 1946a, 5, 246.
———: Interaction of serum albumin, free and esterified oleic acid and lipase in relation to cultivation of the tubercle bacillus. (45), 1946b, 11, 201.
Davy, P. E., and J. C. Levaditi: Rôle de la centrifugation dans la recherche du bacille de Koch par les procédés d'homogéneization. (29), 1938, 61, 300.
Dawson, M. H., and R. H. P. Sia: *In vitro* transformation of pneumococcal types.

1. A technique for inducing transformation of pneumococcal types *in vitro*. (139), 1931, 54, 681, 701.

Dawson, J. R.: A study of chick-embryo-adapted rabies virus. (17), 1941, 17, 177.

Debré, R., J. Paraf, and L. Dautrebande: La période antéallergique dans la tuberculose expérimentale du cobaye, sa durée varie avec la dose de bacilles injectés. (98), 1920, 83, 986.

Debré, R., A. Saenz, R. Broca, and L. Costil: Intérêt de la recherche du bacille tuberculeux dans le contenu gastrique pour le diagnostic précoce du début de la tuberculose chez l'enfant. (42), 1936, 39, 779.

Dehmel, H.: Über die Technik der Tuberkelbazillenzüchtung und ihre Fehlerquellen als Ursache verschiedener Untersuchungsergebnisse. (245), 1933–1934, 130, 450.

Deinse, F. van: Sur l'emploi du milieu au jaune d'oeuf de Besredka comme milieu de conservation pour le bacille tuberculeux. (29), 1937, 59, 467.

———: Über Lupus- und Todesfälle nach BCG-Schutzimpfung. (242), 1956, 109, 33.

Deinse, F. van, and F. Sénéchal: Le BCG est-il virulent pour le hamster doré de Syrie? (29), 1954, 87, 117.

DeLamater, E. D.: A staining and dehydrating procedure for the handling of microorganisms. (216), 1951, 26, 199.

———, and S. Mudd: The occurrence of mitosis in the vegetative phase of *Bacillus megatherium*. (113), 1951, 2, 499.

Dello Jojo, G.: L'influenza del potere rotatorio del asparagina sullo sviluppo del bacillo di Koch. (70), 1937, 24, 46.

Desbordes, J., and E. Fournier: Contribution à l'étude de la physiologie des bacilles acido-alcoolo-résistants. (29), 1950, 79, 208.

———, and C. Guyotjeannin: Nouvelles applications de l'usage des corps tensio-actifs en physiologie bactérienne. Coloration à froid des bacilles tuberculeux. (29), 1952, 83, 268.

Despeignes, V.: Application au diagnostic de la méningite tuberculeuse des milieux de culture électifs pour le bacille de Koch. (98), 1922, 87, 121.

Dhéré, C.: Sur l'absorption des rayons ultraviolets par l'acide nucléique extrait de la levure de bière. (98), 1906, 60, 34.

———, S. Glücksmann, and L. Rapetti: Sur les applications de la spectroscopie et de la spectrographie de fluorescence en microbiologie. (98), 1933, 114, 1250.

Dienes, L.: Complex reproductive process in bacteria. Cold Spring Harbor symposia on quantitative biology, New York, 1946, 11, 51. U.S.A.

Dingle, J. H., and J. Weinzirl: The biology of tubercle bacillus. 2. The asparagin and glycerol metabolism of tubercle bacillus. (135), 1932, 23, 281.

Dissmann, E., and E. Iglauer: Methoden, Ergebnisse und Bedeutung der Streptomycinresistenzbestimmung des Tuberkelbazillus. (223), 1950, 4, 629.

Dixon, M.: Manometric methods as applied to the measurement of cell respiration and other processes. Cambridge University Press, Cambridge, 1951. England.

Dobell, C. C.: Notes on some parasitic protists. (196), 1908, 52, 121.

Doerr, R., and E. Gold: Zur Frage der "Virulenz" der Tuberkelbazillen. (236), 1932, 74, 7.

Donovick, R.: The use of the mouse in the experimental tuberculosis. (36), 1949, 52, 671.

———, C. M. McKee, W. P. Jambor, and G. Rake: The use of the mouse in a standardized test for antituberculous activity of compounds of natural or synthetic origin. II. Choice of mouse strain. (22), 1949, 60, 109.

Dorset, M.: Egg medium for the cultivation of tubercle bacilli. (212), 1903, 17, 374. (See also American Medicine, 1902, 3, 555.)

Dounce, A. L.: Cytochemical foundation of enzyme chemistry. Academic Press, New York, 1950. U.S.A.

Drea, W. F.: The growth of human tubercle bacilli H37, in synthetic medium with and without agar. (135), 1940, 39, 197.

———: Depth growth of acid-fast bacilli in liquid media. (22), 1946, 53, 353.

— —, and A. Andrejew: The metabolism of the tubercle bacillus. C. C. Thomas, Springfield, Ill., 1953. U.S.A.
Dubois, A.: Action inhibante de dérivés chaulmoogriques sur la culture en milieu liquide du bacille tuberculeux aviaire. (28), 1944a, 24, 1.
———: Méthode de recherche du bacille de Koch: selon Osol-Johansson et Hallberg. (28), 1944b, 24, 279.
Dubos, R. J.: The autolytic system of pneumococci. (139), 1937, 65, 873.
———: Rapid and submerged growth of *Mycobacteria* in liquid media. (191), 1945, 58, 361.
———: Effect of long chain fatty acids on bacterial growth. (191), 1946, 63, 56.
———: The effect of lipids and serum albumin on bacterial growth. (139), 1947, 85, 9.
———: The effect of sphingomyelin on the growth of tubercle bacilli. (139), 1948, 88, 73.
———: The bacterial cell. Harvard University Press, Cambridge, Mass., 1949. U.S.A.
———: Biologic and immunologic properties of tubercle bacilli. (16), 1950a, 9, 573.
———: The effect of organic acids on mammalian tubercle bacilli. (139), 1950b, 92, 319.
———, and B. D. Davis: Factors affecting the growth of tubercle bacilli in liquid media. (139), 1946, 83, 409.
———, G. Middlebrook, and C. Pierce: The effect of water soluble lipids on the growth and biological properties of tubercle bacilli. (22), 1946, 54, 204.
Dubos, R. J., and C. M. MacLeod: The effect of a tissue enzyme upon pneumococci. (139), 1938, 67, 791.
Dubos, R. J., and G. Middlebrook: Media for tubercle bacilli. (22), 1947, 56, 334.
———: The effect of wetting agents on the growth of tubercle bacilli. (139), 1948a, 88, 81.
———: Cytochemical reaction of virulent tubercle bacilli. (22), 1948b, 58, 698.
Dubos, R. J., and H. Noufflard: Milieu semi-synthétique à l'albumine pour la culture des bacilles tuberculeux. (29), 1950, 78, 208.
Dubos, R. J., and C. Pierce: The effect of diet on experimental tuberculosis of mice. (22), 1948, 57, 287.
Dubos, R. J., and R. H. S. Thompson: The decomposition of yeast nucleic acid by a heat-resistant enzyme. (136), 1938, 124, 501.
Duclaux, J.: Centrifuges et ultracentrifuges. Hermann, Paris, 1955. France.
Duguid, J. P.: Expulsion of pathogenic organisms from the respiratory tract. (81), 1946, 1, 265.
Dusch, F.: Über die klinische und epidemiologische Bedeutung des Tuberkelbazillennachweises im Mageninhalt von Kinder. (238), 1936, 58, 479.
Dworetzky, A.: Erfahrungen mit der Spenglerschen Formalinmethode zur Reinzüchtung von Tuberkelbazillen aus Bakteriengemischen. (245), 1904, 37, 626.
Dyar, M. T., and E. J. Ordal: Electrokinetic studies on bacterial surfaces. 1. The effects of surface-active agents on the electrophoretic mobilities of bacteria. (135), 1946, 51, 149.
Earle, W. R.: Methods of cleaning glassware. (153), 1943, 4, 131.
Ebel, J. P.: Participation de l'acide métaphosphorique à la constitution des bactéries et des tissus animaux. (99), 1949, 228, 1312.
Ebert, R. H., J. J. Ashern, and R. G. Bloch: Development of tuberculous infection. *In vivo* observations in the rabbit ear chamber. (191), 1948, 68, 625.
Ebina, T., and T. Nakamura: Über den Stoffwechsel der säurefesten Bazillen. 1. Über Atmung und Glykolyse. (219), 1937, 31, 60.
———, and D. Inomata: Influence des compositions gazières sur la croissance des bacilles acido-résistants. (219), 1938, 32, 1.
Edson, N. L.: The oxidation of lactic acid by *Mycobacterium phlei.* (67), 1947, 41, 145.
———: The intermediary metabolism of the *Mycobacteria.* (61), 1951, 15, 147.
———, and G. J. E. Hunter: Respiration and nutritional requirements of certain members of the genus *Mycobacterium.* (67), 1943, 37, 563.

———: The respiration of *Mycobacterium phlei.* (67), 1947, 41, 139.

Eggerth, A. H.: Growth of *Mycobacterium tuberculosis* in egg yolk mediums. (191), 1950, 73, 542.

———, E. Dresher, and V. C. McOsker: Infection of chick and duck embryos with tubercle bacilli. (22), 1948, 57, 632.

Egli, H.: Der Nachweis von Tuberkelbazillen im direkten Ausstrich, gefärbt nach Osol, betrachtet im Dunkelfeld, als Methode der Wahl. (209), 1942, 72, 166.

Ehrlich, P.: Aus dem Verein für innere Medicin zu Berlin. (103), 1882, 8, 269.

———: Über die Methylenblaureaktion der lebenden Nervensubstanz. (72), 1887, 6, 214.

———: Erinnerungen aus der Zeit der ätiologischen Tuberkuloseforschung Robert Kochs. (103), 1913, 39, 2444.

Eichhorn, E. A.: A technique for the intravenous inoculation of chick embryos. (212), 1940, 92, 245.

Eicke, M.: Zur Frage der Verwendbarkeit des syrischen Goldhamsters (*Mesocricetus auratus*) als Versuchstier. (245), 1952, 158, 114.

Eisenberg, P.: Studien zur Ektoplasmatheorie. (245), 1908a, 47, 415; (245), 1909, 49, 465.

———: Über Fetteinschlüsse bei Bakterien. (245), 1908b, 48, 257.

———: Untersuchungen über halbspezifische Desinfektionsvorgange. 1. Über die Wirkung von Farbstoffen auf Bakterien. (245), 1913, 71, 420.

Eisenstark, A., K. J. McMahon, and R. Eisenstark: A cytological study of a pleomorphic strain of *Azotobacter* with the electron and phase microscopes and the Robinow nuclear-staining technique. (135), 1950, 59, 75.

Ellinger, P.: Fluorescence microscopy in biology. (71), 1940, 15, 323.

Elsden, S. R.: The effect of carbon dioxide on the production of succinic acid by *Bacterium coli commune.* (67), 1938, 32, 187.

Elvehjem, C. A.: Respiratory enzymes. Historical introduction. Burgess, Minneapolis, 1949. U.S.A.

Emmart, E. W.: The tuberculostatic action of streptothricin and streptomycin with special reference to the action of streptomycin on the chorioallantoic membrane of the chick embryo. (194), 1945, 60, 1415.

———, and F. B. Seibert: The effect of tuberculous and sensitized sera and serum fractions on the development of tubercles in chorio-allantoic membrane of the chick. (144), 1945, 50, 143.

Emmart, E. W., and M. I. Smith: The growth and effects of the tubercle bacillus on the chorio-allantoic membrane of the chick embryo. (194), 1941, 56, 1277.

———: The chorio-allantoic membrane of the chick embryo as a medium for testing the virulence of tubercle bacilli. (22), 1943, 47, 426.

Engbaek, H. C.: Growth of *Mycobacterium tuberculosis* determined by direct agar microscopy. (4), 1952, 31, 369.

Engel, P. V.: Der Einfluss der Ernährung auf die jahreszeitlichen Schwankungen der Tuberkulinallergie. (48), 1933, 167, 279.

Epstein, G. V., E. D. Ravitsch-Birger, and A. A. Svinkina: K tsitologii tuberkuleznoi palotschki. (73), 1935, 4, 309.

Ernst, P.: Über Kern- und Sporenbildung in Bacterien. (235), 1889, 5, 428.

Esmarch, E.: Die Bereitung der Kartoffel als Nährboden für Microorganismen. (245), 1887, 1, 26.

Espersen, E.: Morphological studies of the normal growth of a human tubercle strain and the effect of some antibacterial substances on same. (4), 1949, 26, 178.

Evans, B., and J. H. Hanks: Growth of small numbers of acid-fast bacteria in blood and in serum. (191), 1939, 40, 112.

Evans, E. A., and L. Slotin: The utilization of carbon dioxide in the synthesis of α-ketoglutaric acid. (136), 1940, 136, 301.

Fabricant, C. G., J. Fabricant, and G. Knaysi: Effects of the composition of the medium on the growth, morphology, and virulence of *Mycobacterium tuberculosis var. avium.* (22), 1952, 66, 567.

Fallin, J. R., R. A. Patnode, and A. K. Hudgins: Toxic effect of penicillin on the culture of tubercle bacilli. (12), 1952, 22, 703.
Farjot, A.: Étude comparative de différents moyens de préparation des crachats pour l'inoculation au cobaye en vue du diagnostic de la tuberculose. (98), 1933, 112, 987.
Faure, H. P.: La microscopie de fluorescence en lumière ordinaire. (98), 1947, 141, 1219.
Feeney, R. E., J. H. Mueller, and P. A. Miller: Growth requirements of *Clostridium tetani*. 2. Factors exhausted by growth of the organism. (135), 1943, 46, 559.
Feinberg: Über den Bau der Bakterien. (245), 1900, 27, 417.
Feldman, W. H.: The susceptibility of chickens to human and bovine tubercle bacilli. (22), 1934, 29, 400.
———: Avian tuberculosis infection. Williams & Wilkins, Baltimore, 1938. U.S.A.
———, and A. H. Baggenstoss: The occurrence of virulent tubercle bacilli in presumably non-tuberculous lung tissue. (17), 1939, 15, 501.
Feldman, W. H., and H. C. Hinshaw: Effect of streptomycin in guinea pigs. A preliminary report. (192), 1944, 19, 593.
———: Chemotherapeutic testing in experimental tuberculosis. Suggested outline of laboratory procedures for testing antituberculosis substances in experimentally infected animals. (22), 1945, 51, 582.
Feldman, W. H., and H. E. Moses: The effect of Promin (sodium salt of p,p'-diaminodiphenyl-sulfone-N, N'-dextrose sulfonate) on experimental tuberculosis. A preliminary report. (192), 1940, 15, 695.
———: Human tuberculosis in a bovine. (22), 1941, 43, 418.
Fenner, F.: The enumeration of viable tubercle bacilli by surface plate counts. (22), 1951, 64, 353.
Fernbach, E., and G. Rullier: Action du sac gastric artificiel sur la virulence des crachats tuberculeux. (205), 1924, 5, 99.
———: Inactivation de la toxicité de la tuberculine vis-à-vis du cobaye tuberculeux, par action sous vide de quelques substances chimiquement définies. (99), 1941, 213, 214.
Ferrán, J.: Études sur le saprophytisme des bacilles tuberculogènes et sur la vaccination antituberculeuse. (125, Tuberculosis), 1905, 1, 170.
Feulgen, R., M. Behrens, and S. Mahdihassan: Darstellung und Identifizierung der in den pflanzlichen Zellkernen vorkommenden Nukleinsäure. (241), 1937, 246, 203.
Feulgen, R., and H. Rossenbeck: Mikroskopisch-chemischer Nachweis einer Nukleinsäure vom Typus der Thymonucleinsäure und die darauf beruhende elektive Färbung von Zellkern in mikroskopischen Präparaten. (241), 1924, 135, 203.
Feulgen, R., and K. Voit: Über den Mechanismus der Nuclealfärbung. 1. Mitteilung. Über den Nachweis der reduzierenden Gruppen in den Kernen partiell hydrolisierter mikroskopischer Präparate. (241), 1924, 135, 249.
Ficker, M.: Wachstum der Tuberkelbacillen auf sauren Gehirnnährböden. (245), 1900, 27, 504.
———: Genügt die Ziehl'sche Färbung zum Nachweis säurefester Bazillen allen Anforderungen? (58), 1940, 11, 125.
Ficus, H. J.: Vergleichende Untersuchung von Salzsäure, Schwefelsäure und Sputusol als Vorbehandlungsmittel bei tuberculösem Sputummaterial zur Erzielung von Tb.-Reinkulturen. Hanover, 1951. Germany.
Finke, L.: Über den fluoreszenzmikroskopischen Nachweis von Tuberkelbazillen in Ausstrichen und Gewebsschnitten. (51), 1940, 123, 381.
Finlayson, M. K.: Stimulation of growth of *Mycobacteria* by egg yolk. (148), 1946, 58, 88.
Fischer, H., and J. Hilger: Zur Kenntnis der natürlichen Porphyrine. 10. Über Blutfarbstoff in der Hefe, Nachweis von Porphyrin in Pflanzen. (241), 1924, 138, 288.
Fish, C. H., and G. A. Spendlove: Safety measures in a tuberculosis laboratory. (194), 1950, 65, 466.

Fisher, M.: The altered growth characteristics of isoniazid-resistant tubercle bacilli. (22), 1952, 66, 626.

Fisher, M. W., W. F. Kirchheimer, and A. R. Hess: The arithmetic linear growth of *Mycobacterium tuberculosis var. hominis.* (135), 1951, 62, 319.

———: Studies on the growth of *Mycobacteria.* 1. The occurrence of arithmetic linear growth. (22), 1952, 66, 758.

Fisher, R. A., H. G. Thornton, and W. A. Mackenzie: The accuracy of the plating method of estimating the density of bacterial population. (35), 1922, 9, 325.

Fite, G. L., and B. J. Olson: The infectivity of *Mycobacteria* for chorioallantoic membranes of chick embryos. (194), 1944, 59, 1423.

Fitzgerald, R. J., and F. Bernheim: The effect of streptomycin on the metabolism of benzoic acid by certain *Mycobacteria.* (135), 1947, 54, 671.

———: The effect of salicylic acid on the growth, morphology and virulence of *M. tuberculosis.* (22), 1948, 58, 210.

———, and D. B. Fitzgerald: The inhibition by streptomycin of adaptive enzyme formation in *Mycobacteria.* (136), 1948, 175, 195.

Fleming, A.: On the etiology of *Acne vulgaris* and its treatment by vaccines. (161), 1909, 176, 1035.

Florence, H.: Atypical acid-fast (chromogenic) organisms complicating pulmonary disease. (106), 1956, 30, 250.

Floyd, C., H. A. Novack, and C. G. Page: Gastric lavage in healthy adolescents. Bacteriological study of fasting gastric contents for tubercle bacilli. (22), 1942, 46, 622.

Flügge, C.: Über Luftinfection. (235), 1897, 25, 179.

Fluke, D., R. Drew, and E. Pollard: Ionizing particle evidence for the molecular weight of the pneumococcus transforming principle. (188), 1952, 38, 180.

Foley, G. E.: Submerged growth of tubercle bacilli from pathologic material in Dubos' medium. (191), 1946, 62, 298.

———: Further observations on the cultivation of tubercle bacilli from pathologic material in Dubos media. (146), 1947, 32, 842.

Fontes, A.: Estudos sobre a tuberculoze. (167), 1909, 1, 51.

———: Algumas considerações sobre a infeção tuberculoza e o seu respectivo virus. (167), 1910a, 2, 141.

———: Estudos sobre a tuberculoze. (167), 1910b, 2, 186.

———: Sur la distribution de la nucléine dans le virus tuberculeux. (98), 1933, 114, 903.

Forbes, G. B., J. V. Hurford, B. J. D. Smith, and V. H. Springett: The laryngeal swab in early and convalescent cases of pulmonary tuberculosis. (161), 1948, 255, 141.

Fournier, F.: Examen de bactéries par diffraction de rayons X. (99), 1949, 229, 37.

Fränkel, C.: Die Einwirkung der Kohlensäure auf die Lebensthätigkeit der Mikroorganismen. (235), 1889, 5, 332.

———: Beiträge zur Frage der Züchtung des Tuberkelbacillus. (123), 1900, 10, 617.

———, and E. Baumann: Untersuchungen über die Infektiosität verschiedener Kulturen des Tuberkelbazillus. (235), 1906, 54, 247.

Fraenkel, E.: The laryngeal swab. (22), 1944, 49, 363.

Fraenkel-Conrat, H., and R. C. Williams: Reconstitution of active tobacco mosaic virus from its inactive protein and nucleic acid components. (188), 1955, 41, 690.

Francis, J.: Bovine tuberculosis. Staples, London, 1947. England.

———: Tuberculosis in the dog, with special reference to experimental bronchogenic tuberculosis. (22), 1956, 73, 748.

———, J. Madinaveitia, H. M. Macturck, and G. A. Snow: Isolation from acid-fast bacteria of a growth factor for *Mycobacterium johnei* and of precursor of phthiocol. (175), 1949, 163, 365.

Franke, W., Li-Tsoung Lee, and D. Kibat: Zum Stoffwechsel der säurefesten Bakterien. 2. Mitteilung. Über das Verhalten der ungesättigten Fettsäuren. (68), 1949, 319, 263.

Franke, W., and A. Schillinger: Zum Stoffwechsel der säurefesten Bakterien. 1. Mitteilung. Orientierende aerobe Reihenversuche. (68), 1944, 316, 313.
Frei, W.: Atmungssysteme der Bakterien. (245), 1935, 134, 26.
———, L. Riedmüller, and F. Almasy: Über Cytochrom und das Atmungssystem der Bakterien. (68), 1934, 274, 253.
Freiman, D. G., and G. F. Mokotoff: Demonstration of tubercle bacilli by fluorescence microscopy. A comparative evaluation of the fluorescence and Ziehl-Neelsen methods in the routine examination of smears for acid-fast bacilli. (22), 1943, 48, 435.
Freiman, D. G., and M. Pinner: Routine examination of sputum for acid-fast bacilli. (22), 1949, 59, 449.
Fremming, B. D., R. E. Benson, R. J. Young, R. E. Nye, and W. E. Smith: Maintenance of a colony of tuberculous monkeys. American Veterinary Medical Association, Proceedings, 1955, p. 219.
Frey-Wyssling, A.: Submicroscopic morphology of protoplasm. Elsevier, Houston, Texas, 1953. U.S.A.
Fribourg-Blanc, A.: Une technique qui s'impose: La recherche des B. K. par la microscopie en fluorescence. (185), 1950, 58, 1400.
Friedemann, T. E., and F. B. Seibert: Metabolism of the tubercle bacillus in Long's synthetic medium. (191), 1939, 42, 41.
Friedheim, E. A. H.: Pyocyanine, an accessory respiratory enzyme. (139), 1931, 54, 207.
Friedmann, I.: Rapid growth of *M. tuberculosis* in an embryonic tissue medium containing penicillin. (221), 1945, 26, 75.
———, and K. Russel: Serpiginous growth of tubercle bacilli in media containing embryonic tissue. (148), 1953, 65, 495.
Friedrich, P. L., and H. Nösske: Studien über die Lokalisierung des Tuberkelbazillus bei direkter Einbringung desselben in den arteriellen Kreislauf (linken Ventrikel). (64), 1899, 26, 470.
Friis, T., V. Lester, and K. N. Rasmussen: Demonstration of tubercle bacilli in sputum and pleural fluid specimens. (6), 1955, 31, 383.
Frimodt-Möller, J.: Dissociation of tubercle bacilli. Investigations on the mammalian types including BCG. (6), 1939, Supplement 2.
Froman, S., D. W. Will, and E. Bogen: Bacteriophage active against virulent *Mycobacterium tuberculosis*. I. Isolation and activity. (19), 1954, 44, 1326.
———, and J. P. M. Black: The bacteriophage typing of atypical and other acid-fast organisms. (173), 1957, page 33.
Frouin, A.: Action des sels de vanadium et de terres rares sur le développement du bacille tuberculeux. (98), 1912, 72, 1034.
———: Sur la teneur en matières grasses des bacilles tuberculeux des types humain, bovin, aviaire. (98), 1921, 84, 606.
———, and M. Guillaumie: Utilisation des sucres: lactose, maltose, saccharose, tréhalose, par le bacille tuberculeux. (98), 1923a, 88, 1002.
———: Influence de la concentration de glucose sur le développement et le rendement en poids du bacille tuberculeux. (98), 1923b, 88, 1095.
———: Influence de la concentration de la glycérine dans les milieux de culture sur le rendement en poids du bacille tuberculeux. (98), 1924a, 90, 731.
———: Influence des sels de fer sur le rendement en poids du bacille tuberculeux. Action de ces sels sur l'utilisation de la glycérine. (98), 1924b, 90, 831.
———: Culture du bacille tuberculeux sur milieux synthétiques. Essai de généralisation de la notion d'équilibre entre les éléments constitutifs des milieux de culture. (29), 1928, 42, 667.
Fujita, A., and T. Kodama: Untersuchungen über die Atmung und Gärung pathogener Bakterien. 3. Mitteilung. Über Cytochrom und das sauerstoffübertragende Ferment, sowie die Atmungshemmung der pathogenen Bakterien durch CO und HCN. (68), 1934, 273, 186.
Furness, G.: Some factors affecting the destruction of *Bacterium coli* by shaking with glass beads. (140), 1952, 7, 335.

Furth, J.: On the serological relationship of acid-fast bacteria. (144), 1926, 12, 273.
Fust, B.: Zur Minimalinfektion mit Tuberkelbacillen. (235), 1938, 120, 547.
Gad, U.: On the diagnostic value of gastric lavage in adult patients without roentgenographic foci in the lungs. (6), 1937, 11, 189.
Gärtner, K.: Die Sulfonamidwirkung im Lichte der Fluoreszenz- und Elektronenmikroskopie. (245), 1943, 150, 97.
Gaffky: Ein Beitrag zum Verhalten der Tuberkelbacillen im Sputum. (170), 2, 126.
Gale, G. R.: The oxidation of benzoic acid by *Mycobacteria*. 1. Metabolic pathways in *Mycobacterium tuberculosis*, *Mycobacterium butyricum*, and *Mycobacterium phlei*. (135), 1952, 63, 273.
Gallavan, M.: Encephalitis and meningitis in the chick embryo following inoculation of the chorio-allantoic membrane with *H. influenzae*. (17), 1937, 13, 911.
Gamble, C. J., and M. C. Herrick: The utilization of dextrose by the tubercle bacillus. (22), 1922, 6, 44.
Garber, E. D., A. J. Hackett, and R. Franklin: The virulence of biochemical mutants of *Klebsiella pneumoniae*. (188), 1952, 38, 693.
Gardiner, P. A., R. J. W. Rees, and J. M. Robson: Intracorneal infection as a method for testing antituberculous substances. (79), 1949, 4, 209.
Gardner, A. D.: Growth and reproduction of *B. tuberculosis*. (148), 1929, 32, Part II, p. 715.
Gardner, G. M., and R. S. Weiser: A bacteriophage for *Mycobacterium smegmatis*. (191), 1947, 66, 205.
Gates, F. L.: A study of the bactericidal action of ultra violet light. 1. The reaction to monochromatic radiations. (141), 1930, 13, 231, 249.
Gelder, F. W. van: Über die Resistenz säurefester Bazillen gegenüber 10%-ger Schwefelsäure. Tübingen, 1933. Germany.
Gengou, O., P.-E. Grégoire, G. Lagrange, and J. Thomas: Action du citrat sodique sur les composés peu solubles de calcium et de barium. (44), 1950, 81, 61.
Georgi, C. E., W. Militzer, L. Burns, and J. Heotis: On the existence of a cell granule in a thermophilic bacterium. (191), 1951, 76, 598.
Gerlach, A. G.: Über die Impfbarkeit der Tuberkulose und der Perlsucht bei Thieren, sowie über die Übertragbarkeit der letzteren durch Fütterung. (224), 1870, 51, 290.
Gernez-Rieux, C., A. Sevin, and C. Chenet: Sur la valeur du milieu de Dubos pour le diagnostic de la tuberculose à partir de produits pathologiques. (30), 1949, 2, 27.
Gernez-Rieux, C., A. Sevin, and C. Spy: Utilisation du milieu de Dubos pour la culture du *Mycobacterium tuberculosis* à partir de produits pauci-bacillaires. (98), 1948, 142, 327.
Gernez-Rieux, Jacquet, and Fabre: Pouvoir pathogène des bacilles tuberculeux résistant à l'isoniazide. (205), 1954, 18, 1208.
Geronimus, L. H., and J. M. Birkeland: Relationship between virulence of tubercle bacilli and vigor of their oxidative attack upon certain substrates. (22), 1951, 64, 520.
Gerstl, B., and R. Tennant: The cellular response to some methylated long chain fatty acids. (229), 1943, 15, 347.
Gerstl, B., and R. M. Thomas: Experimental tuberculosis in mice. (229), 1940–1941, 13, 679.
Gervois, M.: Le bacille de type bovin. Danel, Lille, 1937. France.
Giemsa, G.: Färbemethode für Malariaparasiten. (Vorläufige Mitteilung). (245), 1902, 31, 429; (245), 1902, 32, 307.
Gifford, D., F. McKinley, and C. A. Hunter: A comparative study of methods of isolating *Mycobacterium tuberculosis*. (19), 1951, 41, 164.
Giroux, M.: Tuberculose expérimentale du hamster doré. (*Cricetus auratus*). (162), 1947, 12, 863.
Gissens-de Cavel, C.: Au sujet des méthodes d'isolement et de culture des bacilles de Koch. (204), 1949, 19, 309.
Gitterman, C. O., and S. G. Knight: Carbon dioxide fixation into amino acids of *Penicillium chrysogenum*. (135), 1952, 64, 223.

Gladstone, G. P., P. Fildes, and G. M. Richardson: Carbon dioxide as an essential factor in the growth of bacteria. (77), 1935, 16, 335.
Glover, R. E.: Infection of mice with *Mycobacterium tuberculosis* (*bovis*) by the respiratory route. (77), 1944, 25, 141.
———: Susceptibility of the golden hamster (*Cricetus auratus*) to *Mycobacterium tuberculosis hominis* and *bovis*. (77), 1946, 58, 107.
Göbel, H.: Über die Züchtung von Tb.-Bakterien in flüssigen Nährböden. Düsseldorf, 1948. Germany.
Goeters, W.: Verhandlungsbericht der 2. Nachkriegstagung der deutschen Tuberkulosegesellschaft. (63), 1950–1951, 104, 35.
Goetz, A.: Application of molecular filter membranes to the analysis of aerosols. (19), 1953, 43, 150.
Gözsy, B., and A. Szent-Györgyi: Über den Mechanismus der Hauptatmung des Taubenbrustmuskels. (241), 1934, 224, 1.
Goldie, H.: Acid-permanganate mixture for cleaning glassware contaminated with tubercle bacilli. (22), 1947a, 56, 59.
———: Use of Dubos medium for culture of *M. tuberculosis* from sputum. (191), 1947b, 65, 210.
Goldman, E. C., and D. S. Goldman: Cording and neutral red reaction of two avirulent strains of *Mycobacterium*. (22), 1956, 73, 674.
Gonzales Prendes, M. A., and A. Fors Carbonell: La microscopía fluorescente en leprología. (126), 1953, 21, 35.
Good, R. M.: Tuberculosis of the stomach. An analysis of cases recently reviewed. (47), 1931, 22, 415.
Goodpasture, E. W.: Use of chick embryo in investigation of certain pathological problems. (215), 1933, 26, 418.
———, and K. Anderson: The problem of infection as presented by bacterial invasion of the chorio-allantoic membrane of chick embryos. (17), 1937, 13, 149.
Goodpasture, E. W., A. M. Woodruff, and G. J. Buddingh: The cultivation of vaccine and other viruses in the chorio-allantoic membrane of chick-embryos. (212), 1931, 74, 371.
Gordonoff, T.: Physiologie und Pharmakologie des Expektorationsvorganges. (110), 1938, 40, 53.
Goth, A.: The antitubercular activity of aspergillic acid and its probable mode of action. (146), 1945, 30, 899.
Gotschlich, E., and J. Weigang: Über die Beziehungen zwischen Virulenz und Individuenzahl einer Cholera-Cultur. (235), 1895, 20, 376.
Gottsacker, E.: Die Kultur des Erregers der Tuberkulose. 5. Mitteilung. Die Differenzierung der Typen auf Eigelbnährböden. (245), 1950, 156, 351.
Goulding, R., M. B. King, R. Knox, and J. M. Robson: Relation between *in-vitro* and *in-vivo* resistance to isoniazid. (161), 1952, 263, 69.
Goyal, R. K.: Influence de la concentration de la glycérine et de l'asparagine sur le rendement en poids du bacille tuberculeux et sur le pH des cultures en milieu de Sauton. (98), 1936, 121, 1165.
Grady, E. D.: Cutaneous inoculation tuberculosis. A review of the literature and a report of eight cases. (22), 1951, 63, 526.
Graham, C. F.: Fluorescence microscopy of *Mycobacterium tuberculosis*. A study of basic factors. (22), 1943, 48, 421.
Granville, G. E., D. E. Jenkins, D. A. Cooley, M. E. DeBakey, F. C. Whitcomb, and B. Halpert: Cultural properties of *M. tuberculosis* in resected pulmonary lesions of patients treated with streptomycin and para-aminosalicylic acid. (22), 1953, 68, 727.
Grass, H.: Erleichterung des Tuberkelbazillennachweises durch Kehlkopfabstrich. (172), 1931, 78, 1171.
Gray, C. T.: The nature of the fatty acid metabolism of tubercle bacilli and other *Mycobacteria*. Ohio State University, Columbus, Ohio, 1949. U.S.A.

Gray, D. F.: Detection of small numbers of *Mycobacteria* in sections by fluorescence microscopy. (22), 1953, 68, 82.

———, and M. W. Mattinson: Detection of small numbers of tubercle bacilli from dispersed cultures, using mice, guinea pigs, and artificial media. (22), 1952, 65, 572.

Green, D. E.: The citric acid cycle and the cyclophorase system, in Respiratory enzymes, H. A. Lardy, ed. Burgess, Minneapolis, 1949. U.S.A.

Griffith, A. S.: Investigation of viruses obtained from cases of human tuberculosis (other than lupus). (208), 1911, Final Report, Vol. 1, Part 2, Appendix.

———. Further investigations of the type of tubercle bacilli occurring in the sputum of phthisical persons. (81), 1914, 1, 1171.

———: The bacteriological characteristics of tubercle bacilli from different kinds of human tuberculosis. (148), 1919–1920, 23, 129.

———: Tuberculosis of the domesticated species of animals. (138), 1928, 41, 53.

———: Die Tuberkelbazillentypen beim Lupus. (242), 1932, 64, 108.

———: The susceptibility of the golden hamster (*Cricetus auratus*) to bovine, humar and avian tubercle bacilli and to the vole strain of acid-fast bacillus (Wells). (143), 1939, 39, 154.

———: Further experiments on the golden hamster (*Cricetus auratus*) with tubercle bacilli and the vole strain of acid-fast bacillus (Wells). (143), 1941, 41, 260.

———, and W. T. Munro: Human pulmonary tuberculosis of bovine origin in Great Britain. (143), 1943, 43, 229.

Griffith, F.: The significance of pneumococcal types. (143), 1928, 27, 113.

Griffith, L. J., and S. A. Denaro: Assay of tuberculous contamination on eating utensils of patients with tubercle bacilli in sputum. (22), 1956, 74, 462.

Grimme, A.: Die wichtigsten Methoden der Bakterienfärbung in ihrer Wirkung auf die Membran, den Protoplasten und die Einschlüsse der Bakterienzelle. (245), 1902, 32, 1, 81, 161, 241, 321.

Gróh, E.: Über das gleichzeitige Vorkommen von humanen und bovinen Bacillen bei der Tuberkulose der Rinder. (235), 1940, 122, 62.

Grove, M. O'L., and A. Walker: Coproporphyrin 3 isolated from the human tubercle bacillus by chromatographic and fluorescence analysis. Fluorescence and absorption spectral data. (77), 1951, 32, 1.

Grün, H., and W. Klinner: Die experimentelle Tuberkulose der weissen Maus. (224), 1952, 322, 311.

Grün, L.: Zur Methodik der Prüfung desinfizierender Bohnerwachse. (172), 1952, 94, 1905.

Grumbach, A.: Der erbliche Einfluss auf Überlebensdauer, Organlokalisation und -manifestation im Tuberkuloseversuch. (210), 1949a, 12, 614.

———: Ergebnisse der Tuberkelbazillen-Typisierung in den Jahren 1946–1949, nebst grundsätzlichen Bemerkungen zur Typisierungsfrage. (211), 1949b, 6, 364.

———: Der erbliche Einfluss auf Überlebensdauer, Organlokalisation und -manifestation im Tuberkuloseversuch an C_3H-Mäusen. (210), 1952, 15, 715.

———: Tuberkuloseversuch an genetisch reinem Mäusematerial (C_3H). (86), 1953, 9, 167.

Guilliermond, A.: Contribution à l'étude cytologique des Bacilles endosporés. (55), 1908, 12, 9.

———: A propos des corpuscles métachromatiques ou grains de volutine. (55), 1910, 19, 289.

———: Nouvelles observations sur la structure des bactéries. (98), 1933, 113, 1095.

Gunn, F. D., W. J. Nungester, and E. P. Hougen: Susceptibility of the white mouse to tuberculosis. (191), 1933–1934, 31, 527.

Gutiérrez-Vázquez, J. M.: Studies on the rate of growth of *Mycobacteria*. 1. Generation time of *Mycobacterium tuberculosis* on several solid and liquid media and effects exerted by glycerol and malachite green. (22), 1956, 74, 50.

Gutstein, M.: Das Ektoplasma der Bakterien. 1. Über eine allgemeine Methode zur Darstellung des Ektoplasmas der grampositiven Bakterien. (245), 1924, 93, 393.

Haag, F. E.: Über die Bedeutung von Doppelbindungen in Paraffin des Handels für das Wachstum von Bakterien. (51), 1926, 97, 28.
———: Die saprophytischen Mykobakterien. (247), 1927, 71, 1.
Häflinger, E.: Untersuchungen über das Zonenwachstum der Tuberkelbazillen im halbstarren Nährboden nach Lange. (245), 1939, 143, 238.
Hagemann, P.: Fluoreszenzmikroskopischer Nachweis von Leprabakterien im Nasenschleim und im Blut. (103), 1937, 63, 514.
———: Fluoreszenzfärbung von Tuberkelbakterien mit Auramin. (172), 1938, 85, 1066.
Hahn, F. E.: Über Kernäquivalente und Reduktionsorte in Bakterien. (176), 1952, 39, 527.
Hailer, E.: Die Einwirkung keimtötender Stoffe auf Tuberkelbacillen des *Typus humanus* und *bovinus*. 1. Die Wirkung von anorganischen Säuren und Säuren der aliphatischen Reihe. (235), 1938, 120, 663.
Haitinger, M., and H. Hamperl: Die Anwendung des Fluoreszenzmikroskops zur Untersuchung tierischer Gewebe. (129), 1933, 33, 193.
Hall, H. E., E. W. Hawthorne, and L. M. Marshall: Carbon dioxide fixation by rat heart muscle *in vivo*. (18), 1953, 173, 335.
Hall, W. H., and D. F. Gleason: A bacteriologic and pathologic study of tuberculous lesions resected from 119 patients after chemotherapy. (220), 1953, 12th Conference, p. 219.
Halvorson, H. O., and N. R. Ziegler: Application of statistics to problems in bacteriology. 1. A means of determining bacterial population by the dilution method. (135), 1933, 25, 101.
Hammarsten, O.: Zur Kenntnis der Nucleoproteide. (241), 1894, 19, 19.
Hammerschlag, A.: Bakteriologisch-chemische Untersuchungen über Tuberkelbacillen. (250), 1891, 12, 9.
Harman, J. W.: Studies on mitochondria. 2. The structure of mitochondria in relation to enzymatic activity. (113), 1950, 1, 394.
Harris, S., and T. N. Harris: Effect of cortisone and some reactions of hypersensitivity in laboratory animals. (191), 1950, 74, 186.
Hart, P. D'A., D. A. Long and R. J. W. Rees: Depression of tuberculin sensitivity in guinea-pigs by certain antituberculous surface-active agents. (81), 1952, 1, 680.
Hart, P. D'A., and R. J. W. Rees: Enhancing effect of cortisone on tuberculosis in the mouse. (161), 1950, 259, 391.
———: Changes in morphology of an avirulent strain of *Mycobacterium tuberculosis* under the influence of non-ionic surface-active agents. (140), 1954, 10, 150.
Hasché, E., and P. Loch: Quantitatives über die Einwirkung von Kurzwellen auf Bakterien. (235), 1938, 120, 209.
Hauduroy, P.: Bacilles tuberculeux et paratuberculeux. Masson, Paris, 1950. France.
———, G. Bouvier, and W. Rosset: Nouvelle technique de découverte des bacilles tuberculeux dans des produits pathologiques. (98), 1945, 139, 354.
Hauduroy, P., and Y. Posternak: Recherche des bacilles tuberculeux dans les expectorations par la microscopie en fluorescence. (98), 1941, 135, 755.
Hauduroy, P., and Y. Posternak-Gallia: Sur une réaction cytochimique en rapport avec la virulence des Mycobactéries. (29), 1949, 77, 91.
Hauduroy, P., and W. Rosset: Culture des différentes variétés de Mycobactéries en milieu de Dubos. (98), 1947, 141, 169.
———: Sensibilité du hamster au bacille BCG. (185), 1951, 59, 121.
Hay, D. R.: Multiple sputum cultures in the assessment of pulmonary tuberculosis. (217), 1956, 11, 209.
Hedvall, E.: Bovine tuberculosis in man. (2), 1941, Supplement 135.
Heidelberger, M., and A. E. O. Menzel: Specific and non-specific cell polysaccharides of a human strain of tubercle bacillus, H-37. (136), 1937, 118, 79.
Henley, R. R.: The influence of iron on the growth of the tubercle bacillus upon glycerinated beef broth. (22), 1925, 12, 246.
———: The reaction and growth curves of cultures of tubercle bacilli. (22), 1926, 13, 107.

———: Dextrose in synthetic media for the tubercle bacillus. (22), 1929, 19, 660.
———, and P. W. LeDuc: Ammonium malate as a source of nitrogen for tubercle bacilli in cultures. (22), 1930, 22, 568.
———: Growth and metabolism of tubercle bacilli. The role of the source and proportion of the nitrogen in the medium. (22), 1939, 40, 313.
Hennessen, W., L. Grünn, and E. Lindner: Der Einfluss des zwischen Nährboden und Kultur liegenden Objektfilms auf das Wachstum von Bakterien. (245), 1950, 156 381.
Henry, G.: Une méthode nouvelle pour le dépistage des expectorations bacillifères (185), 1946, 1, 796.
Henry, H., and M. Stacey: Histochemistry of the Gram-staining reaction for micro-organisms. (175), 1943, 151, 671.
———, and E. G. Teece: Nature of the Gram-positive complex in micro-organisms. (175), 1945, 156, 720.
Henry, R. J.: The mode of action of sulfonamides. (61), 1943, 7, 175.
———, and E. C. Smith: Use of sulfuric acid-dichromate mixture in cleaning glassware. (212), 1946, 104, 426.
Heplar, J. Q.: Respiratory quotients of tubercle bacilli at low oxygen tension. (22), 1953, 67, 669.
———, C. E. Clifton, S. Raffel, and C. M. Futrelle: Virulence of the tubercle bacillus. 1. Effect of oxygen tension upon respiration of virulent and avirulent bacilli. (145), 1954, 94, 90.
Herrmann, W.: Der Nachweis von Tuberkelbazillen mit dem Fluoreszenzmikroskop. (103), 1938, 64, 1354.
———: Beiträge zur Tuberkelbakterienkultur. 2. Die Kultivierung von Tuberkelbakterien mittels flüssiger, modifizierter Kirchner-Substrate. (235), 1949, 129, 146.
Herrold, R. D.: Egg-yolk agar medium for the growth of tubercle bacilli. (145), 1931, 48, 236.
Hershey, A. D., and M. Chase: Independent functions of viral protein and nucleic acid in growth of bacteriophage. (141), 1952–1953, 36, 39.
Hertzberg, G.: The infectiousness of human tuberculosis. (6), 1957. Supplement 38.
Herwerden, M. A. van: Über die Nucleasewirkung auf tierische Zelle. Ein Beitrag zur Chromidienfrage. (50), 1913, 10, 431.
———: Über die Nuklease als Reagens auf die Nukleinsäureverbindungen der Zelle. (26), 1914–1915, 47, 312.
———: On the nature and the significance of volutin in yeast cells. (160), 1918, 20, 70.
Hes, J. W.: Action de l'acide carbonique sur les microbes hétérotrophes. (31), 1938, 4, 547.
Hesse, W.: Über die gasförmigen Stoffwechselproducte beim Wachstum der Bakterien. (235), 1893, 15, 17.
———: Ein neues Verfahren zur Züchtung des Tuberkelbacillus. (235), 1899, 31, 502.
———: Ein neuer elektiver Nährboden für Auswurf-Tuberkelbacillen. (245), 1904, 35, 384.
Hettsche, H. O., and B. Weber: Die Ursache der bakteriziden Wirkung von *Mesentericus* Filtraten. (51), 1940, 123, 69.
Hillier, J., G. Knaysi, and R. F. Baker: New preparation techniques for the electron microscopy of bacteria. (135), 1948, 56, 569.
Hillier, J., S. Mudd, A. G. Smith, and E. H. Beutner: The "fixation" of electron microscopic specimens by the electron beam. (135), 1950, 60, 641.
Hinshaw, H. C.: Cooperative clinical research in tuberculosis. (22), 1953, 68, 263.
———, and W. H. Feldman: Evaluation of chemotherapeutic agents in clinical tuberculosis. A suggested procedure. (22), 1944, 50, 202.
Hirsch, A.: Sur le pouvoir bactériostatique de l'acide oléique et des acides gras non saturés. (98), 1947, 141, 222.
Hirsch, J.: Zur Biochemie pathogener Erreger. Wachstum und Stoffwechselleistungen

des *Vibrio cholerae* auf einfachen, chemisch definierten Nährböden. (235), 1926, 106, 433.
———: Die allgemeinen energetischen und chemischen Grundlagen der bakteriellen Assimilation und Dissimilation. (245), 1931, 122, 32.
———: Zur experimentellen Chemotherapie der Isonicotinsäurehydrazid (I.N.H.)-resistenten Tuberkulose. (176), 1952, 39, 525.
Hirsch, J. G.: Studies on egg-yolk growth factors for tubercle bacilli. (22), 1954, 70, 977.
Hoffman, H.: The cytochemistry of bacterial nuclear structures. The examination of the Feulgen nucleal, Piekarski-Robinow, and ribonuclease technics. (135), 1951, 62, 561.
Hoffman, E.: Die Bedeutung des Dunkelfelds für die Untersuchung des Gelbfieber-, Syphilis- und anderer Spirochäten sowie sonstiger Mikroorganismen und kleinster Gebilde in gefärbten Ausstrichen und Schnitten (Leuchtbildmethode). (66), 1921, 58, 73.
Hoffmann, N.: Fortzüchtung von Tuberkelbacillen auf Glycerinkartoffeln während zwei Jahre. (123), 1904, 14, 305.
Hogeboom, G. H., W. C. Schneider, and G. E. Pallade: The isolation of morphologically intact mitochondria from rat liver. (191), 1947, 65, 320.
Hohn, J.: Kultur der Tuberkelbazillen. (245), 1926, 98, 465.
———: Vier Jahre Kultur des Tuberkelbazillus zur Diagnose der Tuberkulose. (245), 1929, 113, 366.
Hollaender, A., and C. W. Emmons: Induced mutations and speciation in fungi. Cold Spring Harbor symposia on quantitative biology, New York, 1946, 11, 78. U.S.A.
Hollande, A. C., and G. Crémieux: Histochimie du bacille de Koch. (98), 1928, 98, 1529.
Holm, J.: Bacteriologic diagnosis of tuberculosis. (111), 1950, 3, 175.
———, and V. Lester: Diagnostic demonstration of tubercle bacilli. Comparison between cultivation and inoculation of guinea-pigs. (6), 1942, 16, 310.
Holmgren, N. B., and G. P. Youmans: Studies on the metabolism of virulent and avirulent *Mycobacteria.* (22), 1952, 66, 416.
Horvath, A.: Über den Einfluss der Ruhe und der Bewegung auf das Leben. (180), 1878, 17, 125.
Hotchkiss, R. D.: Bacterial transformation. (137), 1955, 45, Supplement 2, p. 1.
Hounslow, A. G., and G. Usher: Examination for tubercle bacilli by gastric lavage and by laryngeal swab: A comparative study. (221), 1948, 29, 25.
Howard, J. W.: Action lytique des extraits pancréatiques, spléniques et ganglionaires sur le bacille de Koch. (98), 1930, 104, 1028.
Hudgins, A., and R. A. Patnode: Effect of age of eggs on sensitivity of modified Löwenstein medium. (12), 1952, 22, 809.
Hudson, W. A., and H. A. Jarre: Cin-ex camera studies of the tracheobronchial tree (47), 1929, 19, 1236.
Hüne: Die Tuberkelbazillen-Anreicherung mittels Antiformin. (103), 1909, 35, 1791.
Hüppe, F.: Über Blutserum-Culturen. (245), 1887, 1, 607.
———: Über die Verwendung von Eiern zu Kulturzwecken. (245), 1888, 4, 80
Hughes, G. C.: An improved stain for fluorescence microscopy. (221), 1946, 27, 91.
Hughes, W. H.: Risk in routine tuberculosis investigations. (161), 1952, 263, 762.
Hurni, H., R. Hirt, and L. Ragaz: Die Wirkung von PAS (p-Aminosalicylsäure) und PAS Derivaten auf die experimentelle Mäusetuberkulose. Zugleich ein Beitrag zur Methodik der experimentellen Mäusetuberkulose. (210), 1951, 14, 17.
Hurwitz, C., and M. Silverman: Measurement of growth of tubercle bacilli by means of a spectrophotometer. (22), 1950, 62, 87.
Husemann, E., and H. Ruska: Die Sichtbarmachung von Molekülen des p-Iodobenzoyd glycogens. (176), 1940, 28, 534.
Hussel, L.: Über die Eignung des Goldhamsters als Versuchstier bei der Tuberkulose Diagnostik. (245), 1950, 156, 445.

Hylkema, B., and P. C. Onvlee: The addition of trisodiumphosphate solution to gastric lavages for the cultivation of *Mycobacterium tuberculosis.* (39), 1951, 17, 159.
Ibarra, J. P.: Valor de la baciloscopía negativa en clínica. (122), 1948, 8, 280.
Iland, C. N.: The effect of penicillin on the tubercle bacillus. (148), 1946, 58, 495.
Illemann-Larsen, G.: Resistance determination on tubercle bacilli in sputa with special reference to the Pryce method. (6), 1953, 28, 325.
Imšenecki, A.: Die Feulgen'sche Nuklealreaktion bei Bakterien und Hefen. (247), 1936, 94, 330.
Ingraham, M. A.: The bacteriostatic action of gentian violet and its dependence on the oxidation-reduction potential. (135), 1933, 26, 573.
———, and H. Steenbock: The relation of micro-organisms to carotenoids and vitamin A. 2. The production of carotenoids by *Mycobacterium phlei.* (67), 1935, 29, 2533.
Iterson, W. van: Some electron-microscopical observations on bacterial cytology. (69), 1947, 1, 527.
Ivánovics, G.: Unter welchen Bedingungen werden bei der Nährbodenzüchtung der Milzbrandbazillen Kapseln gebildt? (245), 1937, 138, 449.
Jackson, S., and T. W. Burrows: The virulence-enhancing effect of iron on non-pigmented mutants of virulent strains of *Pasteurella pestis.* (77), 1956, 37, 577.
Jacqué, L.: A propos des procédés de Hesse et de Spengler, pour la culture du bacille de la tuberculose. (245), 1904, 36, 461.
Jeener, R., and J. Brachet: Recherches sur la synthèse de l'acide pentosenucléique par les levures. Relations avec la fermentation et la respiration. (84), 1943, 29, 476.
Jennison, M. W., and G. P. Wadsworth: Evaluation of the errors involved in estimating bacterial numbers by the plating method. (135), 1940, 39, 389.
Jensen, K. A.: Reinzüchtung und Typenbestimmung von Tuberkelbazillenstämmen. Eine Vereinfachung der Methoden für die Praxis. (245), 1932, 125, 222.
———: Humane und bovine Formen der Tuberkelbazillen. (210), 1949, 12, Supplement 435; (91), 1949, 2, 299.
———, and J. Bindslev: Studies on the virulence and germinating percentage of tubercle bacilli in sputum. (6), 1946, 20, 46.
Jensen, K. A., G. Bindslev, and J. Holm: Experimental studies on the development of tuberculous infection in allergic and non-allergic animals. 1. Development of tuberculous infection in the lungs after inhalation of virulent tubercle bacilli. (6), 1935, 9, 27.
Jensen, K. A., and J. Frimodt-Möller: 1. Studies on the types of tubercle bacilli isolated from man. (6), 1934, 8, 153.
———: 2. Strains with attentuated virulence. (6), 1936a, 10, 83.
———: 3. Transformation of some atypical strains, non-pathogenic for rabbits, into bovine type through rabbit passages. (6), 1936b, 10, 217.
Jensen, K. A., and I. Kiaer: Tuberkuloseprophylaxe und -Therapie in experimenteller Beleuchtung. 1. Mitteilung. (4), 1943, 20, 133.
Jessen, F.: The eradication of tuberculosis. With special reference to its early diagnosis. (22), 1927, 16, 234.
Johannson, A.: Die Grundlagen einiger Bakterienfärbung. (245), 1938, 141, 424.
Johansson, K. R., and D. H. Ferris: Photography of airborne particles during bacteriological plating operations. (145), 1946, 78, 238.
Johnson, F. H.: Observations on the electron microscopy of *B. cereus,* and tyrothricin action. (135), 1944, 47, 551.
Jones, O. R., W. D. Platt, Jr., and L. A. Amill: Miliary tuberculosis caused by intravenous self-injection of tubercle bacilli, treated successfully with streptomycin therapy. (22), 1949, 60, 514.
Joseph, A. F. M.: Vergleichende Untersuchungen über neuere Färbeverfahren für Tuberkelbacillen. Inaugural-Dissertation, 1936. Münster, Germany.
Joussaume, Mornand, and Yalcin: La surveillance bactériologique des lésions tuberculeuses minimes du poumon. (185), 1952, 60, 1622.
Kabler, P., and R. Lundholm: Culture of tubercle bacilli from specimens of gastric juice. (12), 1949, 19, 685.

Bibliography

Kabuki, Y.: Über einen operativen Fall von Magentuberkulose. (105), 1942, 355, 1309.

Kahn, M. C.: A development cycle of the tubercle bacillus as revealed by single-cell studies. (22), 1929, 20, 150.

Kaiserling, C.: Über die Unterscheidung von Tuberkelbazillen in Luminiszenzmikroskop. (242), 1917, 27, 156.

Kallós, P., and L. Kallós-Deffner: Über den Nachweis der Tuberkulosebacillämie im Kultur- und Tierversuch. Kritische Übersicht. (248), 1932, 39, 145; (248), 1934, 41, 145.

Kallós, P., and E. Nathan: Über die Einwirkung menschlicher Sera auf humane Tuberkulosebazillen in der Kirchnerschen Tiefenkultur. (236), 1932, 76, 343.

Kamen, M. D., and L. P. Vernon: Comparative studies on bacterial cytochromes. (69), 1955, 17, 10.

Kaplan, A., J. Traum, and R. A. Bankowski: Correlation of the radioactivity of suspensions of tubercle bacilli with their turbidity. (Method of estimating of weight in doses of tubercle bacilli). (22), 1948, 58, 102.

Kaplan, E. H., J. Kennedy, and J. Davis: Effects of salicylate and other benzoates on oxidative enzymes of the tricarboxylic acid cycle in rat tissue homogenates. (45), 1954, 51, 47.

Karlson, A. G., and W. H. Feldman: The use of guinea pigs in studying chemotherapy of experimental tuberculosis. (36), 1949, 52, 637.

Karlson, A. G., and Y. Ikemi: Effect of isonicotinic acid hydrazide (isoniazid) on survival time of mice infected with tubercle bacilli resistant to the drug *in vitro*. (192), 1952, 27, 373.

———: Comparison of the virulence for mice and guinea pigs of an isoniazid-sensitive tubercle bacillus and its isoniazid-resistant variant. (192), 1954, 29, 119.

Kassel, R., and S. Levitan: A jugular technique for the repeated bleeding of small animals. (212), 1953, 118, 563.

Katunuma, N., and H. Nakasato: A study of the mechanism of the development of streptomycin resistant organisms by addition of the desoxyribonucleic acid prepared from resistant bacilli. (156), 1954, 29, 19. Abstract, (111), 1954, 7, 564.

Kaufmann, G., J. Wanner, and H. Amsler: Tuberkelbazillen in resezierten Lungenherden. (211), 1954, 11, 322.

Kausche, G. A., E. Pfankuch, and H. Ruska: Die Sichtbarmachung von pflanzlichen Virus im Übermikroskop. (176), 1939, 27, 292.

Keil, R., E. Botta, and I. Stephan: Über Aggressivitätssteigerung des Tuberkuloseerregers durch Mucin beim Goldhamster. (102), 1953, 8, 729.

Keilin, D.: On cytochrome, a respiratory pigment, common to animals, yeast and higher plants. (190), 1925, 98, 312.

———: Cytochrome and intracellular respiratory enzymes. (109), 1933, 2, 239.

———, and E. F. Hartree: Cytochrome and cytochrome oxidase. (190), 1939, 127, 167.

Keilty, R. A.: A study of the cultivation of tubercle bacillus directly from the sputum by the method of Petroff. (139), 1915, 22, 612.

Kellenberger, E., and G. H. Werner: L'action antibiotique de la streptomycine étudiée au microscope électronique. (112), 1948, 4, 440.

Keller, C. J.: Vereinfachter Nachweis von Tuberkelbazillen im Fluoreszenzlicht. (172), 1938, 85, 2024.

Kempner, W.: Oxygen tension and the tubercle bacillus. (22), 1939, 40, 157.

Kendall, A. I., A. A. Day, and A. W. Walker: The metabolism of saprophytic human tubercle bacilli in plain, dextrose, mannite and glycerin broths. Studies in acid-fast bacteria. (145), 1914, 15, 417, 423, 433.

Kennedy, E. P., and A. L. Lehninger: Intracellular structures and the fatty acid oxidase system of rat liver. (136), 1948, 172, 847.

———: Oxidation of higher fatty acids by isolated rat liver mitochondria. (114), 1949, 8, 213.

Khodukin, N. I.: Elektronnaia mikroskopia v mikrobiologii. (225), 1948, 26, 599.

King, H. K., and H. Alexander: The mechanical destruction of bacteria. (140), 1948, 2, 315.

Kirby, W. M. M., and R. J. Dubos: Effect of penicillin on the tubercle bacillus *in vitro*. (191), 1947, 66, 120.

Kirchensteins, A.: Sur la structure et le mode de développement des bactéries. (98), 1921, 85, 787.

———: Sur la structure et le mode de développement du bacille tuberculeux. (29), 1922, 36, 416.

Kirchheimer, W. F., A. R. Hess, E. M. Williston, and G. P. Youmans: Isolation of tubercle bacilli from feces and gastric contents of intravenously infected mice. (22), 1950, 62, 481.

Kirchheimer, W. F., and S. Malkiel: Tuberculin shock in mice infected with tubercle bacilli. (22), 1953, 68, 629.

Kirchner, M.: Experimentelles zur Prüfung der Frage, inwieweit der Lupus auf humaner oder boviner Infektion beruht. (242), 1922, 36, 482.

Kirchner, O.: Die Fortzüchtung wenig virulenter Tuberkelbacillen, insbesondere des BCG in der Cornea. (63), 1928, 69, 180.

———: Besitzen Tuberkulose- und Nichttuberkulosesera ein bakterizides Vermögen gegenüber dem Tuberkelbazillus? (236), 1932a, 74, 56.

———: Die Leistungsfähigkeit der Tiefenkultur des Tuberkelbazillus bei Verwendung besonders geeigneter flüssinger Nährboden. (245), 1932b, 124, 403.

———, and B. D. Li: Erfahrungen mit der Bestimmung der Keimzahl in Tuberkelbacillenaufschwemmungen. (63), 1932, 80, 454.

Kirkpatrick, P.: An approach to X-ray microscopy. (175), 1950, 166, 251.

Kitasato, S.: Gewinnung von Reinculturen der Tuberkelbacillen und anderer pathogener Bacterien aus Sputum. (235), 1892, 11, 441.

Kite, J. H., Jr., R. A. Patnode, and T. Read, Jr.: Distinguishing saprophytic from virulent *Mycobacteria* by intracutaneous inoculation of guinea pigs. (12), 1952, 22, 250.

Klebs: Zur Geschichte der Tuberkulose. (224), 1870, 49, 291.

Kleiber, M.: The tidal air of laboratory animals. (212), 1944, 99, 542.

Klein, G. C., M. Maltz, M. M. Cummings, and C. H. Fish: Efficacy of centrifugation as a method of concentrating tubercle bacilli. (12), 1952, 22, 581.

Klein, D. T., and R. M. Klein: Transmittance of tumor-inducing ability to avirulent crown-gall and related bacteria. (135), 1953, 66, 220.

Klieneberger, E.: Natural occurrence of pleuropneumonia-like organisms in apparent symbiosis with *Streptobacillus moniliformis* and other bacteria. (148), 1935, 40, 93.

Klieneberger-Nobel, E.: Morphological appearances of various stages in *B. proteus* and *coli*. (143), 1947, 45, 410.

———: Methods for the study of the cytoplasm of bacteria and pleuropneumonia-like organisms. (196), 1950, 91, 340.

Kligler, I. J.: A study of the antiseptic properties of certain organic compounds. (139), 1918, 27, 463.

Klose, F., H. Knothe, and R. Schürmann: Die Züchtung des *Mycobacterium tuberculosis* (*Typ. humanus* und *bovinus*) im bebrüteten Hühnerei. (60), 1951, 6, 881.

———: Über die Einwirkung von Antibiotika und Chemoterapeutika auf das *Mycobacterium tuberculosis typ. humanus* im bebrüteten Hühnerei. (60), 1952, 7, 102.

Knaysi, G.: The cytology and microchemistry of *Mycobacterium tuberculosis*. (145), 1929, 45, 13.

———: Cytology of bacteria. (75), 1938, 4, 83.

———, and R. F. Baker: Demonstration, with the electron microscope, of a nucleus in *Bacillus mycoides* grown in a nitrogen free medium. (135), 1947, 53, 539.

Knaysi, G., J. Hillier, and C. Fabricant: The cytology of an avian strain of *Mycobacterium tuberculosis* studied with the electron and light microscopes. (135), 1950, 60, 423.

Knöll, H.: Zur Anwendung der Phasenkontrastmikroskopie in der Bakteriologie. (230), 1944, 5, 38.

———, and K. Zapf: Untersuchungen zum Problem des Bakterienzellkerns. (245), 1951, 157, 389.

Koch, R.: Die Aetiologie der Tuberculose. (66), 1882, 19, 221; (170), 1884, 2, 1.

———: Über neue Tuberkulinpräparate. (103), 1897, 23, 209.

———: Das Verhältnis zwischen Menschen- und Rindertuberkulose. (66), 1908, 45, 2001.

———: Die Bekämpfung der Tuberkulose unter Berücksichtigung der Erfahrungen, welche bei der erfolgreichen Bekämpfung anderer Infektionskrankheiten gemacht sind. Vortrag . . . Britischer Tuberkulosecongress, 1901. Gesammelte Werke (collected works), Vol. 1, p. 566. Georg Thieme, Leipzig, 1912a. Germany.

———, and Schütz: Vortrag. Gesammelte Werke (collected works), Vol. 2, Part 2, p. 1064. Georg Thieme, Leipzig, 1912b. Germany.

Köhler, A.: Mikrophotographische Untersuchungen mit ultraviolettem Licht. (243), 1904, 21, 129, 273.

———, and W. Loos: Das Phasenkontrastverfahren und seine Anwendung in der Mikroskopie. (176), 1941, 29, 49.

Kölbel, H.: Quantitative Untersuchungen über die Farbstoffspeicherung von Acridinorange in lebenden und toten Hefezellen und ihre Beziehung zu den elektrischen Verhältnissen der Zelle. (239), 1947, 2b, 381.

———: Untersuchungen am *Mycobacterium tuberculosis.* 1. Säurefestigkeit, Vermehrung und Granulationen. (235), 1951, 133, 45.

———: Die fluoreszenzmikroskopische Methode für die Darstellung und den Nachweis des *Mycobacterium tuberculosis.* (243), 1952, 61, 142.

———: 2. Mitteilung. Granulum und Vakuole bei licht- und elektronenmikroskopischer Abbildung. (239), 1953, 86, 631.

König, H.: Erfahrungen mit der Erstzüchtung von Tb.-Bazillen auf dem Dubosschen Nährmedium. (1), 1948, 7, 1.

———, and A. Winkler: Über Einschlüsse in Bakterien und ihre Veränderung im Elektronenmikroskop. (176), 1948, 35, 136.

König, J.: Über den Tuberkelbakteriennachweis in Gewebeausstrichen mit Hilfe der Färbung nach Osol und der Auraminfluoreszenzmethode. (168), 1951, 6, 286.

Königstein, R. P., P. S. Cheng, L. Königstein, and I. D. Suen: Zur Objektträgerkultur des Tuberkelbazillus. (226), 1951, 63, 723.

Kohn, H. J., and S. S. Harris: On the mode of action of the sulfonamides. 1. Action on *Escherichia coli.* (149), 1941, 73, 343.

Kolle, W., and H. Schlossberger: Chemotherapeutische Versuche bei Tuberkulose. (235), 1923, 100, 107.

———, and W. Pfannenstiel: Tuberkulose-Studien. 4. Über die Tierpathogenität der Gruppe der säurefesten Bakterien. Tierpassagen, Virulenzsteigerung und kulturelles Verhalten. (103), 1921, 47, 437.

Kondo, S.: Der Verwendungsstoffwechsel säurefester Bakterien. 3. Mitteilung: Die Nahrungsbedürfnisse des Hühnertuberkelbazillus; sein Wachstum beim Aufbau aus einfachen chemischen Verbindungen. (68), 1924, 153, 302.

———: Der Verwendungsstoffwechsel säurefester Bakterien. 4. Mitteilung: Der Verwendungsstoffwechsel der Tuberkelbazillen des *Typus humanus* und *Typus bovinus.* (68), 1925, 155, 148.

Kopper, P. H.: Studies of bacterial reducing activity in relation to age of culture. (135), 1952, 63, 639.

Korns, J. H., and G. Y. C. Lu: Susceptibility of the hamster to tuberculous infection. (191), 1927, 24, 807.

———: The diagnosis of tuberculosis by means of the hamster. (22), 1928, 17, 279.

Kossel, A.: Über die Nucleinsäure. (54), 1893, p. 157.

Kostenitsch, J., and M. Wolkow: Contribution à l'étude de la tuberculose aviaire chez le lapin. (43), 1893, 5, 169.

Kotani, S., T. Tsujimoto, K. Takeuchi, and T. Seki: Investigations of a modified slide cell culture method for quantitative studies on tuberculosis immunity. (111), 1954, 7, 563.

Kourilsky, R., and E. Coulaud: Effets des réinfections tuberculeuses sur l'allergie tuberculinique du cobaye. (98), 1952, 146, 197.
Kramer, C. H.: Effect of human gastric juice on tubercle bacilli. With special reference to the diagnosis of active pulmonary tuberculosis. (22), 1946, 53, 385.
Krebs, H. A.: Intermediate metabolism of carbohydrates. (175), 1936, 138, 288.
———: Carbon dioxide assimilation in heterotrophic organisms. (37), 1943, 12, 529.
———: Cyclic processes in living matter. (108), 1946, 12, 88.
———, and L. V. Eggleton: Biological synthesis of oxalacetic acid from pyruvic acid and carbon dioxide. (67), 1940, 34, 1383.
Krebs, H. A., and W. A. Johnson: The rôle of citric acid in intermediate metabolism in animal tissues. (108), 1937, 4, 148.
Kresling, K.: Über die Fettsubstanz der Tuberkelbazillen. (245), 1901, 30, 897.
Kretschmer, O. S.: The Gram property of the acid-fast form of the tubercle bacillus. (146), 1934, 19, 350.
Krieg, A.: Nachweis von Kernäquivalenten bei Bakterien *in vivo*. 4. Mitteilung: *Corynebacterium* und *Mycobacterium*. (235), 1954a, 139, 64.
———: Personal communication, 1954b.
Kröger, E.: Versuche zur Verbesserung des bakteriologischen Nachweises und zur Resistenzprüfung von Tuberkelbakterien. (227), 1950, 100, 586.
———, and M. Rosarius: Zur Verwendung von schnellen Zentrifugieren in der Methodik des Tuberkelbazillennachweises. (245), 1949, 154, 213.
Krönig, B., and T. Paul: Die chemischen Grundlagen der Lehre von der Giftwirkung und Desinfection. (235), 1897, 25, 1.
Krompecher, E., and K. Zimmerman: Untersuchungen über die Virulenz der aus verschiedenen tuberkulösen Herden des Menschen reingezüchteten Tuberkelbacillen. (245), 1903, 33, 580.
Krumwiede, C., Jr., and J. S. Pratt: Observations on the growth of bacteria on media containing various anilin dyes. (139), 1914, 19, 20, 501.
Krzyzanowska, S.: De la centrifugation des bactéries en suspension dans l'eau. Bern, 1899. Switzerland.
Kubica, G. P., H. M. Randall, and D. W. Smith: A chemical comparison of recently isolated strains of *Mycobacterium tuberculosis var. hominis*. A preliminary report. (173), 1955.
Kühne, W.: Erfahrungen über Albumosen und Peptone. (232), 1892, 29, 1.
———: 5. Weitere Untersuchungen über die Proteine des Tuberkulins. (232), 1894, 30, 221.
Kuei-Chh'ing, C. L., Shih-Hsuan, and C. Tsung-Yu: A study of the liquid media for growth of *Mycobacterium tuberculosis* by the slide culture method. (100), 1955, 73, 15.
Künzel, K. E.: Beitrag zum kulturellen Nachweis von Tuberkelbazillen. (245), 1950, 156, 235.
Kürsteiner, E.: Zur Frage der bakteriologischen Diagnose der Tuberkulose durch das Kulturverfahren, mit besonderer Berücksichtigung des Dubosschen Nährbodens. (210), 1950, 13, 340.
Kuhn, R., and D. Jerchel: Über Invertseifen. 8. Mitteilung. Reduktion von Tetrazolium-Salzen durch Bakterien, gärende Hefe und keimende Samen. (65), 1941, Abteilung B, 949.
Kull, F. C., and M. R. Grimm: Growth of *Mycobacterium tuberculosis var. hominis* in agitated culture. (135), 1952, 64, 431.
Kulpe, W.: Beitrag zur fluoreszenzmikroskopischen Untersuchung lebender Organe. (224), 1955, 327, 252.
Kunitz, M.: Crystalline ribonuclease. (141), 1940, 24, 15.
———: Isolation of crystalline desoxyribonuclease from beef pancreas. (212), 1948, 108, 19.
Kurnick, N. B.: Methylgreen-pyronin. 1. Basis of selective staining of nucleic acids. (141), 1950, 33, 243.

Lagergren, B., and A. R. Frisk: Evaluation of an improved Dubos medium for routine diagnostic examination of tubercle bacilli. (6), 1950, 25, 86.
Laki, K., F. B. Straub, and A. Szent-Györgyi: Über die Atmungskatalyse durch C_4-Dikarbonsäuren. (Vorlänfige Mitteilung). (241), 1937, 247, I.
Lamanna, C., and M. F. Mallette: The relation of the Gram stain to the cell wall and the ribonucleic acid content of the cell. (135), 1950, 60, 499.
Lange, B.: Untersuchungen über die experimentelle Tuberkulose bei weissen Mäusen. (235), 1922, 98, 229.
———: Die Feststellung der Zahl lebender Tuberkelbazillen in einer Bazillenaufschwemmung durch das Kulturverfahren und Vergleich dieser Ergebnisse mit dem Infektionserfolg. (242), 1926, 46, 455.
———: Zur Frage der Virulenz der bei menschlicher und tierischer Tuberkulose vorkommenden Tuberkelbazillen. Versuch an Meerschweinchen, Mäusen und Kaninchen. (242), 1930, 57, 129, 209.
———: Zur Frage der Virulenz der Tuberkelbazillen. (236), 1932, 74, 7.
———: Die Bakteriologie der tuberkulösen Meningitis. (63), 1939, 93, 273.
———, and K. H. Keschischian: Experimentelle Untersuchungen über die Bedeutung der Tröpfeninfektion bei der Tuberkulose. (235), 1925, 104, 256.
Lange, B., and W. Nowosselsky: Experimentelle Untersuchungen über die Bedeutung der Staubinfektion bei der Tuberkulose. (235), 1925, 104, 286.
Lange, L., and P. Nitsche: Eine neue Methode des Tuberkelbazillennachweises. (103), 1909, 35, 435.
———: Die Tuberkelbazillen. (245), 1932, 127, 10.
Langecker, H.: Das Schicksal der Citronensäure im Organismus des Kaninchens. (68), 1934, 273, 43.
Langer, H.: Die Abgrenzung der offenen Tuberkulose im frühen Kindesalter. (246), 1933, 111, 253.
Laporte, R.: Contribution à l'étude des bacilles paratuberculeux. 1. Propriétés pathogènes. (29), 1940, 65, 282.
Larmola, E.: On the pathogenicity and changeability of strains of *Mycobacterium tuberculosis*. (6), 1947, 21, 292.
Larson, L. W., and W. P. Larson: Factors governing the fat content of bacteria and the influence of fat on pellicle formation. (145), 1922, 31, 407.
Larson, W. P.: The influence of the surface tension of the culture medium on bacterial growth. (191), 1921–1922, 19, 62.
———, W. F. Cantwell, and T. B. Hartzell: The influence of the surface tension of the culture medium on the growth of bacteria. (145), 1919, 25, 41.
Larson, W. P., and I. A. Montank: The effect of wetting on the pathogenicity and viability of the tubercle bacillus. (191), 1923, 20, 229.
Laser, H.: Adaptation of *Bacillus subtilis* to fatty acids. (67), 1953, 51, 57.
Laug, E. P.: Retention of bichromate by glassware after exposure to potassium bichromate cleaning solution. (124), 1934, 6, 111.
Lavollay, J.: Les oligo-éléments dans la nutrition et la croissance des microorganismes. (125, Microbiology) Sixth, Rome, 1953, p. 151. Italy.
Lebeurre, R.: L'emploi des isotopes radioactifs pour l'étude expérimentale de la tuberculose. (205), 1956, 20, 813.
Lederberg, J.: Recombination mechanisms in bacteria. (137), 1955, 45, Supplement 2, p. 75.
———, and E. L. Tatum: Sex in bacteria. Genetic studies, 1945–1952.
———: Sex in microorganisms. Symposium. American association for the advancement of science, Washington, D.C., 1954, p. 12. U.S.A.
Lee, H. F.: Use of the chick embryo for preliminary *in vivo* evaluation of tuberculostatic substances. (36), 1949, 52, 692.
———, and A. B. Stavitsky: Intravenous infection of the chick embryo with tubercle bacilli. Inhibitory effects of streptomycin. (22), 1947, 55, 262.
———, and M. P. Lee: A chick embryo technique for intravenous and chemotherapeutic studies. (191), 1946, 61, 143.

Lehmann, H.: Das Luminiszenz-Mikroskop, seine Grundlagen und seine Anwendungen. (243), 1913, 30, 417.

Lehmann, J.: Determination of pathogenicity of tubercle bacilli by their intermediate metabolism. (161), 1946a, 250, 14.

———: Para-aminosalicylic acid in the treatment of tuberculosis. (161), 1946b, 250, 15.

Lembke, A.: Untersuchungen an den Erregern der Tuberkulose. (245), 1947, 152, 239.

———: Haben Bakterien einen Zellkern? (245), 1950–1951, 156, 377.

———, and H. Lück: Strukturuntersuchungen an Mikroorganismen. 2. Organische Inhaltbestandteile der Bakterienzelle. (245), 1950–1951, 156, 39.

Lembke, A., and H. Ruska: Vergleichende mikroskopische und übermikroskopische Beobachtungen an den Erregern der Tuberkulose. (158), 1940, 19, 217.

Léon-Kindberg, M., G. Lapiné, and B. Adida: Recherche du bacille de Koch par le prélèvement direct: cathétèrisme bronchique et division des crachats. (205), 1937, 3, 471.

Lepeshinskaia, O. B.: Razvitie zhiznennykh processov v dokletochnom periode. Akademia Nauk (Academy of Sciences), Moscow, 1952. U.S.S.R.

Lesne, E., G. Dreyfus-See, and A. Saenz: Recherches sur la contagiosité de la tuberculose pulmonaire du jeune enfant. (178), 1938, 26, 69.

Lester, V.: Saprophytic acid-fast bacilli as a source of error in diagnostic work. (6), 1939, 13, 251.

Lester, W., Jr., O. H. Robertson, and T. T. Puck: The rate of bactericidal action of triethylene glycol vapor on microorganisms dispersed into the air in small droplets. (14), 1949, 50, 174.

Leston, J. M., J. B. Gómez, and A. Cetrángolo: Valor de los cultivos e inoculaciones del esputo y contenido gástrico para el tratamiento y el pronóstico de la tuberculosis pulmonar. (24), 1950, 12, 139.

Levaditi, C.: La spirillose des embryons de poulet dans ses rapports avec la tréponémose héréditaire de l'homme. (29), 1906, 20, 924.

———, and A. Vaisman: Méningite tuberculeuse expérimentale de la souris. Effets de la streptomycine. (98), 1948, 142, 306.

———, and L. Barrat: Cavernes tuberculeuses pulmonaires chez les souris contaminées par le *Mycobacterium tuberculosis*. (98), 1950, 144, 1663.

Levaditi, J. C., R. O. Prudhomme, and J. Augier: Comparison des spectres d'absorption des écrans et des spectres d'absorption et d'émission des fluorochromes au cours de la microscopie en fluorescence. (29), 1948, 75, 217.

Levin, W., G. R. Brandon, and S. McMillen: The culture method of laboratory diagnosis of tuberculosis. (19), 1950, 40, 1305.

Levinthal, W.: Tuberkuloseinfektion von Meerschweinchen mit kleinsten Bacillenmengen. (235), 1927, 107, 387.

Lévy, P. P.: Action sur le virage globulaire des bacilles de Koch et des bacilles paratuberculeux cultivés en milieu de Dubos. (98), 1951, 145, 94.

Lewis, I. M.: The cytology of bacteria. (61), 1941, 5, 181.

Ley, H. L., and H. Mueller: On the isolation from agar of an inhibitor for *Neisseria gonorrhoeae*. (135), 1946, 52, 4.

Liborius, P.: Beiträge zur Kenntnis des Sauerstoffbedürfnisses der Bacterien. (235), 1886, 1, 115.

Lieb, F.: Ein Beitrag zum Stickstoff-Stoffwechsel des Typhusbazillus. (245), 1934, 132, 146.

Liebermann, L.: Nachweis der Metaphosphorsäure im Nuclein der Hefe. (180), 1890, 47, 155.

Liener, I. E., and D. L. Buchanan: The fixation of carbon dioxide by growing and nongrowing yeast. (135), 1951, 61, 527.

Limousin, H.: L'isolement des bacilles de Koch à partir des crachats tuberculeux d'après la méthode de Petrof. (29), 1921, 35, 558.

Lind, H. E., and H. J. Shaughnessy: Fluorescent staining technique for detection of acid-fast bacilli. (146), 1942, 27, 531.

Lindegren, C. C., and R. R. Mellon: Nuclear phenomena suggesting a sexual mechanism for the tubercle bacillus. (191), 1932, 30, 110.

Lindsay, M., T. V. O'Donnell, and N. L. Edson: The oxidation of pyruvate and fatty acids by *Mycobacterium ranae.* (67), 1950, 46, 248.

Linell, F., and A. Nordén: *Mycobacterium balnei.* A new acid-fast bacillus occurring in swimming pools and capable of producing skin lesions in humans. (6), 1954, Supplement 33.

Linhart, G. A.: The free energy of biological processes. (141), 1920, 2, 247.

Lipman, J. G., A. W. Blair, and H. C. McLean: Experiments on ammonia formation in presence of carbohydrates and other non-nitrogenous organic matter. (90), 1912, 246, 36.

Lippelt, H.: Experimentelle Studien und theoretische Betrachtungen zum Problem: Tuberkulose und ihre Erkennung durch Kulturverfahren und Tierversuch. (63), 1939, 93, 230.

Liquier-Milward, J.: Electron microscopy of thymonucleic acid. (69), 1953, 10, 5.

Lockemann, G.: Welche Nährstoffe sind für das Wachstum der Tuberkelbazillen unbedingt notwendig? (245), 1919, 83, 420.

Lodge, R. M., and C. N. Hinshelwood: Influence of magnesium on the lag phase in the growth of *Bact. lactis aerogenes* in synthetic media containing phosphate. (152), 1939, p. 1692.

Loebel, R. O., E. Shorr, and H. B. Richardson: The influence of foodstuffs upon the respiratory metabolism and growth of human tubercle bacilli. (135), 1933a, 26, 139.

———: The influence of adverse conditions upon the respiratory metabolism and growth of human tubercle bacilli. (135), 1933b, 26, 167.

Löwenstein, E.: Beitrag zur Leistungsfähigkeit der direkten Züchtung der Tuberkelbazillen aus dem infektiösen Material, mit einem Beitrag zur Geflügeltuberkulose im Menschen. (226), 1924, 37, 231.

———: Über Septikämie bei Tuberkulose. (242), 1925, 42, 177.

———: Die Methodik der Reinkultur von Tuberkelbazillen aus dem Blute. (103), 1930, 56, 1010.

Loll, W.: Über den Nachweis von Tuberkelbazillen im dicken Tropfen. (227), 1922, 72, 295.

Lominski, I., and E. M. Harper: An unidentified acid-fast bacillus (*Mycobaterium* sp., strain Glasgow) found in human sputum and lung lesions. (148), 1953, 65, 253.

Long, D. A., A. A. Miles, and W. L. M. Perry: Action of ascorbic acid on tuberculin-sensitivity in guinea pigs and its modification by dietary and hormonal factors. (161), 1951, 260, 1085.

Long, E. R.: A study in fundamentals of the nutrition of the tubercle bacillus: the utilization of some amino acids and ammonium salts. (22), 1919, 3, 86.

———: The nutrition of acid-fast bacteria. (22), 1921–1922, 5, 857.

———: Experimental mouse tuberculosis. (135), 1934, 27, 102, Abstract.

———: The hazard of acquiring tuberculosis in the laboratory. (19), 1951, 41, 782.

———, R. J. Anderson, D. Rittenberg, M. L. Karnovsky, and H. J. Henderson: The carbon metabolism of the tubercle bacillus. Studies with isotopic carbon. (22), 1955, 71, 609.

Long, E. R., and L. K. Campbell: The lipin content of acid-fast bacilli. (22), 1922–1923, 6, 636.

Long, E. R., and L. L. Finner: The relation of glycerol in culture media to the growth and chemical composition of tubercle bacilli. (22), 1927, 16, 523.

Long, E. R., and S. W. Holley: The origin of the epitheloid cell in experimental tuberculosis of cornea. (17), 1933, 9, 337.

———, and A. J. Vorwald: A comparison of the cellular reaction in experimental tuberculosis of the cornea in animals of varying resistance. (17), 1933, 9, 329.

Long, E. R., and F. B. Seibert: The chemical composition of the active principle of tuberculin. 1. A non-protein medium suitable for the production of tuberculin in large quantity. (22), 1926, 13, 393.

Lowry, H., and J. W. Berry: Further observations on the technic of slide culture of the tubercle bacillus. (12), 1950, 20, 273.
Lowys, P.: Note sur l'utilité et la simplicité du prélèvement laryngé chez l'enfant, pour la recherche du bacille de Koch et du pneumocoque. (205), 1949, 13, 90.
Lubenau, C.: Der Eigelbnährboden als Ersatz des Serums zur Kultur von Diphtherie- und Tuberkelbacillen. (123), 1907, 17, 1456.
Lucet, A.: Nouvelles recherches sur l'influence de l'agitation des bouillons de culture sur le développement du *Bacillus anthracis* et de quelques autres microbes. (197), 1914, 91, 137.
Lurie, M. B.: A comparison of the sodium hydroxide and antiformin methods for cultivating tubercle bacilli. (22), 1923, 7, 332.
———: Experimental epidemiology of tuberculosis. Air-borne contagion of tuberculosis in an animal room. (139), 1930, 51, 743.
———: Experimental epidemiology of tuberculosis. The prevention of natural air-borne contagion of tuberculosis in rabbits by ultraviolet irradiation. (131), 1944, 79, 559.
———: The efficiency of gauze masks in the protection of rabbits against the inhalation of droplet nuclei of tubercle bacilli. (22), 1949a, 59, 1.
———: Use of the rabbit in experimental chemotherapy of tuberculosis. (36), 1949b, 52, 627.
———, and P. Zappasodi: On the mode of action of cortisone on the pathogenesis of tuberculosis and its implications for the nature of genetic resistance to the disease, in Ciba Foundation, Symposium on experimental tuberculosis: Bacillus and Host. Little, Boston, 1955. U.S.A.
Luzzati, D.: Action des savons sur le bacille de Koch. Facteurs physico-chimiques. (99), 1950, 231, 308.
———: Action des agents tensioactifs sur le bacille de Koch. Action des savons sur la croissance. (29), 1952, 82, 744.
———: Action des agents tensioactifs sur le bacille de Koch. Fixation de l'oléate de sodium par les bactéries. (29), 1954, 87, 101.
Lwoff, A.: Étude sur les fonctions perdues. (31), 1936–1937, 2, 419.
———, and J. Monod: L'anhydride carbonique considéré comme substance indispensable aux microorganismes. La biosynthèse des acides dicarboxyliques. (99), 1946, 222, 696.
———: Essai d'analyse du rôle de l'anhydride carbonique dans la croissance microbienne. (29), 1947, 73, 323.
Maassen, W.: Beiträge zur Verträglichkeit und Wirksamkeit von Luftdesinfektionsmitteln. 5. Mitteilung. Zur Eignung von Euphagol zur Desinfektion der Luft. (235), 1954, 139, 195.
———, and H. Dietz: Bietet das Kulturverfahren bei der Untersuchung tuberkulöser Sputen einen Vorteil gegenüber der mikroskopischen Methode? (63), 1954, 112, 5.
MacCallum, P., J. C. Tolhurst, G. Buckle, and H. A. Sissons: A new mycobacterial infection in man. (148), 1948, 60, 93.
McCune, R. M., Jr., R. Tompsett, and W. McDermott: The fate of *Mycobacterium tuberculosis* in mouse tissues as determined by the microbial enumeration technique. 2. The conversion of tuberculous infection to the latent state by the administration of pyrazinamide and a companion drug. (139), 1956, 104, 763.
Macfarlane, M. G.: On the biochemical mechanism of action of gas-gangrene toxins. Mechanisms of microbial pathogenicity. Symposium. London, 1955, p. 57. England.
McGrady, M. H.: The numerical interpretation of fermentation-tube results. (145), 1915, 17, 183.
Machado Filho, J.: Aspétos chímicos do lavado pulmonar. (203), 1945, 11, 147.
McJunkin, F. A.: The solvent action of oleic acid on cultures of tubercle bacilli. (22), 1923–1924, 8, 393.
McKenzie, D., L. Malone, S. Kushner, J. S. Oleson, and Y. Subbarow: The effect of nicotinic acid on experimental tuberculosis of white mice. (146), 1948, 33, 1249.

McKinstry, R. N., and T. le Q. Blampied: Radiological examination of human contacts of the tuberculin positive cow. (221), 1955, 36, 16.

McLean, D. J., N. H. Robinson, and E. F. Purdie: The influence of the metabolic state and of the medium on carbon dioxide fixation by *Serratia marcescens*. (135), 1951, 61, 617.

MacMunn, C. A.: Researches on myohaematin and the histohaematins. (181), 1886, 177, Part 1, p. 267.

McNabb, A. L.: Cultural methods of isolation of tubercle bacilli. (19), 1936, 26, 619.

McNelly, E., and W. A. Riddell: Use of egg embryos in the culture of *Mycobacterium tuberculosis*. (19), 1949, 39, 1463.

McPhedran, F. M., and E. L. Opie: The spread of tuberculosis in families. (14), 1935, 22, 565.

MacVandiviere, H., W. H. Gentry, and H. S. Willis: A rapid chemical test of total viability for suspensions of tubercle bacilli. (22), 1952, 66, 95.

MacVandiviere, H., C. E. Smith, and E. J. Sunkes: An evaluation of four methods of collecting and mailing gastric washings for tubercle bacilli. (22), 1952, 65, 617.

Maffucci, A.: Über die tuberculöse Infection der Hühnerembryonen. Experimentelle Untersuchung. (245), 1889, 5, 237.

Magarão, M. P., H. Linhares, and A. Scorzelli, Jr.: Pesquisas do bacillo de Koch por meio de cultura e de inoculação. (200), 1948, 12, 109.

Magasanik, B., and E. Chargaff: Studies on the structure of ribonucleic acids. (69), 1951, 7, 396.

Malek, I., and J. Malkova: Evolution des cultures de bacilles tuberculeux en milieux additionnés d'acide oléique. (98), 1948a, 142, 1047.

———: Evolution des cultures de bacille tuberculeux en milieux additionnés de Tween 80. (98), 1948b, 142, 1049.

Malek, I., and J. Sterzl: Les substances nucléaires du bacille tuberculeux. (98), 1948, 142, 1053.

Mallett, G. E., H. Koffler, and J. N. Rinker: The effect of shaking on bacterial flagella and motility. (135), 1951, 61, 703.

Malmgren, B., and C.-G. Hedén: Nucleotide metabolism of bacteria and the bacterial nucleus. (175), 1947, 159, 577.

Manceaux, H. L.: Bacilles tuberculeux et sulfate de magnésie. (98), 1924, 91, 255.

Manfredi, L., and B. Frisco: Experimenteller Beitrag zur Kenntnis der Rolle der Lymphdrüsen als Schutzmittel gegen Tuberkulose. (246), 1903, 32, 295.

Mannsfeld, M.: Untersuchung über die Resistenz der Tuberkelbazillen im Abwasser. (5), 1937, 7, 153.

Marchal, J. G., and R. Nicot: Observations sur la méthode de Gram appliquée à des bactéries (Gram positives) après action de la ribonucléase. (98), 1949, 143, 1366.

Marie-Suzanne, Soeur: Culture du bacille de Stefansky sur embryon de poulet. (98), 1948, 142, 35.

Markham, R., and J. D. Smith: The structure of ribonucleic acids. 1. Cyclic nucleotides produced by ribonuclease and by alkaline hydrolysis. (67), 1952, 52, 552.

Marmorek, A.: Beitrag zur Kenntnis der Virulenz der Tuberkelbazillen. (66), 1906, 43, 328.

Marshak, A., and W. B. Schaefer: Comparison of growth and autolysis of two strains of tubercle bacilli. (22), 1952, 65, 75.

Martin, A., and S. G. Tomlin: A technique for the cultivation and preparation of tissue cultures for electron microscopy. (69), 1950, 5, 154.

Martin, A. R.: The use of mice in the examination of drugs for chemotherapeutic activity against *Mycobacterium tuberculosis*. (148), 1946, 58, 580.

———, and G. T. Stewart: The chemotherapy of experimental tuberculosis in mice. (77), 1950, 31, 189.

Martin, H.: Note sur la culture du bacille de la tuberculose. (43), 1889, 1, 77.

Martin, S. P., and S. N. Chaudhuri: Effect of bacteria and their products on migration of leukocytes. (191), 1952, 81, 286.

Martini, P.: Die Gesetze der Prüfung von Heilmitteln bei der Lungentuberkulose. (63), 1933, 84, 86.

———: Wege und Irrwege der therapeutischen Forschung. (103), 1940, 66, 841.

Martius, C., and F. Knoop: Der physiologische Abbau der Citronensäure. (241), 1937, 246, 1.

Massol, L., and M. Breton: Contribution à l'étude de l'alimentation hydrocarbonée du bacille tuberculeux. (98), 1911, 71, 340.

Masur, B. L.: Zur Biologie des Tuberkelbazillus. (245), 1926, 99, 46.

Mattenheimer, H.: Die enzymatische Aufspaltung anorganischer Poly- und Metaphosphate durch Organextrakte und Trockenhefe. (68), 1951, 322, 36.

Maximow, A. A.: Experimentelle Untersuchungen über die entzündliche Neubildung von Bindgewebe. (64), 1902, Supplement 5.

———: Tuberculosis of mammalian tissue *in vitro*. (145), 1924, 34, 549.

Mayer, E., and M. Dworski: The bactericidal action of ultraviolet irradiations of tubercle bacilli. (22), 1932, 26, 105.

Mayer, R. L., and C. Crane: A yellow pigment formed from para-aminobenzoic and para-aminosalicylic acid by various strains of *Mycobacterium*. (175), 1950, 165, 37.

Mazia, D.: Enzyme studies on chromosomes. Cold Spring Harbor symposia on quantitative biology, New York, 1941, 9, 40. U.S.A.

Mazzetti, G.: L'influenza dell'ematina nei terreni di culture per il bacillo tubercolare. (119), 1932, 9, 610.

Medlar, E. M.: The behavior of pulmonary tuberculous lesions. A pathological study. (22), 1955, 71, Part 2, 1.

———, S. Bernstein, and F. C. Reeves: An interpretation of results obtained from cultivation of sputum samples for *M. tuberculosis*. (19), 1951, 41, 292.

Medlar, E. M., S. Bernstein, and D. M. Steward: A bacteriological study of resected tuberculous lesions. (22), 1952, 66, 36.

Meissner, J., and W. Diller: Über die Aufnahme von Ortho- und Metaphosphat durch das *Mycobacterium tuberculosis*. (235), 1953, 137, 518.

Meissner, J., and F. Kropp: Über die Phosphatresorption beim *Mycobacterium tuberculosis*. (235), 1953, 137, 429.

Meltzer, S. J.: On the importance of vibration to cell life. (177), 1892, 56, 708.

Melvin, I., G. C. Klein, W. Jones, and M. M. Cummings: An evaluation of media for diagnostic cultures of tubercle bacilli. (22), 1951, 63, 459.

Menkin, V.: The accumulation of iron in tuberculous areas. (139), 1934, 60, 463.

Menzel, A. E. O., and M. Heidelberger: Specific and non-specific cell polysaccharides of a bovine strain of tubercle bacillus. (136), 1939, 127, 221.

Menzi, H.: Beitrag zur Züchtung und zur Biologie des Tuberkelbacillus. (235), 1902, 39, 407.

Merrill, M. H.: Carbohydrate metabolism of organisms of the genus *Mycobacterium*. (135), 1930, 20, 235.

———: Studies on carbon metabolism of organisms of the genus *Mycobacterium*. 2. Utilization of organic compounds in a synthetic medium. (135), 1931, 21, 361.

Metschnikoff, E.: Über die phagocytäre Rolle der Tuberkelriesenzellen. (224), 1888, 113, 63.

Meunier, H.: Bacilloscopie des crachats extraits de l'estomac pour le diagnostic de la tuberculose pulmonaire de l'enfant. (185), 1898, No. 67, 81.

Meyer, A.: Die Zelle der Bakterien. Fischer, Jena, 1912. Germany.

Meyer, A., R. Galland, and B. Kobrinsky: Résultats comparés de la culture et de l'examen sur lame pour la recherche des bacilles de Koch. (205), 1951, 15, 932.

Meyer, J., and K. A. Jensen: A fatal case of tuberculosis produced by BCG. (22), 1954, 70, 402.

Meyerhof, O.: Untersuchungen über den Atmungsvorgänge nitrifizierenden Bakterien. 1. Die Atmung des Nitratbildners. (180), 1916, 164, 353.

———: Über den Einfluss des Sauerstoffs auf die alkoholische Gärung der Hefe. (68), 1925, 162, 43.

———, R. Shatas, and A. Kaplan: Heat of hydrolysis of trimetaphosphate. (69), 1953, 12, 121.
Meyer-Lie, A. K.: Tuberculous infection. 1. Investigations on air and dust as vehicles for tubercle bacteria in sanatorium wards and offices. (6), 1953, 28, 349.
Meyn, A: Die Tiefenkultur des Tuberkuloseerregers und ihre diagnostische Bedeutung. (235), 1950, 131, 472.
Michaelis, L.: Die vitale Färbung, eine Darstellungsmethode der Zellgranula. (53), 1900, 55, 558.
———: Das Methylenblau und seine Zersetzungsprodukte. (245), 1901, 29, 763.
———: The nature of the interaction of nucleic acids and nuclei with basic dyestuffs. Cold Spring Harbor symposia on quantitative biology, New York, 1947, 12, 131. U.S.A.
Michel, K.: Die Darstellung von Chromosomen mittels des Phasenkontrastverfahrens. (176), 1941, 29, 61.
Middlebrook, G.: Pathogenic components of the tubercle bacillus. (22), 1945, 51, 244.
———: Recent advances in bacteriologic research in tuberculosis. (9), 1950, 3, 124.
———: Sterilization of tubercle bacilli by isonicotinic acid hydrazide and the incidence of variants resistant to the drug *in vitro*. (22), 1952, 65, 765.
———, M. L. Cohn, and W. B. Schaefer: Studies on isoniazid and tubercle bacilli. 3. The isolation, drug-susceptibility, and catalase-testing of tubercle bacilli from isoniazid-treated patients. (22), 1954, 70, 852.
Middlebrook, G., R. J. Dubos, and C. Pierce: Virulence and morphological characteristics of mammalian tubercle bacilli. (139), 1947, 86, 175.
Miehe, H.: Beiträge zur Biologie, Morphologie and Systematik des Tuberkelbacillus. (235), 1909, 62, 131.
Migaki, H., and E. C. McCulloch: Survivor curves of bacteria exposed to surface-active agents. (135), 1949, 58, 161.
Mikhail, J. R., and W. H. Tattersall: Self-inflicted tuberculosis following BCG vaccination. (221), 1954, 35, 220.
Millar, J. W.: An attempt to confirm the growth of *Mycobacterium leprae murium* on chorioallantoic membrane of live chicken embryos. (126), 1953, 21, 40.
Millberger, H., K. Bartmann, and J. Zander: Der Einfluss einiger nicht-ionogener Netzmittel auf das Wachstum von *Mycobacterium tuberculosis var. hominis*. (235), 1954, 139, 285.
Miller, I. L., and W. G. Roessler: Growth of *Mycobacterium tuberculosis* in liquid media. (22), 1956, 73, 716.
Mills, T. J., R. Owen, and E. H. Strach: Early diagnosis of bone and joint tuberculosis in children. (161), 1956, 271, 57.
Milzer, A., and E. R. Levine: A rapid mouse test for laboratory diagnosis of tuberculosis. (191), 1948, 69, 16.
Minck, R., and A. Minck: Sur la constitution du bacille diphtherique: appareil nucléaire et granulations métachromatiques. (99), 1949, 228, 1313.
Mirsky, A. E.: Chromosomes and nucleoproteins. (7), 1943, 3, 1.
Mitscherlich, E.: Die Differenzierung frisch isolierter Stämme von *Mycobacterium tuberculosis hominis* und *bovis* in Kultur- und Kaninchenversuch. (235), 1952, 134, 375.
———, U. Reuss, and S. Gürtürk: Der Einfluss der Vorbehandlung von tuberkulösem Material auf die Sicherheit des Nachweises von Tuberkelbakterien in Kultur- und Tierversuch. (245), 1952, 158, 97.
Mitsuhashi, S., and Y. Kojima: On the production of toxin by *Corynebacterium diphtheriae*. 3. Effect of gases on the toxin production. (131), 1952, 22, 151.
Miura, S.: Über das Verhalten von Äthylenglycol, Propylenglycol und Glycerin im Tierkörper. (68), 1911, 36, 25.
Mizuno, D.: Einfluss der Wasserstoffionenkonzentration auf das Wachstum der mikroskopischen Kolonien der Tuberkelbacillen. (63), 1954, 112, 378.
Model, L. M.: Zur Biochemie des Wachstums und der Ernährung der Tuberkelbacillen. (63), 1929, 71, 685.

———: Über die Ausnutzung der Kohlehydrate für das Wachstum der Tuberkelbacillen. (63), 1933, 83, 214.
———, and A. S. Stcheglova: Vlianie streptomicina na rost i na nekotorye biokhimitscheskie svoistva kultur tuberkuleznykh mikobakterii. (186), 1955, No. 6, 46.
Moeschlin, S., G. Jaccard, and M. Bosshard: Experimentelle Untersuchungen über die Therapie der Tuberkulose durch Kombination von Streptomycin mit PAS oder Sulfon-N-Azetat. (112), 1948, 4, 158.
Mohler, H. K., and E. H. Funk: Gastric function in pulmonary tuberculosis. (174), 1916, 12th Annual Meeting, p. 185.
Mollov, M., I. Hill, and J. Oshinsky: The Dubos medium in routine cultivation of tubercle bacilli: results of a comparative study with Petrik's medium. (12), 1950, 20, 1085.
Molloy, M. E., P. B. Miner, and R. E. Berry: Dubos' solid agar medium in routine laboratory diagnosis of tuberculosis. (15), 1951, 17, 159.
Monod, J.: The growth of bacterial cultures. (38), 1949, 3, 371.
Moore, B., and R. S. Williams: The growth of the *Bacillus tuberculosis* and other micro-organisms in different percentages of oxygen. (67), 1909, 4, 177.
———: The growth of various species of bacteria and other micro-organisms in atmosphere enriched with oxygen. (67), 1911, 5, 181.
Moore, M.: The chorio-allantoic membrane of the developing chick as a medium for the cultivation and histopathologic study of pathogenic fungi. (17), 1941, 17, 103.
———: The chorio-allantoic membrane of chick embryos and its response to inoculation with some *Mycobacteria*. (17), 1942, 18, 827.
Moreau, E.: Application du milieu de Pétroff à la culture du bacille de Koch. (205), 1922, 3, 381.
Morellini, M.: L'influenza esercitata di alcuni idrocarburi sul bacillo tubercolare umano. (33), 1937, 1, 55.
Morrow, G., J. T. Syverton, W. W. Stiles, and G. P. Berry: The growth of *Leptospira icterohaemorrhagiae* on the chorio-allantoic membrane of the chick embryo. (212), 1938, 88, 384.
Morton, H. J., J. F. Morgan, and R. C. Parker: Nutrition of animal cells in tissue culture. 2. Use of Tweens in synthetic feeding mixtures. (191), 1950, 74, 22.
Moureau, M., and C. Gruvel: Essais de culture du bacille tuberculeux dans différents extraits glycérinés d'organes. (98), 1926, 95, 591.
Much, H.: Über die granuläre, nach Ziehl nicht färbbare Form des Tuberkulosevirus. (63), 1907a, 8, 85.
———: Über die nicht säurefesten Formen des Kochschen Tuberkelbazillus. (63), 1907b, 8, 357.
Mudd, E. B. H., and S. Mudd: The surface composition of tubercle bacillus and other acid-fast bacteria. (139), 1927, 46, 167.
Mudd, S.: Changes in the bacterial cell brought about by the action of germicides and antibacterial substances as demonstrated by the electron microscope. (19), 1943, 33, 167.
———: The mitochondria of bacteria. (142), 1953a, 1, 248.
———: Trends and perspectives of bacterial cytology. (125, Microbiology), 1953b, 1.
———, A. F. Brodie, L. C. Winterscheid, P. E. Hartman, E. H. Beutner, and R. A. McLean: Further evidence of the existence of mitochondria in bacteria. (135), 1951, 62, 729.
Mudd, S., and D. B. Lackman: Bacterial morphology as shown by the electron microscope. 1. Structural differentiation within the streptococcal cell. (135), 1941, 41, 415.
Mudd, S., K. Polevitzky, and T. F. Anderson: 4. Structural differentiation within the bacterial protoplasm. (46), 1942, 34, 199.
———, and L. A. Chambers: The bacterial cell-wall in the *genus Bacillus*. (135), 1941, 42, 251.
Mudd, S., and A. G. Smith: Electron and light microscopic studies of bacterial nuclei.

Bibliography

1. Adaptation of cytological processing to electron microscopy. Bacterial nuclei as vesicular structures. (135), 1950, 59, 561.
———, J. Hillier, and E. H. Beutner: Electron and light microscopic studies of bacterial nuclei. 3. The nuclear sites in metal-shadowed cells of *Escherichia coli.* (135), 1950, 60, 635.
Mudd, S., L. C. Winterscheid, E. D. DeLamater, and H. J. Henderson: Evidence suggesting that the granules of *Mycobacteria* are mitochondria. (135), 1951, 62, 459.
Mühlenbach, V., and K. Tomek: Bakteriologische Untersuchungen in der Umgebung Offentuberkulöser. (223), 1952, 6, 174.
Müller, H.: Die Verwendbarkeit der intrakutanen Tuberkulinprobe zur Diagnose der Meerschweinchentuberkulose. (245), 1920, 84, 251.
Müller, H. O.: Die Ausmessung der Tiefe übermikroskopischer Objekte. (159), 1942, 99, 6.
Mueller, J. H.: An unidentified growth factor for certain strains of the diphtheria bacillus. (191), 1939, 40, 632.
———: The influence of iron on the production of diphtheria toxin. (144), 1941, 42, 343.
Muller, H.: On the use of a modification of Pryce's slide culture method for the estimation of the bacteriostatic power of chemicals on the tubercle bacillus. (148), 1944, 56, 429.
Muschel, L. H., and T. Muto: Bactericidal reaction of mouse serum. (212), 1956, 123, 62.
Myers, J. A.: Invited and conquered. Public Health Association, Minneapolis, 1949. U.S.A.
———, and F. E. Harrington: The effect of initial tuberculous infection on subsequent tuberculous lesions. (151), 1934, 103, 1530.
Mylius, K., and F. Sartorius: Über die Einwirkung reinen Darmsaftes auf Tuberkelbazillen. (236), 1924, 39, 12.
Nakamura, T: Über die Atmung der Tuberkelbazillen. (219), 1938, 34, 231.
Nakanishi, K.: Über den Bau der Bakterien. (245), 1901, 30, 97, 193, 225.
Nalbant, J. P.: Tubercle bacilli in sputum and faeces of children without pulmonary tuberculosis. (22), 1934, 29, 481.
Nassau, E.: The culture of tubercle bacilli from laryngeal swabs. (189), 1941, 34, 397.
Nedelkovitch, Y.: Culture directe du bacille de Koch dans les épanchements sérofibrineux de pleurésie commune. (98), 1933, 113, 434.
Neelsen, F.: Ein casuistischer Beitrag zur Lehre von der Tuberculose. (249), 1883, No. 28, 497.
Nelson, C. D., G. Krotkov, and G. B. Reed: Metabolism of radioactive asparagine in wheat leaves and *Lupinus angustifolius* seedlings. (45), 1953, 44, 218.
Nelson, N.: A photometric adaptation of the Somogyi method for the determination of glucose. (136), 1944, 153, 375.
Neumann, F.: Untersuchungen zur Erforschung der Kernverhältnisse bei den Bakterien. (245), 1941, 103, 385.
Neumayr, R. B., P. Z. Morse, and W. C. Morse: Relationship between isoniazid resistance, endogenous catalase activity and guinea pig pathogenicity of *Mycobacterium tuberculosis.* (191), 1955, 89, 468.
Nickerson, W. J., and F. G. Sherman: Metabolic aspects of bacterial growth in the absence of cell division. 2. Respiration of normal and filamentous cells of *Bacillus cereus.* (135), 1952, 64, 667.
Nicod, J.-L., P. Hauduroy, and W. Rosset: Étude anatomo-pathologique des lésions du hamster inoculé avec le bacille de BCG. (185), 1951, No. 30, 605.
Niel, C. B. van: Biochemical problems of the chemo-autotrophic bacteria. (183), 1943, 23, 338.
———: Recent advances in our knowledge of the physiology of microorganisms. (61), 1944, 8, 225.
Nieman, C.: Influence of trace amounts of fatty acids on the growth of microorganisms. (61), 1954, 18, 147.

Nitti, F., and J. P. Jouin: Granulie expérimentale de la souris provoquée par du bacille tuberculeux humain. Essai de traitement par le p-aminophénylsulfamide. (29), 1942, 68, 556.

Nocard, E.: Recherches expérimentales sur la tuberculose des oiseaux. Culture du bacille. (98), 1885, 37, 601.

———: Sur les relations qui existent entre la tuberculose humaine et la tuberculose aviaire. (29), 1898, 12, 561.

Nocard and Roux: Sur la culture du bacille de la tuberculose. (29), 1887, 1, 19.

Noel, R., and Soeur Marie-Suzanne: Du mode de propagation du bacille de Stefansky inoculé dans la membrane chorio-allantoïdienne de l'embryon de poulet. (29), 1949, 76, 535.

Noguchi, H.: Über die Einwirkung von Seifen auf die Lebensfähigkeit und immunisierende Eigenschaft des Tuberkelbazillus. (245), 1909, 52, 85.

Noll, H., and H. Bloch: Studies on the chemistry of the cord factor of *Mycobacterium tuberculosis*. (136), 1955, 214, 251.

Noll, H., E. Sorkin, and H. Erlenmeyer: Über das Verhalten von Tbc-Kulturen gegenüber mit ^{35}S indiziertem Sulfat. (97), 1950, p. 40.

Noufflard, H.: Études sur la virulence des bacilles tuberculeux résistants à l'isoniazide. (29), 1955, 88, 325.

———, and M. Deslandes: Action bactéricide de l'isoniazide (hydrazide de l'acide isonicotinique) sur le bacille de Koch. (29), 1952, 83, 769.

Novy, F. G., and M. H. Soule: Microbic respiration. 2. Respiration of the tubercle bacillus. (145), 1925, 36, 168.

Nowak, J.: Le bacille de Bang et sa biologie. (29), 1908, 22, 541.

Nunno, R. de: Nuovo metodo di concentrazione del contenuto microbico dei liquidi organici per l'esame batterioscopico, culturale e biologico. (206), 1933, 49, 943.

Obrant, O., and O. Sievers: Gastric lavage in tuberculous guinea pigs. (6), 1950, 24, 167.

Odier, M.: Contribution à l'étude de quelques Mycobactéries: métabolites et antibiotiques. (210), 1949, 12, 380.

Oechsli, W. R., E. Kupka, and C. Bush: Classifying the tuberculous for isolation in California mental institutions. (194), 1955, 70, 1194.

Oeding, P.: Detection of tubercle bacilli in a routine material of sputa by means of the micro culture method. (6), 1951, 25, 208.

———, J. Hasselberg, H. Thrap-Meyer, and E. Waaler: Generalized BCG infection in man. (6), 1954, 29, 173.

Oerskov, J.: Eine morphologische Untersuchung über das Initialwachstum des Tuberkelbazillus. (245), 1932, 123, 271.

Oes, A.: Über die Autolyse der Mytosen. (76), 1908, 66, 89.

Östberg, O.: Studien über die Zitronensäureausscheidung der Menschenniere in normalen und pathologischen Zuständen. (213), 1931, 62, 81.

Oginsky, E. L., P. H. Smith, and M. Solotorovsky: The action of streptomycin. 4. Fatty acid oxidation by *Mycobacterium tuberculosis*, avian type. (135), 1950, 59, 29.

Olson, B. J., H. W. Scott, Jr., C. R. Hanlon, and C. F. T. Mattern: Experimental tuberculosis. 3. Further observations on the effects of alteration of the pulmonary arterial circulation on tuberculosis in monkeys. (22), 1952, 65, 48.

Opitz, H.: Zur Frage der offenen Tuberkulose im Kindesalter. (103), 1928, 54, 2139.

———: Neue Forschungen über die Diagnose der Lungentuberkulose durch Bazillennachweis. (103), 1930, 56, 1995.

———: Untersuchungen über die tatsächliche Häufigkeit offener Lungentuberkulose im Kindesalter. (63), 1933, 82, 296.

Ornstein, G. G., and M. M. Steinbach: The resistance of the albino rat to infection with tubercle bacilli. (22), 1925, 12, 77.

Orth, J.: Experimentelle Untersuchungen über Fütterungstuberculose. (224), 1879, 76, 217.

Osol, A. E.: Tuberkelbazillenfärbung im dicken Ausstrich. (103), 1927, 53, 1002.

———: Tuberkelbazillenfärbung im dicken Ausstrich nach Bearbeitung der Untersuchungsobjekte mit Antiformin. (242), 1929, 54, 332.

Pagel, W.: Experimental tuberculosis. Observations on tissue reaction and natural resistance. (22), 1940, 42, 58.

Palladin, W., and E. Lowtschinowskaia: Durch abgetötete Hefe hervorgerufene Oxydation und Reduktion auf Kosten des Wassers. (68), 1914, 65, 129.

Palmer, C. E., S. H. Ferebee, and O. S. Petersen: Studies on pulmonary findings and antigen sensitivity among student nurses. 6. Geographic differences in sensitivity to tuberculin as evidence of nonspecific allergy. (194), 1950, 65, 1111.

Pansy, F. E., W. L. Koerber, H. Stander, and R. Donovick: The inactivation of isoniazid by Dubos medium. (22), 1953, 68, 284.

Pappenheimer, A. M., Jr., and S. J. Johnson: Studies in diphtheria toxin production. 1. The effect of iron and copper. (77), 1936, 17, 335.

Paraf, J., and J. Desbordes: Réaction d'allergie tuberculinique et acide gras α-α-disubstitués. (29), 1945, 71, 297.

———, and F. Fournier: Contribution au problème de la virulence des bacilles acido-alcoolo-résistants grâce aux rayons X. Examen de corps bacillaires par diffraction de rayons X. (99), 1950, 231, 339.

Parish, H. J., and C. C. Okell: Three notes on tuberculin. 3. The development of skin-sensitiveness to old tuberculin in the tuberculous guinea-pig. (148), 1929, 32, 54.

Park, W. H., and C. Krumwiede, Jr.: The relative importance of the bovine and human types of tubercle bacilli in the different forms of human tuberculosis. (147), 1910, 23, 205.

Passini, F.: Kultureller Nachweis des Kochschen Bazillus im Lumbalpunktate von *Meningitis tuberculosa.* (166), 1934, 2, 1196.

Pasteur, L., and Joubert: Étude sur la maladie charbonneuse. (99), 1877, 84, 900.

Patnode, R. A., M. C. Dail, and P. C. Hudgins: Growth characteristics, virulence, and cytochemical properties of tubercle bacilli recovered from patients treated with isoniazid. (19), 1955, 45, 451.

Pauletta, G., and A. Defranceschi: Studies on the amino-acid metabolism of *Mycobacterium tuberculosis.* 1. Preliminary investigation by paper chromatography. (69), 1952, 9, 271.

Pavlovskii, G. T., and N. M. Sokolova: Izutschenie morfologitscheskikh osobennostei tuberkuleznykh bakterii pri pomoschi elektronnogo mikroskopa. (186), 1955, 3, 61.

Pawlowsky, A. D.: Culture des bacilles de la tuberculose sur la pomme de terre. (29), 1888, 2, 303.

Pease, D. C., and R. F. Baker: Sectioning techniques for electron microscopy using a conventional microtome. (191), 1948, 67, 470.

Peizer, L. R., D. Widelock, and S. Klein: Virulence in guinea pigs of isoniazid-resistant cultures isolated from clinical specimens. (22), 1953, 68, 290.

Perla, D.: Experimental epidemiology of tuberculosis. The elimination of tubercle bacilli in the feces, bile and urine of infected guinea pigs. (139), 1927, 45, 1025.

Peshkov, M. A.: The cytology and caryology of the colon-typhoid group. (21), 1945, 2, 342.

Petering, H. G., and F. Daniels: The determination of dissolved oxygen by means of the dropping-mercury electrode, with applications in biology. (150), 1938, 60, 2796.

Peters, E.: Zur Pathogenität der Tuberkelbacillentypen bei Mäusen. (245), 1912, 62, 1.

Peterson, H.: Über den Wert und die Brauchbarkeit des Nährbodens nach A. S. Griffith bei der Tuberkulose-Züchtung aus pathologischem Material. (235), 1952, 133, 481.

Petragnani, G.: Alcune utili modificazioni al mio terreno ed alla tecnica per l'isolamento in coltura pura dei bacilli di Koch dagli escreati e da altri materiali tubercolari. (74), 1926, 5, 173.

Petroff, S. A.: A new and rapid method for the isolation and cultivation of tubercle bacilli directly from the sputum and feces. (139), 1915a, 21, 38.

———: Some cultural studies on the tubercle bacillus. (87), 1915b, 26, 276.

———, and W. Steenken, Jr.: Biological studies of the tubercle bacillus. 1. Instability of the organism-microbic dissociation. (139), 1930, 51, 831.

Petrovskaia, O. A.: Primenenie v biologii metoda fluorescentnoi mikroskopii. (225), 1948, 26, 703.
Pezzangora, F.: La dispersion du bacille de Koch administré per os et la diffusion de l'infection tuberculeuse d'origine digestive. (98), 1936, 123, 476.
Philip, R. W.: On an improved method for the detection of the tubercle bacillus in sputum. (107), 1886–1887, 32, 409.
Philpot, F. J., and A. Q. Wells: Lipids of living and killed tubercle bacilli. (22), 1952, 66, 28.
Piekarski, G.: Cytologische Untersuchungen an Paratyphus- und Colibakterien. (52), 1937, 8, 428.
———: Lichtoptische und übermikroskopische Untersuchungen zum Problem des Bakterienzellkerns. (245), 1939, 144, 140, Beiheft.
———: Haben Bakterien einen Zellkern? (176), 1950, 37, 201.
———, and G. M. Pontieri: Über Feinstrukturen in der kernähnlichen Körpern von *Escherichia coli.* (245), 1956, 165, 242.
Piekarski, C., and H. Ruska: Übermikroskopische Untersuchungen an Bakterien unter besonderer Berücksichtigung der sogenannten Nucleoide. (52), 1939, 10, 302.
Pierce, C. H., R. J. Dubos, and G. Middlebrook: Infection of mice with mammalian tubercle bacilli grown in Tween-albumin liquid medium. (139), 1947, 86, 159.
Pierce, C. H., R. J. Dubos, and W. B. Schaefer: Multiplication and survival of tubercle bacilli in the organs of mice. (139), 1953, 97, 189.
Pinner, M.: Sputum examination in pulmonary tuberculosis. (146), 1932, 17, 611.
———: Atypical acid-fast microorganisms. 3. Chromogenic acid-fast bacilli from human beings. (22), 1935, 32, 424.
Plunkett, R. E.: Report of the committee on tuberculosis in penal and other institutions. (22), 1947, 56, 469.
Pötschke, G., M. Lewandowski, and S. Mauch: Der Nachweis gefärbter Tuberkelbakterien mit dem Phasenkontrastmikroskop. (235), 1954, 138, 442.
Poiré, A. F., and M. Arzeno-Carranza: Comparaison des méthodes de culture et d'isolement du bacille de Koch dans les crachats. (98), 1926, 95, 1174.
Polk, A., G. J. Buddingh, and E. W. Goodpasture: An experimental study of complement and hemolytic amboceptor introduced into chick embryos. (17), 1938, 14, 71.
Pollock, M. R., G. A. Howard, and B. W. Boughton: Long chain unsaturated fatty acids as essential bacterial growth factors. (67), 1949, 45, 417.
Pope, H.: Respiration of pathogenic and non-pathogenic *Mycobacteria.* (173), 1952, 38, 154.
———, and D. T. Smith: Synthesis of B-complex vitamins by tubercle bacilli when grown on synthetic media. (22), 1946, 54, 559.
Popper, H.: Histological demonstration of vitamin A in the human liver by means of fluorescence microscopy. (191), 1940, 43, 234.
Porter, A. E.: The sensitiveness of tubercle bacilli and other acid-fast bacilli to acids. (143), 1917, 16, 66.
Pothmann, F. J.: Vergleichende Untersuchungen mit der Leuchtbildmethode und dem Fluoreszenzmikroskop zum Nachweis der Tuberkelbazillen bei gleichzeitiger Kontrolle im Hellfeld. (103), 1940, 66, 1301.
———: Erfahrungen mit einem flüssigen Tb.-Nährboden. (245), 1949, 154, 152.
Pottenger, J. E.: The demonstration of rare tubercle bacilli in sputum by the dilution-flotation method in conjunction with picric acid. (22), 1931, 24, 583.
Potter, R. van: Cytochrome systems. Respiratory enzymes. Burgess, Minneapolis, 1949. U.S.A.
Potter, T. S.: The survival of tubercle bacilli subjected to a vacuum of high order. (145), 1935, 57, 149.
———: Possibility of prevention of tuberculosis by non-poisonous chemical air disinfection and by killed vaccines. (212), 1944, 99, 406.
Poulsen, V.: Pulmonary tuberculosis in children. Demonstration of tubercle bacilli in gastric lavage. (13), 1931, 41, 783.
———, and A. O. Andersen: Four years' experience with examination of material ob-

tained by gastric lavage. 1. Demonstration of tubercle bacilli and its significance in prognosis, therapy and estimation of danger of infection. (13), 1934, 47, 307.
Powelson, D. M., and J. R. McCarter: Serum albumin as a food for human tubercle bacilli. (135), 1944, 48, 479.
Price, R. M.: Types of tubercle bacilli in human tuberculosis. (95), 1932a, 7, 606.
———: The influence of silica upon the growth of tubercle bacillus. (95), 1932b, 7, 617.
Priesel, R.: Zur Frage der Ansteckungsfähigkeit der Tuberkulose. (63), 1932, 81, 570.
Prigge, R.: Experimentelle Untersuchungen zur Chemotherapie der Tuberkulose. (158), 1940, 19, 1273.
Proskauer, B., and M. Beck: Beiträge zur Ernährungsphysiolgie des Tuberkelbacillus. (235), 1894, 18, 128.
Prowazek, S. von: Das Lezithin und seine biologische Bedeutung. (72), 1908, 28, 382.
———: Über Fluoreszenz der Zellen. (157), 1914, 6, 30.
Prudhomme, R.-O., M. Rouyer, and A. M. Staub: Spectre d'absorption des microbes dans l'ultraviolet. (29), 1946, 72, 347.
Prunell, A.: Rachiculture dans le milieu de Besredka. (98), 1926, 95, 651.
Pryce, D. M.: Sputum film cultures of tubercle bacilli. A method for the early observation of growth. (148), 1941, 53, 327.
Rabinowitsch, L.: Experimentelle Untersuchungen über die Virulenz latenter tuberkulöser Herde. (242), 1909, 15, 217.
Rabinowitsch-Kempner, L.: The types of tubercle bacilli in human tuberculosis. (22), 1927, 15, 225.
Raleigh, G. W., and G. P. Youmans: The use of mice in experimental chemotherapy of tuberculosis. (145), 1948, 82, 197, 205, 221.
Ratcliffe, H. L.: Tuberculosis induced by droplet nuclei infection. (14), 1952, 55, 36.
Raulin, J.: Études chimiques sur la végétation. (32), 1869, 11, 93.
Ravenel, M. P.: The intercommunicability of human and bovine tuberculosis. (138), 1902, 15, 112.
Reed, C. I., S. R. Rosenthal, and B. P. Reed: Étude du bacille tuberculeux (BCG) au microscope électronique par la méthode des ombres portées. (29), 1948, 75, 504.
Reed, G. B., and C. E. Rice: The action of iron and citrate in synthetic media for tubercle bacilli. (135), 1928, 16, 97.
———: The behavior of acid-fast bacteria in oil and water systems. (135), 1931, 22, 239.
Reed, R. W.: Slide culture of tubercle bacilli. 1. Media and methods. (92), 1953, 31, 367.
Rees, R. J. W., and P. D'A. Hart: The inhibition of growth of avirulent strains of *Mycobacterium tuberculosis* by a surface-active polyoxyethylene ether. (140), 1952, 7, 372.
Rees, R. J. W., and J. M. Robson: Additive effect of streptomycin and p-amino-salicylic acid in experimental tuberculous infection. (175), 1949, 164, 351.
———: Experimental tuberculous infections of the cornea of mouse. A screening test for anti-tuberculous substances. (79), 1950, 5, 77.
Reichenow, E.: Untersuchungen an *Haematococcus pluvialis* nebst Bemerkungen über andere Flagellaten. (40), 1909–1910, 33, 1.
Reinberg, S. A.: Roentgen-ray studies on the physiology and pathology of the tracheobronchial tree. (80), 1925, 30, 451.
Renoux, G. E., and A. Français: La recherche du bacille tuberculeux par la culture du prélèvement laryngé. (185), 1950, 58, 392.
Report of the subcommittee for the evaluation of methods to control air-borne infection. Committee on Research on Standards. (19), 1947, 37, 13.
Report of the committee for the examination of germicides and antibacterial agents. (19), 1946, 36, 390.
Reuss, U.: Der syrische Goldhamster als Versuchstier bei der Tuberkulosediagnostik. (235), 1951, 132, 223.
———: Die Vorbehandlung tuberkulöser Gewebsproben zur kulturellen Untersuchung. (223), 1952, 6, 609.

Rich, A. R.: The pathogenesis of tuberculosis: C. C. Thomas, Springfield, Ill., 1951. U.S.A.
———, and R. H. Follis, Jr.: The effect of low oxygen tension upon the development of experimental tuberculosis. (87), 1942, 71, 345.
Richards, O. W.: Demonstration of tubercle bacilli by fluorescence microscopy. (22), 1941, 44, 255.
———: Phase microscopy in bacteriology. (216), 1948, 23, 55.
———: Phase microscopy 1950–1954. (212), 1954, 120, 631.
———, and H. W. Wade: Application of phase microscopy to the examination of the leprosy bacillus. (126), 1948, 16, 297.
Richmond, L., and M. M. Cummings: An evaluation of methods of testing the virulence of acid-fast bacilli. (22), 1950, 62, 632.
Riemsdijk, M. van: Über den Wert des Löwensteinschen Nährbodens anderen Tuberkelbazillennährböden gegenüber und über das Tiefenwachstum des Tuberkelbazillus. (245), 1932, 124, 394.
Rippel, A., and H. Bortels: Vorläufige Versuche über die allgemeine Bedeutung der Kohlensäure für die Pflanzenzelle. (Versuche an *Aspergillus niger*). (68), 1927, 184, 237.
Ris, H., and A. E. Mirsky: Quantitative cytochemical determination of desoxyribonucleic acid with the Feulgen nucleal reaction. (141), 1950, 33, 125.
Robinow, C. F.: A study of the nuclear apparatus of bacteria. (190), 1942, 130, 299.
———: Nuclear apparatus and cell structure of rod-shaped bacteria. Addendum to R. J. Dubos, The bacterial cell. Harvard University Press, Cambridge, Mass., 1949. U.S.A.
Robinson, J. L., and W. T. Dunn: Gastric lavage and sputum cultures. (22), 1943, 47, 413.
Robinson, L., and W. D. Stovall: Factors influencing demonstration of tubercle bacilli by concentration methods. (146), 1941, 27, 84.
Robson, J. M.: Experimental corneal ulcers. (78), 1944, 28, 15 .
Rochaix, A., and E. Banssillon: Milieu de Pétrof et diagnostique bactériologique rapide de la tuberculose des voies urinaires. (98), 1922, 86, 935.
Rockwell, G. E., and J. H. Highberger: Carbon dioxide as a factor in the growth of the tubercle bacillus and of other acid-fast organisms. (145), 1926, 38, 92.
Römer, P.: Ein Beitrag zur Frage der Wachstumgeschwindigkeit des Tuberkelbacillus. (245), 1900, 27, 705.
———: Tuberkelbacillenstämme. 1. (62), 1903, Heft 6, 1.
———: Über intrakutane Tuberkulinanwendung zu diagnostischen Zwecken. (63), 1909, 12, 185.
Rolland, J.: La mystique bactériologique en matiére de diagnostic positif de la tuberculose. (205), 1952, 16, 797.
Rolle, M.: Der Goldhamster (*Mesocricetus auratus*), ein neues Versuchstier. (120), 1949, 2, 492.
———, and H. Mayer: Die Virulenz der Tuberkulosebakterien aus tuberkulösen Prozessen der alten Kühe. (171), 1953, 5, 127.
Rolle, M., and A. Mayr: Koniferenöle als Desinfektionsmittel gegen Tuberkulose. (171), 1952, 4, 421.
———: Untersuchungen über die chronischen Eutererkrankungen der Schlachtkühe unter besonderer Berücksichtigung der Eutertuberkulose. (171), 1953, 5, 75.
Rolle, M., and B. Wochinger: Die Veränderung des Blutbildes als Tuberkulinreaktion zum Nachweis der Impftuberkulose bei Versuchstieren (Meerschweinchen u. Goldhamster). (218), 1951, Nos. 13–14, 236.
Romanowsky, D.: Zur Frage der Parasitologie und Therapie der Malaria. (179), 1891, 16, 297, 307.
Rondoni, P.: A proposito dell'influenza del siero di sangue sullo sviluppo culturale del bacillo di Koch. (74), 1935, 14, 386.
Rosebury, T.: Experimental air-borne infection. Williams & Wilkins, Baltimore, 1947. U.S.A.

Rosenberg, K. S.: Slide culture method for tubercle bacilli. (161), 1943, 1, 615.
Rosenblatt, M. B., E. F. Fullam, and A. E. Gessler: Studies of *Mycobacteria* with electron microscope. (22), 1942, 46, 587.
Ross, H. M., and M. E. Landry: A comparative study of Dubos and Löwenstein media for the routine diagnosis of tuberculosis. (93), 1952, 14, 60.
Roth, W.: Morphologische Studien an Mikrokulturen über die "cord-formation" von Mycobakterien. (210), 1949, 12, 451.
Roulet, F., and E. A. Zeller: Über die Enzyme des *Mycobacterium tuberculosis* und anderer säurefester Bakterien. 3. Mitteilung. Über den enzymatischen Abbau von L-Peptiden durch säurefeste Bakterien. (121), 1948, 31, 1915.
Rous, P., and J. B. Murphy: Tumor implantations in the developing embryo. Experiments with a transmissible sarcoma of the fowl. (151), 1911, 56, 741.
Roux, E., and A. Yersin: Contribution à l'étude de la diphthérie. (29), 1889, 3, 273.
Rubbo, S. D., and B. J. Pierson: A rapid method of screening antituberculous agents in the guinea pig. (22), 1953, 68, 48.
Ruben, S., and M. D. Kamen: Radioactive carbon in the study of respiration in heterotrophic systems. (188), 1940, 26, 418.
Rubinstein, G. R.: Vsegda li obnarushivaemye v promivnykh vodakh zheludka kislotoupornye palotschki popadaiut tuda iz legkikh? (186), 1950, 3, 3.
Rudat, K. D.: Der syrische Goldhamster (*Cricetus, mesocricetus, auratus*) und seine Eignung als Versuchstier. (102), 1953, 8, 417.
Ruska, H.: Übermikroskopische Untersuchungstechnik. (176), 1939, 27, 287.
———: Über Grenzfragen aus dem Gebiet der Strukturforschung und Mikrobiologie. (103), 1941, 67, 281.
———: Über den Einfluss keimschädigender oder keimtötender Massnahmen auf die Bakterienkultur. 1. Mitteilung. Temperatureinwirkung. (235), 1942, 123, 294.
———: Personal communication, 1954.
———, G. Bringmann, I. Neckel, and G. Schuster: Über die Entwicklung sowie den morphologischen und zytochemischen Aufbau v. *Mycobacterium avium* (Chester). (243), 1952, 60, 425.
Ruziczka, O., and E. Orth: An Tuberkelbazillen elektronenoptisch dargestellte Wirkung von Thiosemicarbazonen. (Tb I, Tb VI). (227), 1950, 100, 95.
———: Altérations morphologiques du bacille tuberculeux consécutives à l'action de divers médicaments. Étude au microscope électronique. (29), 1952, 82, 334.
Sabin, F. R., C. A. Doan, and C. E. Forkner: Studies on tuberculosis. (139), 1930, 52, Supplement 3.
Sabrazès, J.: Colorabilité des bacilles de Koch dans les crachats incorporés à diverses substances. (29), 1903, 17, 303.
Sachs, F.: Über die Nuclease. (241), 1905, 46, 337.
Sacktor, B.: Investigation on the mitochondria of the housefly, *Musca domestica, L.* 3. Requirements for oxidative phosphorylation. (141), 1954, 37, 343.
Saenz, A., and L. Costil: Diagnostic bactériologique de la tuberculose. Masson, Paris, 1936. France.
———, and M. Sadettin: Étude de la toxicité comparée des solutions d'acide sulfurique et d'acide acétique pour le bacille de Koch. (98), 1934, 115, 1175.
Salton, M. R. J., and R. W. Horne: Studies on the bacterial cell wall. 1. Electron microscopical observations in heated bacteria. (69), 1951, 7, 19.
Samson, F. E., A. M. Katz, D. L. Harris, and J. Z. Hearon: Some effects of short chain fatty acids on phosphate and carbohydrate metabolism of yeast. (114), 1952, 11, 136.
Sander: Über das Wachstum von Tuberkelbacillen auf pflanzlichen Nährböden. (51), 1893, 16, 238.
Sandison, J. C.: A new method for the microscopic study of living growing tissues by the introduction of a transparent chamber in the rabbit's ear. (25), 1924, 28, 281; (10), 1928, 41, 447.
Sattler, T. H., and G. P. Youmans: The effect of "Tween 80," bovine albumin, glycerol,

and glucose on the growth of *Mycobacterium var. hominis* (H37Rv). (135), 1948, 56, 235.
Sauton, B.: Sur la nutrition minérale du bacille tuberculeux. (99), 1912, 155, 860.
Saxer, E., and H. Vonarburg: Untersuchungen über die Lebensfähigkeit von Tuberkelbazillen. (210), 1951, 14, 532.
Saz, A. K.: The effect of long-chain carbon compounds, particularly hydrocarbons, on the metabolism of tubercle bacilli. (45), 1949, 22, 195.
———, and F. Bernheim: The effect of 2,3,5-triiodobenzoate on the growth of tubercle bacilli. (212), 1941, 93, 622.
Scartozzi, G.: Sull'influenza della centrifugazione nell'isolamento del micobatterio del tubercolo. (119), 1939, 22, 85.
Schaefer, W. B.: Recherches sur la spécifité des protéides des bacilles tuberculeux. Identification sérologique des souches bovines et sérodiagnostique de la tuberculose bovine chez l'homme. (29), 1940, 64, 517.
———: Identification sérologique des bacilles tuberculeux du type bovin. (29), 1947, 73, 1157.
———: Recherches sur la croissance du *Mycobacterium tuberculosis* en culture homogène. (29), 1948, 74, 458.
———: Growth requirements of dysgonic and eugonic strains of *Mycobacterium tuberculosis var. bovis.* (139), 1952, 96, 207.
Schaefer, W. B., A. Marshak, and B. Burkhart: The growth of *Mycobacterium tuberculosis* as a function of its nutrients. (135), 1949, 58, 549.
Schallock, G.: Vereinfachter Nachweis von Tuberkelbazillen in histologischen Schnitten durch die Fluoreszenzmethode nach Hagemann. (172), 1940, 87, 102.
Schatz, A., and S. A. Waksman: Effect of streptomycin and other antibiotic substances on *Mycobacterium tuberculosis* and related organisms. (191), 1944, 57, 244.
Schierholz, H., and R. Jeder: Kinetische Untersuchungen über den durch Bangbakterien verursachten Peroxydzerfall. (245), 1956, 167, 281.
Schmidt, G., L. Hecht, and S. J. Thannhauser: The enzymic formation and the accumulation of large amounts of a metaphosphate in bakers' yeast under certain conditions. (136), 1946, 166, 775.
Schmidt-Lange, W.: Schnellere Zentrifugen ins Laboratorium. (158), 1940, 19, 206.
———, and H. Banning: Verbesserter Tuberkelbazillennachweis durch schnellere Zentrifugen. (158), 1941, 20, 344.
Schneider, C. H.: Untersuchungen über die bakterizide Wirksamkeit von Methyl- und Äthylalkohol auf die Bakterien mit Hilfe der Acridinorange-Methodik. Hanover, 1944. Germany.
Schneider, W. C.: Intracellular distribution of enzymes. 1. The distribution of succinic dehydrogenase, cytochrome oxidase, adenosinetriphosphatase and phosphorous compounds in normal rat tissue. (136), 1946, 165, 585.
Scholer, H. J.: Ersatz des Rinderalbumins (Fraction V) durch Vollserum in Dubosschen Nährböden. (210), 1951, 14, 586; (210), 1952, 15, 1.
Schottelius, M.: Beobachtung kernartiger Körper im Innern von Spaltpilzen. (245), 1888, 4, 705.
Schramek, J., and P. Hegedüs: Die Kultur von Tuberkelbacillen aus Larynxabstrichen. (158), 1935, 14, 237.
Schraufstätter, E.: Über die *in-vitro*-Prüfung tuberkulostatischer Stoffe. (235), 1950, 131, 318.
Schrell, G. M., R. W. Thomas, and W. H. Peterson: Amino acid and unsaturated fatty acid requirements of *Clostridium tetani.* (45), 1949, 20, 227.
Schürmann, R.: Zur Histogenese des Tuberkels in der Chorio-Allantois-Membran des Hühnerembryos. (224), 1952, 321, 395.
Schwabacher, H.: The occurrence of saprophytic and acid-fast bacilli in human or animal blood cultures and their isolation from water, dust, and comedones. (165), 1933, No. 182, Appendix C, p. 124.
———, and G. S. Wilson: The inoculation of minimal doses of tubercle bacilli into guinea pigs, rabbits, mice. (221), 1937, 18, 442.

Schwarting, V. H.: The action of gastric contents on tubercle bacilli. (22), 1948, 58, 123.
Schweinitz, E. A. de, and M. Dorset: Tuberculosis investigations. The growth of the tuberculosis bacillus upon acid media. (83), 1896, No. 13, 7.
Sclavo, A: Della cultura del diplococco di Fraenkel nelle uova. (207), 1894, 5, 254.
Second, L., and R. Chatelain: La gélose-gélatine de Legroux. Milieu de culture de *Mycobacterium tuberculosis.* (29), 1951, 81, 227.
Šedriks, F.: Ricerche comparative sul valore dei terreni Petragnani, Frimodt-Möller e Löwenstein per l'isolamento in coltura dei bacilli tubercolari del tipo bovino. (33), 1937, 1, 59.
Seibert, F. B.: Progress in the chemistry of tuberculin. (9), 1950, 3, 1.
———, E. R. Long, and N. Morley: Two avian tubercle bacillus dissociants and two human tubercle bacillus strains of different virulence. A chemical and biological study. (145), 1933, 53, 175.
Seibert, F. B., and N. Morley: The relationship of the tuberculin proteins of different acid-fast bacilli to sensitization as indicated by their reactivity in sensitized animals. (144), 1933, 24, 149.
Sergejev, G. M.: Izsledovanie vliania biostimulatorov na rost bakterialnykh kultur. (251), 1954, 12, 81.
Shapiro, H.: An analysis of the mechanism of the bacterial filtering action of gauze masks. (14), 1950, 51, 135.
Shaw, J. B., and N. Wynn-Williams: Infectivity of pulmonary tuberculosis in relation to sputum status. (22), 1954, 69, 724.
Sher, B. C., and H. C. Sweany: Chemical factors influencing the growth of tubercle bacilli. 1. Metal catalysts. (135), 1939, 37, 377.
Shiga, K.: Über Gewöhnung der Bakterien an Farbstoffe. (236), 1913, 18, 65.
Siebenmann, C. O.: Effect of BCG vaccination and chemotherapy on experimental tuberculosis in mice. (144), 1951, 67, 137.
Siebert, C.: Zur Biologie der Tuberkelbacillen. (245), 1909, 51, 305.
Silveira, J., E. Darzins, and A. Ventura de Matos: Mycobacteria apatógenas isoladas no escarro, lavado gástrico e lavado bronquico. (59), 1951, 10, 143.
Smith, A. G.: Electron and light microscopic studies of bacterial nuclei. 2. An improved staining technique for the nuclear chromatin of bacterial cells. (135), 1950, 59, 575.
Smith, C. L.: The breakdown of desoxyribonucleic acid under deuteron and electron bombardment. (45), 1953, 46, 12.
Smith, C. R.: A sanatorium program for the bacteriological diagnosis of tuberculosis. The results obtained in cases admitted during a period of ten years. (22), 1949, 59, 589.
———: Clinical comparison of several culture media in the diagnostic demonstration of tubercle bacilli. (22), 1951, 63, 470.
Smith, D. G.: Quantitative measurement of growth of *Mycobacterium tuberculosis.* Effect of streptomycin. (191), 1947, 64, 36.
Smith, H., and J. Keppie: Studies on the chemical basis of the pathogenicity of *Bacillus anthracis* using organisms grown *in vivo.* Mechanisms of microbial pathogenicity, Symposium. Cambridge University Press, Cambridge, 1955, p. 126. England.
Smith, J. W., J. Humiston, W. P. Creger, and W. M. M. Kirby: Evaluation of Dubos' solid medium containing penicillin in the isolation of tubercle bacilli. (191), 1949, 70, 589.
Smith, M. I., and E. W. Emmart: The action of *Penicillium* extracts in experimental tuberculosis. (194), 1944, 59, 417.
Smith, Th.: A comparative study of bovine tubercle bacilli and of human bacilli from sputum. (139), 1898, 3, 451.
———: Studies in mammalian tubercle bacilli. Description of a bovine bacillus from the human body. A culture test for distinguishing the human from the bovine type of bacilli. (147), 1904–1905, 13, 253.
———: The reaction curve of the human and the bovine type of the tubercle bacillus in glycerine broth. (147), 1910, 23, 185.

Smithburn, K. C.: Virulence of tubercle bacilli; its variations attendant on animal passage. (22), 1939, 39, 116.
———, and G. I. Lavin: The effect of ultraviolet radiation on tubercle bacilli. (22), 1939, 39, 782.
Söhngen, N. L.: Benzin, Petroleum, Paraffinöl und Paraffin als Kohlenstoff- und Energiequelle für Mikroben. (247), 1913, 37, 595.
Solomidès, J.: Pouvoir pathogène des cultures tuberculeuses du type humain et bovin additionnées d'huile d'arachide. (29), 1946, 72, 156.
Solotorovsky, M., E. J. Bugie, and B. M. Frost: The effect of penicillin on the growth of *Mycobacterium tuberculosis* in Dubos' medium. (135), 1948, 55, 555.
Solotorovsky, M., H. J. Robinson, and M. Kniazuk: Design and operation of a laboratory for experimental tuberculosis. (22), 1953, 68, 212.
Soltys, M. A.: The effect of penicillin on *Mycobacteria in vitro* and *in vivo.* (221), 1952, 33, 120.
Sommermeyer, L., and M. Frobisher, Jr.: Penicillin as a decontaminant in cultures for tubercle bacilli from undigested sputum. (22), 1953, 67, 530.
Sorkin, E., H. Erlenmeyer, and H. Bloch: Purification of a lipid material (cord factor) obtained from young cultures of tubercle bacilli. (175), 1952, 170, 124.
Spain, D. M., and N. Molomut: Effects of cortisone on the development of tuberculous lesions in guinea pigs and on their modification by streptomycin therapy. (22), 1950, 62, 337.
Spanedda, A.: Ricerche sui mycobatteri non patogeni da materiali patologici. (119), 1951, 43, 396.
Spendlove, G. A., M. M. Cummings, and R. A. Patnode: Toxicity of sputum digestants to tubercle bacilli in water and sputum. (22), 1949, 60, 628.
Spengler, C.: Tuberkelbacillenzüchtung aus Bakteriengemischen und Formaldehydde-sinfection. (235), 1903, 42, 93.
———: Über Splittersputa Tuberkulöser. (235), 1905a, 49, 541.
———: Zur Formaldehyd-Abtötung und Züchtung der Tuberkel- und anderer säurefesten Bacillen. (235), 1905b, 51, 335.
Sperry, J. A., and L. F. Rettger: The behavior of bacteria towards purified animal and vegetable proteins. (136), 1915, 20, 445.
Sprick, M. G., and J. W. Towey: Isolation of *Mycobacterium tuberculosis* from gastric contents neutralized after varying periods. (194), 1946, 61, 648.
Stableforth, A. W.: A bacteriological investigation of cases of tuberculosis in five cats, sixteen dogs, a parrot, and a wallaby. (138), 1929, 42, 163.
Stadnichenko, A., S. J. Cohen, and H. C. Sweany: Stomach lavage in the diagnosis and control of treatment of tuberculosis. (151), 1940, 114, 634.
Stamatin, N., and L. Stamatin: Virulence des trois types de bacilles tuberculeux pour la souris blanche. (29), 1939, 63, 269.
Stanier, R. Y.: The oxidation of aromatic compounds by fluorescent pseudomonas. (135), 1948, 55, 477.
———, B. P. Sleeper, M. Tsuchida, and D. L. Macdonald: The bacterial oxidation of aromatic compounds. 3. The enzymatic oxidation of catechol and protocatechuic acid to β-ketoadipic acid. (135), 1950, 59, 137.
Stanley, W. M., and T. F. Anderson: Electron micrographs of protein molecules. (136), 1942, 146, 25.
Stanley, W. M., G. H. Coleman, C. M. Greer, J. Sacks, and R. Adams: Bacteriological action of certain synthetic organic acids toward *Mycobacterium leprae* and other acid-fast bacteria. (149), 1932, 45, 121.
Starck, H. J., and P. Viehmann: Über die Brauchbarkeit des syrischen Goldhamsters ald Versuchstier bei der Tuberkulose-Diagnose. (245), 1955, 162, 446.
Starkey, H., and E. Aubert: The use of tri-sodium phosphate in techniques for the isolation of *M. tuberculosis.* (94), 1950, 41, 27.
Stavitsky, A. B., and J. Beck: Reaction of the developing chick embryo and the chorio-allantoic membrane to inoculation with various strains of *Mycobacterium paratuberculosis* (Johne's bacillus). (20), 1946, 7, 470.

Steenken, W., Jr., and M. M. Smith: Culture of tubercle bacilli. 1. The effect of sodium hydroxide and sulphuric acid upon acid-fast variants of homologous strains and the influence of the hydrogen ion concentration in different media upon subsequent growth. (22), 1938, 38, 503.

———: A shaking machine and containers for shaking sputums and other body fluids during the process of homogenization. (146), 1942, 27, 1582.

Steenken, W., Jr., and E. Wolinsky: Virulence of tubercle bacilli recovered from patients treated with isoniazid. (22), 1953, 68, 548.

———, L. J. Bristol, and W. J. Costigan: Use of the rabbit in experimental tuberculosis. 1. A visual method of evaluation of antituberculous agents by serial chest roentgenograms. (22), 1953, 68, 65.

Steigner, K. F.: Die bakteriologische Diagnose der Tuberkulose. (245), 1949, 153, 297.

Stempen, H.: Demonstration of the chromatinic bodies of *Escherichia coli* and *Proteus vulgaris* with the aid of the phase contrast microscope. (135), 1950, 60, 81.

Stephenson, M., and M. D. Whetham: Studies in the fat metabolism of the timothy grass bacillus. (190), 1922, 93, 262.

———: The carbon balance-sheet and respiratory quotient. (190), 1924, 95, 200.

Stern, J. R., and S. Ochoa: Enzymatic synthesis of citric acid by condensation of acetate and oxalacetate. (136), 1949, 179, 491.

Sternberg, J., and M. O. Padoski: Recherches faites avec les Mycobactéries marquées. 1. *Mycobacterium phlei* et radiophosphore: technique d'obtention et vitesse d'utilisation du phosphore exogène. (29), 1953, 84, 853.

Stewart, G. T.: The pathogenesis of tuberculosis in mice infected intravenously with human tubercle bacilli. The use of mice in chemotherapeutic tests. (77), 1950, 31, 5.

———: Virulence of human tubercle bacilli. (161), 1951, 261, 562.

———, and M. Tamargo-Sanchez: An experimental basis for estimating the virulence of tubercle bacilli. (143), 1952, 50, 37.

Stief, M., and W. H. Hall: Acid-fast bacilli not pathogenic for guinea pigs. (22), 1956, 74, 478.

Stille, B.: Zytologische Untersuchungen an Bakterien mit Hilfe der Feulgenschen Nuklealreaktion. (52), 1937, 8, 125.

Stilling, J.: Über die Anwendung der Anilinfarbstoffe. (66), 1890, 27, 531.

Stotz, E.: Pyruvate metabolism. (7), 1945, 5, 129.

Strandgaard, E.: Intermittent excretion of bacilli in pulmonary tuberculosis. (6), 1950, 24, 269.

Straus, I.: La tuberculose et son bacille. Rueff, Paris, 1895. France.

———, and R. Wurtz: De l'action du suc gastric sur quelques microbes pathogènes. (43), 1889, 1, 371.

Strauss, W.: Zur Frage der Virulenzsteigerung säurefester Saprophyten durch Tierpassagen. (235), 1922, 98, 243.

Stringer, C. J., and H. E. Cope: Examination of pooled sputum specimens. (22), 1943, 47, 524.

Ström, L., and L. Rudbäck: On labeling tubercle bacteria with radioactive phosphorous. (6), 1949, Supplement 21, 98.

Strugger, S.: Fluoreszenzmikroskopische Untersuchungen über die Aufnahme und Speicherung des Acridinorange durch lebende und tote Pflanzenzellen. (132), 1940, 73, 97.

———: Fluoreszenzsmikroskopie und Mikrobiologie. Schaper, Hanover, 1949. Germany.

Šula, L.: A liquid ascitic medium for the isolation of *Mycobacterium tuberculosis* from pathological material. (194), 1948, 63, 867.

Sulkin, S. E., and R. M. Pike: Survey of laboratory-acquired infections. (19), 1951, 41, 769.

Sumiyoshi, Y.: Beitrag zur Reinzüchtung der Tuberkelbazillen aus dem Sputum. 1. Mitteilung. (242), 1924, 39, 333.

Suter, E.: Multiplication of tubercle bacilli within phagocytes cultivated *in vitro,* and effect of streptomycin and isonicotinic acid hydrazide. (22), 1952a, 65, 775.

———: Multiplication of tubercle bacilli within normal phagocytes in tissue cultures. (139), 1952b, 96, 137.
Svedberg, B.: Studies in experimental tuberculosis. Investigation of some problems of immunity and resistance. (2), 1951, Supplement 254, 1.
Syverton, J. T., A. A. Werder, J. Friedman, F. J. Roth, A. B. Graham, and O. J. Mira: Cortisone and Roentgen radiation in combination as synergistic agents for production of lethal infections. (191), 1952, 80, 123.
Takaro, T., O. T. Clagett, C. H. Hodgson, and D. T. Carr: Pulmonary resection for tuberculosis: a review of 73 cases with a follow-up of one year or longer. (192), 1952, 27, 345.
Tamura, M., G. Ogawa, I. Sagawa, and S. Amano: Observations on an epidemic of cutaneous and lymphatic tuberculosis which followed the use of anti-typhoid vaccine. (22), 1955, 71, 465.
Tarshis, M. S., and A. W. Frisch: Chromogenic acid-fast bacilli from human sources. (22), 1952, 65, 278, 289, 302.
Tatum, E. L., and J. Lederberg: Gene recombination in the bacterium *Escherichia coli.* (135), 1947, 53, 673.
Team of British investigators: Cultivation of *Mycobacterium tuberculosis.* Part 1. Methods of homogenization. (88), 1952, August, 187.
Tegström, A.: A case of accidental laboratory tuberculous eye-infection. (6), 1942, 16, 250.
Theorell, H: Über die chemische Konstitution des Cytochroms C. (68), 1938, 298, 242.
Thiel, W.: Die Maus als Versuchstier bei der Tuberkulosediagnostik. (235), 1956, 142, 545.
Thilo, E., and R. Rätz: Die Konstitution des Natriumtrimetaphosphates $Na_3(P_3O_9)$. (231), 1949, 258, 33.
Thompson, L.: The value of vegetable extracts in culture media. (135), 1929, 17, 379.
Thunberg, T.: Zur Kenntnis der Einwirkung tierischer Gewebe auf Methylenblau. (213), 1917, 35, 165.
———: Occurrence and significance of citric acid in the animal organism. (183), 1953, 33, 1.
Tiffeneau, M., and A. Marie: Sur diverses conditions de culture du bacille tuberculeux. (98), 1912, 72, 48.
Timpe, A., and E. H. Runyon: The relationship of "atypical" acid-fast bacteria to human disease. (146), 1954, 44, 202.
Tison, F.: Les délais de réponse demandés par l'inoculation au cobaye de produits suspects de tuberculose. (29), 1951, 80, 551.
Tobie, W. C.: Nitric and sulphuric acid, a colorless cleaning mixture for glassware. (146), 1941, 26, 1797.
Toda, T.: Vergleichende Prüfung der Pathogenität von Tuberkelbazillenstämmen am Kaninchen durch intrakutane Verimpfung der zu prüfenden Stämme an ein und demselben Tier. 1. Mitteilung. Unterscheidung des *Typus bovinus* und *humanus.* (242), 1930, 55, 302.
Todd, C. M.: Occurrence of cytochrome and coproporphyrin in *Mycobacteria.* (67), 1949, 45, 386.
Tomarkin, E., and S. Peschič: Über die Differenzierung des *Typus humanus* und *Typus bovinus* des Tuberkelbacillus durch Kutaninfektion beim Meerschweinchen. (103), 1912, 38, 1032.
Topley, W. W. C., and G. S. Wilson: The principles of bacteriology and immunity. Williams & Wilkins, Baltimore, 1946. U.S.A.
Treffers, H. P.: Studies on resistance to antibiotics. 1. The action of penicillin on some Gram-positive and Gram-negative organisms and its potentiation by various inhibitors. (229), 1945–1946, 18, 609.
Trommsdorff, R.: Über intravenöse Impfungen mit Menschen- und Rindertuberkelbazillen bei Mäusen. (40), 1909, 32, 568.
Tschertkova, E. I., and N. I. Buinov: Izutschenie deistvia aktivnykh khimiopreparatov

na tuberkuleznuiu palotschku s pomoschiu elektronnogo mikroskopa. (186), 1953, 1, 22.

Tsuji, S. and K. Ito: An *in vivo* method of culturing tubercle bacilli: the chamber method. (22), 1955, 72, 393.

Tulasne, R.: Sur la mise en évidence du noyau des cellules bactériennes. (98), 1947, 141, 411.

———: Sur la cytologie des bactéries vivantes étudiées grâce au microscope à contraste de phase. (98), 1949, 143, 1390.

———, and R. Vendrely: Demonstration of bacterial nuclei with ribonuclease. (175), 1947, 160, 225.

T'ung, T., and S. C. Wong: Rapid multiplication of *Mycobacterium tuberculosis* in Chinese hamsters. (191), 1940, 43, 70.

Turian, G.: Recherches sur la biosynthèse des caroténoïdes chez un bacille paratuberculeux. 2. Identification d'un poluène acide voisin de l'astacine. (121), 1950, 33, 1303.

———: 3. Action plasmogène du fer chez les Mycobactéries. Le bacille de la fléole, indicateur biologique du fer. (121), 1951, 34, 917.

Turner, C. E., M. W. Jennison, and H. E. Edgerton: Public health applications of high-speed photography. (19), 1941, 31, 319.

Uehlinger, E., and R. Siebenmann: Der Einfluss von Cortison auf die Tuberkulinreaktion und auf das Arthus-Phänomen. (86), 1952, 8, 203.

Uga, T.: On the oxygen metabolism of tubercle bacilli and some kinds of acid-fast bacilli. (131), 1935, 13, 167.

Uhlenhuth and Kersten: Eine neue Methode zum culturellen und mikroskopischen Nachweis von Tuberkelbacillen im Sputum und anderem tuberculösen Material. (233), 1909, 6, 759.

Uhlenhuth and Xylander: Antiformin, ein bakterienauflösendes Desinfektionsmittel. (66), 1908, 45, 1346.

Uhlenhuth, P., and W. Seiffert: Das Verhalten schwachvirulenter Tuberkelbazillen im Tierversuch. (236), 1930, 69, 187.

———: Vergleichende Untersuchungen über die Tuberkulinempfindlichkeit nach Infection mit Tuberkelbacillen verschiedener Virulenz. (236), 1932, 74, 101.

Ulmar, D., and G. G. Ornstein: Gastric examination in pulmonary tuberculosis with negative sputum. (151), 1933, 101, 835.

Umbreit, W. W., R. H. Burris, and J. F. Stauffer: Manometric techniques and tissue metabolism. Burgess, Minneapolis, 1951. U.S.A.

Ungar, J.: The golden hamster as a test animal for tubercular infection. (175), 1942, 150, 432.

———, and P. W. Muggleton: The effect of penicillin on the growth of human type of *M. tuberculosis.* (148), 1946, 58, 501.

———: The relationship of the aluminum phosphate precipitation of organisms of *Haemophilus pertussis* strains to their other biological properties. (140), 1949, 3, 353.

Unholtz, K: Der Kirchner-Nährboden in der Tuberkulosediagnostik. (242), 1950, 94, 192.

Utter, M. F.: Interrelation of oxalacetic and L-malic acids in carbon dioxide fixation. (136), 1951, 188, 847.

———, and H. G. Wood: Mechanism of fixation of carbon dioxide by heterotrophs and autotrophs. (7), 1951, 12, 41.

Uyei, N.: The nature of the growth-promoting active principle in the potato in cultivation of bacteria and especially of tubercle bacillus. (22), 1930, 22, 203.

Vaccaro, H., and G. Alonso: El cultivo en lamina del bacilo de Koch. 1. Método de diagnóstico precoz. (199), 1951, 79, 31.

Vagedes: Experimentelle Prüfung der Virulenz von Tuberkelbacillen. (235), 1898, 28, 276.

Vaillant, L.: Sur le bacille tuberculeux cultivé en milieu sucré. (98), 1906, 60, 741.

Valley, G., and L. F. Rettger: The influence of carbon dioxide on bacteria. (135), 1927, 14, 101.

Valtis, J., F. van Deinse, and J. Solomidès: Essais de culture de BK dans le milieu de Dubos. (29), 1948, 74, 134.

Vaudremer, A.: Formes filtrantes des bacilles tuberculeux. (98), 1923, 89, 80.

Vendrely, R., and Y. Lehoult: Les acides ribo- et désoxyribonucléiques de la cellule bactérienne et leur signification. (99), 1946, 222, 1357.

Vendrely, R., and J. Lipardy: Acides nucléiques et noyaux bactériens. (99), 1946, 223, 342.

Vendrely-Randaval, C.: L'acide chlorhydrique, succédané de la ribonucléase dans la localisation de l'acide ribonucléique chez les cellules des êtres supérieurs aussi bien que chez les bactéries; aspect histologique de la question. (99), 1949, 228, 606.

Vennesland, K., R. H. Ebert, and R. G. Bloch: *In vivo* effect of streptomycin and para-aminosalicylic acid (PAS) on the growth of tubercle bacilli. (191), 1948, 68, 250.

Verge, J., P. Davenas, and J. Dabrigeon: Recherches sur la bacillémie dans la tuberculose des bovidés. (205), 1952, 16, 442.

Verzhbovskaia: Report. (186), 1955, 3, 73.

Veterans Administration twelfth conference on the chemotherapy of tuberculosis. Atlanta, Georgia. 1953. U.S.A.

Viallier, J., and J. Tigaud: Coloration de *Mycobacterium tuberculosis* par le rouge neutre et virulence du bacille pour le cobaye. (98), 1952, 146, 281.

Vignais, P.: Structure de l'acide ribonucléique. 2. Mode d'action de la ribonucléase. Influence de ses conditions d'action sur le remaniement possible des liaisons internucléotidiques de l'acide ribonucléique. (29), 1953, 85, 230.

Villemin, J. A.: Cause et nature de la tuberculose. (82), 1865, 31, 211.

———: Études sur la tuberculose. Paris, 1868. France.

Vincent, V., and E. A. Birge: Cultivation of tubercle bacilli from gastric juice. A study of the factors affecting the cultivation of *Mycobacterium tuberculosis* from gastric juice. (22), 1947, 55, 556.

Vischer, E., S. Zamenhof, and E. Chargaff: Microbial nucleic acids: the desoxypentose nucleic acids of avian tubercle bacilli and yeast. (136), 1949, 177, 429.

Voit, K.: Über das Verhalten der Bakterien zur Nuklealfärbung. (234), 1925, 47, 183; (234), 1927, 55, 564.

Volk, W. A., and Q. N. Myrvik: An explanation for the arithmetic linear growth of *Mycobacteria.* (135), 1953, 66, 386.

Vorwald, A. J., and A. B. Delahant: The influence of silica on the natural and acquired resistance to the tubercle bacillus. (22), 1938, 38, 347.

Wagener, K.: Das Problem der bovinen Tuberkulose vom medizinischen und wirtschaftlichen Standpunkt. (63), 1950–1951, 104, 7.

———, and E. Mitscherlich: Fortschritte in der kulturellen Differenzierung der Tuberkelbakterientypen. (245), 1951, 157, 87.

Wagner, J.: Einfluss der p-Aminobenzoesäure und ähnlicher Stoffe auf das Wachstum von Tuberkelbakterien in Kultur. Würzburg, 1951. Germany.

Wagner, W. H.: Über den oxydativen Abbau aromatischer Substanzen durch saprophytäre Mycobakterien. (68), 1951, 322, 121.

Wakabayashi, H.: Einfluss der Fettsäuren auf das Tuberkelbazillen-Wachstum. (131), 1933, 11, 171.

Wallace, T.: Trace elements in plant physiology. Symposium. Waltham, 1950. U.S.A.

Wallgren, A.: On decrease in tuberculous meningitis. (3), 1936, 18, 474.

Wámoscher, L.: Versuche über die Struktur der Bakterienzelle. (235), 1930, 111, 422.

———, and Stöcklin: Infektionsversuche mit einzelnen Tuberkelbazillen, durchgeführt mit der mikrurgischen Methode. (245), 1927, 104, 86.

Warburg, O.: Über die Rolle des Eisens in der Atmung des Seeigeleis nebst Bemerkungen über einige durch Eisen beschleunigte Oxydationen. (241), 1914a, 92, 231.

———: Beiträge zur Physiologie der Zelle, insbesondere über die Oxydationsgeschwindigkeit in Zellen. (110), 1914b, 14, 253.

———: Über die katalytischen Wirkungen der lebendigen Substanz (collected early papers). Springer, Berlin, 1928. Germany.

———: Schwermetalle als Wirkungsgruppen von Fermenten. Saenger, 1948. Germany.
———: Über die Entstehung der Krebszellen. (176), 1955, 42, 401. English translation, (212), 1956, 123, 309.
———, and W. Christian: Über ein neues Oxydationsferment und sein Absorptionsspektrum. (68), 1932, 254, 438.
Warburg, O., and E. Negelein: Direkter spektroskopischer Nachweis des sauerstoffübertragenden Ferments in Essigbakterien. (68), 1933, 262, 237.
Warnery, M.: Sur la résistance des bacilles tuberculeux à l'acide sulfurique suivant l'âge des cultures. (98), 1932, 111, 575.
Watson, M. L.: A new microtome for thin-sectioning for electron microscopy. (69), 1953, 10, 1.
Webb, G. B., C. H. Boissevain, and C. T. Ryder: Gas requirements of the tubercle bacillus. (22), 1924, 9, 534.
Webb, G. B., C. T. Ryder, G. B. Gilbert: The survival and virulence of tubercle bacilli in excised animal lymph nodes. (22), 1921, 5, 388.
Webb, M.: The influence of magnesium on cell division. 3. The effect of magnesium on the growth of bacteria in simple chemically defined media. (140), 1949, 3, 418.
———: Effects of magnesium on cellular division in bacteria. (212), 1953, 118, 607.
Weber, A.: Zur Tuberkulose des Menschen und der Tiere. (245), 1912, 64, 243.
———, and M. Taute: Die Kaltblütertuberkulose. (222), 1904–1905, Heft 3, 110.
Weber, H.: Die Behandlung der Schwindsucht mit Kohlensäure. (66), 1889, 26, 779.
Wedum, A. G.: Glycerol and carbohydrate utilization by *Mycobacterium tuberculosis*. (135), 1936, 32, 599.
Weed, L. A., J. R. McDonald, and G. M. Needham: The isolation of "saprophytic" acid-fast bacilli from lesions of caseous granulomas. (192), 1956, 31, 246.
Weidmann, S.: Die S.P.-Methode nach E. Darzins zur Isolierung von Tuberkelbazillen aus pathologischen Material. (235), 1952, 134, 47.
Weigand, W.: Kulturelle Isolierung von Tuberkelbacillen nach Vorbehandlung mit Schwefelsäure. (235), 1953, 136, 471.
Weinzirl, J., and F. Knapton: The biology of tubercle bacillus. 1. Hydrogen-ion concentration produced by some members of the genus *Mycobacterium*. (22), 1927, 15, 380.
Weitzel, G.: Antituberkuläre Wirkung ungesättigter Fettstoffe *in vitro*. (241), 1952, 290, 252.
Wells, G. H. and E. R. Long: The chemistry of tuberculosis. Williams & Wilkins, Baltimore, 1932. U.S.A.
Wells, W. F.: Airborne contagion and air hygiene; an ecological study of droplet infections. Harvard University Press, Cambridge, Mass., 1955. U.S.A.
———, and M. B. Lurie: Experimental air-borne disease. Quantitative natural respiratory contagion of tuberculosis. (14), 1941, 34, 21, Section B.
Wells, W. F., H. L. Ratcliffe, and C. Crumb: On the mechanics of droplet nuclei infection. 2. Quantitative experimental air-borne tuberculosis in rabbits. (14), 1948, 47, 11.
Wells, W. F., and M. W. Wells: Air-borne infection. (151), 1936, 107, 1698.
Welsch, M., and E. Nihoul: A propos de la mise en évidence du noyau bactérien. (98), 1948, 142, 1449.
Werner, G. H.: La cytologie des bacilles tuberculeux etudiée en relation avec leurs caractères de virulence. (185), 1951, 59, 1043.
Wessel, E.: Übermikroskopische Beobachtungen an Tuberkelbazillen von *Typus humanus*. (242), 1942, 88, 22.
Wessels, C. C.: Tuberculosis in the rat. Gross organ changes and tuberculin sensitivity in rats infected with tubercle bacilli. (22), 1941, 43, 449.
Weyrauch, F., and J. Rzymkowski: Photographien zur Tröpcheninfektion. (235), 1938, 120, 444.
Wherry, W. B., and D. M. Ervin: The necessity of carbon dioxide for the growth of *B. tuberculosis*. (145), 1918, 22, 194.
Wherry, W. B., and W. W. Oliver: Adaptation to certain tensions of oxyyen as shown by gonococcus and other parasitic and saprophytic bacteria. (145), 1916, 19, 288.

Wiame, J. M.: The occurrence and physiological behavior of two metaphosphate fractions in yeast. (136), 1949, 178, 919.
Widelock, D., L. R. Peizer, S. Klein: Public health significance of tubercle bacilli resistant to isoniazid. (19), 1955, 45, 79.
Wieland, H.: Über Hydrierung und Dehydrierung. (65), 1912, 45, 484.
———: Über den Mechanismus der Oxydationsvorgänge. (110), 1922, 20, 477.
Wier, J. A., P. B. Storey, P. Walrath, O. Weiser, and C. W. Tempel: The incidence of smear positive–culturally negative sputum in patients with pulmonary tuberculosis. (220), 1955, 14th Conference, p. 255.
Williams, R. C., and R. W. G. Wyckoff: Electron shadow-micrographs of haemocyanin molecules. (175), 1945, 156, 68.
———: Applications of metallic shadow-casting to microscopy. (134), 1946, 17, 23.
Willis, H. S.: The effect of mechanical grinding on tubercle bacilli. (22), 1932, 25, 224.
———: The effect of animal passage on the virulence of tubercle bacilli. (22), 1933, 28, 884.
———, and R. G. Kelly: Results of intensive study of sputum in pulmonary tuberculosis. (22), 1939, 39, 81.
Wilson, F. J., C. Kalish, and C. H. Fish: Use of oxidation-reduction dyes in the determination of virulence of *Mycobacteria in vitro.* (22), 1952, 65, 187.
Wilson, G. S.: The proportion of viable bacteria in young cultures with especial reference to the technique employed in counting. (135), 1922, 7, 405.
———: Non-pulmonary tuberculosis caused by the bovine type of bacillus. (161), 1950, 259, 255.
———, and H. Schwabacher: The relationship between moist weight and numbers of total and viable organisms in cultures of tubercle bacilli. (221), 1937, 18, 161.
Wilson, M. M.: Fluorescence microscopy in examination of smears for *Mycobacterium tuberculosis.* (22), 1952, 65, 709.
Winder, F. and J. M. Denneny: Metaphosphate in Mycobacterial metabolism. (175), 1954, 174, 353.
———: Phosphorous metabolism of *Mycobacteria*: determination of phosphorous compounds in some *Mycobacteria.* (140), 1956, 15, 1.
Winogradsky, S.: Über Schwefelbakterien. (76), 1887, 45, Nos. 31–37.
Winterscheid, L. C., and S. Mudd: The differential staining of mitochondria and nuclei in *Mycobacteria.* (153), 1952, 13, 243.
———: The cytology of the tubercle bacillus with reference to mitochondria and nuclei. (22), 1953, 67, 59.
Wise, W. S.: The measurement of the aeration of culture media. (140), 1951, 5, 167.
Wissner, B.: La méthode d'Osol dans la recherche des bacilles de Koch. (185), 1947, 55, 181.
Witte, S.: Morphologische und serologische Studien über Tuberkulinwirkungen an Leukocyten *in vitro.* (63), 1950, 104, 252.
Wolinsky, E., and W. Steenken, Jr.: Effect of streptomycin on the tubercle bacillus. The use of Dubos' and other media in tests for streptomycin sensitivity. (22), 1947, 55, 281.
Wollman, E. L., and F. Jacob: Sur le mécanisme du transfert de matériel génétique au cours de la recombinaison chez *Escherichia coli K 12.* (99), 1955, 240, 2449.
Wolters, K. L., and H. Dehmel: Zur Züchtung und Differenzierung der Tuberkelbazillen. (245), 1930, 117, 279.
Wood, H. G., and C. H. Werkman: The utilization of CO_2 in the dissimilation of glycerol by the propionic acid bacteria. (135), 1935, 30, 332; (67), 1936, 30, 48.
———, A. Hemingway, and A. O. Nier: Fixation of carbon dioxide by pigeon liver in the dissimilation of pyruvic acid. (136), 1942, 142, 31.
Wood, L. E., V. B. Buhler, and A. Pollak: Human infection with the "yellow" acid-fast bacillus. A report of fifteen additional cases. (22), 1956, 73, 917.
Woodruff, A. M., and E. W. Goodpasture: The susceptibility of the chorio-allantoic membrane of chick embryos to infection with the fowl-pox virus. (29), 1931, 7, 209.

Woodruff, C. E., and R. G. Kelly: Growth of tubercle bacilli in tissues of normal and allergic guinea pigs. (22), 1940, 42, 782.
Woodruff, H. B., and J. W. Foster: Microbiological aspects of penicillin. 7. Bacterial penicillinase. (135), 1945, 49, 7.
Wrede, F.: Über das Pyocyanin, den blauen Farbstoff des *Bacillus pyocyaneus.* (235), 1930, 111, 90.
Wuhrmann, K., A. Heuberger, and K. Mühlethaler: Elektronenmikroskopische Untersuchungen an Zellulosefasern nach Behandlung mit Ultraschall. (112), 1946, 2, 105.
Wyckoff, R. W. G.: A micro-motion-picture study of the growth of tubercle bacilli from cold-blooded animals. (22), 1934, 29, 389.
———: The electron microscopy of macromolecules. (8), 1951, 6, 1.
———, and A. L. Ter Louw: Some ultraviolet photomicrographs of *B. subtilis.* (139), 1931, 54, 449.
Xalabarder, G.: La biología del *My. tuberculosis* estudiada con el microscopio electrónico. Instituto Antituberculoso Francisco Moragas, Barcelona, 1953. Spain.
Yaoi, H., and H. Tamiya: On the respiratory pigment, cytochrome, in bacteria. (187), 1928, 4, 436.
Yegian, D., and V. Budd: The growth and enumeration of *Mycobacteria* in transparent agar medium. (22), 1951, 64, 81.
———: Toxic effect of sodium hydroxide on tubercle bacilli. (12), 1952, 22, 456.
———: Certain nonpathogenic *Mycobacteria* as a cause of error in diagnosis and drug-susceptibility tests. (22), 1953, 68, 557.
Yegian, D., and J. Kurung: Growth pattern and virulence of tubercle bacilli. (22), 1952, 65, 181.
Yersin, A.: Étude sur le développement du tubercle expérimental. (29), 1888, 2, 246.
Youmans, G. P.: A method for the determination of the culture cycle and growth rate of virulent human type tubercle bacilli. (135), 1946a, 51, 703.
———: The effect of para-aminosalicylic acid *in vitro* and *in vivo* on virulent human type tubercle bacilli. (195), 1946b, 20, 420.
———: The use of the mouse for the testing of chemotherapeutic agents against *Mycobacterium tuberculosis.* (36), 1949, 52, 662.
———, and W. H. Feldman: The sensitivity of tubercle bacilli *in vitro* to streptomycin. (135), 1946, 51, 608.
Youmans, G. P., and J. C. McCarter: A preliminary note on the effect of streptomycin on experimental tuberculosis of white mice. (195), 1945, 19, 210.
Youmans, G. P., and A. S. Youmans: A method for the determination of the rate of growth of tubercle bacilli by the use of small inocula. (135), 1949, 58, 247.
———: The relation between the size of the infecting dose of tubercle bacilli and the survival time of mice. (22), 1951, 64, 534.
———: Studies on the metabolism of *Mycobacterium tuberculosis.* 1. The effect of carbohydrates and alcohols on the growth of *Mycobacterium tuberculosis var. hominis.* (135), 1953, 65, 92.
———: 4. The effect of fatty acids on the growth of *Mycobacterium tuberculosis var. hominis.* (135), 1954a, 67, 731.
———: 5. The effect of amino acids on the growth of *Mycobacterium tuberculosis var. hominis.* (135), 1954b, 67, 734.
Zahn: Ein neues einfaches Anreicherungsverfahren für Tuberkelbazillen. (172), 1910, 57, 840.
Zederbauer, G.: Über die Ansteckungsfähigkeit der verkappten Tuberkelbazillenausscheider. (166), 1935, 31, 1458.
Zernike, F.: Diffraction theory of the knife edge test and its improved form the phase contrast method. (182), 1934, 1, 689.
Zetterberg, B.: Effects on tubercle bacilli of bacteriostatics, respiration inhibitors and bactericides. (4), 1949, Supplement 82, 1.
Zettnow: Romanowski's Färbung bei Bakterien. (235), 1899, 30, 1; (103), 1900, 26, 377.
Ziegler, E.: Experimentelle Untersuchungen über die Herkunft der Tuberkelelemente,

mit besonderer Berücksichtigung der Histogenese der Riesenzellen. Würzburg, 1875. Germany.

Ziehl, F.: Zur Färbung des Tuberkelbacillus. (103), 1882, 8, 451.

Ziemann, H.: Eine Methode der Doppelfärbung bei Flagellaten, Pilzen, Spirillen und Bakterien, sowie bei einigen Amöben. (245), 1898, 24, 945.

Zobell, C. E.: Action of microorganisms on hydrocarbons. (61), 1946, 10, 1.

Zuckermann, A., and L. A. Rantz: The use of a Dubos-type solid medium containing penicillin for the primary isolation of *M. tuberculosis* from human discharges. (22), 1951, 64, 318.

LIST OF PERIODICALS

1. Acta Davosiana. Switzerland
2. Acta Medica Scandinavica. Sweden
3. Acta Paediatrica. Sweden
4. Acta Pathologica et Microbiologica Scandinavica. Denmark
5. Acta Societatis Biologiae Latviae. Latvia
6. Acta Tuberculosea Scandinavica. Denmark
7. Advances in Enzymology. U.S.A.
8. Advances in Protein Chemistry. U.S.A.
9. Advances in Tuberculosis Research. Switzerland
10. American Journal of Anatomy
11. American Journal of Botany
12. American Journal of Clinical Pathology
13. American Journal of Diseases of Children
14. American Journal of Hygiene
15. American Journal of Medical Technology
16. American Journal of Medicine
17. American Journal of Pathology
18. American Journal of Physiology
19. American Journal of Public Health
20. American Journal of Veterinary Research
21. American Review of Soviet Medicine
22. American Review of Tuberculosis and Pulmonary Diseases
23. American Society of Clinical Pathologists. Technical Bulletin
24. Anales de la Cátedra de Patología y Clínica de la Tuberculosis. Argentina
25. Anatomical Record. U.S.A.
26. Anatomischer Anzeiger. Germany
27. Annalen der Physik. Germany
28. Annales de la Société Belge de Médecine Tropicale
29. Annales de l'Institut Pasteur. France
30. Annales de l'Institut Pasteur de Lille. France
31. Annales des Fermentations. France
32. Annales des Sciences Naturelles. Botanique. France
33. Annali dell'Istituto Carlo Forlanini. Italy.
34. Annali d'Igiene Sperimentale. Italy
35. Annals of Applied Biology. England
36. Annals of the New York Academy of Science. U.S.A.
37. Annual Review of Biochemistry. U.S.A.
38. Annual Review of Microbiology. U.S.A.
39. Antonie van Leeuwenhoek. The Netherlands
40. Arbeiten aus dem kaiserlichen Gesundheitsamte (Started 1886). Germany
41. Archives de l'Institut Pasteur de Tunis. Tunisia
42. Archives de Médecine des Enfants. France
43. Archives de Médecine Expérimentale et d'Anatomie Pathologique. France
44. Archives Internationales de Pharmacodynamie et de Thérapie. Belgium
45. Archives of Biochemistry and Biophysics. U.S.A.
46. Archives of Pathology and Laboratory Medicine. U.S.A.

47. Archives of Surgery. U.S.A.
48. Archiv für Dermatologie und Syphilis. Austria
49. Archiv für experimentelle Pathologie und Pharmakologie. Germany
50. Archiv für experimentelle Zellforschung. Germany
51. Archiv für Hygiene und Bakteriologie. Germany
52. Archiv für Mikrobiologie. Germany
53. Archiv für mikroskopische Anatomie und Entwicklungsmechanik. Germany
54. Archiv für Physiologie. Germany
55. Archiv für Protistenkunde. Germany
56. Archivio Italiano di Medicina Sperimentale.
57. Archivio per le Science Mediche. Italy
58. Arquivos do Instituto Biologico. Brazil
59. Arquivos do Instituto Brazileiro para Investigação da Tuberculose. Brazil
60. Ärztliche Wochenschrift. Germany
61. Bacteriological Reviews. U.S.A.
62. Beiträge zur experimentellen Therapie. (E. Behring). Germany
63. Beiträge zur Klinik der Tuberkulose und spezifischen Tuberkulose-Forschung. Germany
64. Beiträge zur pathologischen Anatomie und zur allgemeinen Pathologie. Germany
65. Berichte der deutschen chemischen Gesellschaft. Germany
66. Berliner klinische Wochenschrift. Germany
67. Biochemical Journal. England
68. Biochemische Zeitschrift. Germany
69. Biochimica et Biophysica Acta. The Netherlands
70. Biochimica e Terapia Sperimentale. Italy
71. Biological Reviews and Biological Proceedings of the Cambridge Philosophical Society. England
72. Biologisches Zentralblatt. Germany
73. Biologitscheskii Zhurnal. U.S.S.R.
74. Bolletino dell'Istituto Sieroterapico Milanese. Italy
75. Botanical Review. U.S.A.
76. Botanische Zeitung. Germany
77. British Journal of Experimental Pathology
78. British Journal of Ophthalmology
79. British Journal of Pharmacology and Chemotherapy
80. British Journal of Radiology
81. British Medical Journal
82. Bulletin de l'Academie de Médecine. France
83. Bulletin of the Bureau of Animal Industry. Department of Agriculture. U.S.A.
84. Bulletin de la classe des sciences. 5-e série. Academie Royal de Belgique
85. Bulletin de la Société de Chimie Biologique. France
86. Bulletin der schweizerischen Akademie der medizinischen Wissenschaften. Switzerland
87. Bulletin of the Johns Hopkins Hospital. U.S.A.
88. Bulletin Monthly. Ministry of Health. England
89. Bulletin of the National Tuberculosis Association. U.S.A.
90. Bulletin of the New Jersey Agricultural Experiment Station. U.S.A.
91. Bulletin of the World Health Organization. Switzerland
92. Canadian Journal of Medical Sciences
93. Canadian Journal of Medical Technology
94. Canadian Journal of Public Health
95. Canadian Journal of Research
96. Canadian Medical Association Journal
97. Communications from the Statens Seruminstitut. Denmark
98. Comptes Rendus des Séances et Mémoires de la Société de Biologie. France
99. Comptes Rendus Hebdomadaires des Séances de l'Academie des Sciences. France
100. Chinese Medical Journal. Peking

101. Chromosoma. Germany
102. Deutsche Gesundheitswesen. Germany
103. Deutsche medizinische Wochenschrift. Germany
104. Deutsche tierärztliche Wochenschrift. Germany
105. Deutsche Zeitschrift für Chirurgie. Germany
106. Diseases of the Chest. U.S.A.
107. Edinburgh Medical Journal. Scotland
108. Enzymologia. The Netherlands
109. Ergebnisse der Enzymforschung. Germany
110. Ergebnisse der Physiologie. (Ascher-Spiro). Germany
111. Excerpta Medica. Section 15. (Tuberculosis). The Netherlands
112. Experientia. Switzerland
113. Experimental Cell Research. U.S.A.
114. Federation Proceedings. U.S.A.
115. Flora. Germany
116. Fortschritte der Medizin. Germany
117. Frequenz. Germany
118. Gazette Médicale de Lyon. France
119. Giornale di Batteriologia e Immunologia. Italy
120. Grenzgebiete der Medizin. Germany
121. Helvetica Chimica Acta. Switzerland
122. Hoja Tisiológica. Uruguay
123. Hygienische Rundschau. Germany
124. Industrial and Engineering Chemistry. U.S.A.
125. International Congress of Microbiology or Tuberculosis. Reports
126. International Journal of Leprosy. U.S.A.
127. International Review of Cytology. U.S.A.
128. Izvestia Akademii Nauk. Seria biologitscheskaia. Moscow. U.S.S.R.
129. Jahrbuch für Morphologie und mikroskopische Anatomie. Zweite Abteilung. Germany
130. Jahrbuch für wissenschaftliche Botanik. Germany
131. Japanese Journal of Experimental Medicine
132. Jenaische Zeitschrift für Naturwissenschaft. Germany
133. Journal Médical de Leysin. Switzerland
134. Journal of Applied Physics. U.S.A.
135. Journal of Bacteriology. U.S.A.
136. Journal of Biological Chemistry. U.S.A.
137. Journal of Cellular and Comparative Physiology. U.S.A.
138. Journal of Comparative Pathology and Therapeutics. England
139. Journal of Experimental Medicine. U.S.A.
140. Journal of General Microbiology. England
141. Journal of General Physiology. U.S.A.
142. Journal of Histochemistry and Cytochemistry. U.S.A.
143. Journal of Hygiene. England
144. Journal of Immunology. U.S.A.
145. Journal of Infectious Diseases. U.S.A.
146. Journal of Laboratory and Clinical Medicine. U.S.A.
147. Journal of Medical Research. U.S.A.
148. Journal of Pathology and Bacteriology. England
149. Journal of Pharmacology and Experimental Therapeutics. U.S.A.
150. Journal of the American Chemical Society
151. Journal of the American Medical Association
152. Journal of the Chemical Society. England
153. Journal of the National Cancer Institute. U.S.A.
154. Journal of the Royal Microscopical Society. Series 3. England
155. Journal of Thoracic Surgery. U.S.A.
156. Kekkaku. Japan

157. Kleinwelt. Germany
158. Klinische Wochenschrift. Germany
159. Kolloid Zeitschrift. Germany
160. Koninklijke Akademie van Wetenschappen te Amsterdam. Proceedings. The Netherlands
161. Lancet. England
162. Laval Médical. Canada
163. Lotta contro la Tubercolosi. Italy
164. Medical Research Council. Reports. England
165. Medical Research Council. Special Report Series. England
166. Medizinische Klinik. Germany
167. Memórias do Instituto Oswaldo Cruz. Brazil
168. Mikroskopie. Austria
169. Mitteilungen aus der biologischen Versuchsanstalt der kaiserlichen Akademie der Wissenschaften. Austria
170. Mitteilungen aus dem kaiserlichen Gesundheitsamte. (1881–1884). Germany
171. Monatshefte für praktische Tierheilkunde. Germany
172. Münchener medizinische Wochenschrift. Germany
173. National Tuberculosis Association. Abstracts and Papers. U.S.A.
174. National Tuberculosis Association. Transactions. U.S.A.
175. Nature. England
176. Naturwissenschaften. Germany
177. New York Medical Journal. U.S.A.
178. Nourrisson. France
179. Petersburger (St.) medizinische Wochenschrift. U.S.S.R.
180. Pflüger's Archiv für die gesamte Physiologie des Menschen und der Tiere. Germany
181. Philosophical Transactions of the Royal Society of London. England
182. Physica. The Netherlands
183. Physiological Reviews. U.S.A.
184. Prensa Médica. Argentina
185. Presse Médicale. France
186. Problemi Tuberkuleza. U.S.S.R.
187. Proceedings of the Imperial Academy of Japan
188. Proceedings of the National Academy of Science of the U.S.A.
189. Proceedings of the Royal Society of Medicine. England
190. Proceedings of the Royal Society. Series B. England
191. Proceedings of the Society for Experimental Biology and Medicine. U.S.A.
192. Proceedings of the Staff Meetings of the Mayo Clinic. U.S.A.
193. Protoplasma. Austria
194. Public Health Reports. U.S.A.
195. Quarterly Bulletin of Northwestern University Medical School. U.S.A.
196. Quarterly Journal of Microscopical Science. England
197. Recueil de Médecine Vétérinaire de l'École d'Alfort. France
198. Revista de Tuberculosis de Uruguay
199. Revista Médica de Chile
200. Revista Médica Municipal. Brazil
201. Revista Médico-Cirúrgica do Brasil
202. Revista Paulista de Medicina. Brazil
203. Revista Paulista de Tisiologia. Brazil
204. Revue Belge de Pathologie et de Médecine Expérimentale
205. Revue de la Tuberculose. France
206. Riforma Medica. Italy
207. Rivista d'Igiene e Sanità Publica. Italy
208. Royal Commission on Tuberculosis. England
209. Schweizerische medizinische Wochenschrift. Switzerland

210. Schweizerische Zeitschrift für allgemeine Pathologie und Bakteriologie. Switzerland
211. Schweizerische Zeitschrift für Tuberkulose. Switzerland
212. Science. U.S.A.
213. Skandinavisches Archiv für Physiologie. Sweden
214. Society of American Bacteriologists. Meetings. Abstracts and Papers
215. Southern Medical Journal. U.S.A.
216. Stain Technology. U.S.A.
217. Thorax. England
218. Tierärztliche Umschau. Germany
219. Tôhoku Journal of Experimental Medicine. Japan
220. Transactions of the Conferences of Tuberculosis. Veterans Administration. U.S.A.
221. Tubercle. England
222. Tuberkulose-Arbeiten aus dem kaiserlichen Gesundheitsamte. Germany
223. Tuberkulosearzt. Germany
224. Virchow's Archiv für pathologische Anatomie und Physiologie. Germany
225. Uspekhi Sovremennoi Biologii. U.S.S.R.
226. Wiener klinische Wochenschrift. Austria
227. Wiener medizinische Wochenschrift. Austria
228. Wissenschaftliche Veröffentlichungen aus den Siemens-Werken. Germany
229. Yale Journal of Biology and Medicine. U.S.A.
230. Zeiss-Nachrichten. Germany
231. Zeitschrift für anorganische Chemie. Germany
232. Zeitschrift für Biologie. Germany
233. Zeitschrift für experimentelle Pathologie und Therapie. Germany
234. Zeitschrift für die gesamte experimentelle Medizin. Germany
235. Zeitschrift für Hygiene und Infektionskrankheiten. Germany
236. Zeitschrift für Immunitätsforschung und experimentelle Therapie. Germany
237. Zeitschrift für Infektionskrankheiten der Haustiere. Germany
238. Zeitschrift für Kinderheilkunde. Germany
239. Zeitschrift für Naturforschung. Germany
240. Zeitschrift für Physik. Germany
241. Zeitschrift für physiologische Chemie. (Hoppe-Seyler). Germany
242. Zeitschrift für Tuberkulose. Germany
243. Zeitschrift für wissenschaftliche Mikroskopie und für mikroskopische Technik. Germany
244. Zeitschrift für Zellforschung und mikroskopische Anatomie. Germany
245. Zentralblatt für Bakteriologie, Parasitenkunde, Infektionskrankheiten und Hygiene. Erste Abteilung. Originale. Germany
246. Zentralblatt für Bakteriologie, Parasitenkunde, Erste Abteilung. Referate. Germany
247. Zentralblatt für Bakteriologie, Zweite Abteilung. Originale. Germany
248. Zentralblatt für die gesamte Tuberkuloseforschung. Germany
249. Zentralblatt für die medizinischen Wissenschaften. Germany
250. Zentralblatt für klinische Medizin. Germany
251. Zhurnal Mikrobiologii, Epidemiologii i Immunobiologii. U.S.S.R.
252. Zhurnal Obshchei Biologii. U.S.S.R.

Author Index

Author Index

Author Index

Author Index

Author Index

Author Index

Author Index

Subject Index

Subject Index

Subject Index

Made in the USA
Monee, IL
05 November 2026

67977847R00275